DRUGS FOR PAIN

DRUGS FOR PAIN

Howard S. Smith, MD, FACP

Director of Pain Medicine
Albany Medical Center
Professor of Anesthesiology
Albany Medical College
Albany, New York

HANLEY & BELFUS, INC./Philadelphia

Publisher: HANLEY & BELFUS, INC.
Medical Publishers
210 South 13th Street
Philadelphia, PA 19107
(215) 546-7293; 800-962-1892
FAX (215) 790-9330
Web site: http://www.hanleyandbelfus.com

Note to the reader: Although the information in this book has been carefully reviewed for correctness of dosage and indications, neither the authors nor the editor nor the publisher can accept any legal responsibility for any errors or omissions that may be made. Neither the publisher nor the editor makes any warranty, expressed or implied, with respect to the material contained herein. Before prescribing any drug, the reader must review the manufacturer's current product information (package inserts) for accepted indications, absolute dosage recommendations, and other information pertinent to the safe and effective use of the product described.

Library of Congress Cataloging-in-Publication Data

Drugs for pain / [edited by] Howard S. Smith.
    p. cm.
  Includes bibliographical references and index.
  ISBN 1–56053–511–3 (alk. paper)
  1. Analgesics. I. Smith, Howard S., 1956–
RM319 .D784 2002
615'.783—dc21

                                                    2002068795

DRUGS FOR PAIN   ISBN 1-56053-511-3

Last digit is the print number: 9 8 7 6 5 4 3 2 1

DEDICATION

I dedicate this book:

    In memory of my mother, Arlene Smith—The wind beneath my wings.

    In memory of my grandmother, Helen Friedman.

    In memory of my mother-in-law, Joan Buckley.

    To my wife, Joan, and children Alyssa, Joshua, Benjamin, and Eric, who made this project possible (and who made it all worthwhile).

    To my father and stepmother, Nathan and Priscilla Smith.

    To my aunt and uncle, Corinne and Sheldon Simon.

    To my father-in-law, John Buckley, Jr.

CONTENTS

CONTRIBUTORS

Salahadin Abdi, MD, PhD
Clinical Professor of Anesthesiology and Chief, Division of Pain Medicine, University of Miami Medical School, Miami, Florida

Jonathan E. Alpert, MD, PhD
Assistant Professor of Psychiatry, Harvard Medical School, Boston, Massachusetts; Assistant Psychiatrist, Massachusetts General Hospital, Boston, Massachusetts

Joseph Audette, MA, MD
Instructor, Harvard Medical School, Department of Physical Medicine and Rehabilitation, Boston, Massachusetts; Director of Outpatient Pain Services, Spaulding Rehabilitation Hospital, Boston, Massachusetts

Zahid H. Bajwa, MD
Assistant Professor of Anesthesia (Neurology), Harvard Medical School, Boston, Massachusetts; Director, Education and Clinical Pain Research, Beth Israel Deaconess Medical Center, Boston, Massachusetts

Mark V. Boswell, MD, PhD
Associate Professor, Department of Anesthesiology, Case Western Reserve University, Cleveland, Ohio; University Hospitals of Cleveland, Cleveland, Ohio

Leonard S. Bushnell, BSE, MD
Anesthetist-in-Chief Emeritus, Associate Professor of Anesthesia Emeritus, Department of Anesthesiology and Critical Care, Harvard Medical School, Boston, Massachusetts

Pasarapa Chaiyakul, PhD
Department of Pharmacology, Chulalongkorn University, Bangkok, Thailand

Lucy Chen, MD
Instructor, Massachusetts General Hospital Pain Center, Department of Anesthesia and Critical Care, Massachusetts General Hospital, Harvard Medical School, Boston, Massachusetts

Pradeep Chopra, MD
Assistant Professor, Boston University Medical Center, Boston, Massachusetts; Director, Pain Management Center of Rhode Island, Providence, Rhode Island

Steven P. Cohen, MD
Director, Inpatient Pain Management Service, Department of Anesthesiology, New York University School of Medicine, New York, New York

James C. Crews, MD
Associate Professor, Department of Anesthesiology, Wake Forest University School of Medicine, Winston-Salem, North Carolina

Jennifer A. Elliott, MD
Assistant Professor, Department of Anesthesiology, University of Missouri–Kansas City School of Medicine, Kansas City, Missouri; Staff Pain Physician, St. Luke's Hospital, Kansas City, Missouri

Maurizio Fava, MD
Professor of Psychiatry, Harvard Medical School, Boston, Massachusetts; Psychiatrist and Associate Chief of Psychiatry for Clinical Research, Massachusetts General Hospital, Boston, Massachusetts

Scott M. Fishman, MD
Chief and Associate Professor, Division of Pain Medicine, Department of Anesthesia and Pain Medicine, University of California at Davis Medical Center, Davis, California

Andreas Grabinsky, MD
Fellow, Pain Management, Department of Anesthesiology, Case Western Reserve University, Cleveland, Ohio; University Hospitals of Cleveland, Cleveland, Ohio

David V. Iosifescu, MD
Instructor, Department of Psychiatry, Harvard Medical School, Boston, Massachusetts; Clinical Assistant in Psychiatry, Massachusetts General Hospital, Boston, Massachusetts

Piotr K. Janicki, MD, PhD
Associate Professor, Department of Anesthesiology, Vanderbilt University School of Medicine, Nashville, Tennessee; Attending Anesthesiologist, Vanderbilt University Hospital, Nashville, Tennessee

Wiebke Janson, MD
Department of Anesthesiology and Critical Care Medicine, Freie Universitaet Berlin, Berlin, Germany

Sajid Kahn, MD
Research Assistant, Department of Anesthesia and Critical Care, Beth Israel Deaconess Medical Center, Boston, Massachusetts

Josephine Lai, PhD
Professor, Department of Pharmacology, College of Medicine, University of Arizona, Tucson, Arizona

John Loughrey, MB, BCh, MRCPI, FCARCSI
Consultant Anaesthetist, Department of Anaesthesia, Mater Misercordiae Hospital, Dublin, Ireland

Gagan Mahajan, MD
Assistant Professor and Fellowship Director, Pain Medicine, University of California, Davis, Sacramento, California

Timothy J. Maher, PhD
Sawyer Professor of Pharmaceutical Sciences, Department of Pharmaceutical Sciences, Massachusetts College of Pharmacy and Health Sciences, Boston, Massachusetts

Jianren Mao, MD, PhD
Assistant Professor, Massachusetts General Hospital Pain Center, Department of Anesthesia and Critical Care, Massachusetts General Hospital, Harvard Medical School, Boston, Massachusetts

Gary McCleane, MD, FCARCSI
Consultant in Pain Management, Rampark Pain Centre, Lurgan, North Ireland

Timothy J. Ness, MD, PhD
Associate Professor, Department of Anesthesiology, University of Alabama at Birmingham, Birmingham, Alabama; University of Alabama Hospital, Birmingham, Alabama

Susan E. Opper, MD
Assistant Professor, Department of Anesthesiology, University of Missouri–Kansas City School of Medicine, Kansas City, Missouri; Director of Pain Management, St. Luke's Hospital, Kansas City, Missouri

Michael H. Ossipov, PhD
Research Assistant Professor, Department of Pharmacology, University of Arizona, Tempe, Arizona

Michel Paré PhD
Postdoctoral Fellow, Department of Pharmacology and Therapeutics, McGill University, Montreal, Quebec, Canada

Winston C. Parris, MD, FACPM
Adjunct Professor of Anesthesiology, Vanderbilt University Medical Center, Nashville, Tennessee; Clinical Professor of Anesthesiology, University of South Florida, Tampa, Florida; Pain Consultant, Tampa Pain Relief Center, Tampa Florida

Frank Porreca, PhD
Professor, Department of Pharmacology, University of Arizona, Tucson, Arizona; University Medical Center, Tucson, Arizona

Frank Lambert Rice, PhD
Professor, Center for Neuropharmacology and Neurosciences, Albany Medical College, Albany, New York

Tarek Samad, PhD
Neural Plasticity Research Group, Department of Anesthesia and Critical Care, Massachusetts General Hospital and Harvard Medical School, Boston, Massachusetts

Christine Sang, MD, MPH
Director, Clinical Trials Program, MGH Pain Center, Department of Anesthesia, Massachusetts General Hospital, Boston, Massachusetts

Juan Santiago-Palma, MD
Clinical Pain Fellow, Massachusetts General Hospital, Department of Anesthesia, Boston, Massachusetts

Lee Stuart Simon, MD
Associate Professor, Department of Medicine, Division of Rheumatology, Harvard Medical School, Boston, Massachusetts; Beth Israel Deaconess Medical Center, Boston, Massachusetts

Howard S. Smith, MD, FACP
Director of Pain Medicine, Albany Medical Center; Professor of Anesthesiology, Albany Medical College, Albany, New York

Christoph Stein, MD
Professor and Chairman, Department of Anesthesiology and Critical Care Medicine, Freie Universitaet Berlin, Berlin, Germany

Andrew S. Strassman, PhD
Associate Professor, Department of Anesthesia, Harvard Medical School, Boston, Massachusetts; Staff, Department of Anesthesia and Critical Care, Beth Israel Deaconess Medical Center, Boston, Massachusetts

Wolfgang Ummenhofer, MD
Associate Professor, Department of Anesthesia, Kantonsspital/University Clinics, Basel, Switzerland

Todd W. Vanderah, PhD
Assistant Professor, Department of Anesthesiology, University of Arizona, Tucson, Arizona

K. M. A. Welch, MD
Vice Chancellor for Research, University of Kansas Medical Center, Kansas City, Kansas

Barth L. Wilsey, MD
Director, Northern California Veterans Administration Pain Clinics, Davis, California; Associate Clinical Professor of Anesthesiology and Pain Medicine, University of California at Davis, Davis, California

Alan Witkower, EdD
Assistant Director of Outpatient Pain Services, Spaulding Rehabilitation Hospital, Boston, Massachusetts

YiLi Zhou, MD, PhD
Division of Pain Medicine, University of Miami Medical School, Miami, Florida

ACKNOWLEDGMENTS

I would like to thank Doris Eve Jensen for her enormous efforts in the preparation of this text. I would also like to thank Dr. Lindsay Hough for discussions related to histamine and analgesia, Dr. Ronald Gailey for discussions related to drug biotransformation, and Dr. Sajid Kahn and Michael Ciarmiello for help with figures. I would also like to acknowledge my pain fellows, and all my family, relatives, friends and colleagues for their support. Special thanks also to Christopher Edwards and Jennifer Branik.

PREFACE

This book is intended to give a wide variety of students and practitioners a source to appreciate the analgesics available to treat patients complaining of pain. The material presented here has previously been difficult to find in a single source. There is also a significant amount of information that is available only in this text. The chapter authors are among the major authorities in the world. This text can be used as a reference or as a practical guide to aid practitioners in approaching clinical problems in the pharmacologic practice of pain medicine. Also, it enables the curious a chance to delve into some of the potential proposed mechanisms of various analgesics—how and why they may work.

There is some purposeful overlap of material, as some of these topics are best presented from different vantage points. References are provided both as good sources for more in-depth material and for purposes of standard reference citation.

After many years of presenting didactic lectures for pain fellows, I began to hear many of the same questions when it came to medications: What source can I go to and find all that? Where do you get this stuff? How do you know that? Is there anything I can read that will explain that? I was never able to give them a single reliable source to meet their growing educational needs. This textbook sprang from a need to provide students, trainees/residents/fellows, and practitioners of pain medicine an in-depth look at the exciting world of analgesics.

The book is arranged largely in a bench-to-bedside format, allowing readers to gain some basic science background for the clinical topics presented.

In order to appeal to a wide audience as well as to get certain educational points across, some material may be simplified or modified for educational purposes, and various concepts are illustrated with innovative figures.

Additionally, concepts are presented on issues of *translational analgesia*. I coin this term to refer to the changes (e.g., mood, behavior, function, relationships) that pain relief translates into (e.g., "Ever since my husband has been more comfortable, he is more animated and occasionally helps around the house.")

This text represents an important opportunity to appreciate the past, present, and future of some of the basic science and clinical aspects of analgesia/analgesics and brings a unique flavor to the extremely important topic of analgesics in pain management.

Howard S. Smith, MD

Chapter 1

Introduction

Howard S. Smith, MD

The field of pain medicine and management, although still in its infancy, has seen enormous advances in the clinical arena and in the basic sciences. Currently, although it is still early in the so-called decade of pain (2000–2010), the clinical sciences seem to lag behind the explosion of basic science information. The wealth of animal data generated may or may not be relevant to human pain, and even if it is, it does not currently help clinicians to assess exactly which mechanisms are at play in an individual patient and how to approach optimally the treatment of patients who have failed traditional pain management therapies.

As the field of pain medicine expands, the roots of the interdisciplinary team with strong ties to physical medicine and behavioral medicine should not be ignored. Although there are many exciting pharmacologic therapies on the horizon, it seems that there always will be patients who will not dramatically improve with the administration of medication. Physical medicine and behavioral medicine treatment strategies should be interwoven when appropriate into the total treatment plan. No single approach ever should be used exclusively for all patients.

IS PAIN UNIQUE AS A MEDICAL CONDITION?

The field of pain medicine *crosses* many disciplines; it often deals with mostly subjective issues; and it involves the patient's perception of comfort, suffering, quality of life, and individual goals. When treating patients for localized infection, if the offending pathogen is known, the susceptibility to various antibiotics is reported. The decision of which antibiotic to use often is made with that information. Occasionally the patient's age, specific infection (e.g., bronchitis, pneumonia), medical conditions, and hepatic and renal function are factors that may affect the dose—in general, however, a standard dose is given, and the infection is eradicated. When a similar approach is applied to the management of pain, the pain may not be eradicated for the following reasons: (1) Because the mechanisms of pain are often unknown, specific targets become guesswork (specific mechanisms contributing to an individual's pain are often unknown). (2) Even if the clinician knows that in a particular patient the overexpression of the NaV1.8 sodium channel is a major contributor to the patient's pain, a specific effective treatment may not be available to target this. (3) Assuming a specific treatment that can target the precise mechanisms that are at play leading to pain is available, the proper dose must be achieved. Although antibiotic dosing seems straightforward in treating infections, genetic variability, gender differences, and differences in intrinsic affinity and coupling of receptors and distribution and concentrations of various receptor subtypes make dosing of analgesics for pain relief an extremely complex endeavor. The need to individualize therapy in pain medicine cannot be overemphasized. (4) Even if the clinician can *eradicate nociception*, pain is a sensory and an emotional experience, and the patient still may be experiencing pain and suffering. Also, if the clinician can eradicate pain and suffering, he or she still may not be successful in helping the patient to achieve a similar type of quality of life or lifestyle as the patient had in the premorbid state (e.g. before the patient had chronic pain).

WHY IS THERE PAIN?

It is conceivable that pain (acute pain) may be considered essential for humans to survive as a species; it may be among the crucial perceptions that the brain must evolve for the continued survival of the human organism (e.g., hunger, thirst, and pain). For the organism to perpetuate the species, it must propagate and reproduce. Even much less evolved organisms use *sensing mechanisms* to strive for *environmental comfort* and to avoid toxins, stress, irritability, and extremes of temperature. Although it seems that less is known about the requirement for sleep, this too may be one of the essential *primal drives* or *urges*. Some scientists believe that some of these perceptions (e.g., hunger/satiety, pain/pleasure) may involve similar regions, neurotransmitters and receptors, and systems in the brain. Research efforts centered on the brain may provide some of the key missing links in unlocking some of the mysteries of pain.

DIFFERENCES BETWEEN ACUTE AND CHRONIC PAIN

Some traditional textbooks addressing pain attempted to make distinctions of acute pain versus chronic pain, with acute pain having some potential utility and chronic pain being labeled as *useless*. Subacute pain, cancer pain, and other labels are not dealt with in this discussion (various medical specialists may protest the use of the term *useless*).

The definitions of acute pain versus chronic pain vary as well, with some still using time periods (e.g., >6 months) to characterize chronic pain and others holding to more vague definitions (e.g., pain persisting well beyond the normal or appropriate *healing period* for the particular condition or pathophysiology that the patient has). It may be more useful to separate acute (e.g., postoperative) versus chronic pain on the basis of assessment and treatment approaches and responses and goals. Acute pain tends to be nociceptive (usually somatic), and as such tends to respond reasonably well to one or two medications or modalities (e.g. opioids, nonsteroidal antiinflammatory drugs). The goal for acute pain tends to be complete resolution of pain and complete functional restoration.

Chronic noncancer pain tends to be less responsive (e.g., more difficult to treat) and to have a neuropathic pain component. Multimodal and multimedication treatment regimens seem to be employed more often (in efforts to take advantage of synergy and achieve improved efficacy or fewer side effects).

The treatment controversy of whether to employ one or more medications is not peculiar to therapies of pain medicine and is evident in many other fields. In psychiatry, some clinicians (whom some label as *purists*) stay with one medication when treating depression or other psychiatric diagnoses. They continue to "push the dose higher" until they see efficacy or side effects before switching to a different agent (other psychiatrists often employ more than one medication, especially when the patient is not responding well).

CONTROVERSIES OF LONG-TERM OPIOID THERAPY FOR CHRONIC NONCANCER PAIN

Controversies continue to exist in the use of opioids for chronic noncancer pain and the goals of treatment. From 1996 to 2002, the number of prescriptions for long-acting opioids increased at least fivefold mostly secondary to an increase in prescriptions written for chronic noncancer pain. Pain is a sensory and emotional experience and essentially subjective in nature. Some clinicians who employ opioids seemingly continue to increase opioid dosages to high levels as long as patients are still complaining of pain. These *opioid-generous clinicians* are criticized by other *opioid-stingy clinicians*. In general, a moderate approach seems prudent.

The use of ultra-high-dose opioid therapy for chronic noncancer pain has not been well studied. Anecdotal issues from clinicians that may not be in the literature in terms of side effects (which are different from the ones already well documented, such as itching and nausea) may include: effects on testosterone function and libido, effects on sleep (e.g., altered sleep architecture, insomnia, facilitation or induction of a sleep apnea–type effect), effects on mood, (dysphoria, feeling "hyper" or irritable, depression), effects on coping mechanisms, fatigue, excessive daytime sleepiness, myoclonus, hyperalgesia, worsening of pain or induction of new pain, and an unusual craving for ice cream. (Some of these may occur at low doses too.)

In terms of assessment of pain, different tools may be better suited for acute versus chronic pain. The popular NRS-11 (numerical rating scale) seems to be a reasonable gauge for acute or cancer pain, but it may not be as useful for chronic noncancer pain. Because the NRS-11 is unidimensional, it may not be optimal for the assessment of chronic pain. Other tools may be too cumbersome, costly, or not practical for routine use in a busy clinical practice, however. Many patients in chronic pain clinics describe doing significantly better or worse than during their last visit or their initial visit, but visit after visit they record the same NRS-11 score as they did during the initial visit. Some patients believe they are doing well and wish to attempt to decrease to taper off of their opioids, which may not be reflected in their NRS-11 pain scores.

No consensus exists on when or if to taper patients on stable long-term opioid therapy who seem to be doing reasonably well. Most clinicians are content to *continue present management*, unless things change or the patient requests a change. The NRS-11 does not seem to be especially useful in this situation. A change in the NRS-11 pain score of only 2 (e.g., from a 9 to 7) may seem modest to clinicians but could be significant to the patient. Additionally, this change may seem different (e.g., less important) to the patient than a change from 6 to 4.

The goals of treatment for chronic noncancer pain tend to be different than for acute pain. Currently, it seems that for many patients with chronic noncancer pain complete resolution of pain is unrealistic; however, improved pain control may be attainable. The use of increasing doses of opioids to achieve slightly to mildly improved or essentially no significant change in pain control is controversial. In most fields of medicine, if a clinician is treating a patient's disorder without significant success, the patient should be reassessed and the plan revised. Pain medicine should not be an exception: If after multiple dose escalations of opioid, one cannot document significantly improved pain control, the opioid probably should be tapered to off (unless it is thought to be a useful adjunct at a lower dose). Some patients seem to do better off opioids or on low opioid doses, and some chronic pain in patients seems to be relatively opioid insensitive (e.g., opioid-resistant/opioid unresponsive) or only partially opioid responsive (even at much higher doses than usual).

Various clinicians (a significant majority of "pain experts," by my informal poll) when prescribing opioids for chronic noncancer pain want to see some change in the patient other than purely improved analgesia. These changes include factors generally thought to be associated with an improved quality of life (however, each patient may have his or her own idea of quality of life), improved functionality, increased ambulation; more active lifestyle; an increase in activities and hobbies, increased interest or sense of purpose, improved socialization and recreation, improved coping skills, and improved family life. Some clinicians may believe that lifestyle changes such as smoking cessation or weight loss may be associated goals.

Although it may seem humane to attempt to achieve purely improved analgesia, many clinicians are not comfortable continuing long-term high-dose opioids for patients who report minimal or no improvement in analgesia and continue to live their life without improvement in the above-mentioned lifestyle factors. Return to work seems to be an unrealistic goal for many patients, but whatever goals the patient is to aim for, they should be discussed and mutually agreed on before therapy (with some type of assessment to determine if the goals are attained). Patients may shape or make their own personal goals. A 92-year-old frail woman with multiple advanced medical conditions and severe arthralgias may request to be able to tolerate riding 90 minutes in a car to visit her grandchildren once a month.

Although traditional teachings always have stressed that only the patient can tell you how much pain that they are experiencing (for acute and chronic pain), it seems that for chronic noncancer pain in efforts to achieve goals of improved functionality and quality of life, a clinician-generated assessment tool may have some utility, especially if used in conjunction with a patient generated tool (although this is predicated on the assumptions that the clinican listens carefully to the patient, knows the patient well, and gives appropriately heavy weight to the patient's subjective complaints). The interobserver variability of clinician-generated assessments may be large (especially between opioid-generous clinicians and opioid-stingy clinicians); however, it is hoped that at least the intraobserver variability during multiple visits when the patient is essentially unchanged would be relatively small. It will be interesting in the future to see if the SAFE tool (discussed in Chapter 39) may possess utility as a viable potential assessment alternative).

USE OF POLYPHARMACY

Chronic noncancer pain treatment seems to be approached best in a multimodal fashion, often employing multiple medications. The use of multiple medications to address chronic noncancer pain has been termed by others *rational polypharmacy* or *balanced analgesia*. Although it certainly seems as if certain patients with chronic noncancer pain respond better with fewer side effects to low-dose combinations of multiple medications, it also seems that the medications employed are chosen without much scientific process.

An emphasis on supplementing a disease-based treatment approach with an approach based on the patient's history/physical examination, signs, and symptoms and the underlying mechanisms responsible for the symptoms[4] may facilitate new treatment approaches. This emphasis would allow for the fact that patients with one disease entity (e.g., diabetic neuropathy) may have vastly different symptoms arising from totally different mechanisms and that patients with different diseases may have similar symptoms arising from the same or similar mechanisms.[4] Although largely speculative (there is currently no definitive means of knowing which mechanisms are contributing to an individual patient's pain), a mechanistic approach may provide a future framework from which to tailor an individual patient's *cocktail* of medications based partly on diagnosis, supplemented with the signs, symptoms and putative mechanisms (Tables 1 and 2).[6] By specifically targeting the mechanisms underlying these symptoms, improved therapeutic responses may be realized. I use the terms *educated polypharmacy* or *targeted polypharmacy* to refer to the use of multiple medications specifically chosen based on mechanisms to treat chronic pain.

As one reflects on the enormous advances in pain research, it is interesting to visualize an intern in the early 1980s who suggests to his attending physician that in efforts to enhance analgesia, diminish tolerance, and treat side effects, the addition of an ultra-low dose of

TABLE 1

Mechanism-Based Approach to Signs: Stimulus-Evoked Pain

Sign	Mechanism	Goal of Treatment	Treatment
Mechanical, static, thermal hyperalgesia	Peripheral sensitization	Block peripheral changes	Topical/local anesthetic (capsaicin)
Punctate hyperalgesia	Wind-up central sensitization	Block peripheral sensitization	Topical/local anesthetics Sodium channel blockers
Allodynia	Loss of inhibitory controls central sensitization	Restore inhibitory controls Block central sensitization	Gabapentin NMDA antagonists
	Central root reorganization	Block nerve growth	Nerve growth factor antagonists

Based on Woolf CJ, Mannion RJ: Neuropathic Pain: Aetiology, symptoms, mechanisms, and management. Lancet 353:1959–1964, 1999.

TABLE 2

Mechanism-Based Approach to Symptoms: Stimulus-Independent Pain

Sign	Mechanism	Goal of Treatment	Treatment
Paresthesias Dysesthesias	Ectopic discharges	Block sodium channels	ACDs (CBZ, PHT)
Paroxysmal Shooting Lancinating	Ectopic discharges	Block sodium channels Amitriptyline Gabapentin	ACDs (CBZ, PHT)
Continuous burning pain	Loss of inhibitory controls Peripheral sensitization Ectopic discharges	Restore inhibitory controls Block peripheral changes Block sodium channels	Gabapentin Amitriptyline Topical/local anesthetics (capsaicin) Sodium channel blockers

ACDs, anticonvulsive drugs; CBZ, carbamazepine; PHT, phenytoin.
Based on Woolf CJ, Mannion RJ: Neuropathic pain: Aetiology, symptoms, mechanisms, and management. Lancet 353:1959–1964, 1999.

naloxone may be a useful adjunct to his patient with severe pain being treated with significant doses of morphine. Although one can only imagine the response from the attending physician, it would be safe to assume that the intern would not be rapidly advanced to chief resident track at that moment.

CAN THERAPY BE IMPROVED USING CURRENT CLINICALLY AVAILABLE AGENTS?

Crain and Shen[1] proposed that ultra-low doses of opioid receptor antagonists (e.g., naloxone or nalmefene, a 6-methylene analog of naltrexone) may enhance the analgesic potency of morphine and other opioids and attenuate opioid tolerance. Clinical studies have seemed to lend some support for this concept,[2,3] although conflicting evidence exists. The use of ultra-low-dose opioid antagonists may diminish the severity or incidence of opioid side effects (e.g., pruritus, nausea). If the use of ultra-low-dose opioid antagonists with opioids is completely safe and leads to better analgesia, fewer side effects, and diminished tolerance, it seems that these agents should be used as concomitant therapy with almost all opioid administrations. One hypothetical scenario in which such concomitant therapy may be particularly useful is the administration of nalmefene, 20 μg subcutaneously every 12 hours, whenever an epidural solution is being administered containing an opioid (because itching is often an underappreciated side effect of spinal opioids).

Traditional opioid analgesics (e.g., morphine) exhibit bimodal modulation of the action potential of sensory neurons. One effect is *antianalgesic* via *excitatory* G_s-coupled opioid receptor–mediated effects (e.g., prolongation of the action potential duration) leading to increased neurotransmitter release. This antianalgesic effect is what Crain and Shen[1] proposed is blocked with picomolar concentrations of opioid antagonists (e.g., naloxone, naltrexone, nalmefene). These investigators also showed that cholera toxin B at remarkably low doses (10 ng/kg) selectively blocks hyperalgesic effects elicited by morphine and attenuated opioid tolerance in mice most likely via interference with the binding effects of GM_1 ganglioside on the opioid receptor complex.[5]

The second effect is analgesic via *inhibitory* G_s-coupled opioid receptor–mediated effects leading to decreased neurotransmitter release. This analgesic effect is what is blocked with higher (micromolar) concentrations of opioid antagonists (e.g., naloxone, naltrexone, nalmefene).

The concept could be explained as follows: μ agonists (e.g., morphine) bind to the μ receptor, producing essentially two effects: (1) a mild antianalgesic affect (via G_s coupling) and (2) a stronger proanalgesic effect (via G_i coupling). The addition of a clinical dose of a μ antagonist (e.g., naloxone) functionally blocks proanalgesic effects, whereas the addition of ultra-low doses of a μ antagonist (e.g., naloxone) may block the antianalgesic effects of a μ agonist and not affect the proanalgesic effects. Although these are fascinating ideas and seem to have some clinical support, conflicting evidence exists, and they are far from proven as clinical dogma. Cepeda et al have presented more conflicting evidence.[7]

As understanding of the mechanisms at play leading to pain conditions in individuals expands, the concept of what an analgesic is expands, too. In the future, analgesics may be different; clinicians may choose combinations of agonist or antagonist receptor subtypes, antibodies to various receptor subtypes and mediators, agents with neurotrophic factors, and specific modulators of cytokines or various transcriptional factors or employ gene therapy technology.

CONCLUSIONS

Presently, a variety of drug classes are used to treat chronic noncancer pain, including antidepressants, anticonvulsants, anti-inflammatory agents, muscle relaxants, antiarrhythmics, opioids, local anesthetics, and topical capsaicin. Thus far, these agents primarily have been directed toward the disease state associated with the pain. Treatment of pain may potentially be optimized, however, by supplementing existing information with the signs and symptoms manifested by the patient. By specifically targeting the mechanisms underlying these symptoms, it is hoped that an improved therapeutic response may be realized. The data on the symptom/mechanism/treatment relationship are preliminary, and further investigation is needed to substantiate existing observations. Current knowledge provides a framework, however, with which to begin addressing improved treatment. A relatively large number of neuropathic pain patients fail to find adequate relief with existing practices; these patients often develop significant comorbidity with sizable impact on their quality of life. It seems prudent to at least attempt to begin to focus treatment more directly toward the patient's putative mechanisms with the recognition that as additional data become available, specific therapeutic strategies may be modified.

REFERENCES FOR ADDITIONAL READING

1. Crain SM, Shen KF: Acute thermal hyperalgesia elicited by low-dose morphine in mormal mice is blocked by ultra-low-dose naltrexone, unmasking potent analgesia. Brain Res 888:75–82, 2001.
2. Gan TJ, Ginsberg B, Glass PS, et al: Opioid-sparing effects of a low-dose infusion of naloxone in patient-administered morphine sulfate. Anesthesiology 87:1075–1081, 1997.
3. Joshi GP, Duffy L, Chehade J, et al: Effects of prophylactic nalmefene on the incidence of morphine-related side effects in patients receiving intravenous patient-controlled analgesia. Anesthesiology 90:1007–1011, 1999.
4. Serra J: Overview of neuropathic pain syndromes. Acta Neurol Scand Suppl 173:7–11, 1999.
5. Shen KF, Crain SM: Cholera toxin-B subunit blocks excitatory opioid receptor-mediated hyperalgesic effects in mice, thereby unmasking potent opioid analgesia and attenuating opioid tolerance/dependence. Brain Res 919:20–30, 2001.
6. Woolf CJ, Mannion RJ: Neuropathic pain: Aetiolgy, symptoms, mechanisms, and management. Lancet 353:1959–1964, 1999.
7. Cepeda MS, Africano JM, Manrique AM et al: The combination of low dose of naloxone and morphine in PCA does not decrease opioid requirements in the postoperative period. Pain 96:73–79, 2002.

Chapter 2

Pathophysiology of Pain

Andrew Strassman, PhD

We most commonly think of pain as the unpleasant sensation that normally is evoked by an intense, potentially tissue-damaging stimulus. Pain stands apart from other sensations, however, in the extreme variability that characterizes the relationship between the stimulus and the resulting sensation. Severe injury may occur with no pain, as has been reported by soldiers in battle, whereas intense pain can be present with no detectable injury in the painful region, as occurs in some types of neuropathic pain. The ability of a given stimulus to evoke pain depends not only on the characteristics of the stimulus, but also on the current state of the neural systems that are responsible for the generation and modulation of pain. A major goal of basic pain research is to understand the neural basis for the extraordinary degree of plasticity exhibited by the pain system. This chapter gives an overview of the neural organization of the pain system, with a focus on modulatory mechanisms in primary afferent and dorsal horn neurons. More detailed reviews on specific topics with extensive references to the primary literature can be found in the References for Additional Reading.

It is useful to distinguish between three conditions under which pain may be evoked, based on the state of the tissue and its nerve supply: (1) pain evoked from uninjured tissue, (2) inflammatory pain, and (3) neuropathic pain. In uninjured tissue, pain normally is evoked only by relatively high intensities of stimuli that have the potential to cause injury. Such pain is an example of *nociception*, or the detection of a potentially harmful stimulus, and is initiated by the activation of the peripheral endings of nociceptive neurons. The stimulus intensity required to activate nociceptors and evoke pain in uninjured tissue is below the intensity required to produce actual tissue damage. This type of pain serves as a warning to prevent injury from occurring. It is generally not of any clinical consequence but nonetheless serves an essential protective function, as graphically illustrated by the debilitating injuries suffered by people with congenital inability to feel pain.

When tissue injury has occurred, with the concomitant production of endogenous inflammatory agents, a state of inflammatory pain hypersensitivity may be induced, in which the stimulus-response relationship is radically altered. This hypersensitivity may include *allodynia*, or pain evoked by a normally innocuous stimulus, and *hyperalgesia*, or abnormally intense or prolonged pain evoked by a noxious stimulus. The hypersensitive state results from changes in peripheral and central components of the pain system, including the induction of a state of *sensitization*, or abnormally elevated sensitivity, in primary afferent and dorsal horn neurons. Inflammatory pain hypersensitivity also serves a crucial protective function, in that it promotes healing by preventing use of the injured body part. It typically resolves with healing of the injured tissue.

Neuropathic pain results from injury or disease of the peripheral or central components of the neural systems involved in pain. Such injury induces additional changes in the affected neurons, beyond those produced by inflammation alone, that result partly from the disruption of axonal transport and the consequent loss of tissue-derived neurotrophic factors that regulate the expression of neurotransmitters and membrane components that govern excitability. As with inflammatory pain, neuropathic pain may be characterized by allodynia and hyperalgesia. Neuropathic pain also can occur in combination with partial or complete loss of evoked sensation. In contrast to inflammatory pain, neuropathic pain can persist after all healing from the initial injury has resolved. It does not serve any known adaptive function.

PRIMARY AFFERENT NOCICEPTORS AND THE SPECIFICITY THEORY OF PAIN

The specificity theory holds that the sensation of pain is mediated by a specialized neural system that is distinct from the systems that mediate nonpainful sensory modalities of touch and temperature. The simplest alternative theory would be that nonpainful and painful sensations result from different levels of activity in a single neuronal population. The specificity theory implies that selective activation of the neural systems that mediate non-painful sensations will not result in pain, even with maximal activation. It is instructive to consider to what degree the pain system can be understood within the context of the specificity theory, particularly in light of the phenomena of allodynia and pain hypersensitivity.

As predicted by the specificity theory, the skin is innervated by separate populations of sensory fibers that are specialized for the detection of either noxious or nonnoxious intensities of stimulation. Mechanoreceptors, which are primarily A beta fibers, respond maximally to innocuous mechanical stimulation. Thermoreceptors, which are A delta and C fibers, respond maximally to innocuous thermal stimuli and are subdivided into separate populations of warm and cold receptors. Nociceptors, which also are primarily A delta and C fibers, respond selectively to noxious, potentially damaging intensities of stimulation. Nociceptors can be distinguished from the other primary afferent classes not only by their higher response thresholds, but also by the shape of their stimulus-response curves. Heat-sensitive nociceptors show progressive increases in discharge rates with increasing stimulus temperatures in the noxious range ($>45°$ C), whereas warm receptors do not show such increases and instead may exhibit reduced or no discharge at these higher temperatures.

An additional distinguishing characteristic of nociceptors is their sensitivity to endogenous substances that are produced at sites of tissue injury or inflammation. Such inflammatory mediators in some cases can evoke discharge in nociceptors, although the discharge is typically of short duration and much lower frequency than that evoked by mechanical or thermal stimuli. A far more robust and long-lasting effect of inflammatory mediators is the induction of sensitization, a state of enhanced sensitivity to mechanical or thermal stimuli. This state includes a decreased response threshold and an increased response to normally suprathreshold stimuli. Sensitization of peripheral nociceptors is thought to be partly responsible for the primary hyperalgesia that develops at a site of injury. (The secondary hyperalgesia that develops outside a region of injury is thought to be mediated by central mechanisms, which are discussed subsequently.)

Nociceptors can be subdivided based on their responsiveness to mechanical, thermal, and chemical stimuli. Many nociceptors respond to thermal and mechanical noxious stimuli, whereas others respond only to one modality or the other. Based on their response modality, these classes are termed mechanical-heat, mechanical, and heat nociceptors. A subset of these neurons also responds to noxious cold. Each of these subclasses also includes a percentage of neurons that are responsive to endogenous inflammatory mediators and are said to be chemosensitive as well. Some fibers also have been found that are initially unresponsive to mechanical stimuli but that acquire mechanosensitivity after exposure to inflammatory mediators. Such *silent nociceptors* have been described in a variety of somatic and visceral tissues and are thought to be important contributors to inflammatory pain hypersensitivity.

Visceral tissues receive a sensory innervation from small diameter (A delta and C) fibers that share with cutaneous nociceptors many anatomic and physiologic properties, including a sensitivity to a wide spectrum of inflammatory mediators. Classification of visceral primary afferents as nociceptors is complicated, however, by the fact that the criteria used for defining cutaneous nociceptors are not directly applicable to visceral afferents. This is partly because of the fundamentally different roles served by these neurons and the corresponding differences in the nature of the adequate stimuli for visceral and cutaneous pain. Direct mechanical trauma, such as from cutting, which evokes pain and activates nociceptors in skin, is generally not painful in hollow viscera, although distention can be extremely painful. Conversely, some visceral afferent neurons display a sensitivity to relatively small increases in temperature that would be innocuous in the skin but are potentially harmful to internal organs. There is generally far less information available on pain thresholds for visceral tissues than there is for skin.

More importantly, the existence of a distinct class of visceral primary afferents that are uniquely responsible for nociceptive function is open to question. Although visceral afferents with high response thresholds exist, it has been argued that they represent one end of a single population of neurons with response thresholds distributed throughout the physiologic and supraphysiologic range. Some visceral afferents exhibit a wide-dynamic-range (WDR) type of response, in that they respond with increasing discharge frequency to increases in stimulus intensity from the innocuous to the noxious range. This response contrasts with cutaneous innervation, in which no WDR neurons are present peripherally, and instead innocuous and noxious stimuli are detected by separate populations of afferents. Examination of the stimulus-response functions for visceral afferents in many tissues indicates that progressive increases in stimulus intensity from the innocuous to the noxious range evoke a progressive increase in the discharge of individual neurons along with the recruitment of increasing numbers of neurons with progressively higher thresholds. Such data have led some investigators to suggest that visceral nociception may be subserved in part by summation of inputs from primary afferents with a wide range of response thresholds, rather than (or in addition to) activity in a single population of specific nociceptors.

TRANSDUCTION IN NOCICEPTORS

Great progress has been made recently in understanding the transduction mechanisms by which nociceptors become activated in response to noxious stimuli. The fact that mechanical and thermal sensitivity can be modulated independently in individual nociceptors is evidence for the existence of separate, possibly multiple, transduction mechanisms. The receptor for capsaicin, the active ingredient in chili peppers, was cloned and identified as a nonselective cation channel. The cloned receptor, *VR-1*, is expressed selectively in a population of small-diameter dorsal root ganglion cells, consistent with the selective action of capsaicin *in vivo* on a subpopulation of small-diameter primary afferent nociceptors. The capsaicin receptor is activated by noxious heat and may function as a heat transducer *in vivo*. Another heat-activated nonselective cation current, I_{heat}, has been identified in a subpopulation of dorsal root ganglion cells that seems to be distinguished from the capsaicin-activated current by its lower relative contribution from calcium ions and its insensitivity to the pharmacologic blocker ruthenium red. The activation of VR-1 and I_{heat} is enhanced by bradykinin through a protein kinase C (PKC)–dependent mechanism and by prostaglandin E_2 (PGE_2) through the cyclic adenosine monophosphate (cAMP) cascade. Multiple transduction pathways seem to exist for noxious heat. The molecular basis for mechanotransduction in nociceptors has not yet been identified.

INFLAMMATORY MEDIATORS

Sensitivity to inflammatory mediators is common to small-diameter afferents in somatic and visceral tissues and is fundamental to their function in signaling the state of the tissue and evoking protective responses. As mentioned earlier, such agents may evoke discharge and enhance the neurons' sensitivity to other stimuli. These processes of activation and sensitization may be evoked independently and are mediated by distinct cellular mechanisms.

The excitatory and sensitizing effects of inflammatory mediators can be mediated either by a direct action on the primary afferent terminals or by an indirect action through the release of other agents from the neuron itself or other nonneural tissue elements. The direct actions are mediated by specific membrane receptors that are localized selectively in the primary afferent nerve branches in the innervated tissue. Individual primary afferent fibers typically possess receptors to multiple inflammatory mediators, and each mediator may bind to multiple receptor subtypes. In most cases, the receptor is not itself an ion channel but instead is coupled to an intracellular second-messenger cascade, whose activation results in the modification of ion channels, often through phosphorylation by one of two specific protein kinases: the cAMP-dependent protein kinase A (PKA) or PKC, which is activated by the phospholipase C–generated second messengers diacylglycerol and calcium. One exception is the 5-hydroxytryptamine (5-HT)$_3$ receptor, which is itself a cation channel that mediates the direct excitatory action of 5-HT (serotonin).

Bradykinin, a peptide that is cleaved from circulating precursor proteins by activated kallikreins at sites of tissue injury, directly excites nociceptors and causes sensitization, in part by stimulating release of prostaglandins from sympathetic nerve terminals. In contrast, PGE_2 and other arachidonic acid metabolites generally evoke little or no discharge in most cutaneous and visceral afferents, but they produce sensitization to mechanical and thermal stimuli through a direct action on nociceptors. PGE_2 sensitization is mediated by the cAMP/PKA cascade. Prostaglandins are synthesized by the cyclooxygenase pathway, which is the target of nonsteroidal antiinflammatory drugs. 5-HT is released by activated platelets during inflammation and produces excitation and sensitization of nociceptors. As noted earlier, excitation is through 5-HT_3 receptors, whereas sensitization is through 5-HT_{1A} and 5-HT_4 receptors acting through a cAMP-dependent mechanism. An opposing, inhibitory action is exerted on cAMP synthesis, however, through $5HT_{1D}$ receptors that reduces calcium current and neuropeptide release. These latter actions are thought to be involved in the antimigraine effect of 5-HT_{1D} agonists such as sumatriptan.

Adenosine triphosphate (ATP) is released from cells by tissue damage and excites sensory neurons through an action at the P2X purinoreceptor, which is a nonselective cation channel. A $P2X_3$ purinoreceptor subtype has been identified that is selectively expressed by primary afferent C fiber neurons. Adenosine is a breakdown product of ATP that produces pain and hyperalgesia through a direct cAMP-dependent action at the A_2 adenosine receptor. One of the actions of adenosine, 5-HT, and PGE_2 is to enhance the magnitude of a tetrodotoxin-resistant, voltage-gated sodium current that is expressed only in C fibers.

Inflammatory mediators can exert synergistic effects when applied in combination.

Bradykinin-evoked discharge of small-diameter primary afferents is enhanced greatly by 5-HT. Histamine, which is released by degranulating mast cells, produces only itch sensations when applied alone to skin but produces pain after a conditioning application of bradykinin. This change is paralleled by an increase in the histamine response of C fiber neurons and in the proportion of histamine-responsive neurons. Acidic pH, which is present in inflamed tissues, not only produces activation and sensitization of C fibers, but also enhances the effects of other inflammatory mediators. The excitatory actions of acidic pH seem to be mediated in part through a hydrogen ion–gated nonselective cation channel that is expressed in small-diameter, neuropeptide-containing sensory neurons. Acidic pH also potentiates current flow through the capsaicin receptor.

Evidence has shown that cytokines and neurotrophic factors also play a crucial role in the mediation of inflammatory pain hypersensitivity. Many proinflammatory cytokines are released by macrophages and mast cells after tissue injury, including tumor necrosis factor-α interleukin 1-β, and interleukin-6, that interact with other inflammatory mediators and have either direct or indirect sensitizing actions on nociceptors. Nerve growth factor is up-regulated during inflammation and acts on nociceptors through tyrosine kinase A receptors to increase excitability by altering the expression of a variety of membrane channels and receptors and neuropeptides.

NEUROGENIC INFLAMMATION

Subpopulations of small diameter (A delta and C) primary afferent fibers contain neuropeptides that can have inflammatory effects when released from the peripheral nerve endings. The most abundant are calcitonin gene–related peptide, which mediates vasodilation, and substance P, which degranulates mast cells and causes plasma extravasation. It has not been established clearly whether release of these neuropeptides can produce activation or sensitization of primary afferent nociceptors. The role of neurogenic inflammation in clinical pain states is uncertain, although it has been hypothesized to contribute to the pathogenesis of conditions such as arthritis and migraine.

NOCICEPTIVE ORGANIZATION IN THE SPINAL DORSAL HORN

Anatomic Organization

Primary afferent nociceptors have small to medium-sized cell bodies located in the dorsal root and trigeminal (gasserian) ganglia and, as noted earlier, mostly possess small myelinated (A delta fiber) or unmyelinated (C fiber) axons. The main central axonal termination site of primary afferent nociceptors is the spinal dorsal horn and its trigeminal equivalent, the trigeminal subnucleus caudalis (medullary dorsal horn). Nociceptive primary afferents terminate most heavily in the superficial part of the dorsal horn, laminae I and II (marginal zone and substantia gelatinosa), and in lamina V (the neck or base of the dorsal horn). Additional terminals also are found in lamina X, the area around the central canal. Primary afferent thermoreceptors also terminate in laminae I and II. In contrast, primary afferent mechanoreceptors terminate primarily in laminae III and IV and are segregated spatially from the nociceptor termination zone.

Central terminals of small-diameter primary afferents in the dorsal horn form synaptic contacts on dorsal horn projection neurons, whose axons ascend to specific regions of the brainstem and thalamus, and on local interneurons, whose axons remain within the dorsal horn. Dorsal horn interneurons form synaptic contacts on other dorsal horn neurons and on the central axonal terminals of primary afferent neurons.

Nociceptive projection neurons are concentrated most heavily in laminae I and V, whereas lamina II contains primarily local interneurons. In addition to the axonal projections from primary afferents and local interneurons, dorsal horn neurons receive descending axonal projections from brainstem regions, such as the nucleus raphe magnus, that exert modulatory influences on nociceptive transmission. These brainstem projections descend in part through the dorsolateral funiculus of the spinal cord and terminate heavily in laminae I, II, and V.

Response Properties of Dorsal Horn Neurons

Primary afferent mechanoreceptors, thermoreceptors, and nociceptors each have axonal projections that terminate centrally in the spinal dorsal horn (and its trigeminal equivalent, the nucleus caudalis or medullary dorsal horn). The dorsal horn contains three classes of neurons that each receive their main peripheral sensory input from one of these three classes of primary afferent neurons and are called low-threshold mechanoreceptors, thermoreceptors, and nociceptive-specific neurons. The dorsal horn also contains another type of neuron, the WDR neuron, which receives a convergent input from primary afferent nociceptors and mechanoreceptors. As a result of this convergent input, WDR neurons respond to innocuous and noxious intensities of mechanical stimuli. WDR neurons have higher discharge rates for noxious than nonnoxious mechanical stimulation and are considered to have a nociceptive function. Many lines of indirect evidence support the idea that WDR neurons are involved in the mediation of painful sensations. The axons of WDR neurons project to the thalamus via the ventrolateral quadrant of the spinal white matter, and the ventrolateral quadrant is implicated strongly in the transmission of ascending signals involved in pain. Electrical stimulation of the ventrolateral quadrant with parameters that are effective for activation of WDR axons evokes painful sensations in humans. In addition, the stimulus-response relationship of human pain sensation to noxious heat is matched more closely by the intensity coding of WDR neurons than nociceptive-specific neurons.

If WDR neurons do mediate painful sensations, this raises the question of why activation of WDR neurons by low-threshold mechanoreceptive A beta fibers does not normally evoke pain. The explanation commonly given is that WDR neuron discharge must reach a certain minimal rate before pain is evoked, and the A beta fiber input to WDR neurons normally is not sufficiently strong to produce this required level of activation. This explanation may be incomplete, however. WDR neurons can be made to discharge at substantial rates by nonnoxious mechanical stimuli, such as brush and, especially, pressure, and these rates are often as high or higher than those evoked by mildly noxious heat (46°C). It is not fully understood what factors determine whether a given level of WDR discharge will be associated with pain.

PERIPHERAL VERSUS CENTRAL MECHANISMS OF PAIN HYPERSENSITIVITY

Sensitization can occur not only in primary afferent nociceptors, but also in dorsal horn neurons. Such central sensitization potentially has different consequences for pain hypersensitivity that allow it to be distinguished from peripheral sensitization. Activation of A beta fibers normally evokes only nonpainful, tactile sensations, but in some conditions of pain hypersensitivity, A beta fiber activation evokes pain, resulting in a condition called *A beta–mediated allodynia*. A beta–mediated allodynia can result only from a central alteration, not from peripheral sensitization. The allodynia that results from peripheral sensitization is mediated by C and A delta nociceptive fibers. It results from a lowering of the threshold of fibers that normally evoke pain. In contrast, A beta–mediated allodynia is a condition in which fibers that already have a low threshold acquire the ability to evoke pain.

One way that this condition might occur is through central sensitization of WDR dorsal horn neurons. Central sensitization is a state of increased excitability that is induced by sustained C fiber activity and results in augmented responses to all sensory inputs, including those from A beta fibers. After sensitization, WDR neurons respond to A beta fiber inputs with discharge rates that normally are evoked only by noxious stimuli. Sensitization of nociceptive-specific dorsal horn neurons would not result in A beta–mediated allodynia because these neurons do not receive an input from A beta fibers, and central sensitization only can amplify the existing inputs, not create new ones.

An amplification of A beta inputs to WDR neurons also could result from an alteration in the neurotransmitter that is released from A beta fibers. The neuropeptide substance P normally is synthesized only in A delta and C fibers, but there is evidence that peripheral inflammation can result in the expression of substance P in A beta fibers. Because substance P exerts a more prolonged excitatory action than the transmitters such as glutamate that are normally present in A beta fibers, substance P release from A beta fibers could augment the activity they evoke in WDR neurons through increased temporal summation of excitatory postsynaptic potentials.

One potential mechanism for A beta–mediated allodynia that does not depend on WDR neurons is the sprouting of new axonal branches of A beta fibers within the dorsal horn into areas that normally are reserved for nociceptive (A delta and C) fibers. Normally A beta fiber terminals are restricted to laminae III and IV of the dorsal horn, but peripheral nerve injury can induce A beta fibers to sprout new branches that enter the more superficial layers, which normally receive only A delta and C fiber input. This change might allow A beta fibers to activate nociceptive-specific dorsal horn neurons in laminae I and II. Central sprouting apparently requires peripheral nerve injury and is potentially relevant only for neuropathic but not inflammatory pain.

The three potential mechanisms of allodynia described are examples of three different types of neural plasticity. Central sensitization involves modification of existing proteins through phosphorylation (see subsequently) and requires no new protein synthesis. This is also true of peripheral sensitization. Synthesis of substance P by A beta fibers involves a change in gene expression (*phenotypic change*) that includes synthesis of new proteins. Central sprouting involves not only new protein synthesis, but also actual growth and structural change.

PRIMARY AFFERENT TRANSMITTERS, NMDA RECEPTORS, AND THE CELLULAR MECHANISM OF CENTRAL SENSITIZATION

Stimulation of small-diameter primary afferent fibers evokes excitatory postsynaptic potentials in dorsal horn neurons that exhibit two kinetically and pharmacologically distinct components: (1) a fast, brief excitation resulting from release of glutamate and (2) a slower, more prolonged excitation resulting from the release of the neuropeptide substance P. Glutamate and substance P are colocalized in many small-diameter primary afferents and are thought to be coreleased from their central terminals. The postsynaptic actions of glutamate are mediated by two classes of receptors: *ionotropic*, which are directly coupled to membrane ion channels, and *metabotropic*, which exert their effects by coupling via G proteins to intracellular second-messenger systems. The fast excitation evoked by glutamate in dorsal horn neurons is mediated by ionotropic receptors, of which there are three subtypes: N-methyl-D-aspartate (NMDA), kainate, and AMPA. The ionotropic glutamate receptors all act by opening a Na^+/Ca^{++} cation channel, although the NMDA receptor has a relatively greater permeability to Ca^{++}, which is important in the phenomenon of central sensitization. The slower excitation produced by substance P and the related peptide neurokinin A is mediated by the neurokinin receptors NK1 and NK2 and results from a decrease in K^+ conductance. It is thought that the excitation produced by a brief, acute noxious stimulus is mediated primarily by the non-NMDA (kainate and AMPA) ionotropic glutamate receptors, whereas activation of NMDA and neurokinin receptors occurs with more prolonged noxious stimuli.

The distinctive properties of the NMDA receptor underly the phenomenon of central sensitization. Most ion channels are opened (*gated*) by either ligand binding or a voltage change, but the NMDA receptor is an unusual example of a ligand-gated channel that also has a strong voltage dependence. At resting membrane potentials, ion flow through the NMDA receptor/ion channel is blocked by Mg^{++} ions. This Mg^{++} block is voltage dependent and is removed by depolarization. Glutamate binding to the receptors produces no ion flow unless the cell already is depolarized, such as by corelease of substance P. When the cell has been depolarized, opening of the channel results in influx of Na^{++} and Ca^{++}, which produces further depolarization and in turn causes further Ca^{++} inflow as a result of opening of voltage-dependent Ca^{++} channels. The resulting elevation in intracellular Ca^{++} results in activation of PKC and phosphorylation of the NMDA receptor. Phosphorylation of the receptor partially removes the Mg^{++} block so that glutamate binding produces ion flow even at resting membrane potentials. The phosphorylation-induced increase in glutamate sensitivity results in an increased state of neuronal excitability, or sensitization.

Inhibition

All of the mechanisms of pain hypersensitivity discussed involve augmenting of neuronal excitation. The dorsal horn also contains powerful inhibitory mechanisms, however, and disruption or removal of inhibition also is a potential mechanism of neuronal hyperexcitability. Although the direct effect of primary afferents on their postsynaptic target neurons in the dorsal horn is predominantly excitatory, primary afferents indirectly exert inhibitory effects on dorsal horn neurons through the activation of inhibitory interneurons. In addition to inhibiting other dorsal horn neurons, inhibitory interneurons can suppress the release of transmitters from the central terminals of primary afferent neurons, an effect termed *presynaptic inhibition*. As a result of these inhibitory interneurons, any afferent-evoked excitation in the dorsal horn normally is accompanied by inhibition as well. The inhibition places a limit on the excitatory effects, in terms of amplitude, spatial distribution, and duration.

The most abundant inhibitory transmitter in dorsal horn interneurons is γ-aminobutyric acid (GABA), which is present in approximately 30% of neurons in the superficial dorsal horn. About half of the GABA-containing cells also contain the inhibitory transmitter glycine. GABA, through an action at the $GABA_A$ receptor, and glycine produce inhibition by opening of chloride channels. Acetylcholine, which also exerts inhibitory actions, is present in a subset of the GABAergic neurons that do not contain glycine. Antagonism of spinal glycine,

GABA, or cholinergic receptors by intrathecal administration of strychnine, bicuculline, or atropine can produce hypersensitivity and aversive behavioral responses to nonnoxious mechanical stimuli. Strychnine and bicuculline also reduce the myelinated afferent–induced inhibition of nociceptive dorsal horn neurons. From these observations, it seems that myelinated afferents activate GABA-ergic and glycinergic inhibitory interneurons, which in turn attenuate the responses of nociceptive projection neurons to nonnoxious stimulation.

The opioid peptide enkephalin also is present in a subset of dorsal horn interneurons. Enkephalin has a hyperpolarizing (inhibitory) effect on dorsal horn neurons mediated by μ opiate receptors. μ agonists produce a selective inhibition of nociceptive responses. δ opiate receptors also are present in the dorsal horn but are located predominantly on axons, where they are thought to mediate presynaptic inhibition. A separate subset of dorsal horn neurons contains dynorphin, the endogenous ligand for the κ opiate receptor. The number of dynorphin-containing neurons in the dorsal horn is increased greatly after peripheral inflammation or nerve injury. It has been suggested that spinal dynorphin may antagonize the antinociceptive actions of other opioid peptides.

Peripheral nerve injury produces many changes that could result in a reduced inhibition of dorsal horn neurons, including decreased dorsal horn levels of GABA, GABA receptors, and μ opioid receptors. The ectopic discharge that results from peripheral nerve injury is thought to produce excitotoxic damage and death of inhibitory interneurons in lamina II. Interneurons are the smallest neurons in the dorsal horn and the most likely to be damaged because small neurons have a higher susceptibility to excitotoxicity.

DESCENDING MODULATION

Dorsal horn neurons are influenced not only by sensory inputs from peripheral tissues, but also by descending modulatory projections arising from specific brainstem sites. The power of these descending influences is shown by the profound analgesia that can be produced by electrical stimulation or microinjection of morphine at these sites, most notably the brainstem periaqueductal gray. Periaqueductal gray neurons do not project directly to the spinal cord but instead excite neurons in other brainstem regions, which send axonal projections directly to the spinal dorsal horn. These descending spinal projections arise in part from neurons that contain the biogenic amines 5-HT and noradrenaline. Descending 5-HT projections originate entirely from a subset of neurons in the nucleus raphe magnus, which is located in the rostral ventromedial medulla. Spinal projecting noradrenaline neurons are distributed in specific cell groups of the dorsolateral pontomesencephalic tegmentum, including the locus caeruleus and the A7 region. Spinal actions of noradrenaline on dorsal horn nociceptive transmission are mediated by α_2-receptors and are inhibitory. 5-HT actions in the dorsal horn are mediated by several receptor subtypes, including 5-HT$_{1A}$, 5-HT$_2$, and 5-HT$_3$, and include facilitatory and inhibitory effects. In addition to the biogenic amines, many other transmitters and neuromodulators have been localized in populations of spinal-projecting brainstem neurons, including enkephalin, substance P, and GABA.

Descending modulation can be excitatory and inhibitory. The rostroventral medulla contains two separate classes of spinal-projecting cells, *On cells* and *Off cells*, that are thought to exert excitatory and inhibitory effects on dorsal horn nociceptive transmission. Neither cell type contains 5-HT. On cells, which have μ-opiate receptors, exert a tonic GABA-mediated inhibition of Off cell activity through local axon collaterals. Opioids produce antinociception in part through μ-mediated inhibition of On cells, which in turn results in a removal of the On cell–mediated GABAergic inhibition of Off cells. Opioids inhibit On cells and excite Off cells, and both actions are thought to result in a reduction in dorsal horn activity. Evidence indicates that alterations in the activity of descending modulatory neurons can contribute to inflammatory and neuropathic pain states.

ECTOPIC DISCHARGE AND NEUROPATHIC PAIN

Action potential initiation in peripheral sensory nerve fibers normally is restricted to specialized sites in the peripheral branches within the innervated tissue. These sites contain specific transduction elements that are sensitive to thermal, mechanical, or chemical stimuli. The remainder of the peripheral nerve axon does not contain such transduction elements and normally serves only for the conduction of action potentials, not for their initiation. Peripheral nerve injury can induce changes in the neuronal membrane, however, that result in the generation of ectopic discharge. Such changes may occur at the neuroma or injury site and in the cell body in the dorsal root ganglion. These changes include the abnormal expression of α-adrenoreceptors, alterations in the number and type of sodium channels, and the development of ectopic mechanosensitivity. Adrenoreceptor expression renders the neurons sensitive to activation by circulating catecholamines and noradrenaline released from local sympathetic nerve terminals and may be the basis for the phenomenon of sympathetically maintained pain that is present in a subset of neuropathic pain patients. The abnormal sodium channel expression apparently can lower the firing threshold sufficiently to produce spontaneous discharge. Of importance in the generation of ectopic discharge is the accumulation of the tetrodotoxin-resistant class of sodium channels that are present only in C fibers and exhibit distinctive kinetic and pharmacologic properties. Suppression of these abnormal sodium currents may be part of the basis for the therapeutic actions in neuropathic pain of systemically administered local anesthetics and anticonvulsants. Spontaneous discharge of injured nociceptive peripheral nerve fibers potentially could contribute not only to spontaneous pain, but also to the establishment and maintenance of a sensitized state in dorsal horn neurons that could underly the persistent allodynia and hyperalgesia.

REFERENCES FOR ADDITIONAL READING

1. Devor M, Seltzer Z: Pathophysiology of damaged nerves in relation to chronic pain. In: Wall PD, Melzack R (eds): Textbook of Pain, 4th ed. New York: Churchill Livingstone, 1999, pp 129–164.
2. Doubell TP, Mannion RJ, Woolf CJ: The dorsal horn: State-dependent sensory processing, plasticity and the generation of pain. In: Wall PD, Melzack R (eds): Textbook of Pain, 4th ed. New York: Churchill Livingstone, 1999, pp 165–182.
3. Fields HL, Basbaum AI: Central nervous system mechanisms of pain modulation. In: Wall PD, Melzack R (eds): Textbook of Pain, 4th ed. New York: Churchill Livingstone, 1999, pp 309–329.
4. Levine J, Reichling DB: Peripheral mechanisms of inflammatory pain. In: Wall PD, Melzack R (eds): Textbook of Pain, 4th ed. New York: Churchill Livingstone, 1999, pp 59–84.
5. Millan MJ: The induction of pain: An integrative review. Prog Neurobiol 57:1–164, 1999.
6. Rafa SN, Meyer RA, Ringkamp M, Campbell JN: Peripheral neural mechanisms of nociception. In: Wall PD, Melzack R (eds): Textbook of Pain, 4th ed. New York: Churchill Livingstone, 1999, pp 11–58.
7. Urban MO, Gebhart GF: Supraspinal contributions to hyperalgesia. Proc Natl Acad Sci U S A 96:7687–7692, 1999.
8. Woolf CJ: Windup and central sensitization are not equivalent. Pain 66:105–108, 1996.
9. Woolf CJ, Mannion RJ: Neuropathic pain: Aetiology, symptoms, mechanisms, and management. Lancet 353:1959–1964, 1999.

Chapter 3

Acetaminophen (Bench)

Howard S. Smith, MD

Acetaminophen (known in the United Kingdom as *paracetamol*) is an aniline derivative. Aniline derivatives (occasionally referred to as *coal tar analgesics*) are strong antipyretics that may exert their antipyretic effects on the thermoregulatory center of the hypothalamus. Aniline can lead to formation of methemoglobin and methemoglobinemia in large doses. The hydroxylated anilines (ortho, meta, and para) are known as the *aminophenols*. p-Aminophenol (a metabolite of aniline) is the least toxic of the three. Early attempts to reduce toxicity of p-aminophenol involved the acetylation of the amine group, yielding N-acetyl-p-aminophenol (APAP) (Fig. 1). This compound has seemed to be the safest; however, it still contains the free amino group, and the production of methemoglobin is possible if acetaminophen is ingested in supraphysiologic doses.

MECHANISM OF ACTION

Although the mechanism of action of acetaminophen is uncertain, significant data have accumulated suggesting a central mechanism of action. It seems rational that acetaminophen should exert some of its actions in the central nervous system because it would be expected to present in significant concentrations there. Acetaminophen has a high lipid solubility,[25] it binds weakly to plasma proteins,[18] and it crosses the human and rat blood-brain barrier.[3] Acetaminophen accumulates in the central nervous system of the rat after oral administration.[5]

Carlsson and Jurna[15] concluded that acetaminophen diminished (but did not abolish at any dose) thalamic evoked potentials in rats, elicited by nociceptive electrical stimulation of the sural nerve. The evoked activity was diminished to 60% of the controls (the same by all three doses), and the effect was unchanged by naloxone. Morphine sulfate completely blocked thalamic activity.[15] Piguet et al[51] did not find a ceiling effect. Directly stimulating the sural nerve with suprathreshold stimuli, Bustamante et al[14] showed that acetaminophen exerted an inhibitory effect on a rat C fiber–evoked reflex.

Pilleta et al[52] concluded that acetaminophen-induced analgesia is centrally mediated. These investigators showed that 2 g of propacetamol (a prodrug of acetaminophen that yields half the amount, i.e., 1 g of acetaminophen) induced a significant increase in the RIII reflex and pain threshold. The *RIII reflex* (a direct stimulation of the sural nerve while recording electromyographic response in the biceps femoris) generally is used as an index of central pain modulation by drugs.[52] The effect of 1 g of aspirin did not differ significantly from placebo. The maximal effect was delayed for 2 hours, which coincides with the peak cerebrospinal fluid acetaminophen concentrations. Ketoprofen might be expected to have effects intermediate between aspirin and acetaminophen because it is relatively lipophilic and crosses the blood-brain barrier to some extent. It may be clinically useful to employ aspirin (acetylsalicylic acid [ASA]) and acetaminophen together for analgesia (taking advantage of

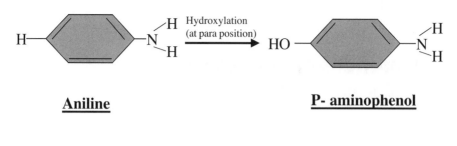

Figure 1. Chemical structure of acetaminophen.

peripheral [ASA] and central [APAP] mechanisms of action). A potential key mechanism of action for the central effects of APAP seems to involve the serotoninergic system.[50,67,69]

Peripheral action of acetaminophen is present and may contribute to the overall analgesic effects of acetaminophen.[12] Greenberg et al[27] suggested that single or multiple doses of acetaminophen reduce prostacyclin synthesis (although less so than indomethacin) and that single doses but not multiple doses of acetaminophen mildly reduce thromboxane synthesis (although much less so than indomethacin).

Flower and Vane[24] advanced the theory that acetaminophen had a high sensitivity for central cyclooxygenase (COX). This theory was not confirmed in later studies, however.[39] Another possible contributing mechanism of acetaminophen is that it could exert effects on COX-1 indirectly via free radical uptake *scavenging* (free radicals seem to be needed for COX activity).

Although not available in the United States, intravenous administration of propacetamol may be used in other countries (where generally intravenous N-acetylcysteine also is available). Luthy et al[42] using healthy volunteers compared the analgesic effects (using the RIII reflex) of a continuous infusion of propacetamol (total dose, 8 mg/24 h) with four short 10-minute infusions (2 g/dose) every 6 hours for 24 hours. Each bolus dose (2 g) yielded significant analgesia (maximum at 2 hours postinjection) for about 5 hours.[42] No significant analgesic effects could be detected after a continuous infusion, although the area under the curve (AUC) of APAP concentrations at steady-state were equivalent. It is conceivable that transient high plasma concentrations of paracetamol are required to achieve a *critical analgesic concentration* across the blood-brain barrier.

Different antinociceptive mechanisms seem to be present for aspirn (ASA) versus acetaminophen. (APAP).[17] ASA and APA reduced nociceptive behavior in glutamate pain models.[17] In a formalin pain model, ASA produced an antinociceptive effect during the second phase (20 to 40 minutes) but not during the first phase (0 to 5 minutes), whereas APAP was antinociceptive in both phases. In the substance P–induced nociceptive response, APAP but not ASA yielded antinociceptive effects in a dose-dependent fashion.[17]

Hoffer et al[23] theorized that glucosamine sulfate may be beneficial in osteoarthritis by contributing sulfate, which is required for glycosaminoglycan synthesis. If this theory holds true, factors that can reduce sulfate (e.g., APAP therapy, poor diet, altered renal function) potentially may adversely affect osteoarthritis or glucosamine sulfate treatment, and non-sulfate salts of glucosamine would not be predicted to have efficacy.

Acetaminophen plus caffeine exhibited synergistic effects on the inhibition of prostaglandin E_2 synthesis in rat microglial cells.[20] Acetaminophen only inhibited COX enzyme activity, but caffeine inhibited COX-2 protein synthesis as well.

Raffa et al[58] showed strong antinociceptive synergism between acetaminophen and phentolamine, revealing a potential role for ion channel subtypes or spinal cord adrenoceptors with acetaminophen-induced antinociception. Muth-Selbach et al[47] proposed that the antinociceptive effects of acetaminophen are due at least partly to inhibition of spinal prostaglandin E_2 release.

Botting[9] proposed the existence of a COX-2 variant or new COX, which she referred to as COX-3. Acetaminophen could inhibit COX-3 selectively and effectively, and this may account for differential actions of APAP in different tissues and partially explain acetaminophen's mechanism of action for analgesia.[9] An alternative explanation for the known tissue selectivity of acetaminophen may be that its effects vary dramatically depending on the local redox milieu. Acetaminophen may act to reduce the active oxidized form of COX to the resting form.[49] If this is the case, acetaminophen-induced COX inhibition would be more effective under conditions of low peroxide concentration.

Previous studies indicated that some nonsteroidal antiinflammatory drugs (NSAIDs) seem to exhibit central opioid receptor-mediated effects.[7] Pini et al[53] showed that naloxone is able to prevent the antinociceptive activity of acetaminophen in the hot-plate test and in the first phase of the formalin test. Sandrini et al[66] examined the rat brain for immunoreactive dynorphin A levels in rats subjected to the hot-plate and formalin tests. They hypothesized that a relationship exists between the dynorphinergic system and acetaminophen-induced antinociception because dynorphin was generated as soon as the inflammatory process started, and blockade of the κ receptors alone is enough to reverse the acetaminophen-induced antinociceptive effects.[66]

Raffa et al[57] proposed a *self-synergistic interaction* of acetaminophen's actions at the spinal and supraspinal levels to account for the antinociceptive activity of APAP. APAP induced spinally mediated antinociception, which was augmented significantly with the presence of supraspinal acetaminophen. Supraspinal APAP alone (e.g., in the intracerebral ventricle) had no antinociceptive effects. Potential mechanisms for spinal action include inhibition of nitric oxide mechanisms[8]; indirect effects on spinal cord hydroxytryptamine receptors[50]; and decreasing spinal prostaglandin E_2 release mechanism, which may *cross-talk* with endogenous opioid systems.[57] Additionally, it is conceivable that acetaminophen may possess direct scavenging activity of reactive oxygen species, similar to indomethacin, etodolac, and loxoprofen.[50] The analgesic mechanisms of acetaminophen remain unknown but are probably multiple.

Acetaminophen may act spinally to inhibit prostaglandin E_2 release via direct action on a COX-2 variant/COX-3–type isoenzyme and may act spinally to inhibit nitric oxide generation, which could impair the nociceptive potential of N-methyl-D-aspartate (NMDA) or NK-1 activation. Acetaminophen also may act supraspinally to alter the descending inhibitory pathways via indirect effects on serotoninergic pathways or indirect and direct effects on opioidergic systems predominantly by modulating dynorphin release and κ receptor function. APAP-induced antinociception may involve a complex interplay with synergism of spinal and supraspinal effects (Fig. 2).

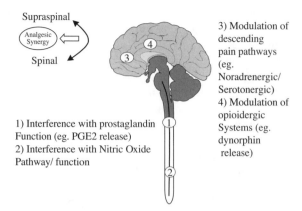

Figure 2. Potential analgesic mechanisms of acetaminophen.

ACETAMINOPHEN TOXICITY

The liver receives the major insult from acetaminophen toxicity, with the predominant lesion being acute centrilobular hepatic necrosis. Severe liver damage (arbitrarily defined as elevated plasma alanine or aspartate aminotransferase activity from >1,000 U/L) may result from a single dose of 150 to 250 mg/kg, but there is marked individual variation.

Mechanisms of Toxicity

A minor route of acetaminophen metabolism by cytochrome P-450–dependent mixed-function oxidase yields a reactive arylating metabolite, N-acetyl-p-benzoquinone imine (NAPQI) (Fig. 3). NAPQI can be produced by direct two-electron oxidation of acetaminophen by cytochrome P-450 or by a one-electron oxidation to N-acetyl-p-benzo-semi-quinone imine by peroxidase, prostaglandin H synthetase, or cytochrome P-450.[54] NAPQI

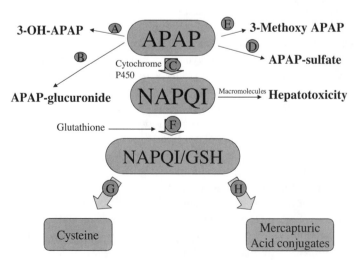

Figure 3. APAP metabolism.

may deplete the mitochondrial and cytosolic pools of reduced glutathione. Without reduced glutathione present, NAPQI directly arylates and oxidizes cellular proteins, leading to inhibition of enzyme activities. Glutathione peroxidase and thiol transferase are two specific enzymes inhibited in acetaminophen-treated animals.

In vivo, oxidants released from macrophages and neutrophils may alter protein thiols in tissues rendered vulnerable after the inhibition of glutathione peroxidase and thiol transferase. Calcium homeostatic disturbances may activate calcium-dependent catabolic activity (e.g., degradation of phospholipids and proteins) and cytoskeleton disruption. Metabolites of acetaminophen (e.g., 1,4-benzoquinone) may trigger calcium release from liver microsome from activation of calcium-releasing channels via direct interaction of 1,4-benzoquinone with the ryanodine-binding protein (ryanodine receptor).[71]

Acetaminophen hepatotoxicity traditionally has been viewed to depend on the balance between the rate of formation of NAPQI versus the rate of glutathione conjugation (Fig. 4). Additionally the NAPQI rate of formation is determined in part by the rate of absorption of acetaminophen, the environmental and genetic determinants of oxidative drug-metabolizing machinery, and the elimination of acetaminophen (glucuronide and sulfate conjugation). Toxicity is diminished by inhibiting acetaminophen oxidation and stimulation of glutathione synthesis. Alternatively, toxicity is augmented by increased acetaminophen oxidation (e.g., increased levels of isoenzymes P-450 2E1 or P-450 1A2) and depletion of hepatic glutathione stores (e.g., low-protein diet). Alcoholics and diabetic patients who do not respond well to insulin may possess increased levels of hepatic cytochrome P-450 2E1. It is conceivable that small amounts of ethanol ingested acutely at the time of overdose may offer protection against acetaminophen toxicity by increasing the NADH to NAD ratio. Alcoholics generally have decreased concentrations of glutathione because ethanol decreases hepatic reduced glutathione.[77] Ethanol, in addition to promoting diminished glutathione levels, leads to increases in levels of CYP2E1 (mostly via posttranscriptional processes), yielding stabilization against degradation.[35] Any process that increases CYP2E1, which generates reactive oxygen species, promotes hepatotoxicity. The generation of reactive oxygen species from ethanol-induced CYP2E1 in the liver Kupffer cell may be a major contributing mechanism to ethanol-induced hepatic insult. Additionally, ethanol tends to increase iron, the increased presence of which yields more powerful oxidants, contributing further to oxidative stress.[35]

Hepatotoxicity also may be promoted in the presence of any processes (e.g., stimulation of tumor necrosis factor receptor 1) that lead to Fas stimulation (bile acids that are elevated secondary to impaired secretion in cholestasis may build up enough to translocate intracellular Fas bearing vesicles to the plasma membrane, where they apparently self-aggregate, e.g., in the absence of a ligand).[35] Activated Fas receptor complexes on the plasma mem-

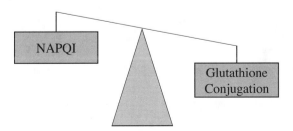

Figure 4. Acetaminophen toxicity. Mechanisms of APAP hepatotoxicity (old paradigm).

brane or if stimulated via other processes (e.g., tumor necrosis factor-α) may lead to caspase 8 activation and an apoptotic cascade.[35] Large doses of acetaminophen do not seem to be an attractive therapeutic option in these settings.

Various factors may reduce the toxicity of acetaminophen; however, none are proven. Cimetidine, calcium channel blocking agents, antioxidants, and NSAIDs and steroids are some possibilities. Bessems and Vermeulen[6] classified the numerous agents proposed to have some protective activity against APAP hepatotoxicity by proposed mechanism.

The basic paradigm of glutathione depletion tipping the scales toward a functional oversupply of the toxic metabolite NAPQI, which results in APAP hepatotoxicity, seems to be far from the whole story of APAP hepatotoxicity. Numerous mechanisms have been advanced to explain APAP toxicity. A partial list includes enzyme dysfunction owing to arylation of critical cell protein[4]; disruption of calcium homeostasis with activation of calcium-dependent degradative pathways[68]; oxidative stress with overproduction of reactive oxygen species and oxygen radicals[1]; enhanced lipid peroxidation[75]; inhibition of cell regeneration and repair[10]; production of cytotoxic mediators by activated Kupffer, reticuloendothelial, and immune cells[40]; mitochondrial dysfunction (respiratory chain insult)[13]; and induction of apoptosis.[61] Because many of these processes are inextricably linked, it becomes difficult to separate out the precise key determinants of APAP hepatotoxicity. APAP hepatotoxicity may be extremely complex and almost certainly multifactorial. The severity of APAP-induced damage seems to be reduced markedly by a wide variety of interventions, including pretreatment with calcium antagonists[60] or macrophage inhibitors (e.g. gadolinium chloride).[45] A new paradigm of APAP hepatotoxicity may be more appropriate (Fig. 5). Insult from oxidative stress seems to play a crucial role. Michael et al[45] showed significant increases in heme-adducted proteins and in nitrotyrosine adducts. The nitrotyrosine adducts are the result of the action of peroxynitrite, which is formed as a by-product of the oxidative burst of activated macrophages that infiltrate the APAP intoxicated liver.

Hepatocytes themselves seem to exhibit diminished ability to withstand oxidative stress in the APAP-intoxicated liver. Hepatocytes seem to be less capable of detoxifying oxidants

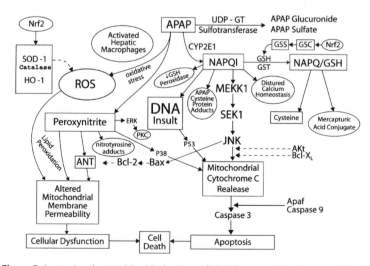

Figure 5. Acetaminophen toxicity. Mechanisms of APAP hepatotoxicity (new paradigm).

via mitochondrial glutathione peroxidase because this enzyme is a significant target of NAPQI.[56]

At low doses, most APAP is readily conjugated with glucuronic acid and sulfate via the action of UDP-glucuronosyltransferase and sulfotransferases, then eliminated. A small amount of APAP is acted on by the cytochrome P-450 system, which yields an electrophilic quinoneimine (NAPQI) that reacts nonenzymatically with glutathione and is excreted. Exposure to high APAP doses overwhelms the glucuronidation and sulfation pathways and depletes the glutathione pool. Excess NAPQI, which is not detoxified by glucuronidation, sulfation, or conjugation with glutathione, is capable of binding to intracellular macromolecules and resulting in cytotoxicity. Glutathione provides a protein measure against NAPQI. The rate-limiting step in the production of reduced glutathione is glutamylcysteine synthetase. Glutamylcysteine synthetase and glutathione synthetase and many other antioxidant enzymes are regulated by antioxidant-responsive elements–mediated gene expression. In glutathione-depleted states, the risk of hepatotoxicity seems to be greater. NAPQI, which may lead to hepatic glutathione depletion by 90%,[46] also may diminish levels of glutathione peroxidase—an enzyme that helps dampen the effects of oxidative stress.

In acetaminophen hepatotoxicity, inducible nitric oxide synthase is up-regulated, yielding nitric oxide, which scavenges superoxide to produce peroxynitrite leading to protein nitration and tissue insult.[35] It does not seem to lead to S-nitrosylation (inhibition) of various caspases, however, which may occur with exogenously administered nitric oxide (e.g., nitric oxide–releasing substances); instead, caspases seem to be activated. In nitric oxide synthase knockout mice, nitration is prevented, but unscavenged superoxide production can lead to toxic lipid peroxidation instead.[35]

In addition to the activation of apoptotic cascades, induction of permeabilization (mitochondrial permeability transition) can lead to mitochondrial failure, adenosine triphosphate depletion, and hepatic necrosis.[35] Another potential point of attack in APAP hepatotoxicity may be the direct action of peroxynitrite and other substances (e.g., nitric oxide) on the adenine nucleotide translocator (ANT). ANT is a key element in the permeability transition pore complex, and by causing ANT to undergo thiol oxidation, peroxynitrite may alter the permeability of the mitochondrial membrane (see Fig. 5).[74]

It seems that nitric oxide may exhibit hepatotoxicity and hepatoprotective effects. Although nitric oxide evolved from inducible nitric oxide synthase, it seems hepatotoxic.[32, 45] Nitric oxide produced from nitric oxide donors may exhibit hepatoprotective effects.[23, 44]

Serum and other factors and conditions can significantly alter the redox state. The local redox environment may affect signal transduction dramatically.[16]

It is conceivable that certain genetic polymorphisms may play a part in determining the susceptibility of individuals to drug-induced hepatitis. The degree of expression of antiinflammatory factors, such as the cytokine interleukin-10, versus the expression of proinflammatory cytokines (e.g., tumor necrosis factor-α, interleukin-1) may protect from or predispose to hepatic insult.[11]

A promising variant of acetaminophen, NCX-701 (nitroparacetamol or nitroacetaminophen), is a nitric oxide–releasing derivative of acetaminophen that seems to possess at least 20 times more potent analgesic effects, significant antiinflammatory activity, and no hepatotoxic effects.[26] NCX-701 seems to be potentially promising in seeming to exhibit at least equal or better analgesic efficacy (especially in certain models) to APAP but without hepatotoxicity.[2, 21, 64] It is conceivable that NCX-701 may possess hepatoprotective characteristics, with nitric oxide causing the S-nitrosylation (e.g., inhibition) of various caspases (e.g., caspase 1 [the interleukin-1β converting enzyme], caspase 8).[22] These caspases seem to be important in contributing to Fas-mediated liver injury and apoptosis, and nitric oxide inhibition of caspases may play a role in hepatoprotection.[22] Additionally, because nitric oxide donors may diminish the gastrointestinal toxicity of NSAIDs, the combination of NCX-701 with a NSAID or COX-2 agent may offer superior analgesia with an extremely low risk of gastrointestinal insult.

The mechanisms of APAP hepatotoxicity are not completely understood. Agents that seem to provide protection against APAP hepatotoxicity include clofibrate, a hypolipidemic drug that can induce peroxisome proliferation via stimulation of the peroxisome proliferator–activated receptor and may provide protection through antioxidant activity (e.g., increased catalase) or through inducing antiapoptotic transcription factors or protective factors (e.g., annexins)[43]; Articum lappa, a perennial herb that may provide protection through antioxidant activity[41]; chlorpromazine, which modulates DNA fragmentation[59]; poly (ADP-ribase) polymerase, which functions in repair of DNA)[59]; 4-aminobenzamide, which can inhibit oxidative stress[59]; stiripentol, an anticonvulsant drug that inhibis various cytochrome P-450 isoenzymes[72]; gadolinium chloride or dextran sulfate, inhibitors of hepatic macrophage functioning[45]; and S-(1,2-dicarboxyethyl) glutathione triester, which may provide protection via elevation of glutathione levels.[76]

Nephrotoxicity is a potential hazard of ingestion of large doses (>4 g/d) of acetaminophen for long periods. Potential mechanisms for this may involve APAP arresting many cells in late G_1 and S phases.[63] APAP via inhibition of ribonucleotide reductase may lead to chromosomal aberrations and inhibit the synthesis of DNA. Acetaminophen can produce a mixed form of cell death—oncosis (swollen cells and nuclei) and apoptosis.[63] APAP also can lead to deterioration of tubular function perhaps by impairing activity of key enzymes (e.g., alkaline phosphatase, Na^+, K^+-ATPase) at the basolateral membrane.[73]

The mechanisms of renal toxicity of acetaminophen and whether chronic acetaminophen nephrotoxicity exists remain obscure. Acute nephrotoxicity may be mediated in part via the formation of NAPQI formed during cytochrome P-450–catalyzed oxidation of acetaminophen in renal microsomes. This oxidation most likely would occur in the cortex and affect proximal tubules, leading to diminished glomerular filtration rates. Also, it is conceivable that the renal medulla may catalyze prostaglandin endoperoxide synthase/N-deacetylase reactions leading to p-aminophenoxy free radical/p-aminophenol production, which may contribute to nephrotoxicity as well.[6] Ray et al[62] showed in vivo protection against acetaminophen-induced nephrotoxicioty in mice pretreated with IH636 grapeseed proanthocyanidin extract.

The diagnosis of acetaminophen intoxication is confirmed with a plasma acetaminophen concentration. The mass units (mg/L) are still used; however, some laboratories may report SI units (1 mmol/L = 151 mg/L). Nonspecific methods should not be used because they may overestimate plasma acetaminophen concentration (PAC), as they also measure metabolites.[70]

The patient with acetaminophen toxicity may exhibit nausea and vomiting (within a few hours of ingestion); abdominal pain and tenderness secondary to swelling of Glisson's capsule (18 to 72 hours); oliguria, renal failure, and back pain (24 to 48 hours), and fulminant hepatic failure (third to sixth day). Other potential complications of acetaminophen intoxication include disseminated intravascular coagulation, acute pancreatitis, impaired carbohydrate tolerance, myocarditis, and hypophosphatemia.[37]

In the United States, some centers use the Rumack and Matthew[65] nomogram treatment line to decide when to treat; however, generally a plasma level of a 1 mmol/L (150 mg/L) or more at 4 hours (PAC) after ingestion is treatable. Patients with high PACs may not develop overt liver damage, and severe liver damage can occur at PACs of 0.083 mmol/L (125 mg/L) at 4 hours. Serial measurements of prothrombin time may be a reasonable prognostic guide.[29]

Patients who ingest 100 mg/kg or more of acetaminophen generally require treatment. Treatment with sulfhydryl donors should begin as soon as possible, especially within 8 hours of ingestion if possible; treatment still should be given for large ingested doses even at 24 hours afterward or if hepatic failure already is established.

Treatment

Prescott et al[55] suggested the use of the glutathione precursor of N-acetylcysteine for the treatment of acetaminophen intoxication in efforts to maintain hepatic reduced glutathione concentrations (reduced GSH cannot be given because it does not cross the plasma membrane). N-acetylcysteine may be beneficial in acetaminophen intoxication via multiple mechanisms:

1. Conjugation with or reduction of NAPQI, leading to the formation of other nucleophiles (e.g., cysteine, reduced glutathione) also capable of detoxifying NAPQI
2. Decrease of the toxic effects of activated oxygen and reduction of oxidixed thiol groups on enzymes
3. Decrease of the amount of acetaminophen bound covalently to proteins (through dissociation of the covalently bound acetaminophen from proteins or facilitating degradation of arylated proteins)

Optimal treatment time seems to be 8 hours or less from ingestion; the clinician should not wait past 8 hours for the results of plasma concentrations. N-acetylcysteine may have theoretical advantages over other therapeutic options, such as oral methionine. N-acetylcysteine has a therapeutic effect in established acetaminophen liver failure. Treatment definitely should be instituted 25 hours after ingestion and probably 50 hours after ingestion (although there are essentially no formal data from 24 hours to 50 hours). In patients who are vomiting and patients who have been given emetics or oral activated charcoal, intravenous N-acetylcysteine may be considered. There is a small incidence of anaphylactoid reactions to intravenous N-acetylcysteine (N-acetylcysteine is available only orally in the United States). It may be prudent to treat chronic alcoholics at a lower threshold than usual. Jones et al[38] addressed the question of whether it would help diminished clinical hepatotoxicity seen in the United Kingdom if methionine were added to every acetaminophen tablet (e.g., combination in the same tablet) and concluded that it would not be wise because the risks (e.g., long-term effects) are not well known.

Significant covalent binding of NAPQI to cellular macromolecules (e.g., DNA) results in hepatic cell death; however, this is not expected until hepatic glutathione concentrations are depressed to 20% of control values or lower.[19, 30, 31] This can occur with buthionine sulfoximine (a glutathione synthesis inhibitor) or diethylmaleate (a glutathione depletor). The most common scenarios of relative glutathione depletion include liver disease (e.g., hepatic cirrhosis), alcohol abuse (although values do not usually decrease to 20% of control—as a general rule, chronic consumption of 3 alcoholic drinks per day may result in significant glutathione depletion and one probably should not ingest 4 g of acetaminophen per day on a long-term basis in this situation), acetaminophen abuse, or use of α-adrenergic agonists. α-

Adrenergic agonists may lower hepatic glutathione significantly.[28] Many over-the-counter cold and allergy preparations contain sympathomimetic drugs, and many prescription drugs and stress may lead to adrenergic effects, which may potentiate hepatotoxicity from acetaminophen (e.g., as in overdose). Conversely, α-adrenergic antagonists may offer some degree of protection from hepatotoxicity.[36] Consumption of green tea (via induction of the microsomal detoxification enzymes, UDP-glucuronosyltransferase)[19] may offer hepatoprotection and may be worthwhile studying as an adjunct for patients taking 4 g/d of acetaminophen for many years.

REFERENCES FOR ADDITIONAL READING

1. Adamson GM, Harman AW: Oxidative stress in cultured hepatocytes exposed to acetaminophen. Biochem Pharmacol 45:2289–2294, 1993.
2. al-Swayeh OA, Futter LE, Clifford RH, et al: Nitroparacetamol exhibits anti-inflammatory and antinociceptive activity. Br J Pharmacol 130:1453–1456, 2000.
3. Bannwarth B, Netter P, Lapicque F, et al: Plasma and cerebrospinal fluid concentrations of paracetamol after a single intravenous dose of propacetamol. Br J Clin Pharmacol 24:79–81, 1992.
4. Bartelone JB, Cohen SD, Khairallah EA: Immunohistochemical localization of acetaminophen-bound liver proteins. Fund Appl Toxicol 13:859–862, 1989.
5. Besse D, Courade JP, Delchambre C, et al: Distribution of acetaminophen in rat central nervous system. Presented at 9th World Congress on Pain, Vienna, Austria, August 22–27, 1999.
6. Bessems JGM, Vermeulen NPE: Paracetamol (acetaminophen)-induced toxicity: Molecular and biochemical mechanisms, analogues and protective approaches. Crit Rev Toxicol 31:55–138, 2001.
7. Bjorkman R: Central antinociceptive effects of non-steroidal anti-inflammatory drugs and paracetamol. Experimental studies in the rat. Acta Anaesthesiol Scand 103:1–44, 1995.
8. Bjorkman R, Hallman KM, Hender T, et al: Acetaminophen blocks spinal hyperalgesia induced by NMDA and substance P. Pain 57:259–264, 1994.
9. Botting RM: Mechanism of action of acetaminophen: Is there a cyclooxygenase 3? Clin Infect Dis 31:S202–S210, 2000.
10. Boulares HA, Giardina C, Navarro CL, et al: Modulation of serum growth factor signal transduction in Hepa 1–6 cells by acetaminophen: An inhibition of c-myc expression, NF-kappa B activation, and Raf-1 kinase activated. Toxicol Sci 48:264–274, 1999.
11. Bourdi M, Masubuchi Y, Reilly TP, et al: Protection against acetaminophen-induced liver injury and lethality by interleukin 10: Role of inducible nitric oxide synthase. Hepatology 35:289–298, 2002.
12. Brune K, Beck WS, Geisslinger G, et al: Aspirin like drugs may block pain independently of prostaglandin synthesis inhibition. EXS (Basel) 46:257–261, 1991.
13. Burcham PC, Harman AW: Acetaminophen toxicity results in site-specific mitochondrial damage in isolated mouse hepatocytes. J Biol Chem 26:5049–5054, 1992.
14. Bustamante D, Paeile C, Willer JC, et al: Effects of intravenous non-steroidal anti-inflammatory drugs on a C-fibre reflex elicited by a wide range of stimulus intensities in the rat. J Pharmacol Exp Ther 276:1232–1243, 1996.
15. Carlsson KH, Jurna I: Central analgesic effect of paracetamol manifested by depression of nociceptive activity in thalamic neurons of the rat. Neurosci Lett 77:339–343, 1987.
16. Chan ED, Riches DW, White CW: Redox paradox: Effect of N-acetylcysteine and serum on oxidation reduction–sensitive mitogen-activated protein kinase signaling pathways. Am J Respir Cell Mol Biol 24:627–632, 2001.
17. Choi SS, Lee JK, Suh HW: Antinociceptive profiles of aspirin and acetaminophen in formalin, substance P and glutamate pain models. Brain Res 921:233–239, 2001.
18. Clissold SP: Paracetamol and phenacetin. Drugs 32(suppl 4):46–59, 1986.

19. Embola CW, Sohn OS, Fiala ES, et al: Induction of UDP-glucuronosyl transferase 1 (UDP-GT1) gene complex by green tea in male F344 rats. Food Chem Toxicol 40:841–844, 2002.

20. Fiebich BL, Lieb K, Hull M, et al: Effects of caffeine and paracetamol alone or in combination with acetylsalicylic acid on prostaglandin E (2) synthesis in rat microglial cells. Neuropharmacology 39:2205–2213, 2000.

21. Fiorucci S, Antonelli E, Mencarelli A, et al: A NO-releasing derivative of acetaminophen spares the liver by acting at several checkpoints in the Fas pathway. Br J Pharmacol 135:589–599, 2002.

22. Fiorucci S, Mencarelli A, Palazetti B, et al: An NO derivative of ursodeoxycholic acid protects agains Fas-mediated liver injury by inhibiting caspase activity. Proc Natl Acad Sci U S A 98:2652–2657, 2001.

23. Fiorucci S, Santucci L, Antonelli E, et al: NO-aspirin protects from T cell-mediated liver injury by inhibiting caspase dependent processing of Th1-like cytokines. Gastroenterology 118:404–421, 2000.

24. Flower RJ, Vane JR: Inhibition of prostaglandin synthetase in brain explains the antipyretic activity of paracetamol (4-acetamino-phenol). Nature 240:410–411, 1972.

25. Forrest JAM, Clements JA, Prescott LF: Clinical pharmacokinetic of paracetamol. Clin Pharmacokinet 7:93–107, 1982.

26. Futter LE, al-Swayeh OA, Moore PK: A comparison of the effect of nitroparacetamol and paracetamol on liver injury. Br J Pharmacol 132:10–12, 2001.

27. Greenberg HE, Schwartz JI, Waldman SA, et al: Acetaminophen inhibits prostacyclin synthesis in vivo. Poster presentation, American College of Rheumatology 63rd Annual Scientific Meeting, November 14, 1999.

28. Harbison RD, Jones RC, Roberts SM: Hepatic glutathione suppression by the α-adrenoreceptor stimulating agents phenylephrine and clonidine. Toxicology 69:279–290, 1991.

29. Harrison PM, O'Grady JG, Keays RT, et al: Serial prothrombin time as prognostic indicator in paracetamol induced fulimant hepatic failure. BMJ 301:964–966, 1990.

30. Hinson JA: Biochemical toxicology of acetaminophen. Rev Biochem Toxicol 69:279–290, 1980.

31. Hinson JA, Nelson SD, Mitchell JR: Studies on the microsomal formation of arylating metabolites of acetaminophen and phenacetin. Mol Pharmacol 13:625–633, 1977.

32. Hinson JA, Pike SL, Pumford NR, et al: Nitrotyrosine-protein adducts in hepatic centrilobular areas following toxic doses of acetaminophen in mice. Chem Res Toxicol 11:604–607, 1998.

33. Hoffer LJ, Kaplan LN, Hamadeh MJ, et al: Sulfate could mediate the therapeutic effect of glucosamine sulfate. Metabolism 50:767–770, 2001.

34. Ikeda Y, Matsumoto K, Dohi K, et al: Direct superoxide scavenging activity of nonsteroidal anti-inflammatory drugs: Determination by electron spin resonance using the spin trap method. Headache 41:138–141, 2001.

35. Jaeschke H, Gores GJ, Cederbaum AI, et al: Mechanisms of hepatotoxicity. Toxicol Sci 65:166–176, 2002.

36. James RC, Schieffer MA, Roberts SM, et al: Antagonism of cocaine-induced hepatotoxicity by the alpha adrenergic antagonists phentolamine and yohimbine. J Pharmacol Exp Ther 242:726–732, 1987.

37. Jones AF, Harvey JM, Vale JA: Hypophosphataemia and phosphaturia in paracetamol poisoning. Lancet 2:608–609, 1989.

38. Jones AL, Hayes PC, Proudfoot AT, et al: Should methionine be added to every paracetamol tablet? BMJ 315:301–304, 1997.

39. Lanz R, Polster P, Brune K: Antipyretic analgesic inhibit prostaglandin release from astrocytes and macrophages similarly. Eur J Pharmacol 130:105–109, 1986.

40. Laskin DL, Gardner CR, Price VF, et al: Modulation of macrophage functioning abrogates the acute hepatotoxicity of acetaminophen. Hepatology 21:1045–1050, 1995.

41. Lin SC, Chung TC, Lin CC: Hepatoprotective effects of Arctium lappa on carbon tetrachloride- and acetaminophen-induced liver damage. Am J Chin Med 28:163–73, 2000.

42. Luthy CS, Collart L, Stribemi R, et al: The rate of administration influences the analgesic effect of paracetamol. Clin Pharmacol Ther 32:151, 1992.

43. Mehendale HM: PPAE-alpha: A key to the mechanism of hepatoprotection by clofibrate. Toxicol Sci 57:187–190, 2000.

44. Michael SL, Mayeux PR, Bucci TJ, et al: Acetaminophen-induced hepatotoxicity in mice lacking inducible nitric oxide synthase activity. Nitric Oxide 5:432–441, 2001.

45. Michael SL, Pumford NR, Mayeux PR, et al: Pretreatment of mice with macrophage inhibitors decreases acetaminophen hepatotoxicity and the formation of reactive oxygen and nitrogen species. Hepatology 30:186–195, 1999.

46. Mitchell JR, Jollow DJ, Potter WZ, et al: Acetaminophen-induced necrosis: IV. Protective role of glutathione. J Pharmacol Exp Ther 187:211–217, 1973.

47. Muth-Selbach US, Tegeder I, Brune K, et al: Acetaminophen inhibits spinal prostaglandin E2 release after peripheral noxious stimulation. Anesthesiology 91:231–239, 1999.

48. Orrenium S, McConkey DJ, Nicotera P: Role of calcium in toxic and programmed cell death. Adv Exp Med Biol 283:419–425, 1991.

49. Ouellet M, Percival MD: Mechanism of acetaminophen inhibition of cyclooxygenase isoforms. Arch Biochem Biophys 387:273–280, 2001.

50. Pelissier T, Alloui A, Caussade F, et al: Paracetamol exerts a spinal antinociceptive effect involving an indirect interaction with 5-hydroxytryptamine 3 receptors: In vivo and in vitro evidence. J Pharmacol Exp Ther 278:8–14, 1996.

51. Piguet V, Desmeules J, Dayer P, et al: Lack of acetaminophen ceiling effect on RIII nociceptive flexion reflex. Eur J Clin Pharmacol 53:321–324, 1998.

52. Pilleta P, Porchet HC, Dayer P: Central analgesic of acetaminophen but not of aspirin. Clin Pharmacol Ther 49:350–354, 1991.

53. Pini LA, Vitale G, Ottani A, et al: Naloxone reversible antinociception by paracetamol in the rat. J Pharmacol Exp Ther 280:934–940, 1997.

54. Potter DW, Hinson JA: Mechanisms of acetaminophen oxidation to N-acetyl-P-benzoquinone imine by horseradish peroxidase and cytochrome P-450. J Biol Chem 262:966–973, 1987.

55. Prescott LF, Park J, Ballantyne A, et al: Treatment of paracetamol (acetaminophen) poisoning with N-acetylcysteine. Lancet 2:432–434, 1977.

56. Qiu Y, Benet LZ, Burlingame AL: Identification of the hepatic protein targets of reactive metabolities of acetaminophen in vivo in mice using two-dimensional gel electrophoresis and mass spectrometry. J Biol Chem 273:17940–17953, 1998.

57. Raffa RB, Stone DJ Jr, Tallarida RJ: Discovery of "self-synergistic" spinal/supraspinal antinociception produced by acetaminophen (paracetamol). J Pharmacol Exp Ther 295:291–294, 2000.

58. Raffa RB, Stone DJ Jr, Tallarida RJ: Unexpected and pronounced antinociceptive synergy between spinal acetaminophen (paracetamol) and phentolamine. Eur J Pharmacol 412:R1–2, 2001.

59. Ray SD, Balasubramanian G, Bagchi D, et al: Ca(2+)-calmodulin antagonist chlorpromazine and poly (ADP-ribose) polymerase modulators 4-aminobenzamide and nicotinamide influence hepatic expression of BCL-XL and P53 and protect against acetaminophen-induced programmed and unprogrammed cell death in mice. Free Radic Biol Med 31:277–291, 2001.

60. Ray SD, Kamendulis LM, Gurule MW, et al: Ca2+ antagonists inhibit DNA fragmentation and toxic cell death induced by acetaminophen. FASEB J 7:453–463, 1993.

61. Ray SD, Mumaw VR, Raje RR, et al: Protection of acetaminophen induced hepatocellular apoptosis and necrosis by cholesteryl hemisuccinate pretreatment. J Pharmacol Exp Ther 279:1470–1483, 1996.

62. Ray SD, Patel D, Wong V, et al: In vivo protection of DNA damage associated apoptotic and necrotic cell deaths during acetaminophen-induced nephrotoxicity, amiodarone-induced lung toxicity, and doxorubicin-induced cardiotoxicity by a novel IH636 grape seed proanthocyanidin extract. Res Commun Mol Pathol Pharmacol 107:137–166, 2000.

63. Rocha GM, Michea LF, Peters EM, et al: Direct toxicity of nonsteroidal anti-inflammatory drugs for renal medullary cells. Proc Natl Acad Sci U S A 98:5317–5322, 2001.

64. Romero-Sandoval EA, Mazario J, Howat D, et al: NCX-701 (nitroparacetamol) is an effective antinociceptive agent in rat withdrawl reflexed and wind-up. Br J Pharmacol 135:1556–1562, 2002.
65. Rumack BH, Matthew H: Acetaminophen poisoning and toxicity. Pediatrics 55:871–876, 1975.
66. Sandrini M. Romualdi P, Capobianco A, et al: The effect of paracetamol on nociception and dynorphin A levels in the rat brain. Neuropeptides 35:110–116, 2001.
67. Sandrini M, Vitale G, Ottani A, et al: The potentiation of analgesic activity of paracetamol plus morphine involved the serotoniergic system in the rat brain. Inflamm Res 48:127, 1999.
68. Shen W, Kamendulis LM, Ray SD, et al: Acetaminophen-induced cytotoxicity in cultured mouse hepatocytes: Effects of $Ca(2+)$—endonuclase, DNA repair, and glutathione depletion inhibitors on DNA fragmentation and cell death. Toxicol Appl Pharmacol 112:32–40, 1992.
69. Srikiatkhacor A, Tarasub N, Govitrapong P: Acetaminophen-induced antinociception via central 5-HT (2A) receptors. Neurochem Int 34:491–498, 1999.
70. Stewart MJ: Drug analyses in poisoned patients—the need to be specific. Ann Clin Biochem 19: 254–257, 1982.
71. Stoyanovsky DA, Cederbaum AI: Metabolites of acetaminophen trigger $Cz2+$ release from liver microsomes. Toxicol Lett 106:23–29, 1999.
72. Tran A, Treluyer JM, Rey E, et al: Protective effect of stirpentol on acetaminophen-induced hepatotoxicity in rat. Toxicol Appl Pharmacol 170:145–152, 2001.
73. Trumper L, Coux G, Elias MM: Effect of acetamionphen on $Na(+)$, $K(+)$ ATPase and alkaline phosphatase on plasma membranes of renal proximal tubules. Toxicol Appl Pharmacol 164:143–148, 2000.
74. Vieira HL, Belzacq AS, Haouzi D, et al: The adenine nucleotide translocator: A target of nitric oxide, peroxynitrite, and 4—hydroxynonenal. Oncogene 20:4350–4416, 2001.
75. Wendel A, Feuerstein S: Drug-induced lipid peroxidation in mice: I. Modulation by monooxygenase activity, glutathione and selenium status. Biochem Pharmacol 30:2513–2520, 1981.
76. Yasuda M, Matsumoo S, Matsushima S: Mechanism of protection by S-(1,2-dicarboxyethyl) glutathione triester against acetaminophen-induced hepatotoxicity in rat hepatocytes. Biol Pharm Bull 24:749–753, 2001.
77. Zhou Z, Sun X, James Kang Y: Metallothionein protection against alcoholic liver injury through inhibition of oxidative stress. Exp Biol Med (Maywood) 227:214–222, 2002.

Chapter 4

Acetaminophen (Bedside)

Howard S. Smith, MD

Acetaminophen is one of the most widely used of all drugs and still is considered as a first-line analgesic agent for treating many mild-to-moderate acute and chronic pain states. Acetaminophen has been the overwhelming favorite first-line drug for the pain of osteoarthritis, although currently more therapeutic options exist.[7] It often is used as a sole agent for pain relief and in conjunction with other analgesics (e.g., opioids, nonsteroidal antiinflammatory drugs [NSAIDs]). Clinicians also tend to favor acetaminophen over aspirin or NSAIDs in patients with aspirin-sensitive asthma or history of aspirin or NSAID hypersensitivity, patients at significant increased risk of gastrointestinal mucosal insult, patients at increased risk of bleeding, patients with multiple concurrent drug therapy, and patients at increased risk of renal insult.

Clinical research has shown efficacy for acetaminophen in the following pain states: arthritis pain, headache, post–oral surgery pain, episiotomy pain, orthopedic surgery pain, menstrual pain or dysmenorrhea, postimmunization muscle aches and pain, cancer pain, and sore throat pain. The American College of Rheumatology guidelines for the medical management of osteoarthritis recommend acetaminophen as the preferred first-line therapy in patients with symptomatic osteoarthritis of the knee.[11] The American Geriatrics Society Clinical Practice Guidelines for the management of chronic pain in older persons recommend acetaminophen as the drug of choice for relieving mild-to-moderate musculoskeletal pain. (No dose adjustment is necessary in the elderly; maximum daily dose [MDD] is 4,000 mg).[1]

Acetaminophen is available for oral administration in multiple forms (liquid and solid). Tablets, caplets, and capsules are available. The capsules contain tasteless granules that can be emptied onto a teaspoon containing a small amount of applesauce. Care should be taken to ensure full dissolution of drug if the capsule is emptied into a glass of liquid because large numbers of granules may adhere to the side of the glass. The liquid should be at room temperature because mixing the granules with a hot beverage can yield a better taste.

The recommended adult dosage of acetaminophen is 325 to 650 mg every 4 hours, 325 to 500 mg every 3 hours, or 650 to 1,000 mg every 6 hours with a maximum daily dose of 4 g in 24 hours. Acetaminophen is absorbed rapidly and almost completely from the gastrointestinal tract. The concentration in plasma reaches a peak in 30 to 60 minutes, and the plasma half-life is approximately 2 hours after administration. Rectal bioavailability of acetaminophen is roughly half that of the oral dose. If using a suppository and it is soft, cold water should be run over it while it is still in foil or it should be refrigerated for 30 minutes. The foil is removed, the suppository is moistened with cold water, and the suppository is pushed well up into the rectum with a finger while on the patient lies on his or her side.

In the United States, adult acetaminophen generally comes in regular-strength 325-mg tablets or caplets or extra-strength 500-mg gel caps, gel tabs, caplets, or tablets. Tylenol Arthritis Extended Relief is a 650-mg caplet. Tylenol adult liquid is alcohol-free, and each 15 mL (0.5 fluid oz. or 1 tablespoonful) contains 500 mg of acetaminophen (also comes in honey lemon and cherry flavors and multiple other forms (e.g., pediatric). The various pediatric preparations include Tylenol Infants' Drops (80 mg/0.8 mL), Children's Tylenol elixir (160 mg/5 mL), Children's Tylenol suspension liquid (160 mg/5 mL), Children's Tylenol chewable tablets (80 mg), Tylenol Junior Strength chewable tablets (160 mg), and Tylenol Junior Strength caplets (160 mg). Of the forms mentioned, only regular-strength Tylenol tablets, Tylenol Arthritis Extended Relief caplets, and maximum-strength Tylenol sore throat honey-lemon–flavored adult liquid do not contain FD&C Red #40 in the inactive ingredients, which may be important for individuals known to be allergic to FD&C Red #40.

Acetaminophen is used mainly as an antipyretic and analgesic. Equal doses of acetaminophen and aspirin administered by the same route produce an equal degree of analgesia.[19] Acetaminophen also seems to possess weak antiinflammatory activity.

In the treatment of acute pain, onset time is an issue, so rectal administration is suboptimal because there is slow and ongoing absorption that does not peak within 4 hours after administration.[9] Although not available in the United States, the time of onset with effervescent acetaminophen, 1,000 mg (single dose), is significantly faster than with tablet acetaminophen, 1,000 mg. Median time to onset of analgesia is 20 minutes (effervescent) versus 45 minutes (tablet), and median time to meaningful pain relief is 45 minutes (effervescent) versus 60 minutes (tablet).[23] This difference may be due to significantly faster absorption with the effervescent form.[36]

The duration was longer with the tablet at 4 hours after administration, and the pain relief was significantly better with tablet acetaminophen than with effervescent acetaminophen.[23] In treatment regimens for chronic pain, sustained-release preparations seem well suited for many patients. Acetaminophen has been formulated in controlled-release sprinkles, which currently are not available in the United States, and the extended-release Tylenol Arthritis Extended Relief caplets, which are available in the United States. This 650-mg caplet is a unique, patented bilayer; the first layer dissolves quickly (roughly about half the dose, e.g., similar to taking a regular-strength Tylenol, 325 mg), whereas the second layer is time released to provide 8 hours of relief. If an overdose of this caplet is taken, it may be appropriate to repeat an additional plasma acetaminophen level 4 to 6 hours after the initial level.

In vitro data suggest that two 650-mg extended-release caplets (1,300 mg of acetaminophen) release 88% and 95% of the drug within 3 and 5 hours.[40] After one dose of two 650-mg extended-release caplets, the average maximal plasma concentrations occurred with 0.5 to 3 hours after ingestion.

The package label instructs patients not to take acetaminophen for more than 10 days (for fever, $\leq$ 5 days) unless directed by their physician; however, clinical experience has bourne out that with appropriate monitoring and caution, acetaminophen can be used long-term for chronic conditions. The use of 4,000 mg of acetaminophen in adults with osteoarthritis of the knee was evaluated for 4 weeks.[6] Williams et al[41] evaluated treatment with acetaminophen in doses of 2,600 mg/d for 2 years. In these studies, acetaminophen was well tolerated.

McQuay and Moore[18] did a systematic review looking at acetaminophen for analgesia in moderate-to-severe acute pain states. A total of 37 acceptable studies (with 2,530 patients given paracetamol and 1,594 given placebo) were analyzed. Combining data across conditions, the pooled relative benefits for all doses of paracetamol versus placebo were significant.[18] At a dose of 500 mg, acetaminophen had numbers to treat (NNT) for at least, 50% pain relief compared with placebo in a single-dose administration of 5.6 (95% confidence interval [CI], 3.9 to 9.5); at 600 mg or 650 mg, the NNT was 5.3 (95 CI, 4.1 to 7.2); at 1,000 mg, the NNT was 4.6 (95 CI, 3.9 to 5.4); and at 1,500 mg, the NNT was 5.0 (95 CI, 3.3 to 11), with overlap between the CIs.[18]

Acetaminophen, 1,000 mg, has on overall NNT of 4.6 for at least 50% pain relief compared with placebo in single-dose administration.[18] This means that one out of every five patients with pain of moderate-to-severe intensity obtains at least 50% pain relief who would not have done had they been given a placebo.[18] The equivalent NNT at 600 mg or 650 mg was 5.3 and at 1,500 mg was 5.0, indicating a lower efficacy, although the dose response was not significant.

Moore et al,[24] in a more recent update of the *Cochrane Review*, published data that were essentially unchanged but based on 40 trials (4,717 patients) of acetaminophen versus placebo for moderate-to-severe acute pain. Through all these studies and data, the safety of acetaminophen in appropriate dosing was shown, and there were no serious adverse events that necessitated withdrawal from any study.

The results confirm that acetaminophen is an effective and safe analgesic and that for single-dose administration for moderate-to-severe pain, 1,000 mg may be the optimal dose for most patients. In a prospective open, single-blind randomized study, intravenous propacetamol, tramadol and diclofenac were equally efficacious for emergency analgesic treatment of single peripheral trauma.[12]

Acetaminophen ($C_8 H_9 NO_2$) is a white crystallin powder with a molecular weight of 151.16 and a pKa of 9.51 at 25°C (it is stable at a pH between 4 and 7 at 25°C) and is generally stable for 3 years in solid formulations and 2 years in liquid formulations. Oral acetaminophen is absorbed rapidly and almost completely from the gastrointestinal tract by passive transport primarily in the small intestines. The relative bioavailabilty ranges from 85% to 98%.[17]

A relatively small amount of acetaminophen (10% to 25%) is bound to plasma proteins.[21] Acetaminophen seems to be widely distributed with most body fluids except fat. Acetaminophen's low protein binding and low molecular weight permit easy access through the blood-brain barrier. The peak concentration of acetaminophen in cerebrospinal fluid is attained after 2 to 3 hours.[2]

Acetaminophen primarily is metabolized in the liver by first-order kinetics and involves three principal separate pathways: conjugation with glucuronide; conjugation with sulfate; and oxidation via the cytochrome P-450–dependent, mixed-function oxidative enzyme pathways. The cytochrome P-450 system forms a reactive intermediate metabolite, which conjugates with glutathione and is metabolized further to form cysteine and mercapturic acid conjugates.[22] The principal cytochrome P-450 isoenzyme involved seems to be CYP2E1.[28] CYP3A4 and CYP1A2 provide additional pathways.[28]

Acetaminophen is distributed relatively uniformly throughout most of the body fluids. Plasma protein binding may be variable. Of the drug, 90% to 100% may be recovered in the urine within the first day after administration.

The primary metabolic pathway is via hepatic conjugation with glucuronic acid (about 55%) conjugation with sulfuric acid (about 35%) or conjugation with cysteine (about 3%). Mercapturate and free acetaminophen comprise roughly 3% and 4% of urine metabolites. Small amounts of hydroxylated and deacetylated metabolites have been found in the urine. Children seem to have less capacity for glucuronidation than adults.

Two other minor metabolic pathways that may be available are hydroxylation to form 3-hydroxy-acetaminophen and methoxylation to for M3-methoxy-acetaminophen. These metabolites are conjugated further with glucuronide or sulfate, producing the minor metabolites (sulfate and glucuronide conjugates) 3-methoxy-acetaminophen, 3-hydroxy-acetaminophen, and 3-methyl-thioacetaminophen.[25]

In adults, most acetaminophen is conjugated with glucuronic acid (a lesser extent is conjugated with sulfate). The glucuronide-derived, sulfate-derived; and glutathione-derived metabolites lack biologic activity.[14] In premature infants, newborns, and young infants, the sulfate conjugate predominates.[20] The biologic half-life of acetaminophen in normal adults is roughly 2 to 3 hours with usual therapeutic dosing.[31] It tends to be less in children and more in neonates and patients with cirrhosis.[16] The elimination half-life is about 3 hours for the extended-release product. The elimination half-life of acetaminophen in the cerebrospinal fluid is 3.2 hours according to pooled data.[2]

Acetaminophen generally is safe to use with most medical conditions. Some brands of acetaminophen contain aspartame, which potentially could worsen phenylketonuria. Acetaminophen should be used with caution in patients who have been fasting, have active alcohol abuse, or have significant renal or hepatic disease.

Acetaminophen crosses the placenta; it generally is considered safe for use during pregnancy if a medication is believed to be required. After maternal ingestion of therapeutic doses, acetaminophen crosses the placenta to the fetal circulation in 30 minutes (serum concentration differences between maternal and cord blood are not statistically significant).[26] Acetaminophen is metabolized effectively via sulfate conjugation in the fetus.[34]

The American Academy of Pediatrics considers acetaminophen use to be compatible with breast-feeding. Amounts in milk range from 0.1% to 1.85% of the ingested maternal dose.[4, 5, 27] The nursing infant receives less than 2% of the maternal dose even at the moment of peak acetaminophen concentration.

Acetaminophen was thought to interfere with some blood glucose tests in the past; however, at recommended doses, it does not seem to interfere with glucose analysis using currently marketed blood glucose meters. At therapeutic doses, acetaminophen may interfere with the determination of 5-hydroxyindoleacetic acid, leading to false-positive results. False determinations should be eliminated by avoiding acetaminophen administration for several hours before and during the collection of the urine specimen.[13]

Acetaminophen has essentially no major clinically significant drug interactions. It may produce a small rise in the international normalized ratio (INR) in patients taking anticoagulation medication and in patients with acetaminophen poisoning without hepatic injury, which appears to be caused by inhibition of vitamin K–dependent activation of coagulation factor (i.e., reducing functional factor VII).[42]

Acetaminophen should be used, but perhaps with more caution and with a short-term duration, with zidovudine in patients with clinical manifestations of human immunodeficiency virus infection. Richman et al[32] thought that the concurrent administration of acetaminophen and zidovudine led to an increased incidence of bone marrow suppression. Subsequent studies showed that short-term concurrent use of zidovudine and acetaminophen does not increase plasma levels of zidovudine, does not impair zidovudine clearance and metabolism, and does not increase the risk of bone marrow suppression.[37, 39]

Concomitant administration of acetaminophen with diflunisal produces about a 50% increase in the plasma levels of acetaminophen in normal volunteers. Isoniazid probably has no clinically significant effects on acetaminophen; however, it is possible that some acetylation genotypes may alter the activity of CYP2E1 (which primarily metabolized acetaminophen), and theoretically inhibition or induction of CYP2E1 may occur on discontinuation of isoniazid after concomitant administration of isoniazid and acetaminophen. The only other potential drug interaction is when acetaminophen is given concomitantly with chloramphenicol (an older antibiotic that currently is not used clinically in any significant fashion); the plasma chloramphenicol half-life is prolonged five-fold.

Although an infrequent occurrence, severe adverse reactions (including anaphylactic-type reactions) can occur with acetaminophen. An IgE-mediated mechanism seems to be responsible, and these patients can tolerate aspirin and other NSAIDs.[8]

The hepatotoxicity of acetaminophen is a well-recognized possibility after supranormal doses (i.e., > 4 g/d). Acetaminophen should be used with caution in patients with preexisting hepatic injury potential for glutathione storage depletion (e.g., prolonged fasting, consumption of ≥3 alcoholic drinks per day) and chronic alcohol abusers. The variety of factors that may influence acetaminophen hepatotoxicity could include dose, concomitant use of microsome-inducing agents and other drugs, underlying disease, malnutrition, fasting, acute and chronic alcohol intake, ethnicity, and age.[30] None of these factors has been well studied in humans.[30]

Benson[3] found no adverse reactions or abnormalities of liver function in a double-blind, two-period crossover study evaluating the use of acetaminophen for 13 days in patients with stable chronic liver disease. In a drug detoxification facility, 201 alcoholics in a randomized double-blind, placebo-controlled trial received 2 consecutive days of placebo or 4 g/d of acetaminophem immediately after discontinuing alcohol use with no evidence of liver toxicity.[15] There does not seem to be any absolute contraindication for the use of a short course of appropriately dosed acetaminophen under cautious medical direction in patients with mild preexisting liver disease.

Although hepatotoxicity is recognized in patients taking a major acetaminophen overdose, the incidence of adverse events with its proper use is low, particularly when considering the enormous volume of drug use.[36] Although conflicting data exist suggesting an association between long-term acetaminophen use and renal insult, there is no hard evidence linking long-term acetaminophen use as a causal agent for renal insult. In the study by Perneger et al[29] that reported *heavy users* of acetaminophen (> 366 pills per year) had an increased risk of end-stage renal disease, the index date was the date of initiation of long-term dialysis and not the date of the start of renal disease. Perneger et al later concluded that analgesic use was measured imprecisely in the study (telephone calls to patients relying on their memory recall). Acetaminophen was not established as a cause of end-stage renal disease.

Acute nephrotoxicity has been reported after massive overdose.[35] Additionally, there are potential theoretical mechanisms of renal insult secondary to acetaminophen[33]; however, a National Kidney Foundation position paper noted that there is negligible clinical evidence to suggest that the habitual appropriate use of acetaminophen alone causes analgesic nephropathy.[10] Long-term use of acetaminophen combined with other pharmaceutical agents (e.g., aspirin, caffeine, codeine) in large doses may be associated with an increased risk of renal papillary necrosis resulting in analgesic nephropathy.[10] The panel that authored the National Kidney Foundation's position paper concluded that acetaminophen has been recommended preferentially by physicians to patients with renal failure and that there is no strong evidence that the occasional use of acetaminophen causes renal injury.[10] The National Kidney Foundation position paper recommended acetaminophen as the nonnarcotic analgesic of choice for episodic use in patients with preexisting kidney disease.[10] Clinical data seem to support the notion that acetaminophen in appropriate doses is not nephrotoxic.

In the future, saliva may be the optimal means for determinations of plasma concentrations in patients in whom toxicity is a concern or issue. Anectdotal guidelines concerning the adjustments of MDD in various situations have been advanced. One such recommendation is as follows:

Acute pain (short term): MDD = 4 g/d
Chronic pain (long term): MDD = 3 g/d
Preexisting organ damage: MDD = 2 g/d

Although downward adjustments of dosage/MDD may be appropriate in certain patients or clinical situations, no specific guidelines have been presented out in the literature, and there remains no significant evidence to support the above-listed or any other guidelines.

The American College of Rheumatology has updated their original 1995 Guidelines for Osteoarthritis designed to provide suggestions on an approach to the management of osteoarthritis of the knee and hip.[38] Members of the Ad Hoc Committee on Osteoarthritis Guidelines followed an evidence-based approach by reviewing the guidelines by reviewing an extensive literature search of the Cochrane and Medline databases, published abstracts, and input from expert rheumatologists regarding the evidence.[38] Goals of the guidelines are to provide recommendations to control patient's osteoarthritis pain, improve functions, and improve health-related quality of life without therapeutic toxicity.[38] The pharmacologic algorithm was updated to include currently available medications, especially cyclooxygenase-2-selective inhibitors.[38] Acetaminophen remains first-line pharmacologic therapy because of its cost, efficacy, and safety profiles.

CONCLUSION

Acetaminophen has a wealth of clinical experience (in terms of years of usage and volume of usage), broad tolerability, and efficacy in a wide variety of mild-to-moderate painful conditions. With appropriate use, acetaminophen seldom causes adverse effects and rarely causes serious side effects. More research is needed in efforts to understand better the mechanisms of analgesia and toxicity and investigations of other possible future clinical utility.

REFERENCES FOR ADDITIONAL READING

1. American Geriatrics Society Panel on Chronic Pain in Older Persons: Clinical practice guidelines: The management of chronic pain in older persons. J Am Geriatr Soc 46:635–651, 1998.
2. Bannwarth B, Netter P, Lapicque F, et al: Plasma and cerebrospinal fluid concentrations of paracetamol after a single intravenous dose of propacetamol. Br J Clin Pharmacol 34:79–81, 1992.
3. Benson GD: Acetaminophen in chronic liver desease. Clin Pharmacol Ther 33:95–101, 1983.
4. Berlin CM Jr, Yaffe SJ, Ragni M: Disposition of acetaminophen in milk, saliva, and plasma of lactating women. Pediatr Pharmacol 1:135–141, 1980.
5. Bitzen PO, Gustafsson B, Jostell KG, et al: Excretion of paracentamol in human breast milk. Eur J Clin Pharmacol 20:123–125, 1981.
6. Bradley JD, Brandt KD, Katz BR, et al: Comparison of an anti-inflammatory dose of ibuprofen, an analgesic dose of ibuprofen, and acetaminophen in the treatment of patients with osteoarthritis of the knee. N Engl J Med 325:87–91, 1991.
7. Creamer P: Curr Opin Rheumatol 12:450–455, 2000.
8. De Paramo BJ, Gancedo SQ, Cuevas M, et al: Paracetamol (acetaminophen) hypersensitivity. Ann Allergy Asthma Immunol 85:508–511, 2000.

9. Hahn TW, Mogensen T, Lund C, et al: High-dose rectal and oral acetaminophen in post-operative patients—serum and saliva concentrations. Acta Anaesthesiol Scand 44:302–306, 2000.

10. Henrich WL, Agodoa LE, Barrett B, et al: Analgesics and the kidney: Summary and recommendations to the Scientific Advisory Board of the National Kidney Foundation from an Ad Hoc Committee of the National Kidney Foundation. Am J Kidney Dis 27:162–165, 1996.

11. Hochberg MC, Altman RD, Brandt KD, et al: Guidelines for the medical management of osteoarthritis: Part I. Osteoarthritis of the hip. Part II. Osteoarthritis of the knee. Arthritis Rheum 38:1535–1546, 1995.

12. Hoogewiji J, Diltoer MW, Hubloue I, et al: A prospective, open, single blind, randomized study comparing four analgesics in the treatment of peripheral injury in the emergency department. Eur J Emerg Med 7:119–23, 2000.

13. Jones TA, Walwick ER: Interference of Tylenol with liquid chromatography of urinary catacholamines (letter). Clin Chem 27:1951, 1981.

14. Koch-Weser J: Drug therapy: Acetaminophen. N Engl J Med 295:1297–1300, 1976.

15. Kuffner EK, Dart RC: Acetaminophen used in patients who drink alcohol: Current study evidence. Am J Managed Care 7:5592–5596, 2001.

16. Levy G: Comparative pharmacokinetics of aspirin and acetaminophen. Arch Intern Med 141:279–281, 1981.

17. McGilveray IJ, Mattock GL, Fooks JR, et al: Acetaminophen II: A comparison of the physiological availabilities of different commercial dosage forms. Can J Pharmaceut Sci 6:38–42, 1971.

18. McQuay HJ, Moore RA: An Evidence-Based Resource for Pain Relief. New York, Oxford University Press, 1998.

19. Mehlisch DR: Review of the comparative analgesic efficacy of salicylates, acetaminophen, and pyrazolones. Am J Med 75:47–52, 1983.

20. Miller PP, Roberts RJ, Fischer LJ: Acetaminophen elimination kinetics in neonates, children, and adults. Clin Pharmacol Ther 19:284–294, 1976.

21. Milligan TP, Morris HC, Hammond PM, et al: Studies on paracetamol binding to serum proteins. Ann Clin Biochem 31:492–496, 1994.

22. Mitchell JR, Thorgeirsson SS, Potter WZ, et al: Acetaminophen-induced hepatic injury: Protective role of glutathione in man and rationale for therapy. Clin Pharmacol Ther 16:676–684, 1974.

23. Moller PL, Norholt SE, Ganry HE, et al: Time to onset of analgesia and analgesic efficacy of effervescent acetaminophen: 1000 mg compared to tablet acetaminophen 1000 mg in post-operative dental pain: A single-dose, double blind, randomized, placebo controlled study. J Clin Pharmacol 40:370–378, 2000.

24. Moore A, Collins S, Carroll D, et al: Single dose paracetamol (acetaminophen) with and without codeine, for post operative pain. Cochrane Review, in: The Cochrane Library, vol 4. Oxford, Update Software, 2001.

25. Mrochek JE, Katz S, Christie WH, et al: Acetaminophen metabolism in man, as determined by high-resolution liquid chromatography. Clin Chem 20:1086–1096, 1974.

26. Naga Rani MA, Joseph T, Narayanan R: Placental transfer of paracetamol. J Indian Med Assoc 87:182–183, 1989.

27. Notarianni LJ, Oldham HG, Bennett PN: Passage of paracetamol into breast milk and its subsequent metabolism by the neonate. Br J Clin Pharmacol 24:63–67, 1987.

28. Patten CJ, Thomas PE, Guy RL, et al: Cytochrome P450 enzymes involved in acetaminophen activation by rat and human liver microsomes and their kinetics. Chem Res Toxicol 6:511–518, 1993.

29. Perneger TV, Whelton PK, Klag MJ: Risk of kidney failure associated with the use of acetaminophen, aspirin and nonsteroidal anti-inflammatory drugs. N Engl J Med 331:1675–1679, 1994.

30. Prescott LF: Therapeutic misadventure with paracetamol: Fact or fiction? Am J Ther 7:99–114, 2000.

31. Rawlins MD, Henderson DR, Hijab AR: Pharmacokinetics of paracetamol acetaminophen after intravenous and oral administration. Eur J Clin Pharmacol 11:283–286, 1997.

32. Richman DD, et al: The toxicity of azidothymidine (AZT) in the treatment of patients with AIDS and AIDS-related complex: A double-blind, placebo controlled trial. N Engl J Med 317:192–197, 1987.

33. Rocha GM, Michea LF, Peters EM, et al: Direct toxicity of nonsteroidal anti-inflammatory drugs for renal medullary cells. Proc Natl Acad Sci U S A 98:5317–5322, 2001.

34. Rollins DE, von Bahr C, Glaumann H, et al: Acetaminophen: Potentially toxic metabolite formed by human fetal and adult live microsomes and isolated fetal liver cells. Science 205:1414–1416, 1979.

35. Rumack BH, Matthew H: Acetaminophen poisoning and toxicity. Pediatrics 55:871–876, 1975.

36. Rygnestad T, Zahlsen K, Samdal FA: Absorbtion of effervescent paracetamol tablets relative to ordinary paracetamol tablets in healthy volunteers. Eur J Clin Pharmacol 56:141–143, 2000.

37. Sattler FR, et al: Acetaminophen does not impair clearance of zidovudine. Ann Intern Med 114:937–940, 1991.

38. Schnitzer TJ: Update of ACR Guidelines for Osteoarthritis: Role of the Coxibs. J Pain Symptom Manage 23:524–530, 2002.

39. Steffe EM, et al: The effect of acetaminophen on zidovudine metabolism in HIV-infected patients. J Acquir Immune Defic Synr Hum Retrovirol 3:691–694, 1990.

40. Temple AR, Mrazik TJ: More on extended-release acetaminophen (letter). N Engl J Med 333:1508–1509, 1995.

41. Williams HJ, Ward JR, Egger MJ, et al: Comparison of naproxen and acetaminophen in a two-year study of treatment of osteoarthritis of the knee. Arthritis Rheum 36:1196–1206, 1993.

42. Whyte IM, Budkley NA, Reith DM, et al: Acetaminophen causes an increased international normalized ratio by reducing functional factor VII. Ther Drug Monit 22:742–748, 2000.

Chapter 5

Nonsteroidal Anti-inflammatory Drugs and Cyclooxygenase-2 Selective Inhibitors

Lee S. Simon, MD

Nonsteroidal antiinflammatory drugs (NSAIDs) are antiinflammatory, analgesic, and antipyretic agents. They are used widely to reduce pain, decrease gel phenomenon, and improve function in patients with osteoarthritis and rheumatoid arthritis and to treat pain, including headache, dysmenorrhea, and postoperative pain. Whether their efficacy is due solely to their antiinflammatory or analgesic effects or other possible properties is not known. There are at least 20 different NSAIDs currently available in the United States. Cyclooxygenase-2 (COX-2)–specific inhibitors (e.g., celecoxib, rofecoxib, valdecoxib) have similar efficacy, but risks for gastrointestinal toxic effects are significantly decreased. These selective COX-2 inhibitors also have no effect on the platelet.

NSAIDs are one of the most commonly used classes of drugs in the world. It has been estimated that more than 17 million Americans use these agents on a daily basis. With the aging of the U.S. population, the Centers for Disease Control predicts a significant increase in the prevalence of painful degenerative and inflammatory rheumatic conditions and an increased use of NSAIDs. Approximately 60 million NSAID prescriptions are written each year in the United States; the number for elderly patients exceeds that for younger patients by approximately 3.6-fold. Aspirin (acetylsalicylic acid [ASA]) ibuprofen, naproxen, and ketoprofen are available over-the-counter. At equipotent doses, the clinical efficacy and tolerability of the various NSAIDs are similar; however, individual responses are highly variable. Anecdotally, it is believed that if a patient fails to respond to one NSAID of one class, it is reasonable to try another NSAID from a different class; however, no one has studied this in a prospective controlled manner.[3,19]

Sodium salicylic acid was discovered in 1763. Impure forms of salicylates had been used as analgesics and antipyretics throughout the 1600s to 1700s. When purified and synthesized, the acetyl derivative of salicylate, ASA, was found to provide more antiinflammatory activity with better tolerability than salicylate alone. Because of the toxicity of ASA, particularly related to the potential for upper gastrointestinal intolerance, phenylbutazone, an indoleacetic acid derivative, was introduced in the early 1950s. This was the first nonsalicylate NSAID developed for use in patients with painful and inflammatory conditions. This drug, a weak prostaglandin synthase inhibitor, induced uricosuria and was found to be useful in patients with ankylosing spondylitis and gout. Because of concerns related to bone marrow toxicity, particularly in women older than age 60, this compound rarely is prescribed now. Indomethacin, another indoleacetic acid derivative, subsequently was developed in the 1960s. It had significant toxicity as well, and the search for safer (particularly gastrointestinally safer) and at least equally effective NSAIDs followed.

MECHANISM OF ACTION

The primary mechanism of action of the NSAIDs is the inhibtion of prostaglandin synthesis.[6,11] Differential effects also have been attributed to variations in the enantiomeric state of the agent and its pharmacokinetics, pharmacodynamics, and metabolism. Although variability can be explained in part by absorption, distribution, and metabolism, potential differences in mechanism of action must be considered an important explanation for their variable effects.[24] These other effects of NSAIDs are seen variably with the different products, typically in in vitro experiments, and it is not clear how important any of them are in the context of clinical applicability.

Inhibition of Prostaglandin Synthesis

NSAIDs are primarily antiinflammatory and analgesic by decreasing the production of prostaglandins of the E series. These prostanoic acids are proinflammatory and increase vascular permeability and sensitivity to the release of bradykinins. NSAIDs also have been shown to inhibit the formation of prostacyclin and thromboxane, resulting in complex effects on vascular permeability and platelet aggregation.[28]

Polyunsaturated fatty acids, including arachidonic acid, which are constituents of all cell membranes, are in ester linkage in the glycerols of phospholipids and are converted to prostaglandins or leukotrienes initially through the action of phospholipase A_2 or phospholipase C. Free arachidonic acid, when released by the phospholipase, acts as a substrate for the prostaglandin H (PGH) synthase complex, which includes COX and peroxidase. These enzymes catalyze the conversion of arachidonic acid to the unstable cyclic-endoperoxide intermediates, PGG_2 and PGH_2. These arachidonic acid metabolites are converted to the more stable PGE_2 and PGF_2 compounds by specific tissue prostaglandin synthases. NSAIDs specifically inhibit COX and reduce the conversion of arachidonic acid to PGG_2. ASA acetylates the COX enzyme, whereas all of the other nonsalicylate NSAIDs are reversible inhibitors maintaining an effect based on serum half-life and drug availability.[26]

There are at least two isoforms of the COX enzymes.[16,28] Although they share 60% homology in the amino acid sequences considered important for catalysis of arachidonic acid, they are products of two different genes. They differ most importantly in regulation and expression. COX-1 or prostaglandin synthase H_1 is a *housekeeping enzyme*, which typically regulates normal cellular processes and is stimulated by hormones or growth factors. It is constitutively expressed in most tissues and is inhibited by all NSAIDs to varying degrees depending on the applied experimental model system used to measure drug effects. COX-1 is important in maintaining the integrity of the gastric and duodenal mucosa, and many of the toxic effects of NSAIDs on the gastrointestinal tract are attributed to its inhibition. Similarly, COX-1 is important in modulating renal plasma flow, particularly in patients who are relatively dehydrated or who have clinically significant congestive heart failure, cirrhosis with or without ascites, or intrinsic kidney disease such as systemic lupus erythematosus or diabetes (Table 1).

The other isoform, COX-2 or prostaglandin synthase H_2, is an inducible enzyme and is usually undetectable in most tissues. Its expression is increased during states of inflammation or experimentally in response to mitogenic stimuli. This isoform also is constitutively expressed in the brain, specifically cortex and hippocampus; in the female reproductive tract associated with ovulation and implantation of a fertilized ovum; in the male vas def-

TABLE 1

Cyclooxygenases

COX-1	COX-2
Constitutive	Inducible
Only enzyme in platelet	Up-regulated by cytokines and mitogens
Important in vascular endothelium	Increased in synovitis including RA and OA, other inflammation
Kidney, glomerulus	Up-regulated in some cancers
Skin, mucous membranes	Constitutive: brain/CNS, kidney (tubule), vas deferens, bone, ovulation, implantation of fertilized ovum, lung
Gastrointestinal mucosa	
Lung	

RA, rheumatoid arthritis; OA, osteoarthritis; CNS, central nervous system.

erens; in bone; and at least in some models in human kidney associated with the macula densa and thick ascending limb of Henle. It is has been shown that COX-2 activity is important in modulating renal electrolyte and water balance in the normal kidney. It seems that in patients whose kidneys are stressed COX-2 also is up-regulated, similar to COX-1 activity (Table 1).[7,9]

The activity of COX-1 and COX-2 is inhibited by all of the presently available NSAIDs to a greater or lesser degree. The clinical effectiveness of these drugs is believed to be due to the effects on COX-2, whereas many of the mechanism-based toxic effects are thought to be secondary to inhibition of COX-1. The expression of COX-2 is inhibited by glucocorticoids. Evidence has accumulated that several NSAIDs are more selective for COX-2 enzyme effects than COX-1. In vitro effects of etodolac and meloxicam show approximately a 10-fold inhibition of COX-2 compared with COX-1, at low dose.[28] At higher antiinflammatory doses, however, this specificity seems to be mitigated because both enzymes begin to be affected to variable degrees. Specific COX-2 inhibitors (or COX-1-sparing agents) that are at least 300 times more effective at inhibiting COX-2 activity than COX-1 and have no measurable effect on COX-1-mediated events at any efficacious therapeutic dose are now available: celecoxib, rofecoxib, and valdecoxib.[16] These COX-2-selective (specific) inhibitors have been shown as effective at inhibiting osteoarthritis pain, dental pain, and the pain and inflammation associated with rheumatoid arthritis, as naproxen at 500 mg twice a day, ibuprofen at 800 mg three times day, and diclofenac at 75 mg twice a day, without endoscopic evidence of gastroduodenal damage and without affecting platelet aggregation.[22] Large gastrointestinal outcome trials showed that celecoxib and rofecoxib at two to four times the normal treatment doses for rheumatoid arthritis and osteoarthritis have a two to three fold decreased incidence of important gastrointestinal bleeding, perforation, or obstruction compared with ibuprofen, diclofenac, or naproxen at normal treatment doses.[4, 20] Owing to the design of the randomized controlled trials, many of the important questions regarding the renal effects of the specific COX-2 inhibitors remain unanswered.

It has been described that prostaglandins inhibit apoptosis (programmed cell death) and that NSAIDs, via inhibition of prostaglandin synthesis, may reestablish more normal cell cycle responses. There also is evidence suggesting that some NSAIDs may reduce PGH synthase gene expression, supporting the clinical evidence of differences in activity in NSAIDs in sites of active inflammation.[7]

Other Potential Mechanisms (Non–Prostaglandin-Mediated) Effects

NSAIDs are lipophilic and become incorporated in the lipid bilayer of cell membranes and may interrupt protein-protein interactions important for signal transduction. Stimulus response coupling, which is crucial for recruitment of phagocytic cells to sites of inflammation, has been shown in vitro to be inhibited by some NSAIDs. NSAIDs also have been shown to inhibit activation and chemotaxis of neutrophils and to reduce toxic oxygen radical production in stimulated neutrophils. NSAIDs scavenge superoxide radicals.[1, 21]

Salicylates have been shown to inhibit phospholipase C activity in macrophages, inhibiting the arachidonic cascade earlier than the COX enzymes. Some NSAIDs have been shown to affect T lymphocyte function experimentally by inhibiting rheumatoid factor production in vitro. Interference with neutrophil endothelial cell adherence has been described, which is crucial to migration of granulocytes to sites of inflammation, and expression of L-selectins is decreased.[1, 8, 21] NSAIDs have been shown in vitro to inhibit NF-κB (nitric oxide transcription factor)–dependent transcription, inhibiting inducible nitric oxide synthetase.[2] Antiinflammatory levels of ASA have been shown to inhibit expression of inducible nitric oxide synthetase and subsequent production of nitrite in vitro. At pharmacologic doses, sodium salicylate, indomethacin, and acetaminophen have been studied and had no effect, but at suprapharmacologic dosages, sodium salicylate inhibited nitrite production. Although nonacetylated salicylates have been shown in vitro to inhibit neutrophil function and to have equal efficacy in patients with rheumatoid arthritis,[15] clinically there is no evidence to suggest that these biologic effects are more important than prostaglandin synthase inhibition.

PHARMACOLOGY

Bioavailability

All NSAIDs are absorbed completely after oral administration. Absorption rates may vary in patients with altered gastrointestinal blood flow or motility and with certain NSAIDs when taken with food. Enteric coating may reduce direct effects of NSAIDs on the gastric mucosa but also may reduce the rate of absorption.

Most NSAIDs are weak organic acids; when absorbed, they are greater than 95% bound to serum albumin. This is a saturable process. Clinically significant decreases in serum albumin levels or institution of other highly protein bound medications may lead to an increase in the free component of NSAID in serum. This increase may be important in patients who are elderly or are chronically ill with associated hypoalbuminemic states. Because of increased vascular permeability in localized sites of inflammation, this high degree of protein binding may result in delivery of higher levels of NSAIDs.

METABOLISM

NSAIDs are metabolized predominantly in the liver by the cytochrome P-450 system, most commonly the CYP2C9 isoform, and excreted in the urine. This metabolism must be taken into consideration when prescribing NSAIDs for patients with hepatic or renal dysfunction. Some NSAIDs, such as oxaprozin, have two metabolic pathways, whereby some portion is secreted directly into the bile and another part is metabolized further and excreted in the urine. Others (e.g., indomethacin, sulindac, and piroxicam) have prominent enterohepatic circulation, resulting in a prolonged half-life, and should be used with caution in the elderly. In patients with renal insufficiency, some inactive metabolites may be resynthesized in *vivo* to the active compound. Diclofenac, flurbiprofen, celecoxib, and rofecoxib are metabolized in the liver and should be used with care and at lowest possible doses in patients with clinically significant liver disease; this would mean patients with significant liver dysfunction, such as patients with cirrhosis with or without ascites, prolonged prothrombin times, falling serum albumin levels, or marked elevations in liver transaminases in blood. As noted, most of the NSAIDs and celecoxib are metabolized through the P-450 CYP2C9 isoenzyme, whereas rofecoxib is not. The exact mechanism to explain the metabolism of rofecoxib is unknown.

Salicylates are the least highly protein bound NSAIDs: approximately 68%. Zero-order kinetics are dominant in salicylate metabolism. Increasing the dose of salicylates is effective over a narrow range, but when the metabolism is saturated, incremental dose increases may lead to high serum salicylate levels. Changes in salicylate doses need to be considered carefully at chronic steady-state levels, particularly in patients with altered renal or hepatic function.

Plasma Half-Life

Significant differences in plasma half-lives of the NSAIDs may be important in explaining their diverse clinical effects. NSAIDs with long half-lives typically do not attain maximal plasma concentrations quickly, and clinical responses may be delayed. These drugs with delayed onset but long half-lives may not be ideal choices for acute pain relief. Plasma concentrations can vary widely because of differences in renal clearance and metabolism. Piroxicam has the longest serum half-life of currently marketed NSAIDs, 57 ± 22 hours, whereas diclofenac has one of the shortest, 1.1 ± 0.2 hours. Although drugs have been developed with long half-lives to improve patient compliance, the fact that piroxicam has such a long half-life is not advantageous for elderly patients at risk for specific NSAID-induced toxic effects. In older patients in the treatment of chronic conditions, it sometimes is preferable to use drugs of shorter half-life so that when the drug is discontinued the unwanted effects may disappear more rapidly.

Sulindac and nabumetone are *prodrugs*, in which the active compound is produced after first-pass metabolism through the liver. Prodrugs were developed to decrease the exposure of the gastrointestinal mucosa to the local effects of NSAIDs. With adequate inhibition of COX-1, the patient is placed at substantial risk of an NSAID-induced upper gastrointestinal event as long as COX-1 activity is inhibited.

Other pharmacologic properties may be important clinically. NSAIDs that are highly lipid soluble in serum penetrate the central nervous system more effectively and occasionally produce striking changes in mentation, perception, and mood. Indomethacin has been associated with many of these side effects, even after a single dose, particularly in the elderly.

ADVERSE EFFECTS

NSAIDs may produce toxic effects in any organ system. There are effects that are unique to these drugs through effects mediated by their main mode of action of inhibition of prostaglandin synthesis. There are other effects mediated by unknown mechanisms.

Hepatotoxicity

Elevation in hepatic transaminase levels is common, although it occurs more often in patients with juvenile rheumatoid arthritis or systemic lupus erythematosus. Although there are many reports indicating that elevated serum transaminases are common in patients taking NSAIDs, unless elevations exceed two to three times the upper limits of normal[12] or serum albumin or prothrombin times are altered, these effects usually are not considered clinically significant. Nonetheless, overt liver failure has been reported after use of many NSAIDs, including diclofenac, flurbiprofen, and sulindac. Of all NSAIDs, sulindac has been associated with the highest incidence of cholestasis in certain countries.[12] It is recommended that patients at risk for liver toxicity be followed carefully. When initiating NSAID treatment, all patients should be evaluated again within 8 to 12 weeks and consideration given to doing a blood analysis for serum transaminase changes.

Mechanism-Based (Prostaglandin-Related) Adverse Effects

Many adverse reactions attributed to NSAIDs are due to inhibition of prostaglandin synthesis in local tissues. Patients with allergic rhinitis, nasal polyposis, or a history of asthma, in whom all NSAIDs effectively inhibit prostaglandin synthetase, are at increased risk for anaphylaxis. In high doses, even nonacetylated salicylates may decrease prostaglandin synthesis sufficiently to induce an anaphylactic reaction in sensitive patients. Although the exact mechanism for this effect is unclear, it is known that E prostaglandins serve as bronchodilators. When COX activity is inhibited in patients at risk, a decrease in synthesis of prostaglandins that contribute to bronchodilation results. Another explanation implicates the alternate pathway of arachidonate metabolism, whereby shunting of arachidonate into the leukotriene pathway occurs when COX is inhibited. This explanation implies that large stores of arachidonate released in certain inflammatory situations lead to excess substrate for leukotriene metabolism; this results in release of products that are highly reactive, such as the SRSA pathway, which stimulate anaphylaxis.

Platelet Effects

Platelet aggregation and the ability to clot are induced primarily through stimulating thromboxane production with activation of platelet COX-1. There is no COX-2 in the platelet. NSAIDs and aspirin inhibit the activity of COX-1, but the COX-2 inhibitors (COX-1–sparing agents) have no effect on COX-1 at clinically effective therapeutic doses.

The effect of the nonaspirin NSAIDs on platelet function is reversible and related to the half-life of the drug, whereas the effect of ASA is to acetylate the COX-1 enzyme, serving to inactivate it permanently. The individual platelet cannot make new COX-1 enzyme so that for the life span of the platelet after exposure to ASA, the platelet does not function appropriately. Only with repopulation of platelets unexposed to ASA can normal platelet aggregation return. Patients who are awaiting surgery should be able to stop nonaspirin NSAIDs at a time determined by four to five times their serum half-life, whereas ASA needs to be discontinued 1 to 2 weeks before the planned procedure to allow a normal platelet population to reestablish itself with platelets unexposed to ASA.

ASA has been shown to decrease the risk of recurrent thromboembolic disease in patients with a history of cerebrovascular or cardiovascular disease. It is useful partly because it decreases platelet aggregation through inhibition of COX-1. Because the COX-2 selective inhibitors do not affect platelets, in that there is no COX-2 in the platelet, patients at risk for a thromboembolic event who are to be treated with a COX-2–specific inhibitor must be treated with concomitant low-dose ASA. Whether patients who are risk for cerebrovascular or cardiovascular thromboembolic disease are at increased risk from unbalanced inhibition of COX-2 without concomitant effects on COX-1 with exposure to the COX-1–sparing agents remains unknown. The randomized clinical trials of rofecoxib and celecoxib were not designed to address this question; we have to await postmarketing surveillance to help resolve this problem. We have little information that shows that the long-acting nonselective NSAIDs are as effective as low-dose ASA in preventing further thromboembolic events in patients at risk. Only ASA has been studied prospectively, and low-dose aspirin should be given concomitantly with either nonselective NSAIDs or specific COX-2 inhibitors in patients at risk for thrombosis. Given the decreased incidence of upper and lower gastrointestinal damage with COX-2 inhibitors, when possible, low-dose aspirin should be prescribed with COX-2 inhibitors rather than nonselective NSAIDs when appropriate.

Gastrointestinal Tolerability

The most clinically significant adverse effects after use of NSAIDs occur in the gastrointestinal tract. NSAIDs cause a wide range of gastrointestinal problems, including abdominal pain, dyspepsia, nausea, vomiting, esophagitis, esophageal stricture, gastritis, mucosal erosions, hemorrhage, peptic ulceration or perforation, obstruction, and death.[30] The cause of NSAID-induced gastrointestinal symptoms, such as abdominal pain, dyspepsia, or diarrhea, is unknown. The structural changes, beginning with ulcers, are due to systemic inhibition of prostaglandin synthesis. In addition to the known effects on gastric and duodenal mucosa, there is increasing evidence that the mucosa of the large bowel and the small bowel is affected. These agents also may induce stricture formation. These strictures may manifest as diaphragms, which precipitate small or large bowel obstruction, and may be difficult to detect on contrast radiographic studies. There also is evidence to suggest that NSAIDs induce dysfunction in gastrointestinal mucosal permeability.[17,30]

NSAIDs rapidly penetrate the gastrointestinal mucosa in the presence of stomach acid. The lipophilic and weakly acidic NSAIDs penetrate the superficial lining cells of the thick mucus layer, leading to oxidative uncoupling of cellular metabolism, which leads to local tissue injury and cell death. This damage consists of local erosions and hemorrhages, which with further damage can lead to formation of clinically significant ulcers.[17]

The magnitude of risk for clinically important gastrointestinal adverse events is controversial. The U.S. Food and Drug Administration reports an overall risk of 2% to 4% per year for NSAID-induced gastric ulcer development and its complications.[10,30] In general, the relative risk as summarized in multiple clinical trials ranges from 4.0 to 5.0 for the development of gastric ulcer; from 1.1 to 1.6 for the development of duodenal ulcer; and from 4.5 to 5.0 for the development of clinically significant gastric ulcer with hemorrhage, perforation, or death. There are data that suggest the risk of hospitalization for adverse gastrointestinal effects may be 7 to 10 fold greater in patients with rheumatoid arthritis treated with NSAIDs compared with patients who are not receiving these agents.

Epidemiologic studies suggest that the safest NSAIDs are nonacetylated salicylates. There are controversial data about their efficacy at safe doses, however. NSAIDs with prominent enterohepatic circulation and significantly prolonged half-lives, such as sulindac and piroxicam, have been linked to increased gastrointestinal toxicity as a result of reexposure of gastric and duodenal mucosa to bile reflux and the active moiety of the drug. As noted, other sites in the gastrointestinal tract, including the esophagus and small and large bowel, also may be affected. Exposure to NSAIDs is probably a major factor in the development of esophagitis and subsequent stricture formation.

Endoscopic studies showed that NSAID administration results in shallow erosions or submucosal hemorrhage, which although occurring at any site in the gastrointestinal tract are observed more commonly in the stomach near the prepyloric area and the antrum. Typically, these lesions are asymptomatic, making prevalence data difficult to determine, although there are data showing that by endoscopy NSAID-induced ulcers greater than 3 mm in diameter with obvious depth are found in upward of 15% to 31% of patients so treated. The number of lesions that spontaneously heal or that progress to ulceration, frank perforation, gastric or duodenal obstruction, serious gastrointestinal hemorrhage, or subsequent death is not known. Risk factors for development of gastrointestinal toxicity in patients receiving NSAIDs include age greater than 60, prior history of peptic ulcer disease, prior use of antiulcer therapies for any reason, concomitant use of glucocorticoids particularly in patients with rheumatoid arthritis, comorbidities such as significant cardiovascular disease, and severe rheumatoid arthritis. Other risk factors include increasing dose of specific and singular NSAIDs (Table 2).

Endoscopic data from large numbers of patients treated with COX-2–specific inhibitors showed that induction of ulcers occurs at the same rate as in patients who received placebo, whereas the active comparators induced ulcers greater than 3 mm in diameter with obvious depth from 15% (diclofenac, 75 mg twice a day; ibuprofen, 800 mg three times a day) to 19% (naproxen, 500 mg twice a day) after 1 week of treatment in healthy volunteers and after 12 weeks of treatment in 26% (naproxen, 500 mg twice a day) of patients with osteoarthritis and rheumatoid arthritis.[15,23] In addition, the complications of ulcers, such as obstruction, perforation, or bleeds, are two or three times less frequent with the COX-2–specific inhibitors than with the active comparators (e.g., diclofenac, ibuprofen, naproxen).[4,20] It is possible that patients with an ulcer secondary to low-dose aspirin administration for cardiovascular prophylaxis or who are infected with *Helicobacter pylori* may show delay in healing of ulcers when treated with COX-2–specific inhibitors, but this was not observed in the long-term outcome trials.

TABLE 2

Risk Factors for NSAID-Induced Gastroduodenal Toxic Effects

Increasing patient age (>60)
Past history of peptic ulcer, bleeding, or perforation of any cause
Extent of current and past disease (extent of frailty)
Dose of NSAID (higher dose more likely to cause risk)
Combinations of NSAID
Concomitant use of glucocorticoids
History of gastrointestinal toxicity with NSAIDs

APPROACH TO THE PATIENT AT RISK FOR NONSTEROIDAL ANTIINFLAMMATORY DRUG–INDUCED GASTROINTESTINAL ADVERSE EVENTS

The approach to the patient who requires long-term NSAID treatment and has developed or is at risk for an NSAID-induced gastrointestinal event is controversial (Table 3). Many patients with dyspepsia or upper gastrointestinal distress while treated with nonselective NSAIDs typically manifest superficial erosions by endoscopy, which often heal spontaneously without change in therapy. More difficult to evaluate is whether agents documented as cytoprotective alter NSAID-induced symptoms that may or may not predict significant gastrointestinal events. Clinical studies showed that greater than 80% of patients who develop significant NSAID-induced endoscopic abnormalities are asymptomatic.[25] Prospective observational trials showed, however, that patients are surprisingly more symptomatic when they develop NSAID-induced toxicities than previously thought.

Patients who develop a gastric or duodenal ulcer while taking NSAIDs should have treatment discontinued and therapy for ulcer disease, either H_2-antagonist or proton-pump inhibitors, instituted. If NSAIDs must be continued, the patient needs to receive antiulcer therapy for a longer time. Diagnostic tests to determine if the patient is H. pylori positive should be done, and if the patient has measurable antibodies, specific antibiotic therapy to eradicate the infection should be administered.

Prophylaxis to prevent NSAID-induced gastric or duodenal ulcers is more complicated. To date, there has been no evidence that agents other than misoprostol therapy prevent NSAID-

---

TABLE 3

Prophylaxis and Treatment of NSAID-Induced Gastrointestinal Toxic Effects

Antacids
No data show utility, although may decrease symptoms
Sucralfate
No data shows prevention of ulcer formation
H_2-antagonists
Regular dose
Prevent duodenal ulcers but not gastric ulcers
Heal over time gastric and duodenal ulcers
Improve symptoms
High dose
Prevent gastric and duodenal ulcers
Proton-pump inhibitors
Prophylaxis against gastric and duodenal ulcers
Improves symptoms
Heal gastric and duodenal ulcers
Misoprostol
Prevents gastric and duodenal ulcers
Decreases incidence of ulcer complications
Heals gastric and duodenal ulcers
Does not improve symptoms
May lead to increased gut motility; increase in diarrhea at full dose

induced gastric ulceration and its complications. Although H_2-antagonists or proton-pump inhibitors have been shown to prevent NSAID-induced duodenal ulcers, prevention of gastric ulcerations has not been shown. An endoscopy study showed that famotidine at twice the approved dose (40 mg twice a day) significantly decreased the incidence of gastric and duodenal ulcers. Similarly an endoscopy study showed that treatment with omeprazole decreased gastroduodenal ulcers. H_2-antagonists and proton-pump inhibitors decrease NSAID-induced dyspeptic symptoms effectively, but these agents have not been studied to determine if they decrease the incidence of ulcer complications.

Misoprostol is a prostaglandin analog, which locally replaces the prostaglandins normally synthesized in the gastric mucosa but whose synthesis is inhibited by NSAIDs. A large prospective trial evaluated 8,843 patients with rheumatoid arthritis on various NSAIDs. Misoprostol successfully inhibited the development of ulcer complications such as bleeding, perforation, and obstruction with a 40% reduction in patients treated with misoprostol versus patients receiving placebo. Further analysis showed that patients with health assessment questionnaire scores greater than 1.5 (worse disease) had an 87% reduction in risk for a NSAID-induced toxic event if concomitantly treated with misoprostol.

These data suggest that high-risk patients may benefit from concomitant misoprostol therapy if NSAID treatment is indicated. Gabriel and others showed the pharmacoeconomic utility of such therapy in high-risk patients. The major adverse event causing withdrawal in approximately 10% of patients was diarrhea, and 30% of patients complained of diarrhea.

The COX-2–specific inhibitors are another choice in that there is clearly less risk for important gastrointestinal damage and associated complications with this form of therapy. These drugs induce less nonspecific gastrointestinal complaints than do the nonselective NSAIDs, however, still more than observed with placebo in the randomized controlled trials.

RENAL ADVERSE EFFECTS

The effects of NSAIDs on renal function include retention of sodium, changes in tubular function, interstitial nephritis, and reversible renal failure owing to alterations in filtration rate and renal plasma flow.[29] Prostaglandins and prostacyclins are important for maintenance of intrarenal blood flow and tubular transport of electrolytes and water. All NSAIDs, including the COX-2–specific inhibitors, except nonacetylated salicylates have the potential to induce reversible impairment of glomerular filtration rate; this effect occurs more frequently in patients with congestive heart failure; established renal disease with altered intrarenal plasma flow, including diabetes, hypertension, or atherosclerosis; and induced hypovolemia (salt depletion or significant hypoalbuminemia) (Table 4). Triamterene-containing diuretics, which increase plasma renin levels, may predispose patients receiving NSAIDs precipitously to develop acute renal failure.

NSAID-associated intersitial nephritis typically is manifested as nephrotic syndrome, characterized by edema or anasarca, proteinuria, hematuria, and pyuria. The usual stigmata of drug-induced allergic nephritis, such as eosinophilia, eosinophiluria, and fever, typically are absent. Interstitial infiltrates of mononuclear cells are seen histologically with relative sparing of the glomeruli. Phenylproprionic acid derivatives, such as fenoprofen, naproxen, and tolmetin, and the indoleacetic acid derivative indomethacin are associated most commonly with the development of interstitial nephritis. Indomethacin has been suggested as a treatment to decrease proteinuria in patients with nephrotic syndrome from other causes.

Inhibition of prostaglandin synthesis intrarenally by NSAIDs decreases renin release and

TABLE 4

Risk Factors for NSAID-Induced Renal Insufficiency

High risk
   Volume depletion states
   Severe congestive heart failure
   Hepatic cirrhosis with or without ascites
   Clinically significant dehydration
   Creatinine clearance <30 mL/min
Low to moderate risk
   Intrinsic renal disease
      Diabetic nephropathy
      Nephrotic syndrome
      Hypertensive nephropathy
   Induction of anesthesia
Questionable risk
   Older age

produces a state of hyporeninemic hypoaldosteronism with resulting hyperkalemia. Physiologically, this effect may be amplified in patients taking potassium-sparing diuretics. Salt retention precipitated by some NSAIDs, which may lead to peripheral edema, is likely due to inhibition of intrarenal prostaglandin production, which decreases renal medullary blood flow and increases tubular reabsorption of sodium chloride, and direct tubular effects. The frequency of such peripheral edema with standard doses of the nonselective NSAIDs and the COX-2–specific inhibitors is about 2% to 3% in normal patients, but in patients at risk the rate may increase. With several of the NSAIDs, as there is increased dose, there is an increased incidence of peripheral edema, although this is not seen with celecoxib. NSAIDs also have been reported to increase the effect of antidiuretic hormone, reducing excretion of free water and resulting in hyponatremia. Thiazide diuretics may produce an added effect on the NSAID-induced hyponatremia. All NSAIDs have been shown to interfere with medical management of hypertension and heart failure by inhibiting the clinical effects of angiotensin-converting enzyme inhibitors, β-blockers, and diuretics. All NSAIDs except for the nonacetylated salicylates have been associated with increases in mean blood pressure. Patients receiving antihypertensive agents, including β-blockers, angiotensin-converting enzyme inhibitors, and thiazide and loop diuretics, must be checked regularly when initiating therapy with a new NSAID to ensure that there are no significant continued and sustained rises in blood pressure.

The mechanism of acute renal failure induced in the *at*-risk patient treated with NSAIDs is believed to be prostaglandin mediated. The role of COX-2 in maintenance of renal homeostasis in humans is unclear, however. COX-2 activity is notably present in the macula densa and tubules in animals and humans and is up-regulated in salt-depleted animals. In humans, COX-1 is an important enzyme for control of intrarenal blood flow. At this time, there is sufficient evidence to indicate that the new COX-2 inhibitors are not safer than traditional NSAIDs in terms of renal function. Until further appropriate clinical trials are done, any patient at high risk for renal complications should be monitored carefully. No patient with a creatinine clearance of less than 30 mL/min should be treated with either a NSAID or a COX-2 inhibitor.

IDIOSYNCRATIC ADVERSE EFFECTS

Many of the untoward effects of NSAIDs are related to their mechanism of action, via prostaglandin inhibition, but they also have important idiosyncratic effects. A typical non-specific reaction includes skin rash and photosensitivity, associated with all currently available NSAIDs and particularly phenylproprionic acid derivatives. The phenylpropionic acid derivatives also may induce aseptic meningitis, especially in patients with systemic lupus erythematosus. The underlying mechanism of action is unknown. This class of NSAIDs also has been associated with a reversible toxic amblyopia.

Tinnitus is a common problem with higher doses of salicylates and nonsalicylate NSAIDs. The mechanism is unknown. The very young and the elderly may not complain of tinnitus but only of hearing loss. Decreasing the dose usually alleviates the effect. In all circumstances, tinnitus is reversible with discontinuation of medication.

Because of the antiplatelet effects of all NSAIDs except nonacetylated salicylates, con-comitant therapy with warfarin puts patients at great risk for bleeding. Because concomitant NSAID therapy would displace warfarin from its albumin binding sites, the prothrombin time may be prolonged; in addition, given the increased relative risk for NSAID-induced gas-troduodenal ulcers and bleeding, there is an increased risk for bleeding when NSAIDs are used concomitantly with warfarin. In that the COX-2–specific inhibitors do not cause ulcers of the gastrointestinal tract and they do not alter platelet function, the patient on warfarin would have less risk for a significant gastrointestinal bleed when treated with these drugs than with traditional NSAIDs. Effects such as these also may be seen with phenytoin or other highly protein bound drugs such as antibiotics. NSAIDs inhibit the renal excretion of lithium and should be used with caution in patients taking this drug. Cholestyramine, an anion-exchange resin, reduces the rate of NSAID absorption and its bioavailability.

The central nervous system side effects of NSAIDs include aseptic meningitis, psychosis, and cognitive dysfunction.[14] Cognitive changes are seen more commonly in elderly patients treated with indomethacin, whereas the phenylproprionic acid derivatives are associated more commonly with the development of aseptic meningitis and toxic amblyopia.

Although there are a few case reports of reversible infertility associated with the use of NSAIDs, given the large numbers of patients who regularly use NSAIDs, there does not seem to be a generalized epidemic of infertility. There is ample evidence that traditional use of NSAIDs does not lead to osteoporosis. Although inflammation in the joint leads to juxtaar-ticular osteopenia, this is the result of increased prostglandin synthesis in the inflammed joint, which likely is related directly to increased COX-2 activity.

Some of the early available NSAIDs were associated with an increased risk for bone mar-row failure.[27] This is particularly true of phenylbutazone and indomethacin. In a case-controlled study done using Medicaid claims data, the adjusted odds ratio for neutropenia for patients treated with a NSAID is 4.2 (confidence interval, 2.0 to 8.7). When patients treated with either phenylbutazone or indomethacin were excluded, the odds ratio for the development of neutropenia was still quite robust at 3.5 (confidence interval, 1.6 to 7.6). There were no specific risks associated with specific NSAIDs. In general, the NSAIDs are com-monly used drugs yet the incidence of neutropenia is small.

There are few data documenting the effects of NSAIDs on pregnancy or the fetus. In ani-mal models, the NSAIDs were shown to increase the incidence of dystocia, postimplantation loss, and delay of parturition. The effect of prostaglandin inhibition may result in premature closure of the ductus arteriosus. ASA has been associated with smaller infants and neonatal bruising; however, it has been used for many years in the treatment of patients who require NSAIDs while pregnant. In animals, there is no evidence that ASA is a teratogen. NSAIDs are excreted in breast milk. Salicylates in normally recommended doses are not considered dangerous to nursing infants.[18]

A potential pulmonary toxic reaction is the development of pulmonary infiltrates with eosinophilia. Each patient with the untoward reaction presented with a pneumonia-like picture, short of breath and at times with a high fever. Peripheral blood eosinophilia was noted. Glucocorticoids were required and discontinuance of the drug to reverse the process. It is unknown whether this is associated with specific NSAIDs or due to the general class.[13]

SUMMARY AND CONCLUSIONS

Although NSAIDs are known to decrease pain, including acute and chronic in nature, to decrease inflammation, and to be antipyretic, they have not been shown to decrease erosions in rheumatoid arthritis, to retard osteophyte formation in osteoarthritis, or to protect cartilage from mechanical or inflammatory injury. Pretreatment with NSAIDs repeatedly has been shown to decrease heterotopic bone formation after joint replacement. Specific NSAIDs have been shown in vitro to inhibit chondrocyte proteoglycan synthesis. A few case reports suggest that the long-term use of some NSAIDs accelerated cartilage damage in osteoarthritis, and some investigators believe the data to be compelling enough to preclude the use of NSAIDs in standard therapy for osteoarthritis. Although this effect may have profound implications clinically, the evidence is inferential that chronic use of NSAIDs damage cartilage in humans or worsen the clinical course of osteoarthritis.

All in all, these drugs are popular with patients and physicians. Their benefit-to-risk ratio continues to be debated as we learn more about their actions and toxic effects. COX-2– selective drugs are safer gastrointestinally than the nonselective NSAIDs, but their overall safety profiles are similar. In that context, these drugs are equally efficacious.

REFERENCES FOR ADDITIONAL READING

1. Abramson SB, Leszczynska-Piziak J, Clancy RM, et al: Inhbition of neutrophil function by aspirin-like drugs (NSAIDs): Requirement for assembly of heterotrimeric G proteins in bilayer phsopholipid. Biochem Pharmacol 47:563–572, 1994.
2. Amin AR, Vyas P, Attur M, et al: The mode of action of aspirin-like drugs: Effect on inducible nitric oxide synthase. Proc Natl Acad Sci U S A 92:7926–7930, 1995.
3. Baum C, Kennedy DL, Forbes MB: Utilization of nonsteroidal anti-sinflammatory drugs. Arthritis Rheum 28:686–691, 1985.
4. Bombardier C, Laine L, Reicin A, et al: Comparison of upper gastrointestinal toxicty of rofecoxib and naproxen in patients with rheumatoid arthritis. N Engl J Med 343:1520–1528, 2000.
5. Bombardier C, Peloso PM, Goldsmith CH: Salsalate, a nonacetylated salicylate, is as efficacious as diclofenac in patients with rheumatoid arthritis: Salsalate-diclofenac study group. J Rheumatol 22:617–624, 1995.
6. Brooks PM, Day RO: Nonsteroidal antiinflammatory drugs: Differences and similarities. N Engl J Med 324:1716–1725, 1991.
7. Crofford LJ, Lipsky PE, Brooks P, et al. Cyclooxygenase-2 (Cox-2): Basic biology and clinical application of specific COX-2 inhibitors. Arthritis Rheum
8. Díaz-González F, González-Alvero I, Companero MR, et al: Prevention of in vitro neutrophil-endothelial attachment through shedding of L-selectin by nonsteroidal antiinflammatory drugs. J Clin Invest 95:1756–1765, 1995.

9. DuBois RN, Abramson SB, Crofford L, et al: Cyclooxygenase in biology and disease. FASEB J 12:1063–1073, 1998.

10. Fries J: NSAID gastropathy: The second most deadly rheumatic disease? Epidemiology and risk appraisal. J Rheumatol 18:6–10, 1991.

11. Furst DE: Are there differences among nonsteroidal antiinflammatory drugs? Comparing acetylated salicylates, nonacetylated salicylates, and nonacetylated nonsteroidal antiinflammatory drugs. Arthritis Rheum 37:1–9, 1994.

12. Garcia Rodriguez LA, Williams R, Derby LE, et al: Acute liver injury associated with nonsteroidal antiinflammatory drugs and the role of risk factors. Arch Intern Med 154:311–316, 1994.

13. Goodwin SD, Glenny RW: Nonsteroidal anti-inflammatory drug–associated pulmonary infiltrates with eosinophilia. Arch Intern Med 152:1521–1524, 1992.

14. Hoppmann RA, Peden JG, Ober SK: Central nervous system side effects of nonsteroidal antiinflammatory drugs: Aseptic menengitis, psychosis, and cognitive dysfunction. Arch Intern Med 151:1309–1313, 1991.

15. Laine L, Harper S, Simon T, et al: A randomized trial comparing the effect of rofecoxib, a cyclooxygenase-2 specific inhibitor, with that of ibuprofen on gastroduodenal mucosa of patients with osteoarthritis. Gastroenterology 117:776–783, 1999.

16. Lipsky PE, Abramson SB, Crofford L, et al: The classification of cyclooxygenase inhibitors (editorial). J Rheumatol 25:2298–2303, 1998.

17. Mahmud T, Rafi SS, Scott DL, et al: Nonsteroidal antiinflammatory drugs and uncoupling of mitochondrial oxidative phosphorylation. Arthritis Rheum 39:1998–2003, 1996.

18. Ostensen M, Ostensen H: Safety of nonsteroidal anti-inflammatory drugs in pregnant patients with rheumatic disease. J Rheumatol 23:1045–1049, 1996.

19. Phillips AC, Simon LS: NSAIDs and the elderly: Toxicity and the economic implications. Drugs Aging 1996.

20. Silverstein FE, Faich G, Goldstein JL, et al: Gastrointestinal toxicity with celecoxib vs nonsteroidal anti-inflammatory drugs for osteoarthritis and rheumatoid arthritis. JAMA 284:1247–1255, 2000.

21. Simon LS: Nonsteroidal Antiinflammatory Drugs and Their Effects: The importance of COX selectivity. J Clin Rheum 2:135–140, 1996.

22. Simon LS: Are the biologic and clinical effects of the COX-2-specific inhibitors an advance compared with the effects of traditional NSAIDs? Curr Opin Rheum 12:163–170, 2000.

23. Simon LS, Weaver AL, Graham DY, et al: The anti-inflammatory and upper gastrointestinal effects of celecoxib in rheumatoid arthritis: A randomized, controlled trial. JAMA 282:1921–1928, 1999.

24. Simon LS, Strand V: Clinical resposne to nonsteroidal antiinflammatory drugs. Arthritis Rheum 40:1940–1943, 1997.

25. Singh G, Ramey DR, Morfeld D, et al: Gastrointestinal tract complications of nonsteroidal antiinflammaotry drug treatment in rheumatoid arthritis: A prospective observational study. Arch Intern Med 156:1530, 1996.

26. Smith WL: Prostanoid biosynthesis and mechanisms of action. Am J Physiol 263:F181–F196, 1992.

27. Strom BL, Carson JL, Schinnar R, et al: Nonsteroidal anti-inflammatory drugs and neutropenia. Arch Intern Med 153:2119–2124, 1993.

28. Vane JR, Bakhle YS, Botting RM: Cyclooxygenase 1 and 2. Annu Rev Pharmacol Toxicol 38:97–120, 1998.

29. Whelton A: Nephrotoxicity of nonsteroidal anti-inflammatory drugs: Physiologic foundations and clinical implications. A J Med 106:13S–24S, 1999.

30. Wolfe MM, Lichtenstein DR, Singh G: Gastrointestinal toxicity of the nonsteroidal antiinflammatory drugs. N Engl J Med 340:1888–1899, 1999.

Chapter 6

A Basic Science Aspect of COX-2 Inhibitors

Tarek Samad PhD / Salahadin Abdi, MD, PhD

Prostanoids are a group of fatty acid derivatives that exert their effects in autocrine and paracrine manners in a wide variety of physiologic processes. In the central nervous system, prostanoids are well recognized as mediators in many processes, including fever generation, modulation of the stress response, sleep/wake cycle, control of cerebral blood flow, and hyperalgesia. Arachidonic acid liberated from phospholipids in the cell membrane is converted into prostanoids by the action of phospholipase A_2. Cyclooxygenase (COX) is the enzyme that catalyzes the first two reactions of the prostaglandin pathway, leading to the formation of PGH_2. Tissue-specific isomerases further metabolize PGH_2 into other prostaglandin isoforms (PGE_2, PGD_2, and PGF_2), prostacyclin (PGI_2), or thromboxane (TxA_2),[15, 35] which then exert their biologic actions via seven transmembrane domain receptors classified as DP, EP, FP, IP, and TP receptors according to their respective prostanoid ligand.[6, 27]

The two rate-limiting steps in prostaglandin synthesis are the regulation of arachidonic acid release from membrane phospholipids by phospholipase A_2 (PLA_2) and the conversion of arachidonic acid to the prostanoid precursor PGH_2 by COX. Prostanoid production requires free arachidonic acid and COX enzyme. The standard therapy for inflammatory pain is the use of nonsteroidal antiinflammatory drugs (NSAIDs), which are shown to reduce prostanoid levels in vitro and in vivo.[35, 41] COX are of particular interest because they are the major targets of NSAIDs. The existence of an inducible COX isoform whose expression was regulated by endogenous cytokines and glucocorticoids was long suggested, but it was not until the early 1990s when a new COX isoenzyme (COX-2) was cloned successfully.[19] This finding marked the beginning of a new era in the treatment of pain and inflammation. The recognition that two isoforms of COX exist has led to intense efforts to characterize the relative contribution of each isoform to prostanoid production in specific systems to develop specific antagonists that provide antiinflammatory action with minimal side effects compared with currently used NSAIDs.

COX-1 is expressed constitutively and generally produces prostanoids in response to fine-tuned physiologic processes requiring instantaneous, continuous regulation (e.g., hemostasis)[35]; in contrast, COX-2 is inducible and typically produces prostanoids that mediate responses to physiologic stress, such as injury, infection, and inflammation.[35] The two COX isoforms reveal a differential gene expression profile and distinct kinetic properties, subcellular compartmentation, and interactions with phospholipases and synthases.[14, 35]

COX-1 and COX-2 are membrane-associated enzymes with a 60% amino acid sequence homology.[15] The major sequence differences between COX isoforms occur in the membrane binding domains.[35] Structure-function studies of COX isoforms revealed a homodimer profile structurally and functionally.[35] The general consensus is that COX-1 is present in many cell types and is constitutively expressed, whereas COX-2 is induced as an immediate early gene and is strongly regulated at transcriptional and translational levels.[28] Studies have described an induction of COX-1 expression in stress conditions, such as nerve injury,[33] and the constitutive expression of COX-2 in many tissues, including the central nervous system and the kidney, is well established.[40]

PROSTANOIDS IN PATHOLOGIC PAIN

Pain symptoms comprise two categories: physiologic and pathologic. Multiple mechanisms control the occurrence of neural plasticity, the cellular basis of painful sensation manifested in the ability of neurons to change their function, chemical profile, or structure.

Physiologic pain is an essential early alert to the presence in the environment of damaging stimuli. Pathologic pain can be divided into two groups: inflammatory pain, initiated by tissue damage or inflammation, and neuropathic pain, initiated by nervous system lesions. Both groups of pathologic pain are characterized by hypersensitivity at the site of damage and in adjacent normal tissue. Pain may occur spontaneously or after a stimulus that normally does not produce pain (allodynia). Noxious stimuli may evoke a greater and more prolonged pain (hyperalgesia).[42]

Inflammatory pain hypersensitivity usually returns to normal if the disease process is controlled. Neuropathic pain persists long after the initiating event has healed and is an expression of pathologic operation of the nervous system rather than reaction pathology.

Inflammatory Pain

Soon after their initial isolation, the ability of prostanoids to influence inflammation and immune responses was recognized. Administration of prostanoids alone or in combination with proinflammatory cytokines could reproduce the major signs of inflammation, including pain. Although prostanoid levels are generally low in uninflamed tissues, they increase immediately in acute inflammation. As immune cells infiltrate the tissues, further increases in prostanoid levels are observed. The profile of prostanoids that are produced can vary during the course of inflammatory response. In the carrageenan-induced pleurisy model, elevated PGE_2 levels are observed only during the early stages of inflammation, whereas PGD_2 levels become pronounced during the late stages.

Arthritis Model. Rheumatoid arthritis is a disease that is characterized as an exudative inflammatory response, a proliferative inflammatory response or pannus formation, bone destruction, and pain. Induction of COX-2 and prostanoids in these responses is well established and documented, indicating an involvement of these molecules in arthritis.[23]

In rat adjuvant arthritis, marked edema of the hind footpad was associated with local PGE_2 generation and up-regulation of COX-2 mRNA and protein in the affected paw.[1] The involvement of PGE_2 also was confirmed by the observation that therapeutic administration of anti-PGE_2 antibody substantially reversed edema in the affected paws and decreased levels of interleukin (IL)-6 in the paw and the serum.[29]

COX-2 expression has been shown to be increased in rheumatoid synovial explant cultures by stimulation with IL-1β.[7] Following peripheral inflammation, COX-2 mRNA and protein levels are up-regulated at many levels in the spinal cord and the brain.[31] This induction, followed by increases in prostaglandin levels, suggests that central COX-2 could be an important mediator in the associated central inflammatory response. The time course of the increase in prostaglandin levels corresponds well with the development of allodynia and hyperalgesia, a process that is part of the central adaptive response to intraplantar CFA administration. Pharmacologic analysis using COX inhibitors has shown the involvement of central COX-2 and prostanoids in inflammatory pain hypersensitivity.[31] The involvement of peripheral and central COX-2 in arthritis and the effectiveness of its selective inhibitors have been shown in various animal models of peripheral inflammation, using different inflammatory agents, such as CFA, carrageenan, zymosan, and formalin.[4, 17, 18, 31]

Induction of COX-2 in the spinal cord and the brain has been shown to occur as a response to interleukins, acute peripheral inflammation, and chronic inflammation. This induction is more widespread than the spinal projection of the inflamed tissue, in neuronal and non-neuronal cells of the central nervous system.

Neuropathic Pain Models

In general, pharmacotherapy for neuropathic pain has been disappointing. Chronic neuropathic pain is a significant clinical problem and is poorly relieved by conventional analgesics.[44] The mechanisms of neuroplasticity associated with neuropathic pain are not clear. Partial nerve injury is much more likely to produce pain in humans than complete transection of the nerve. Several animal models of neuropathic pain have been developed, which involve lesioning some of the fibers of the sciatic nerve. In the most frequently used models, a mixture of intact and injured fibers is created by loose ligation of the sciatic nerve (chronic constriction injury of the sciatic nerve [CCI] model[5]) or a tight ligation of a part of the sciatic nerve.[34] Another neuropathic pain model is produced by a tight ligation of an entire spinal segmental nerve (segmental spinal injury (SSI]25). An interesting neuropathic pain model was shown by Decosterd and Woolf[8] involving a lesion of two of the three terminal branches of the sciatic nerve (tibial and common peroneal nerves), leaving the remaining sural nerve intact. A major characteristic of this model is that the commingling of distal intact axons with degenerating axons is restricted, and it permits behavioral testing of the non-injured skin territories adjacent to the denervated areas. These models have improved understanding of the basic mechanisms underlying neuropathic pain. It is generally accepted that hyperalgesia is due to sensitization of peripheral afferent fibers and to increased responsiveness of spinal interneurons or central sensitization.[43]

Experimental neuropathy points to an important contribution of central mechanisms.[37] The role of spinal COX in nociception has been implicated in several studies (as discussed earlier), mainly by intrathecal administration of prostanoids causing hyperalgesia in the rat or by administration of COX inhibitors to reduce allodynia and hyperalgesia. COX-2 (but not COX-1) mRNA and protein levels in the dorsal spinal cord and thalamus increase significantly 1 day after L5–L6 spinal nerve ligation in the rat.[44] Intrathecal administration of a COX inhibitor (indomethacin) was shown to attenuate the development of tactile allodynia.[44] Behavioral assays hypothesized that spinal COX-2 and prostaglandins may play an important role in the early development, but not the maintenance, of neuropathic pain caused by spinal nerve ligation. In another study, in which the Seltzer model was used, subcutaneous administration of either COX-2 inhibitors or EP1 prostaglandin receptor antagonist produced significant attenuation of mechanical and thermal hyperalgesia.[37] EP1 receptor antagonist also has been shown to reduce hyperalgesia, allodynia, and c-*fos* gene expression in the CCI rat model.[24] Studies are still under way in our laboratory and in other groups to characterize the contribution of COX-2 and prostanoids to neuropathic pain.

COX-2 KNOCKOUT MODELS

COX-1 and COX-2 physiologic roles have been investigated using genetic approaches such as knockout and transgenics. In addition to other features unrelated to pain pathophysiology, such as renal dysplasia, COX-2-deficient mice showed an involvement of prostanoids generated by COX-2 in promoting inflammation in several animal models of disease; however, normal inflammatory responses to a few tests, including ear edema after phorbol ester or AA treatment and paw edema after carrageenan injection, were obtained in COX-2-deficient mice.[38] These results point to a compensation mechanism by COX-1 to provide prostanoids.[2] Tumor necrosis factor-α and lipopolysaccharide effects were reduced markedly in the mutant mice, however, and produced fewer prostaglandins.[38] Studies using COX-deficient mice and selective COX-1 and COX-2 inhibitors showed that COX-1-generated prostanoids also may contribute to hyperalgesia in acetic acid, stretching, hot plate, and formalin pain models.[2]

NONSTEROIDAL ANTIINFLAMMATORY DRUGS AND COX-2 INHIBITION

The existence of an inducible COX isoform whose expression was regulated by endogenous cytokines and glucocorticoids has long been suggested, but it was not until the early 1990s when a new COX isoenzyme (COX-2) was cloned successfully.[28] This finding marked the beginning of a new era in the treatment of pain and inflammation. The recognition that two isoforms of COX exist led to intense efforts to characterize the relative contribution of each isoform to prostanoid production in specific systems, to develop specific antagonists that provide antiinflammatory action with minimal side effects compared with the currently used NSAIDs.

COX-1 is expressed constitutively and generally produces prostanoids in response to fine-tuned physiologic processes requiring instantaneous, continuous regulation (e.g., hemostasis).[18] In contrast, COX-2 is inducible and typically produces prostanoids that mediate responses to physiologic stress, such as injury, infection, and inflammation.[18] The two COX isoforms reveal a differential gene expression profile and distinct kinetic properties, subcellular compartmentation, and interactions with phospholipases and synthases.[4] COX-1 and COX-2 are membrane-associated enzymes with a 60% amino acid sequence homology.[35] The major sequence differences between COX isoforms occur in the membrane binding domains.[35] Structure-function studies of COX isoforms[35] revealed a homodimer profile structurally and functionally. The general consensus is that COX-1 is present in many cell types and is constitutively expressed, whereas COX-2 is induced as an immediate early gene and is strongly regulated at the transcriptional and the translational levels.[28] Studies[23, 33] described an induction of COX-1 expression in stress conditions, such as nerve injury. The constitutive expression of COX-2 in many tissues, including the central nervous system and the kidney, is well established.[40]

The regulation of COX-2 mRNA was shown to represent a key mechanism for the control of COX-2 levels. Since its discovery, COX-2 expression has been shown to be induced by numerous factors, including neurotransmitters, growth factors, proinflammatory cytokines, lipopolysaccharide, calcium, phorbol esters, and small peptide hormones.[28] The antiinflammatory and analgesic benefits of NSAIDs have been proposed to derive from the inhibition of COX-2 isoforms induced at the site of injury or inflammation.[39] Prostanoids contribute to the development of peripheral sensitization by acting on sensory nerve terminals, more specifically by contributing to a protein kinase–mediated phosphorylation of sodium channels in nociceptor terminals, increasing excitability, reducing the pain threshold, and potentiating the action of pain-producing molecules such as bradykinin.[16] New knowledge about the functional properties of COX-1 and COX-2 has had a major impact on the development of compounds that specifically target and inhibit COX-2 activity, while sparing COX-1 at therapeutic doses. COX-2-specific inhibition would alleviate pain and inflammation without disrupting the homeostatic functions mediated by COX-1-derived prostanoids, suggesting that many of the deleterious side effects of conventional NSAIDs, which cannot distinguish between COX-1 and COX-2 isoforms, could be avoided.

SELECTIVE COX-2 INHIBITORS

On the basis of their biochemical and pharmacologic properties, in vitro and in vivo, COX inhibitors can be classified into four categories: COX-1-specific inhibitors, COX nonspecific inhibitors, COX-2 preferential inhibitors, and COX-2-specific inhibitors.[23] Preferential COX-2 inhibitors also may inhibit COX-1 but with reduced potency. Nimesulide may be 5 to 16 times more potent at inhibiting COX-2 than COX-1.[23] COX-2-specific inhibitors, such as celecoxib (SC58635) and rofecoxib (MK0966), are 375-fold and 800-fold selective for COX-2 over COX-1.[23]

The first COX-2-selective compounds to be identified were DuP697 and NS398,[9] before the cloning of COX-2. They were developed for their gastrointestinal-sparing properties in animal models. They were shown to be 80-fold and 1000-fold selective for the inhibition of COX-2.[9] The group of diarylheterocyclic compounds related to DuP697, the most diverse class of inhibitors and the first to be approved for human use, includes the two COX-2 inhibitors on the market, celecoxib and rofecoxib.

An examination of the structure-function relationship revealed that the presence of a 4-methylsulfone substituent on the stilbene framework is crucial for the activity of members of this class of inhibitors.[9, 13] The selectivity of these compounds was assessed in vitro and in vivo (animal models) as the ratio of IC_{50} values for COX-1 and COX-2.[9, 23] Good selectivity and in vivo activity (bioavailability) with favorable metabolic properties constitute a prerequisite for the choice of a COX-2 inhibitor.

Structurally the COX enzyme is composed of three independent folding units: an epidermal growth factor–like domain, a membrane-binding motif, and an enzymatic domain. The active site of this enzyme consists of a long hydrophobic channel with the amino acids tyrosine 385 and serine 530 at its apex.[13]

The COX-2 x-ray structure shows that it closely resembles that of COX-1, and the binding sites for arachidonic acid in the two enzymes isoforms are comparable. NSAIDs block the COX substrate–binding pocket by binding to an arginine residue at position 120, preventing the arachidonic acid from reaching the binding site. This arginine residue also is a binding site for the carboxyl group of arachidonic acids and is the site for competitive interaction with NSAIDs, which all contain carboxylic groups.[13]

The main structural feature that confers specificity to the inhibition by selective NSAIDs is several amino acid changes that increase the size and chemical environment of the COX-2 substrate binding pocket. Most important among these is the substitution of valine in COX-2 for isoleucine 523, an amino acid that lines the surface of the COX-1 active site.[9] Because valine is smaller than isoleucine, it leaves a gap in the long hydrophobic channel, providing access to a side channel, believed to be the site of binding of COX-2-selective agents.[9]

NS-398 was the first compound with high selectivity for COX-2 over COX-1 that was shown to have antiinflammatory and analgesic properties similar to indomethacin, with reduced side effects on the kidney and gastric mucosa at antiinflammatory doses.[9, 12, 13, 32] Subsequently, many compounds selective for COX-2 have been developed by the pharmaceutical industry. Many COX-2-selective and preferential inhibitors have been developed, and clinical trials on some COX-2 inhibitors already have been conducted.

The two COX-2 inhibitors commonly used in the United States differ not only in their doses, but also in the indications approved by the Food and Drug Administration. Celecoxib and rofecoxib are classified as COX-2-specific inhibitors because they do not cause any clinically significant inhibition of COX-1 at maximal therapeutic doses; This has been supported by the results of clinical trials and early postmarketing experience in the treatment of inflammation and pain. The Food and Drug Administration approved the two compounds for slightly different indications: Celecoxib is indicated for rheumatoid arthritis and osteoarthritis, whereas rofecoxib is indicated only for the signs and symptoms of osteoarthritis, dysmenorrhea, and acute pain.[23]

Celecoxib generally is used at a dose of 200 mg/d or 100 mg twice a day. Rofecoxib is given at an average dose of 25 mg/d for osteoarthritis, whereas for acute pain such as dysmenorrhea or after surgery, 50 mg/d for a few days is commonly used. Both COX-2 inhibitors are used not only as antiinflammatory drugs, but also as analgesics. Rofecoxib has a quicker onset of action (30 minutes versus 60 minutes for celecoxib) and a longer duration of action than celecoxib because of its longer half-life (17 hours versus 11 hours for celecoxib).[30] One thing the two agents have in common is their analgesic ceiling effect.[36]

When COX-2 inhibitors are used for pain, they can be combined with acetaminophen, opioids, or other adjuvant pain medications to potentiate their analgesic effects. Care should be taken, however, when prescribing these drugs to patients with history of allergic reaction to aspirin or other NSAIDs. Celecoxib (Celebrex) is contraindicated in patients with sulfa allergy.

MECHANISM OF ACTION: PERIPHERAL VERSUS CENTRAL

Many reports showed that NSAIDs, in addition to their peripheral action, have antinociceptive effects by acting central nervous system structures, including the spinal cord.[10, 11, 26] It was shown that the central administration of prostanoids potentiates and enhances peripheral nociception.[21, 22] The finding that both COX are constitutively expressed in the central nervous system and that COX-2 expression is up-regulated after a variety of peripheral and central stimuli, such as acute and chronic peripheral inflammation, interleukins, peripheral and central nerve injury, enhanced synaptic transmission, and cerebral ischemia, supported the hypothesis of a central action of NSAIDs.[20, 40]

A direct action of NSAIDs in the central nervous system has been established firmly in studies[26, 31, 36] in which pain hypersensitivity was reduced by the direct application of NSAIDs to the central nervous system. At present, the permeability of the blood-brain barrier to currently used NSAIDs and COX-2 inhibitors has not been elucidated fully. Inhibitors of COX-2 that penetrate the blood-brain barrier more effectively may represent more efficient painkillers, working to block the oversensitivity to pain that is coordinated by the brain.[3]

A peripheral inflammation induces a widespread increase in COX-2 expression in the spinal cord and many regions in the brain, including the thalamus and the hypothalamus. The up-regulation of IL-1s in the central nervous system has been shown to constitute a major inducer of central COX-2 up-regulation.[31] Consequently the administration of either COX-2 or IL-1s synthesis inhibitors into the subarachnoid space of the spinal cord reduces inflammation-induced central prostaglandin E_2 levels and mechanical hyperalgesia without altering basal pain sensitivity.[3, 31] The modulation of COX-2 up-regulation after tissue injury and inflammation, in addition to inhibiting COX-2 activity, may be a powerful tool to prevent inflammatory pain.

SUMMARY

The COX enzymes catalyze arachidonic acid and produce prostanoids, which play a significant role in inflammation and pain. There is enough evidence to show that the COX isoenzyme, COX-2, specifically is involved in various types of pain, including inflammatory and neuropathic pain syndromes. Experiments in basic science show that selective COX-2 inhibitors play a pivotal role in attenuating pain behaviors in animals and in human pain models.

REFERENCES FOR ADDITIONAL READING

1. Anderson GD, Hauser SD, McGarity KL, et al: Selective inhibition of cyclooxygenase (COX)-2 reverses inflammation and expression of COX-2 and interleukin 6 in rat adjuvant arthritis. J Clin Invest 97:2672–2679, 1996.
2. Ballou LR, Botting RM, Goorha S, et al: Nociception in cyclooxygenase isozyme-deficient mice. Proc Natl Acad Sci U S A 97:10272–10276, 2000.
3. Bartfai T: Immunology: Telling the brain about pain. Nature 410:425–427, 2001.
4. Beiche F, Brune K, Geisslinger G, Goppelt-Struebe M: Expression of cyclooxygenase isoforms in the rat spinal cord and their regulation during adjuvant-induced arthritis. Inflamm Res 47:482–487, 1998.
5. Bennett GJ, Xie YK: A peripheral mononeuropathy in rat that produces disorders of pain sensation like those seen in man. Pain 33:87–107, 1988.
6. Breyer RM, Bagdassarian CK, Myers SA, Breyer MD: Prostanoid receptors: Subtypes and signaling. Annu Rev Pharmacol Toxicol 41:661–690, 2001.
7. Crofford LJ, Wilder RL, Ristimaki AP, et al: Cyclooxygenase-1 and -2 expression in rheumatoid synovial tissues: Effects of interleukin-1 beta, phorbol ester, and corticosteroids. J Clin Invest 93:1095–1101, 1994.
8. Decosterd I, Woolf CJ: Spared nerve injury: An animal model of persistent peripheral neuropathic pain. Pain 87:149–58, 2000.
9. Dewitt DL: COX-2-selective inhibitors: The new super aspirins. Mol Pharmacol 55:625–631, 1999.
10. Dirig DM, Isakson PC, Yaksh TL: Effect of COX-1 and COX-2 inhibition on induction and maintenance of carrageenan-evoked thermal hyperalgesia in rats. J Pharmacol Exp Ther 285:1031–1038, 1998.
11. Dirig DM, Konin GP, Isakson PC, Yaksh TL: Effect of spinal cyclooxygenase inhibitors in rat using the formalin test and in vitro prostaglandin E2 release. Eur J Pharmacol 331:155–160, 1997.
12. Emery P: Cyclooxygenase-2: A major therapeutic advance? Am J Med 110:S42–S45, 2001.
13. Everts B, Wahrborg P, Hedner T: COX-2-specific inhibitors—the emergence of a new class of analgesic and anti-inflammatory drugs. Clin Rheumatol 19:331–343, 2000.
14. Fitzpatrick FA, Soberman R: Regulated formation of eicosanoids. J Clin Invest 107:1347–1351, 2001.

15. Garavito RM, Dewitt DL: The cyclooxygenase isoforms: Structural insights into the conversion of arachidonic acid to prostaglandins. Biochim Biophys Acta 1441:278–287, 1999.

16. Gold MS: Tetrodotoxin-resistant Na$^+$ currents and inflammatory hyperalgesia. Proc Natl Acad Sci U S A 42:111–112, 1999.

17. Hay C, de Belleroche J: Carrageenan-induced hyperalgesia is associated with increased cyclooxygenase-2 expression in spinal cord. Neuroreport 8:1249–1251, 1997.

18. Hay CH, de Belleroche JS: Dexamethasone prevents the induction of COX-2 mRNA and prostaglandins in the lumbar spinal cord following intraplantar FCA in parallel with inhibition of oedema. Neuropharmacology 37:739–744, 1998.

19. Herschman HR, Fletcher BS, Kujubu DA: TIS10, a mitogen-inducible glucocorticoid-inhibited gene that encodes a second prostaglandin synthase/cyclooxygenase enzyme. J Lipid Mediat 6:89–99, 1993.

20. Hoffmann C: COX-2 in brain and spinal cord implications for therapeutic use. Curr Med Chem 7:1113–1120, 2000.

21. Hori T, Oka T, Hosoi M, Aou S: Pain modulatory actions of cytokines and prostaglandin E$_2$ in the brain. Ann N Y Acad Sci 840:269–281, 1998.

22. Hori T, Oka T, Hosoi M, et al: Hypothalamic mechanisms of pain modulatory actions of cytokines and prostaglandin E$_2$. Ann N Y Acad Sci 917:106–120, 2000.

23. Katori M, Majima M: Cyclooxygenase-2: Its rich diversity of roles and possible application of its selective inhibitors. Inflamm Res 49:367–392, 2000.

24. Kawahara H, Sakamoto A, Takeda S, et al: A prostaglandin E2 receptor subtype EP1 receptor antagonist (ONO-8711) reduces hyperalgesia, allodynia, and c-fos gene expression in rats with chronic nerve constriction. Anesth Analg 93:1012–1017, 2001.

25. Kim SH, Chung JM: An experimental model for peripheral neuropathy produced by segmental spinal nerve ligation in the rat. Pain 50:355–363, 1992.

26. Malmberg AB, Yaksh TL: Cyclooxygenase inhibition and the spinal release of prostaglandin E2 and amino acids evoked by paw formalin injection: A microdialysis study in unanesthetized rats. J Neurosci 15:2768–2776, 1995.

27. Minami T, Nakano H, Kobayashi T, et al: Characterization of EP receptor subtypes responsible for prostaglandin E2-induced pain responses by use of EP1 and EP3 receptor knockout mice. Br J Pharmacol 133:438–444, 2001.

28. O'Banion MK: Cyclooxygenase-2: molecular biology, pharmacology, and neurobiology. Crit Rev Neurobiol 13:45–82, 1999.

29. Portanova JP, Zhang Y, Anderson GD, et al: Selective neutralization of prostaglandin E2 blocks inflammation, hyperalgesia, and interleukin 6 production in vivo. J Exp Med 184:883–891, 1996.

30. Reuben SS, Connelly NR: Postoperative analgesic effects of celecoxib or rofecoxib after spinal fusion surgery. Anesth Analg 91:1221–1225, 2000.

31. Samad TA, Moore KA, Sapirstein A, et al: Interleukin-1beta-mediated induction of COX-2 in the CNS contributes to inflammatory pain hypersensitivity. Nature 410:471–475, 2001.

32. Schnitzer TJ: Cyclooxygenase-2-specific inhibitors: Are they safe? Am J Med 110:46S–49S, 2001.

33. Schwab JM, Brechtel K, Nguyen TD, Schluesener HJ: Persistent accumulation of cyclooxygenase-1 (COX-1) expressing microglia/macrophages and upregulation by endothelium following spinal cord injury. J Neuroimmunol 111:122–130, 2000.

34. Seltzer Z, Dubner R, Shir Y: A novel behavioral model of neuropathic pain disorders produced in rats by partial sciatic nerve injury. Pain 43:205–218, 1990.

35. Smith WL, Dewitt DL, Garavito RM: Cyclooxygenases: Structural, cellular, and molecular biology. Annu Rev Biochem 69:145–182, 2000.

36. Sunshine A: A comparison of the newer COX-2 drugs and older non-narcotic oral analgesics. J Pain 1(3 suppl 1):10S–13S, 2000.

37. Syriatowicz JP, Hu D, Walker JS, Tracey DJ: Hyperalgesia due to nerve injury: Role of prostaglandins. Neuroscience 94:587–594, 1999.

38. Tilley SL, Coffman TM, Koller BH: Mixed messages: Modulation of inflammation and immune responses by prostaglandins and thromboxanes. J Clin Invest 108:15–23, 2001.

39. Vane J, Botting R: Inflammation and the mechanism of action of anti-inflammatory drugs. FASEB J 1:89–96, 1987.

40. Vanegas H, Schaible H: Prostaglandins and cyclooxygenases in the spinal cord. Prog Neurobiol 64:327–363, 2001.

41. Verburg KM, Maziasz TJ, Weiner E, et al: COX-2-specific inhibitors: Definition of a new therapeutic concept. Am J Ther 8:49–64, 2001.

42. Woolf CJ, Mannion RJ: Neuropathic pain: Aetiology, symptoms, mechanisms, and management. Lancet 353:1959–1964, 1999.

43. Woolf CJ, Salter MW: Neuronal plasticity: Increasing the gain in pain. Science 288:1765–1769, 2000.

44. Zhao Z, Chen SR, Eisenach JC, et al: Spinal cyclooxygenase-2 is involved in development of allodynia after nerve injury in rats. Neuroscience 97:743–748, 2000.

Chapter 7

Nonsteroidal Antiinflammatory Drugs: Bedside

Howard S. Smith, MD

NONSTEROIDAL ANTIINFLAMMATORY DRUGS

Nonsteroidal antiinflammatory drugs (NSAIDs) have been classified into different classes based on their basic chemical structures (Table 1). NSAIDs differ in potency with respect to their analgesic, antiinflammatory, and antipyretic properties. Doses needed for antiinflammatory activity are generally higher than doses to produce analgesia.

There seem to be wide variations between the analgesic activity of various NSAIDs—even ones in the same class (family; e.g., acetic acids). Large individual differences may exist. One NSAID may not work at all for an individual patient, and another may work well. Theoretically, looking at efficacy in populations (although not always true in reality), equal efficacy between agents should be able to be achieved with increased dosing.

Although differences may exist between NSAIDs, it is not generally thought that one particular NSAID would be the drug of choice for a specific medical condition with perhaps one exception. Although many would not agree, it is conceivable that indomethacin may have advantages for particular medical conditions (e.g., chronic paroxysmal hemicrania) over other NSAIDs. The structural similarity of indomethacin to serotonin could be what may set it apart from other NSAIDs. This structural similarity also may account for the relatively high incidence of central nervous system adverse effects, such as vertigo, headaches, and nausea. The relatively high rate at which indomethacin crosses the blood-brain barrier also could contribute to the aforementioned effects.

Salicylates are classified into two groups: acetylated and nonacetylated. Aspirin and benorylate are from the acetylated group; drugs in the nonacetylated group include choline salicylate (Arthropan), choline magnesium trisalicylate (a combination of choline salicylate and magnesium salicylate; Trilisate), and salsalate or salicylsalicylic acid (hydrolyzed to two molecules of salicylate; Disalcid).[1] Nonacetylated salicylates are converted to salicylic acid and are much less potent inhibitors of cyclooxygenase (COX) than aspirin in vitro, and this may explain partially why they seem to cause less gastrointestinal mucosal insult and may affect platelets only slightly, although they exhibit comparable efficacy with in vivo models of inflammation.[2] Additionally, salicylic acid inhibits COX-2 somewhat more than COX-1; (roughly similar to etodolac)—both agents have COX-2/COX-1 inhibitor ratios in the range of 7–10 (meloxicam is higher and COX-2 selective inhibitors [e.g., celecoxib, rofecoxib] are much higher). The weaker the degree of in vitro COX inhibition, the less apt the agent is to cause bronchospasm, which is sometimes associated with NSAIDs.[3] Some aspirin-sensitive asthmatic patients may be able to use a nonacetylated salicylate without a problem, but asthma has been induced by a nonacetylated salicylate in at least one patient.[4] In a series of dog experiments, it seemed evident that NSAIDs that affect prostaglandin E_2 (PGE_2) synthesis the least may be the best to use

TABLE 1

Classification of Nonsteroidal Antiinflammatory Drugs by Chemical Structure Classes

Class	Drug: Generic Name (Brand Name)
Propionic acids	Naproxen (Naprosyn, Anaprox, Alleve) Flurbiprofen (Ansaid) Oxaprozin (Daypro) Ibuprofen (Motrin) Ketoprofen (Orudis, Oruvail) Ketorolac (Toradol)
Indoleacetic acids	Sulindac (Clinoril) Indomethacin (Indocin) Etodolac (Lodine)
Phenylacetic acids	Diclofenac (Cataflam, Voltaren)
Salicylic acids (nonacetylated)	Salsalate (Disalcid) Choline magnesium trisalicylate (Trilisate)
Naphthylalkanone	Nabumetone (Relafen)
Oxicam	Piroxicam (Feldene)
Anthranilic acid	Mefenamic acid (Ponstel) Meclofenamate
Pyrroleacetic acid	Tolmetin (Tolectin)
Pyrazolone	Phenylbutazone

in patients with borderline or impaired renal function.[5] For weak inhibitors of COX, although efficacy may decline, side effects seem to decline as well.

Choline magnesium trisalicylate is available as 500-mg, 750-mg, and 1,000-mg tablets and as 500 mg/5 mL oral suspension. The usual adult dose is 500 to 750 mg orally three times a day (1,500 to 2,250 mg/d).

Etodolac

Etodolac is available in an extended-release form. It is absorbed rapidly from the gastrointestinal tract, and peak concentrations occur within 1 to 2 hours.[6] The protein binding of etodolac is greater than 99% at concentrations of 10 to 100 μg/mL.[7] Plasma concentrations are slightly higher after multiple doses than after a single dose.[6] The elimination half-life of etodolac is 6 to 7 hours.[6] Maximal analgesia usually occurs about 1 hour after administration and may last 6 to 12 hours.[7] Etodolac is metabolized extensively by the liver (glucuronidation and hydroxylation).[8] After oral dosing, roughly 73% of the dose is excreted in the urine, and about 16% is excreted in the feces.[7] Etodolac is a racemic mixture of S ($-$) and R ($+$) enantiomers. The S ($-$)

enantiomer is 100-fold more active as COX inhibitor than the R(+) enantiomer and has faster clearance but is not clinically available in the United States (chiral inversion does not occur).[9]

The usual adult doses of etodolac are 400 to 1,200 mg/d. Etodolac is available in 200-mg and 300-mg capsules and 400-mg and 500-mg tablets. Etodolac XL is available in 400-mg, 500-mg, and 600-mg tablets.

Oxaprozin

Oxaprozin is a propionic acid with a pKa of 4.3. Oxaprozin has a bioavailability of roughly 95% with peak concentrations occurring 3 to 5 hours after dosing (food slows rate but not extent of absorption).[10] Its protein binding is 99%—largely to albumin. Of oxaprozin, 97% is metabolized by the liver, and the rest is excreted unchanged in the urine. There does not seem to be any significant enterohepatic recirculation. The elimination half-life ranges from 50 to 60 hours after repeated doses.

Oxaprozin is available as 600-mg scored tablets. The usual adult dose is 600 to 1,200 mg/d. On initiation of acute therapy, the clinician can give three tablets (1,800 mg) for a loading dose.

Ketoprofen

Ketoprofen is a propionic acid derivative that potently inhibits prostaglandin synthesis and may inhibit lipoxygenase and decrease polymorphonuclear neutrophil activation.[4] (Meclofenamate, which inhibits 5-lipoxygenase potently, may be tolerated better by patients with aspirin-induced asthma). Ketoprofen is absorbed rapidly and reaches peak serum concentrations in 0.5 to 2 hours.[11] The rate of absorption, but not the extent, is delayed by food.[12] Ketoprofen is marketed as a racemic mixture and does not undergo interconversion *in vivo*. Ketoprofen is 99% protein bound—largely to albumin[11]—and concentrations are detectable in the cerebrospinal fluid within about 15 minutes. Ketoprofen is glucuronidated and hydroxylated extensively by the liver, and the half-life is about 1.4 to 3.3 hours in healthy volunteers.[13] After a single oral dose, roughly 70% to 80% is excreted in the urine, with less than 10% excreted as unchanged drug.[11] Protein binding of ketoprofen is diminished in liver disease (e.g., hepatic cirrhosis). The clearance is reduced by about half in the elderly.[14]

The sustained-release formulation of ketoprofen (Oruvail) yields lower peak plasma concentrations and a longer time to peak concentrations.[13] Ketoprofen is available as 25-mg, 50-mg, and 75-mg capsules and as a 200-mg sustained-release capsule.

Naproxen

Naproxen is marketed as the (+) isomer. It is 97.6% to 99.5% protein bound at doses less than 500 mg.[15] It is essentially completely absorbed from the gastrointestinal tract.[15] The rate of absorption, but not the extent, is increased by sodium bicarbonate and decreased by magnesium carbonate, magnesium oxide, aluminum hydroxide, and food. The elimination half-life of naproxen is 12 to 15 hours.[15] Naproxen is available in a salt form, naproxen sodium (Anaprox, Aleve) and naproxen base (Naprosyn). The main difference is that the salt form is absorbed more rapidly (naproxen sodium, 275 mg, *equals* naproxen base, 250 mg).

Prescription naproxen sodium is available as 275-mg and 550-mg (Anaprox DS) tablets. Naproxen base is available as 250-mg, 375-mg, and 500-mg tablets and as a 125 mg/15 mL oral suspension.

Naproxen also has been marketed as an enteric-coated (EC) formulation and as a long-acting formulation (Naprelan). Naprelan is available in 375-mg and 500-mg controlled-release tablets and uses the proprietary IPADS (Intestinal Protective Drug Absorption System) technology. This technology entails a rapidly disinterating tablet system combining an immediate-release component and a sustained-release component of microparticles that are widely dispersed, which allows for absorption of the NSAID throughout the gastrointestinal tract. This system is able to keep relatively stable plasma levels for about 24 hours.

Tolmetin

Tolmetin is absorbed rapidly orally with peak concentrations between 20 and 65 minutes.[4] Tolmetin is 99% bound to plasma proteins.[16] The elimination half-life is 2.1 to 6.8 hours. Tolmetin undergoes extensive metabolism in the liver to inactive oxidative metabolites and conjugates of tolmetin with 99% of a dose excreted in the urine.[16]

Tolmetin is available as 200-mg and 600-mg tablets and Tolectin DS 400-mg capsules. The usual adult dose is 400 mg orally every 8 hours.

Diclofenac

Diclofenac is a phenylacetic acid. In addition to inhibiting COX, (diclofenac) diminishes the availability of arachidonic acid by stimulating its uptake and inhibiting its release.[17] It is absorbed completely from the gastrointestinal tract after fasting, but during first-pass metabolism the bioavailability is 30% to 70%.[18] Diclofenec has a pKa of 4 and is highly protein bound (99%).[19] It is metabolized to inactive metabolites (95%) via hydroxylation and conjugation and has a half-life of about 75 minutes.[19]

Diclofenac sodium is available in an enteric-coated formulation (Voltaren) and as a potassium salt (Cataflam). Voltaren is available in the United States as 25-mg, 50-mg, and 75-mg enteric-coated tablets, and the adult dose is 75 to 225 mg/d. A combination tablet containing diclofenac, 50 mg (Arthotec 50) or 75 mg (Arthrotec 75), in an inner enteric coated core and misoprostol (200 μg) in the outer mantle, is available. Misoprostol, a prostaglandin E_1 analog, is added in an attempt to minimize gastrointestinal mucosal insult. Although misoprostol, 800 μg/d, may offer maximal gastrointestinal protection, it is not tolerated well by many patients. The dose of 400 μg/d seems to be a reasonable compromise, offering reasonable tolerability and gastrointestinal mucosal protection. Misoprostol should be avoided in women who are considering pregnancy. The major side effects are gastrointestinal, especially diarrhea, which may be explosive in nature.

Indomethacin

Indomethacin is an indole acetic acid that seems to inhibit membrane-bound phospholipase A_2 and C in polymorphonuclear (PMN) cells in addition to inhibiting COX.[20] Indomethacin also may lead to a variety of other effects, including increasing Interleukin-2 and interferon responses,[21] decreasing T- and B-lymphocyte proliferative responses[22] (decreasing leukotriene B_4–induced polymorphonuclear leukocyte neutrophil migration),[23] and increasing lymphokine-activated natural killer cell activity.[24] Penetration of the blood-brain barrier is relatively rapid and high with concentrations in cerebrospinal fluid exceeding serum concentrations within 2 hours after intramuscular administration.[25] Some of these charcteristics may set indomethacin apart from other NSAIDs, contributing to its unique ability to ameliorate chronic paroxysmal hernicrania.

Indomethacin is highly bioavailable, being well absorbed from the gastrointestinal tract with peak plasma concentrations 0.5 to 4 hours after administration.[26] Protein binding is 99%.[26] Food taken in conjunction with indomethacin retards the absorption rate (but not the extent of absorption).[27] Indomethacin is demethylated (largely by the CYP450 system), then undergoes extramicrosomal deacylation.[28] The half-life of indomethacin is 2.2 to 11.2 hours.[28] A relatively high enterohepatic circulation may contribute to the incidence of gastrointestinal mucosal insult.

Indomethacin is the only NSAID in the United States approved for use in patent ductus arteriosus, in which it is used as the sodium trihydrate salt intravenously. Indomethacin is available as 25-mg and 50-mg capsules, 75-mg sustained release capsules (25-mg uncoated pellets for immediate absorption and 50-mg coated pellets for extended release),[29] 50-mg suppositories, and an oral suspension (25 mg/0.5 mL). The usual dose is 75 to 150 mg/d.

Ketorolac

Ketorolac is available for parenteral use or orally as the tromethamine salt. It is available as a racemic mixture with the S(−) enantiomer responsible for its pharmacologic actions.[30] Ketorolac has a high bioavailability and is rapidly and well absorbed. Ketorolac tromethamine dissociates into its active form, ketorolac anion, at physiologic pH. Protein binding is 90% to 99%, and the half-life is 4 to 6 hours.[31] The acyl-glucuronide conjugate is the major metabolite (roughly 75%) and is essentially inactive. A less major metabolite, p-hydroxy-ketorolac (about 12%), possesses about 20% of the antiinflammatory activity and 1% of the analgesic activity of ketorolac.[32]

The parenteral formulation is available as 15 mg/1 mL, 30 mg/1 mL, or 60 mg/2 mL, and the oral formulation is available as 10-mg tablets. It is suggested that ketorolac be given only for a period of 5 days total. Guidelines suggest that oral therapy should be used only as a continuation of parenteral therapy (e.g. 2 days parenteral, then 3 days oral). The parenteral formulation contains alcohol and should not be used for spinal administration. The parenteral maximal daily dose should be 120 mg/day. Oral dosing usually is 10 mg four times a day.

Nabumetone

Nabumetone is a nonacidic naphthylalkanone similar in structure to naproxen.[33] It is a prodrug and undergoes hepatic metabolism to its active metabolite, 6-methoxy-2-naphthylacetic acid (6MNA).[34] The half-life of 6MNA is roughtly 24 hours.

Nabumetone is available as 500-mg and 750-mg tablets. The usual adult dose range is 1,000 to 2,000 mg/d; in the elderly, dosing should be 1,000 mg or less because of kinetic differences.[33] There do not seem to be any significant enterohepatic circulation issues with nabumetone.

Sulindac

Sulindac is an indene-acetic acid derivative chemically related to indomethacin.[8] It is a sulfoxide prodrug with a sulfide (reversible) metabolite that exhibits 500 times more antiinflammatory activity than the parent drug.[2]

The sulfide is metabolized irreversibly to an inactive sulfone.[8] Two enzymes facilitate the *reverse* conversion from sulfide to sulfoxide: a flavoprotein-monooxygenase leading to the less active R(+) parent and a heme-related COX leading to the S(−) patent.[8] Differences exist between cis and trans forms (the cis form being a better COX inhibitor). The overall activity of sulindac in individual patients is difficult to predict.[9] After oral administration, about 90% of the dose is absorbed, with fasting peak levels reached in 1 hour for sulindac and 2 hours for the sulfide metabolite.[35] The protein binding of sulindac is 93%, and all forms of the drug undergo enteroheptaic recirculation.[8]

Sulindac is extensively metabolized in the liver with roughly 50% of a single dose excreted in the urine and 30% recovered in the feces.[8] The mean half-life for sulindac is 7.8 hours, and the mean half-life for the active sulfide metabolite is 16 to 18 hours.[2] The explanation proposed for the controversial idea that sulindac may have a slightly gentler renal profile versus other NSAIDs[36] was that sulindac may inhibit renal COX to a lesser extent than other NSAIDs because the kidney can reoxidize the sulfide back to the inactive sulfoxide prodrug.[37]

Sulindac is available as 150-mg and 200-mg tablets. The usual adult dose is 150 to 200 mg orally twice a day (300 to 400 mg/d) Doses should be reduced significantly (e.g., about ≤ 200 mg/d) in the elderly and patients with impaired hepatic or renal function.

Ibuprofen

Ibuprofen is a propionic acid with a pKa of 4.4.[8] It is more than 90% absorbed from the gastrointestinal tract[2] and more than 90% protein bound. Ibuprofen is administered as a racemic mixture with 56% to 69% of inactive R enantiomer converting irreversibly to the active S form *in vivo*.[38] The American Academy of Pediatrics states that ibuprofen can be administered safely to women who breast-feed their infants.[39] Ibuprofen yields four urinary metabolites, formed by hydroxylation and by further oxidation of the primary alcohol to a carboxyl group.[40] The half-life of ibuprofen has been reported to be 2 to 2.5 hours after multiple dosing.[41]

Ibuprofen is available over-the-counter as 200-mg tablets and by prescription as 300-mg, 480-mg, 600-mg, and 800-mg tablets and 100 mg/5 mL oral suspension. The usual adult dose is 1,200 to 2,400 mg/d.

Meloxicam

Meloxicam is an oxicam derivative and a member of the enolic group of NSAIDs. It has some COX-2 selectivity (e.g., preferential inhibition of COX-2 over COX-1) (most pronounced at lower doses), but meloxicam is not considered a selective COX-2 inhibitor by the U.S. Food and Drug Administration (FDA).

After oral administration of 30-mg meloxicam capsules, the absolute bioavailability is 89%.[42,43] The mean C_{max} (maximum concentration) is reached in 4 to 5 hours after administration of a 7.5-mg tablet.[42,43] A second peak occurs at 12 to 14 hours after dosing, suggesting gastrointestinal recirculation.[42,43] Meloxicam exhibits linear pharmacokinetics and reaches steady-state within 5 days of multiple dosing.[42] Meloxicam can be given without regard to meals.[42] The mean volume of distribution is 10 L with approximately 99.4% bound to plasma proteins (mostly albumin).[42,43] Meloxicam concentrations in the synovial fluid are greater than in the plasma, but the significance of this is unknown.[42] Metabolism to four inactive metabolites occurs in the liver. Cytochrome P-450 2C9 plays a major role, with 3A4 having a minor role in metabolism.[42,43] Meloxicam is excreted predominantly in the form of inactive metabolites in the urine and the feces.[42,43] The elimination half-life is 15 to 20 hours.[42,43]

The Meloxicam Large-scale International Study Safety Assessment (MELISSA) trial is a large-scale, double-blind, randomized international, prospective trial. For 28 days, patients with symptomatic osteoarthritis were given either meloxicam, 7.5 mg (n = 4,635), or diclofenac, 100 mg sustained release (n = 4,688). Patients taking meloxicam experienced fewer gastrointestinal adverse events (dyspepsia, nausea, vomiting, abdominal pain, and diarrhea) than the diclofenac group (13% versus 19%; P < 0.001).[44] More patients discontinued meloxicam compared with diclofenac because of lack of effectiveness (80 of 4,635 versus 49 of 4,688, P < 0.01).[44]

The Safety and Efficacy Large-scale Evaluation of COX-Inhibiting Therapies (SELECT) trial is a large-scale, prospective, international, multicenter, double-blind, double-dummy, randomized, parallel-group study.[45] Meloxicam was compared with piroxicam for the treatment of patients with signs and symptoms of osteoarthritis; 4,320 patients were treated with meloxicam, 7.5 mg, and 4,335 patients were treated with piroxicam, 20 mg, for 28 days.[45] The results of the SELECT trial support the concept that the toxicity of NSAIDs is related to the inhibition of COX-1, and the efficacy is related to the inhibition of COX-2.[45] The incidence of gastrointestinal side events was lower in the meloxicam group compared with the piroxicam group (10.3% versus 15.4%, P < 0.001), whereas the efficacy of both drugs was the same.[45] Individual gastrointestinal adverse events occurred less frequently in the meloxicam group than the piroxicam group: dyspepsia (3.4% versus 5.8%, P < 0.001), nausea and vomiting (2.5% versus 3.4%, P < 0.05), and abdominal pain (2.1% versus 3.6%, P < 0.001).[45]

Meloxicam is available in 7.5-mg tablets. The recommended starting and maintenance dose for osteoarthritis is 7.5 mg orally once a day with a maximal daily dose of 15 mg. Meloxicam may be given without regard to meals.

No significant dose adjustments are required for mild-to-moderate hepatic or renal (creatinine clearance >15 mL/min) insufficiency.[42] The use of meloxicam in severe hepatic or renal impairment has not been studied. Use of meloxicam in patients with severe renal impairment is not recommended.[13]

The most common adverse effects are gastrointestinal in nature and include abdominal pain, diarrhea, dyspepsia, flatulence, and nausea. Meloxicam does not usually increase the prothrombin time of patients while taking warfarin but can, and monitoring is suggested. Cholestyramine given for 4 days before treatment with meloxicam increased its clearance by about 50%.[42,43] Lithium concentrations increased with concomitant use of meloxicam because of an increase in levels and a reduction in clearance.[42,43] The antihypertensive effect of angiotensin-converting enzyme inhibitors may be diminished slightly.[42,43]

CYCLOOXYGENASE-2 SELECTIVE INHIBITORS

The International Consensus Meeting on the Mode of Action of COX-2 Inhibition (ICMMAC) served as a forum for experts from different disciplines (e.g., rheumatology, gastroenterology, pharmacology) to assess the significance of differential inhibition of COX-1 and COX-2 (Brookes). ICMMAC suggested an agent be considered COX-2-selective if it inhibits COX-2 but not COX-1 across the entire therapeutic dose range based on whole blood assays. (Brooks P, et al: Rheumatology (Oxford) 38:779, 1999.)

COX-2 is present under basal conditions in the brain, renal cortex, pancreas, and uterus; however, in most tissues, it is essentially considered *inducible*—increasing by 10 to 80 fold with inflammation.[46,47] Although the CLASS and VIGOR trial controversies are not discussed here, it seems prudent to encourage patients on COX-2 agents with cardiac risk factors to use low-dose aspirin therapy in conjunction with the COX-2 agent. These COX-2 selective agents may possess less gastrointestinal toxicity than traditional nonselective NSAIDs.

Valdecoxib

Valdecoxib (Bextra) is a selective inhibitor of COX-2. The bioavailability after an oral dose is 83%, and the extent of absorption is unaffected by food or aluminum/magnesium–containing antacids. Valdecoxib is 98% protein bound. Valdecoxib's initial response after oral administration is within 1 hour, and peak effects occur within 3 hours. It is extensively metabolized in the liver, primarily via the cytochrome P-450 (CYP) system (largely CYP3A4 and CYP2C9) and non–CYP-dependent pathways, including glucuronidation. Inhibitors of CYP-3A4 and CYP-2C (e.g., fluconazide) may increase valdecoxib levels. Valdecoxib is a moderate inhibitor of CYP-2C19 and a weak inhibitor of CYP-3A4 and CYP-2C9. At least one active metabolite has been identified, but it does not seem to contribute to any great extent to clinical actions probably because of low plasma levels. The plasma elimination half-life is 8 to 11 hours. Urinary excretion of unchanged drug is minimal (<5% of an oral dose). The levels of valdecoxib may increase with significant hepatic disease and probably should be avoided in these patients.

The FDA has approved valdecoxib for osteoarthritis, rheumatoid arthritis, and dysmenorrhea. Valdecoxib is available as 10-mg and 20-mg tablets. A once-daily dose of 10 mg is effective in osteoarthritis and rheumatoid arthritis.[48–50] In primary dysmenorrhea, doses of 20 mg or occasionally 40 mg are often effective.[51] There is some evidence that a dose of 20 mg orally twice a day (40 mg/d) may achieve greater efficacy in the treatment of dysmenorrhea.[51]

Celecoxib

Celecoxib (Celebrex) is a selective COX-2 inhibitor. The tablet is reasonably well absorbed; after 200 mg was given orally with a high-fat meal, absorption was delayed, but bioavailability was increased about 40%. Total protein binding is 97%, and it takes about 3 hours to achieve peak plasma concentration. Celecoxib is metabolized extensively in the liver predominantly via cytochrome P-450 2C9 to three inactive metabolites. The elimination of celecoxib is via the kidney (27%) and feces (57%) with less than 3% eliminated as unchanged drug. The half-life is 11 hours.

Celecoxib is available as 100-mg and 200-mg tablets and can be given once or twice a day. The usual adult dose is 100 to 400 mg/d.

Rofecoxib

Rofecoxib (Vioxx) is a selective inhibitor of COX-2. The bioavailability is about 93%. Rofecoxib has a time to peak concentration after oral administration of approximately 2 to 3 hours. Rofecoxib is 87% bound to plasma proteins. Rofecoxib is metabolized extensively in the liver via reduction of cytosolic enzymes with less than 10% of a dose undergoing oxidative reduction. The two major inactive metabolites are a cis dihydro derivative and a trans dihydro derivative. Elimination is via the kidney (72%) and the feces (14%) with less than 1% eliminated in the urine as unchanged drug. The elimination half-life is 17 hours. Rofecoxib is available as 12.5-mg, 25-mg, and 50-mg tablets and an oral suspension and is dosed once daily. The initial recommended dose for osteoarthritis is 12.5 mg once daily, which may need to be increased to 25 mg once daily. For rheumatoid arthritis, the usual adult dose is 25 mg once daily, and for acute pain or dysmenorrhea, the initial recommended dose is 50 mg. This dose may be repeated once daily as needed for 5 days.

Parecoxib

Parecoxib is a water-soluble prodrug of the COX-2 inhibitor valdecoxib and is not yet clinically available in the United States. *In vivo*, it undergoes rapid hydrolysis to the active drug valdecoxib. Parecoxib is the first COX-2-selective inhibitor formulated for intravenous or intramuscular injection, which allows for greater flexibility of administration.[52] Ketorolac (Toradol) is currently the only available injectable NSAID in the United States. Parecoxib has a fast onset of analgesia, which allows for treatment of acute pain. Parecoxib is being considered for use preoperatively to prevent or reduce hyperalgesia and inflammation and in the perioperative period.[53,54] The use of parecoxib possibly could reduce the need for opioids and consequently their associated side effects. Advantages of parecoxib include no observed effect on platelet aggregation, fewer gastrointestinal adverse effects, and availability in a dosage form for patients who cannot ingest or tolerate oral administration. Traditional NSAIDs have had limited use preoperatively because of their increased risk of bleeding, so parecoxib may be useful in the perioperative period.

Etoricoxib

Etoricoxib (Arcoxia) is a novel selective COX-2 inhibitor being developed by Merck for use in osteoarthritis, rheumatoid arthritis, and pain.[55] Etoricoxib is not yet available clinically in the United States, but it is hoped that it may offer advantages because it seems that it would be the most COX-2 selective agent available in the United States, and it is long lasting (e.g., long half-life) relative to clinically available COX-2 selective inhibitors. The selectivity ratio (COX-1 to COX-2) for the inhibition of COX-2 by etoricoxib in human whole-blood assay was 106 compared with 35, 30, 7.6, 7.3, 2.4, and 2.0 for rofecoxib, valdecoxib, celecoxib, nimesulide, etodolac, and meloxicam.[56] Etoricoxib has the lowest potency of inhibition of COX-1 compared with other reported selective agents.[56]

Lumiracoxib (COX-189)

Lumiracoxib (COX-189) is in phase III clinical trials and may be useful for the treatment of osteoarthritis, rheumatoid arthritis, and pain. It is a highly selective COX-2 inhibitor developed by Novartis and is expected to be at least as effective as nonselective NSAIDs with an improved side-effect profile. Compared with diclofenac, (COX-189) has substantially reduced affinity for COX-1, being 300-fold less potent[57]; this may be beneficial for pain relief in sites of metastatic bone lesions where the local environment is acidic in nature. The pKa of (COX-189) is 4.3.[57]

COX-189 is absorbed rapidly with a median time to C_{max} (maximum concentration) of 2 hours after single or multiple doses.[57] Administration of (COX-189) with a high-fat meal did not alter the bioavailability significantly and it can be given without regard to meals.[57] The protein binding of (COX-189) is greater than 99% and is independent of concentration.[57] (COX-189) is a substrate for cytochrome P-450 2C9 and is metabolized extensively by hydroxylation.[57] After a single dose of (COX-189), 32% of drug-related material was excreted in the urine and 50% in the feces.[57] The amount of unchanged drug excreted in the urine is 1% to 3% and in the feces is 5%.[57] The elimination half-life is 3 to 6 hours, and the apparent volume of distribution is approximately 0.1 L/kg.[57]

ROLE OF CYCLOOXYGENASE

Arachidonic acid is generated from cellular membrane phospholipids mainly via the action of phospholipase A (PLA_2) but also via phospholipase C (PLC). Arachidonic acid generated in nonneuronal cells is evolved predominantly via PLA_2. Although not every phospholipase A enzyme needs calcium, activated G protein, and urokinase to function, the PLA_2 enzyme in certain tissues seems to function optimally with all of these factors. Unesterfied free arachidonic acid may be reincorporated back into being a cellular membrane phospholipid[58] (Figure 1). The arachidonic acid generated may enter one of four major pathways (Figure 2). The various end products of each pathway may have different physiologic effects (e.g., mediators of inflammatory, vasoconstriction/vasodilation, platelet antiaggregation). Eicosanoid actions may include intercellular signaling (as primary messengers), intracellular signaling (as secondary messengers), regulation of ion gradients and ion channels and secretion of hormones and neurotransmitters, modulation of the cellular cytoskeleton, and modulation of the endothelial barrier function.

During the reduction of PGG_2, a reactive oxygen singlet is produced that can inactivate COX. This has been termed *suicide* inactivation and occurs about once every 1,200 turn-

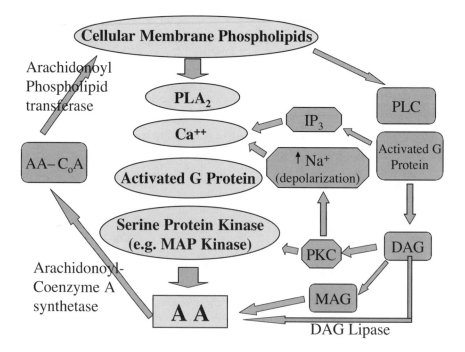

Figure 1. From membrane to arachidonic acid and back.

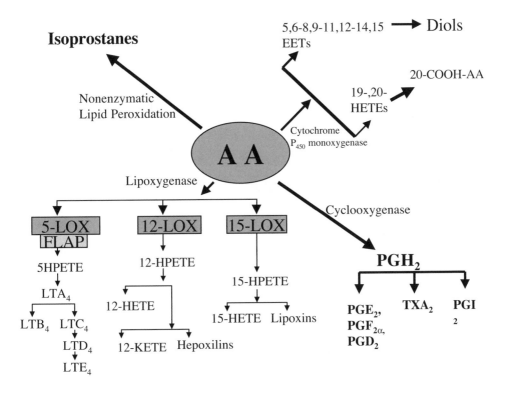

Figure 2. Arachidonic acid metabolism.

overs.[59] This inactivation may be a mechanism to constrain prostaglandin synthesis.[59,60] Reduced glutathione may increase synthesis of PGE_2 through activation of its isomerase, affording more turnover cycles of COX before deactivation. Thromboxane synthase may be inhibited by lipid hydroperoxides, which can be reversed by free radical scavengers.

The arachidonic acid generated in sensory neurons seems to be predominantly via PLC. PLC leaves substrate membrane lipids (e.g., PIP_2) to generate two intracellular messengers, diacylglycerol (DAG) and inositol-1,4,5 triphosphate (IP3) through activation of a pertussis toxin–sensitive G protein.[61] DAG via excitation of sensory neurons stimulates protein kinase C (PKC) to phosphorylate permeable cation channels, which leads to their opening with subsequent neuronal depolarization. Additionally, PKC activates the serine kinase (mitogen-activated protein) via phosphorylation.[62] PKC also enhances the calcium sensitivity of PLA_2. DAG lipase hydrolyzes DAG to form monoacylglycerol and arachidonic acid.[61] Distinct bradykinin receptors mediate stimulation of prostaglandin synthesis by endothelial cells and fibroblasts.[63] Increases in intracellular calcium (which could lead to increases in nitric oxide formation and eventually potentially contribute to hyperalgesia) are evolved in two major ways: (1) via IP3 and (2) via cell depolarization through PKC actions (Figure 3).

The structure of COX is a large globular protein with three major domains: the membrane binding site; the epidermal growth factor; and the two separate active catalytic sites, COX site (CAS) and perioxidase active site (PAS) (Figure 4).[64,65] COX catalyzes two reactions: (1) the addition of molecular oxygen to arachidonic acid at C-9, C-11, and C-15 to yield the

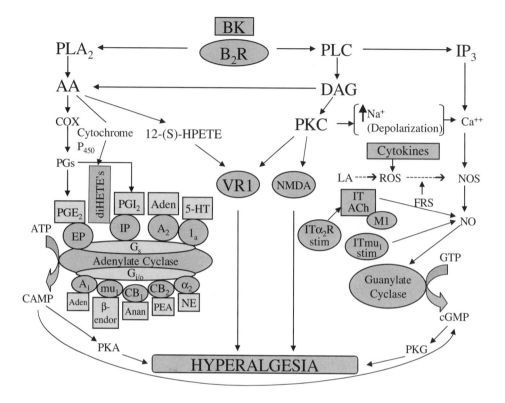

Figure 3. The many roads leading to hyperalgesia.

cyclic endoperoxide PGG_2 at the CAS site and (2) reduction of the C-15 peroxide of PGG_2 to a hydroxyl group to yield PGH_2 at the PAS site.[66,67] The endoperoxides PGG_2 and PGH_2 are unstable (half-life about 4 minutes) and yield other stable prostanoids. The active site (CAS) is located at the end of a long tunnel that is able to accept the long folded structure of lipidic acid precursors.[65] It is believed that COX inhibitors act by preventing access of the lipids acid to the active site (Figure 5).

In the case of aspirin (acetylsalicylicacid [ASA]), when ASA irreversibly acetylates serine 530[65] of COX, conformational changes take place, which impede access to the CAS (Figure 6). Also the sialic acid residue may block access to CAS (Figure 6). Because COX is irreversibly inhibited, enzyme synthesis is required before more prostanoids can be produced. In cells without capability for protein synthesis (e.g., platelets), new cells must be formed before more prostanoids can be produced. Although ASA irreversibly inhibits the COX enzymes, most traditional NSAIDs (e.g., ibuprofen) are reversible enzyme inhibitors of COX that are competitive inhibitors of arachidonic acid binding.

Indomethacin is in between ASA and ibuprofen in terms of interaction with COX.[68–70] Indomethacin causes irreversible inactivation of COX activity without covalent modification of the enzyme.[71,72] It is conceivable that by repetitive interaction between indomethacin and COX, the conformation of COX is changed permanently (irreversibly), perhaps the way that a new shoe may change its shape to accommodate a person's foot after many days of wearing the shoe.

COX

Endoplasmic Reticulum (3 Domains)

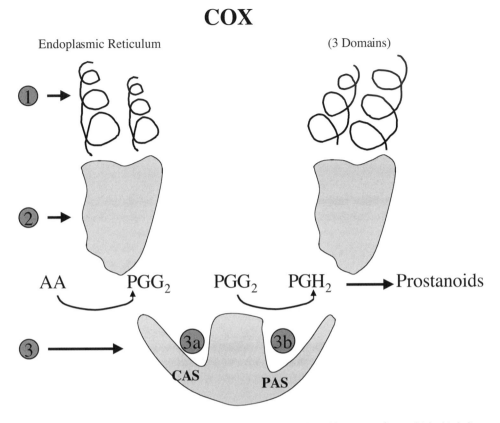

AA PGG_2 PGG_2 PGH_2 ⟶ Prostanoids

Figure 4. Cyclooxygenase features. (1) The membrane-binding site (mouth) consists of 4 amphiphathic helices with hydrophobic residues facing outwards. (2) Epidermal growth factors. (3) The 2 separate active catalytic sites— (3a) cyclooxygenase active site (CAS) and (3b) peroxidase active site (PAS).

Additionally, NSAIDs may increase the activity of hepatic tryptophan 2,3-dioxygenase in certain pain states. This increased tryptophan 2,3-dioxygenase activity may lead to increased levels of kynurenic acid, which may act as a endogenous broad-spectrum excitatory amino acid antagonist.

Therapies to diminish the gastrointestinal toxicity of traditional NSAIDs include the addition of proton-pump inhibitors (e.g., omeprazole), prostaglandin analogs (e.g., misoprostol), nitric oxide donors (NO-NSAIDs) (Fiorucci S, et al: Gastroenterology 68:1089, 1999), or zwitterionic phospholipids (to coat the gastrointestinal mucosa). Additionally, using R-ketoprofen instead of the racemate (R-S) ketoprofen may reduce toxicity. Also, as inhibitors of COX-2 become more superselective [e.g., (5,5-dimethyl-3-(2-propoxy)-4-methanesulfonylphenyl)-2(5H)-furanone)[74]] issues of gastric mucosal protection may be less important.

Endothelin-1 and depletion of sensory neuropeptides or inhibition of nitric oxide synthesis may modulate the gastric mucosal microcirculation, which may lead to mucosal damage. Calcitonin gene–related peptide, vasodilator prostanoids (PGE_2), and NO donors may offer mucosal protection.

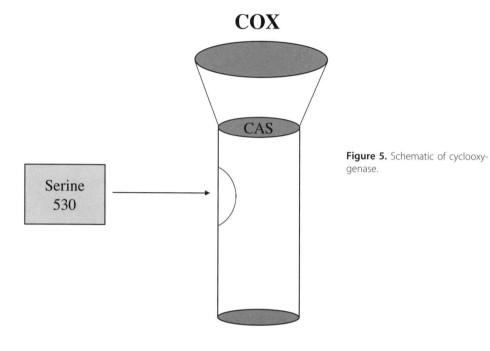

Figure 5. Schematic of cyclooxygenase.

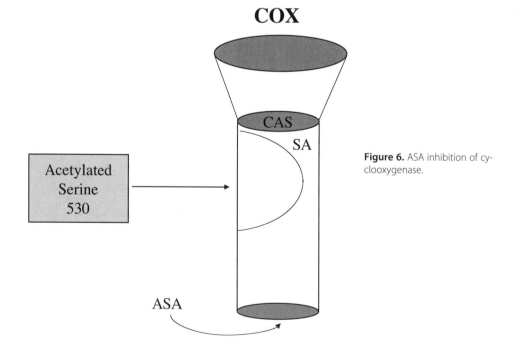

Figure 6. ASA inhibition of cyclooxygenase.

Antiinflammatory agents found in plants such as *Harpagophytum* (devil's claw), whose active ingredient is a compound called *harpagoside*, and *Urtica dioica* (stinging nettle), whose active ingredient is a compound called *caffeoyl malic acid*, may prove useful in providing analgesia in the future.

Arachidonic acid metabolism contributes to only one small part of inflammation and nociceptive input. A major inducer of central COX-2 up-regulation is interleukin-1β. Interleukin-1β–mediated induction of COX-2 in the central nervous system contributes to inflammatory pain hypersensitivity.[75] There are many other inflammatory mediators and receptors (see Figure 3) and inflammatory cells and cytokines that may play a role in analgesia and hyperalgesia related to inflammation.

Once inflammation has evolved, the body apparently possesses endogenous mechanisms to begin to "turn off" proinflammatory signals and dampen the inflammation.

ASA, via acetylation of COX-2, prevents the formation of prostanoids, but the acetylated enzyme remains active *in situ* to generate bioactive lipoxins epimeric at carbon 15 (15-epi-LX, also termed *aspirin-triggered lipoxin*). It is conceivable that some of the beneficial effects of low-dose aspirin therapy (indomethacin, other NSAIDs, and acetaminophen also permit lipoxin generation) and mega-3 polyunsaturated fatty acid therapy may be related to locally evolved lipoxins that possess potent antiinflammatory activity (including inhibition of human polymorphonuclear leukocyte transendothelial migration and infiltration) and an apparent ability to *clean up* local inflammation.[73]

Work by Levy et al[73] contributed the mechanisms of this *cleanup*, or processes involved in the resolution of inflammation. It seems that when inflammation is produced, immune cells (e.g., neutrophils) rush into the area of inflammation and produce leukotriene B$_4$, which is *proinflammatory* and leads to the recruitment of more neutrophils to the area.[73] Subsequently the neutrophils also produce the enzyme COX-2, which evolves PGE$_2$. PGE$_2$ enables a shift to an antiinflammatory arm of events.[73] The PGE$_2$ does this via the induction of 15-lipoxygenase (not normally present in the circulating neutrophils of healthy people). The 15-lipoxygenase induced then leads to the production of lipoxin A$_4$, which exhibits *antiinflammatory* properties, dampening inflammation and stimulating the resolution of inflammation and impeding neutrophils from entering the area of inflammation.[73] It is conceivable that by quelling prostaglandin production with the use of COX-2 selective inhibitors, the natural processes of resolution may be delayed or dampened.[73]

REFERENCES FOR ADDITIONAL READING

1. Dromgoole SH, Furst DE: Salicylates. In Evans WE, Schentag JJ, Jusko WJ (eds): Applied Pharmacokinetics. 3rd ed. Spokane, WA, Applied Therapeutics, 1992, pp 1–34.
2. Furst DE, Paulus HE: Aspirin and other nonsteroidal anti-inflammatory drugs. In McCarty DJ, Koopman WJ (eds): Arthritis and Allied Conditions. 12th ed. Philadelphia, Lea & Febiger, 1993, pp 567–602.
3. Dromgoole SH, Furst DE, Paulus HE. Rational approaches to the use of salicylates in the treatment of rheumatoid arthritis. Semin Arthirits Rheum 11:257–283, 1982.
4. Chudwin DS, Strub M, Golden HE, et al: Sensitivity to non acetylated salicylates in a patient with asthma, nasal polyps, and rheumatoid arthritis. Ann Allergy 57:133–134, 1986.
5. Zambraski EJ, Atkinson DC, Dramond J: Effects of salicylate vs. aspirin on renal prostaglandins and function in normal and sodium-depleted dogs. J Pharmacol Exp Ther 247:96–103, 1988.
6. Brater DC, Lasseter KC: Profile of etodolac: Pharmacokinetic evaluation in special populations. Clin Rheum 8:25–35, 1989.

7. Sanda M, Jacob GB, Fliedner L Jr, et al: Etodolac. In Lewis AH, Furst DE (eds): Nonsteroidal Anti-inflammatory Drugs: Mechanisms and Clinical Uses. New York, Marcel Dekker, 1987, pp 349–370.
8. Nishihara KK, Furst DE: Aspirin and other nonsteroidal anti-inflammatory drugs. In Koopman WJ (ed): Arthritis and Allied Conditions: A Textbook of Rheumatology. 13th ed. Balitmore, Williams & Wilkins, 1997, pp 611–654.
9. Williams KM: Enantiomers in arthritic disorders. Pharmacol Ther 46:273–295, 1990.
10. Janssen FW, Jusko WJ, Chiang ST, et al: Metabolism and kinetics of oxaprozin in normal subjects. Clin Pharmacol Ther 27:352–363, 1980.
11. Ishizaki T, Sasaki T, Saganuma T, et al: Pharmacokinetics of ketoprofen following single oral, intramuscular and rectal doses and after repeated oral administration. Eur J Clin Pharmacol 18: 407–414, 1980.
12. Bannwarth B, Lapicque F, Netter P, et al: The effect of food on the systemic availability of ketoprofen. Eur J Clin Pharmacol 33:643–645, 1988.
13. Williams RL, Upton RA: The clinical pharmacology of ketoprofen. J Clin Pharmacol 28(suppl): S1–S22, 1988.
14. Advenier CA, Rouk A, Gobert C, et al: Pharmacokinetics of ketoprogen in the elderly. Br J Clin Pharmacol 16:65–70, 1983.
15. Brogden RN, Heel RC, Speight TM, Avery GS: Naproxen up to date: A review of its pharmacological properties and therapeutic efficacy and use in rheumatic disease and pain states. Drugs 18: 241–277, 1979.
16. Dromgoole SH, Furst DE: Tolmetin. In Paulus HE, Furst DE, Dromgoole SH (eds): Drugs for Rheumatic Disease. New York, Churchill-Livingstone, 1987, pp 365–377.
17. Liauw HL, Moscaritola JD, Burcher J: Diclofenac sodium (Voltaren). In Lewis AJ, Furst DE (eds): New Anti-Inflammatory Agents. New York, Marcel Dekker, 1987, pp 329–347.
18. Brune K, McCormack K: The over-the-counter use of nonsteroidal anti-inflammatory drugs and other antipyretic analgesics. In Lewis AJ, Furst DE (eds): Nonsteroidal Anti-inflammatory Drugs: Mechanisms and Clinical Uses. 2nd ed. New York, Marcel Dekker, 1994, pp 97–126.
19. Riess W, Stierlin H, Degen P, et al. Pharmacokinetics and metabolism of the anti-inflammatory agent Voltaren. Scand Rheumatol 22(suppl):17–29, 1978.
20. Shakir KMM, Simpkins CO, Gartner SL, et al: Phospholipase activity in human PMN: Partial characterization and effect of indomethacin. Enzyme 42:197–208, 1989.
21. Kim B, Warnaka P: Indomethacin-enhanced immunotherapy of pulmonary metastases using IL-2 and IFN-gamma. Surgery 106:248–256, 1989.
22. Seng GF, Benesohn J, Bayer BM: Changes in T and B lymphocyte proliferative responses in adjuvant arthritic rats: Antagonism by indomethacin. Eur J Pharmacol 178:267–273, 1990.
23. Villa ML, Valenti F, Mantovani M: Modulations of natural killing by cyclo- and lipo-oxygenase inhibitors. Immunology 63:93–97, 1988.
24. Manning LS, Bowman RV, Davis MR, et al: Indomethacin augments lymphokine activated killer cell generation by patients with malignant mesothelioma. Clin Immunol Immunopathol 53:68–77, 1989.
25. Bannwarth B, Netter P, Lapicque F, et al: Plasma and cerebrospinal fluid concentrations of indomethacin in humans relationship to analgesic activity. Eur J Clin Pharmacol 38:343–346, 1990.
26. Hvidberg E, Lausen HH, Jansen JA: Indomethacin: Plasma concentrations and protein binding in man. Eur J Clin Pharmacol 4:119–124, 1972.
27. Wallusch WW, Nowak H, Leopold G, et al: Comparative bioavailability: Influence of various diets on the bioavailability of indomethacin. Int J Clin Pharmacol Ther Toxicol 16:40–44, 1978.
28. Duggan DE, Logans AF, Kwan KC, et al: The metabolism of indomethacin in man. J Pharmacol Exp Ther 181:563–557, 1972.
29. Yeh KC: Indomethacin and indomethacin sustained release—a comparison of their pharmacokinetic progiles. Semin Arthritis Rheum 12(suppl 1):136–141, 1982.
30. Young JM, Yee JP: Ketorolac. In Lewis AJ, Furst DE (eds): Newer Anti-inflammatory Agents: Clinical Implications. New York, Marcel Dekker, 1987, pp 247–266.

31. Wischnik A, Manth SM, Lloyd J, et al: The excretion of ketorolac tromethamine into breast milk after multiple oral dosing. Eur J Clin Pharmacol 36:521–524, 1989.

32. Mroszczak EJ, Lee FW, Combs D, et al: Ketorolac tromethamine absorption, distribution, metabolism, excretion, and pharmacokinetics in animals and humans. Drug Metab Dispos 15:618–626, 1987.

33. Fridel HA, Todd PA: Nabumetone: A preliminary review of its pharmacodnamic and pharmacokinetic properties, and therapeutic efficacy in rheumatic diseases. Drugs 35:504–524, 1988.

34. Blower PR: The unique pharmacologic profile of nabumetone. J Rheumatol 19(suppl 36):13–19, 1992.

35. Brogden RN, Heel RC, Speight TM, et al: Sulindac: A review of its pharmacological properties and therapeutic efficacy in rheumatic diseases. Drugs 16:97–114, 1978.

36. Ciabattoni G, Cinotti GA, Pierucci A, et al: Effects of sulindac and ibuprofen in patients with chronic glomerular disease: Evidence for the dependence of renal function on prostacyclin. N Engl J Med 310:279–283, 1984.

37. Miller MJS, Bednar MM, McGiff JC: Renal metabolism of sulindac, a novel non-steroidal antiinflammatory agent. Adv Prostaglandin Thromboxane Leukot Res 11:487–491, 1983.

38. Cheng H, Rogers JD, Demetriades JL, et al: Pharmacokinetics and bioinversion of ibuprofen enantiomers in humans. Pharm Res 11:824–830, 1994.

39. American Academy of Pediatrics Committee on Drugs: The transfer of drugs and other chemicals into human breast milk. Pediatrics 72:375, 1983.

40. Brooks CJW, Gilbert MT: Studies of urinary metabolites of 2-(4-isobutylphenyl) propionic acid by gas-liquid chromatography–mass spectrometry. J Chromatogr 99:541–551, 1974.

41. Bennett WM, Porter GA, Bagby SP, et al: Drugs and Renal Disease. Vol. 2 New York, Churchill-Livingstone, 1978.

42. Boehringer Ingelheim Pharma/Abbott Laboratories: Mobic (meloxicam) package insert. Ridgefield, CT, 2000.

43. Davies NM, Skjodt NM: Clinical pharmacokinetics of meloxicam, a cyclooxygenase-2 preferential nonsteroidal anti-inflammatory drug. Clin Pharmacokinet 36:115–126, 1999.

44. Hawkey C, Kahan A, Steinbruck K, et al: Gastrointestinal tolerability of meloxicam compared to diclofenac in osteoarthritis patients. Br J Rheumatol 37:937–945, 1998.

45. Dequeker J, Hawkey C, Kahan A, et al: Improvement in gastrointestinal tolerability of the selective cyclooxygenase (COX)-2 inhibitor, meloxicam compared with poroxicam: Results of the safety and efficacy large-scale evaluation of COX-inhibiting therapier (SELECT) trial in osteoarthritis. Br J Rheumatol 37:937–945, 1998.

46. DeWitt D, Meade E, Smith W: PGH synthase isoenzyme selectivity: The potential for safer nonsteroidal anti-inflammatory drugs. Am J Med 95(suppl 2A):40–43, 1993.

47. Kujubu D, Reddy S, Fletcher B, Herschman H: Expression of the protein product of the prostaglandin synthase-2/TIS10 gene in mitogen-stimulated Swiss 3T3 cells. J Biol Chem 268: 5425–5430, 1993.

48. Bensen W, Weaver A, Espinoza L, et al: Valdecoxib, a new COX-2 specific inhibitor, is effective in treating the signs and symptoms of rhematoid arthritis (abstr). Presented at the American College of Rheumatology (ACR) 65th Annual Scientific meeting, November 2001, San Francisco, CA.

49. Fiechtner JJ, Sikes D, Recker D, et al: A double-blind, placebo-controlled dose ranging study to evaluate the efficacy of valdecoxib, a novel COX-2 specific inhibitor, in treating the signs and symptoms of osteoarthritis of the knee (abstr). Presented at the European Congress of Rheumatology (EULAR 2001), June 2001, Prague, Czech Republic.

50. Kivitz A, Eisen G, Zhao WW, et al: The COX-2 specific inhibitor valdecoxib is as effective as the conventional NSAID naproxen in treating symptomatic osteoarthritis of the knee and demonstrates reduced gastrointestinal ulceration (abstr). Presented at the American College of Rheumatology (ACR) 65th Annual Scientific Meeing, November 2001, San Francisco, CA.

51. Torri S, Kuss ME, Talwalker SC, et al: The cyclooxygenase (COX)-2 specific inhibitor valdecoxib effectively treats primary dysmenorrhea (abstr) Fertil Steril 76:S95, 2001.

52. Cheer SM, Goa KL: Parecoxib (parecoxib sodium). Drugs 61:1133–1141, 2001.

53. Desjardins PJ, Grossman EH, Kuss ME, et al: The injectable cyclooxygenase-2 specific inhibitor parecoxib sodium has analgesic efficacy when administered preoperatively. Anesth Analg 93: 721–727, 2001.

54. Stoltz RR, Harris SI, Kuss ME, et al: Upper GI mucosal effects of parecoxib sodium in healthy elderly subjects. Am J Gastroenterol 97:65– 71, 2002.

55. Agrawal NGB, Porras AG, Matthews CZ, et al: Dose proportionality of oral etoricoxib, a highly selective cyclooxygenase-1 inhibitor, in healthy volunteers. J Clin Pharmacol 41:1106–1110, 2001.

56. Riendeay D, Percival MD, Brideau C, et al. Etoricoxib (MK-0663): Preclinical profile and comparison with other agents that selectively inhibit cyclooxygenase-2. J Pharmacol Exp Ther 296: 558–566, 2001.

57. Data on File with Novartis Pharmaceuticals (2001), East Hanover, NJ.

58. Chilton FH, Hadley JS, Murphy RD: Incorporation of arachidonic acid into 1-acyl-2-lyso-sn-glycero-3-phosphocholine of the human neutorphil. Biochim Biophys Acta 917:48–56, 1987.

59. Kent RS, Diedrich SL, Whorton AR: Regulation of vascular prostaglandin synthesis by metabolites of arachidonic acid in perfused rabbit aorta. J Clin Invest 72:455–465, 1983.

60. Marshall PJ, Kulmacz RJ, Lands WEM: Constraints of prostaglandin biosynthesis in tissues. J Biol Chem 262:3510–3517, 1987.

61. Gammon CM, Allen AC, Morrell P: Bradykinin stimulates phosphoinositide hydrolysis and mobilization of arachidonic acid in dorsal root ganglion neurons. Neurochem 53:95–101, 1989.

62. Lin LL, Wartmann M, Lin AY, et al: cPLA2 is phosphorylated and activated by MAP kinase. Cell 72:269–278, 1993.

63. Conklin BR, Burch RM, Steranka LR, Axelrod J: Distinct bradykinin receptors mediate stimulation of prostaglandin synthesis by endothelial cells and fibroblasts. J Pharmacol Exp Ther 244:646–649, 1988.

64. Garavito RM, Picot D, Loll PJ: Preliminary x-ray investigations into NSAID-binding to cyclooxygenase-1. Am J Ther 2:611–615, 1995.

65. Picot D, Loll PJ, Garavito M: The x-ray crystal structure of the membrane protein prostaglandin H2 synthase-1. Nature 367:243–249, 1994.

66. Ohki S, Ogino N, Yamamoto S, Hayaishi O: Prostaglandin hydroperoxidase, an integral part of prostaglandin endoperoxide synthetase from bovine vesicular gland microsomes. J Biol Chem 254:829–836, 1979.

67. Pagels WR, Sachs RJ, Marnett LJ, et al: Immunochemical evidence for the involvement of prostaglandin H synthase in hydroperoxide-dependent oxidations by ram seminal vesicle microsomes. J Biol Chem 258:6517–6523, 1983.

68. Mizuno K, Yamamoto S, Lands WE: Effects of non-steroidal anti-inflammatory drugs on fatty acid cyclooxygenase and prostaglandin hydroperoxidase activities. Prostaglandins 23:743–757, 1982.

69. Smith WL, Lands WE: Stimulation and blockade of prostaglandin biosynthesis. J Biol Chem 246: 6700–6702, 1971.

70. Volterra A: Arachidonic acid metabolites as mediators of synaptic modulation. Cell Biol Int Rep 13:1189–1199, 1989.

71. Rome LH, Lands WE: Structural requirements for time-dependent inhibition of prostaglandin biosynthesis by anti-inflammatory drugs. Proc Natl Acad Sci U S A 72:4863–4865, 1975.

72. Stanford N, Roth GJ, Shen TY, Majerus PW: Lack of covalent modification of prostaglandin synthetase (cyclo-oxygenase) by indomethacin. Prostaglandins 13:699–675, 1977.

73. Levy BD, Clish CB, Schmidt B, et al: Lipid mediator class switching during acute inflammation: Signals in resolution. Nat Immun 2:612–619, 2001.

74. Leblanc Y, Roy P, Boyce S, et al: SAR in the alkoxy lactone series: The discovery of DFP, a potent and orally active COX-2 inhibitor. Bioorg Med Chem Lett 9:227–212, 1999.

75. Samad TA, Moore KA, Sapirstein A, et al: Interleukin-1β-mediated induction of COX-2 in the CNS contributes to inflammatory pain hypersensitivity. Nature 410:471–475, 2001.

Chapter 8

Opioids (Bench)

Timothy J. Maher, PhD / Pasarapa Chaiyakul, PhD

HISTORY OF OPIOIDS

The juice from the opium plant has long been recognized for its important medicinal properties and social uses. Although many accounts of its uses may be found in ancient Egyptian, Greek, and Roman writings, the earliest accounts generally are credited to the Sumerian cultures from Mesopotamia in Asia Minor dating back to 3500 B.C., which refer to opium as Hul Gil or the joy plant. Opium, from the Greek word opos meaning juice, is derived from the unripe seed pods of the poppy plant, Papaver somniferum. During the Middle Ages, the English apothecary Sydenham wrote that of the "remedies which it has pleased Almighty God to give to man to relieve his sufferings, none is so universal and so efficacious as opium." Although there are more than 20 distinct alkaloids in the crude opium extract, Sertürner, a German pharmacist, first reported in 1806 the isolation of a pure substance that he named "morphine", after Morpheus, the Greek god of dreams.[1] During the 19th century, many derivatives of the crude opium extract, in addition to the synthesis of novel morphine analogs, appeared for medicinal use. Other important alkaloids found in opium also were isolated during this time, including papaverine, thebaine, and codeine.

The term opioid refers to all agonists with morphine-like pharmacologic activity that can be antagonized by an opioid antagonist such as naloxone.[2] Opioids include morphine-like compounds derived from opium alkaloids, synthetic and semisynthetic congeners, and the more recently discovered endogenous peptides that normally interact with opioid receptors. Although the older terms opiates (compounds derived from opium) and narcotics (from the Greek meaning to cause stupor) no longer are widely used in pharmacology, the generic term endorphin, referring to any of the endogenous opioid peptides (enkephalins, dynorphins, and β-endorphin), still is used.

Opioid drugs can be classified as full agonists, partial agonists, and antagonists. Full agonist opioids also are known as high-efficacy or strong agonists. These compounds are thought typically to require only a small percentage (e.g., 10% to 20%) of the available receptors to be occupied to produce a maximum pharmacologic response.[3] Partial agonist opioids are compounds that require close to full receptor occupancy (e.g., 75% to 100%) to produce a maximum response. Although these latter agents can evoke agonist effects, they also may compete with or displace full agonists from opioid binding sites and reduce the full agonist's biologic effect. In this way, partial agonists may act as agonists or antagonists depending upon the conditions in which they are used. Because there are different subtypes of opioid receptors, it is possible for a compound to have an agonist effect at one opioid receptor subtype and a partial agonist or antagonist effect at another. Such compounds are known as mixed agonist-antagonists. Pure antagonists are compounds that bind to the receptor (i.e., they have affinity); however, they fail to activate the receptor (i.e., they lack intrinsic activity). Examples include morphine analogs that are closely related structurally to morphine and frequently synthesized from it, such as agonists (e.g., morphine, diacetylmorphine [heroin], and codeine), partial agonists (e.g., nalorphine and levallorphan), and antagonists (e.g., naloxone). Additionally, synthetic derivatives structurally unrelated to morphine have been developed and are available, including the phenylpiperidines (e.g., fentanyl), methadone-related compounds (e.g., methadone and dextropropoxyphene), benzomorphans (e.g., pentazocine and cyclazocine), and the semisynthetic thebaine derivatives (e.g., etorphine and buprenorphine).[4]

Numerous other organic molecules have been developed that interact with the various opioid receptors. By carefully manipulating their structures, compounds with greatly improved selectivity for a specific receptor subtype, potency, or reduced adverse effect potential have been developed. One such example is loperamide, an opioid that because of its physicochemical properties is not well absorbed orally, and much of an administered dose appears in the feces. Although the small amount of systemically absorbed loperamide is capable of crossing the blood-brain barrier, there is an active efflux mechanism via a p-glycoprotein system that pumps loperamide out of the brain at a rate estimated to be approximately 10 times greater than the rate of transport into the brain.[5] This mechanism helps to explain the lack of analgesic and respiratory depressant activities of this compound. Loperamide is extremely useful therapeutically for the control of diarrhea, however, as a result of its ability to decrease gastrointestinal peristalsis and increase overall smooth muscle tone. Abuse potential also is decreased greatly because of loperamide's limited aqueous solubility and difficulty of administering this agent intravenously.

ENDORPHINS: ENDOGENOUS OPIOID PEPTIDES

The observation that the administration of an exogenously derived compound such as morphine could produce specific, highly reproducible, and potent pharmacologic actions suggested the existence of specific binding sites or receptors that were required to mediate the actions of the opioids. Additionally, minor structural modifications in the morphine molecule were found to lead to dramatic changes in binding affinities in vitro and pharmacologic actions in vivo. This strict stereochemical requirement is consistent with the existence of a receptor-mediated action. Because these receptors or binding sites normally were found in animals, including humans, the existence of an endogenous ligand was postulated. The hunt for such an endogenous ligand led to the discovery of the opioid peptides.[6]

The endogenous opioid peptides generally are classified according to their precursor peptides from which they derive[7] (Fig. 1). There are four known precursor peptides in mammalian systems: proopiomelanocortin, proenkephalin, prodynorphin, and pronociceptin/orphanin FQ (N/OFQ), all of which have been cloned (Table1). Although the precursor peptides are synthesized in the nucleus of the neuronal cell, they must be transported down the axon to the nerve terminal, where they are cleaved enzymatically by processing proteases to the active peptides and stored in vesicles awaiting depolarization-induced release.

Proopiomelanocortin, besides containing within its structure the 31-amino acid opioid peptide β-endorphin, contains the stress-induced mediator adrenocorticotropic hormone, in addition to α-melanocyte-stimulating hormone (α-MSH), and β-lipotropin. Numerous studies have supported a common physiologic pathway between many of the responses to stress and pain, which may help to explain the colocalization of these stress and pain homeostatic mediators in the same precursor peptide.[8]

Although there exists within the structure of β-endorphin the pentapeptide methionine-enkephalin (Met-enkephalin), this endogenous opioid is not believed to be derived from

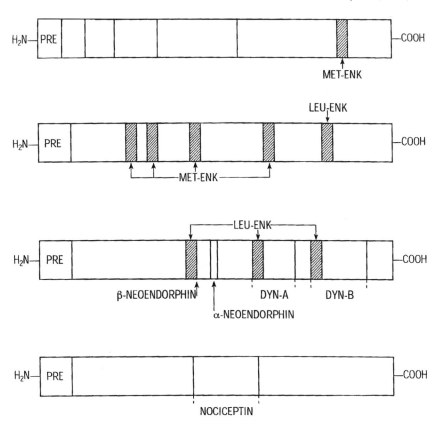

Figure 1. Endogenous opioid peptides

TABLE 1

ENDOGENOUS OPIOID PEPTIDES

Precursor Peptide	Endogenous Peptide	Receptor Activity
Proopiomelanocortin	β-Endorphin	μ and κ
Prodynorphin	Dynorphin-A	κ > μ
	Dynorphin-B	κ > μ
	α-Neodynorphin	κ > μ
	β-Neodynorphin	κ > μ
Proenkephalin	Leu-enkephalin	δ > μ > δ
	Met-enkephalin	δ > μ > δ
Pronociceptin/OFQ	Nociceptin	N/OFQ
Proendomorphin*	Endomorphin-1	μ
	Endomorphin-2	μ

*Not not yet identified but presumed to exist.
N/OFQ = nociceptin/orphanin FQ.

this precursor. Met-enkephalin and its closely related congener leucine-enkephalin (Leu-enkephalin) are found within and believed normally to derive from preproenkephalin, also known as *preproenkephalin A*. Dynorphin A and dynorphin B, in addition to α-neoendorphin and β-neoendorphin, all of which begin their N-termini with the pentapeptide sequence of Leu-enkephalin (Tyr-Gly-Gly-Phe-Leu), derive from prodynorphin, also known as preproenkephalin B. Pronociceptin /OFQ is the precursor for the peptide nociceptin, also named *orphanin* FQ, or N/OFQ, a compound reported by some to be capable of lowering pain threshold to produce a hyperalgesic response.[9] A yet to be discovered precursor peptide is believed to exist that contains endomorphin-1 and endomorphin-2.

Although most investigators in the opioid field consider the above-described opioid peptides to be the normal endogenous ligands for the various opioid receptors, there have been some reports of the isolation of compounds such as morphine, codeine, and related morphine analogs in various tissues of some mammals, such as the rat, that have never received these compounds exogenously.[10] Found in opioid-naïve animals, these compounds typically are conjugated to protein. Others have shown the existence of the necessary enzymes for such endogenous synthesis.[11] Although these observations are intriguing, there seems to be little enthusiasm for accepting such compounds as the normal endogenous opioid ligands because so much is known about the role the endogenous opioid peptides play.

OPIOID RECEPTORS: NOMENCLATURE AND FUNCTION

Opioid receptors have been cloned and generally are divided into three major subtype families: μ, δ, and κ (Table 2).[12] Each family typically can be divided further into at least two subtypes that have unique binding and pharmacologic characteristics. Previously a σ receptor, which was bound by phencyclidine, generally was thought to be a member of the opi-

TABLE 2

OPIOID RECEPTORS AND PHARMACOLOGIC ACTIVITY

Opioid Action	Receptors Involved
Analgesia	
Supraspinal	$\mu_1, \delta_1, \delta_2, \kappa_3$
Spinal	μ_2, δ_2, κ
Respiratory depression	μ_2
Sedation	μ_1, κ_1
Gastrointestinal motility ($\downarrow$)	μ_2, κ_1
Feeding ($\uparrow$)	$\mu_1, \delta_1, \kappa_1$
Diuresis	κ
Antidiuresis	μ
Euphoria	μ_1
Dysphoria	κ_1
Prolactin release ($\uparrow$)	μ_1
Growth hormone release ($\uparrow$)	μ_2, δ_1
Miosis	κ, μ
Emesis	μ_1
Tolerance/dependence	μ_1
Immune suppression	μ_1
Hyperalgesia	N/OFQ

oid family of receptors. This receptor since has been classified as nonopioid, however. More recently a fourth family of receptors was identified and termed simultaneously the *nociceptin* and *orphanin FQ receptor*; this generally is referred to as the N/OFQ *receptor*. Although there is some pharmacologic evidence for the existence of other less well characterized opioid receptors termed ϵ, λ, ι, and ζ, much investigation is needed before these putative receptors might become generally accepted.[13]

The best-characterized family, the μ receptor, can be divided further into μ_1 and μ_2 subtypes. The μ_1 receptor is believed to mediate supraspinal analgesia, whereas the μ_2 receptor is thought to mediate spinal analgesia.[14] Knockout mice lacking the μ receptor, as defined by a lack of binding of the specific μ agonist DAMGO, failed to show analgesia, dependence and withdrawal, or reward behaviors, indicating that at least in this species analgesia is μ receptor–mediated. The μ_1 receptor also mediates euphoria, immune suppression, emesis, tolerance, prolactin release, increased feeding behaviors, sedation, and decreased acetylcholine release from certain neurons. In addition to spinal analgesia, respiratory depression, decreased gastrointestinal motility, and increased growth hormone release are thought to be μ_2 receptor–mediated. Relatively selective μ agonists include DAMGO, morphine, methadone, and fentanyl. A useful experimental selective antagonist is CTOP.

The μ receptor is a member of the G_i/G_o superfamily of seven membrane–spanning, pertussis toxin–sensitive, heterotrimeric guanine nucleotide binding protein (G-protein)–coupled receptors (GPCR) (Fig. 2). Agonist binding of the μ receptor leads to GTP binding, which results in the intracellular dissociation of the α-subunit from $\beta\gamma$-subunits. The α-subunit interacts with an effector system to cause activation of receptor-operated K^+ currents, sup-

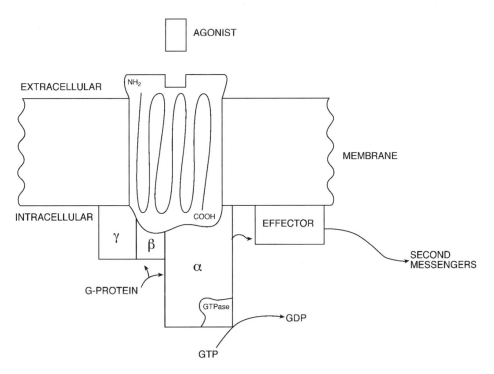

Figure 2. G-protein–coupled receptor structure.

pression of voltage-gated Ca^{2+} currents, or inhibition of adenylyl cyclase activity.[15,16] The activation of K^+ currents causing hyperpolarization and the suppression of Ca^{2+} currents may be the mechanism by which the inhibitory actions of opioids on neurotransmitter release, which are thought to be responsible for their analgesic actions, occur. To date, there are no useful therapeutic agents that effectively differentiate between the μ_1 and μ_2 receptor subtypes.

Endomorphin-1 and endomorphin-2 have been shown to bind potently and selectively to the μ receptors.[17] These two peptides differ from the remaining peptides structurally in having a C-terminal tyrosyl-proline. The remaining peptides all have a tyrosyl-glycyl-glycyl-phenylalanine C-terminal. The terminal amino acid is either methionine (e.g., β-endorphin and Met-enkephalin) or leucine (e.g., Leu-enkephalin, dynorphin A and B, and the neoendorphins). This combination of 5 amino acids seems to be the opioid "motif" most commonly present in endogenous peptides.[18]

The δ receptor, which is thought to be endogenously activated by the enkephalins, seems to have two subtypes, δ_1 and δ_2.[19] The suggestion of two subtypes initially was based on the selective activation of the δ_1 receptor by the synthetic peptides DPDPE and DADLE, whereas the δ_2 receptor was selectively activated by DSLET and deltorphin II.[20] Naltrindole is a selective δ receptor antagonist. The δ_1 receptor mediates supraspinal analgesia and probably stimulation of feeding and growth hormone release. A decrease in neuronal dopamine release also has been attributed to this receptor subtype. The δ_2 receptor is thought to mediate supraspinal and spinal analgesia. The δ receptor is a GPCR that uses similar effector mechanisms to that of the μ receptor, K^+ and Ca^{2+} currents, in addition to adenylyl cyclase coupling.[21]

The κ-receptor family includes at least three subtypes. The κ_1 receptor, which is selectively activated by U50 488, and dynorphin A and antagonized by nor-binaltorphimine (nor-BNI), mediates spinal analgesia, miosis, and possibly an increase in diuresis.[22] The κ_1 receptor also may be responsible for the occasionally observed dysphoric responses after opioid administration. Butorphanol also binds tightly to the κ_1 receptor, with little affinity for the other receptor subtypes. Although little is known about the characteristics of the κ_2 receptor, the κ_3 receptor is thought to mediate supraspinal analgesia. No outstanding κ_3 receptor selective or specific agonists or antagonists have been identified. Ethylketocyclazocine binds all three subtypes with high affinity. Besides their involvement in analgesic responses, the κ receptors as a group probably also mediate increased feeding behaviors, decreased gastrointestinal transit, and sedation. Similar to the μ and the δ receptors, the κ receptor also is a classic GPCR.

The N/OFQ receptor is a poorly understood opioid receptor that seems to be selectively activated by the endogenous peptide nociceptin.[23] This receptor may mediate the hyperalgesia (nociception) observed in some experiments in which nociceptin was administered intracerebroventricularly to rats. Some studies showed the ability of N/OFQ receptor activation to cause an increase in the release of substance P, an effect that would be expected to lower pain threshold and possibly precipitate pain responses.

The degree of selectivity of the endogenous peptides for the different identified opioid receptor subtypes varies significantly. Of these peptides, nociceptin displays the greatest degree of selectivity for a particular receptor subtype, the N/OFQ receptor. Nociceptin is the only endogenous opioid peptide that lacks a C-terminal tyrosine because it has a phenylalanine in this position. Nociceptin has little or no affinity for the μ, κ, or δ receptors. Similarly, none of the other endogenous peptides have significant affinity for the N/OFQ receptor.

The structural homology between the μ, δ, and κ receptors is overall about 65%, with the greatest similarity in the seven transmembrane portions and the least similarity in the extra-cellular amino terminus, the third and final extracelluar loop, and the cytosolic carboxyl ter-minus.[24] The N/OFQ receptor shares less homology with the aforementioned three opioid re-ceptors, especially at the extracellular amino terminus, where there is essentially no similarity.

The opioid receptors, similar to many other receptor families, are not static proteins an-chored in the cell membrane but rather are extremely dynamic. Many receptors change in number or conformation after agonist/antagonist interactions, which may help to explain some of the seemingly perplexing observations made in standard experimental systems. Many of the opioid receptors are desensitized or internalized into the cytoplasm after activation, which may account for the observed acute tolerance frequently seen.[25] Desensitization of the μ and δ receptors involves phosphorylation by protein kinase C, GPCR kinases, or other ki-nases inside the cell.[26] When phosphorylated, a conformational change occurs rendering the receptor sensitive to the action of β-arrestins, peptides that promote internalization of recep-tors. Receptors can be internalized rapidly via an endocytotic pathway operating within the cell membrane. Although internalization of the μ and δ receptors seems to require specific endocytotic processes, the κ receptor does seem to be subject to internalization. Experiments in transgenic mice deficient in β-arrestin 2 show an enhanced analgesic response to morphine and a lack of tolerance.[27] After long-term agonist exposure, tolerance may occur as a result of a compensatory overstimulation of adenylyl cyclase activity.

There also has been some evidence to indicate that opioid receptors may exist as dimers in intact biologic systems, similar to some other receptor systems. The opioid receptors may be subject to RNA splice variations during synthesis, in addition to posttranslational modifica-tions, leading to phenotypic consequences that could help explain findings that do not fit the traditional theories of opioid receptor function. Studies have shown a tremendous amount of polymorphism associated with the μ receptor in humans, which might help explain individ-ual differences regarding the analgesic and dependence attributes of opioids. Attempts to help explain why some individuals are more prone than others to abuse and become dependent on opioids have not been linked successfully to μ receptor polymorphism.

OPIOIDS AND PAIN

Although the analgesic properties of opium have been recognized for centuries, newly syn-thesized organic compounds suspected of possessing analgesic activity require testing in in vitro and in vivo settings. Initially, new compounds typically are tested in an in vitro competitive binding assay for affinity at the μ, δ, and κ receptors. Radiolabeled naloxone, which binds all three major opioid receptors, is incubated with brain tissue homogenates, then the nonla-beled new compound is added. A compound that has affinity for one of the opioid receptors competes for binding and displaces the previously bound naloxone. Additional studies can be done using the agonists DAMGO, DSLET, and U50,488 or the antagonists CTOP, naltrindole and nor-BNI, which more selectively bind the μ, δ, and κ receptors. Promising candidates can be screened for intrinsic activity by incubating with tissue homogenates, and the inhibi-tion of adenylyl cyclase can be determined. In this way, an indication as to whether the com-pound is an agonist or an antagonist can be determined. Further preclinical screening in vivo typically uses experimental animals (e.g., mice, rats, dogs, or nonhuman primates) in a vari-ety of analgesia/pain models. Rodents can be used to test quickly for supraspinal analgesic potential of a new compound by determining paw withdrawal responses when animals are placed on a heated plate (50°C to 52°C). Spinal analgesia typically is determined by measuring latency to move or "flick" the tail when thermally stimulated. More sophisticated experiments in dogs measure responses to electrical stimulation of the tooth pulp. Clinical studies in humans typically involve administration of the compound to individuals experiencing pain (e.g., after a standard surgical procedure), and their ratings using a visual analog scale or some similar way of quantifying the analgesia are determined. Together the in vitro and in vivo screening can help to characterize new chemical entities that someday might improve the arsenal of analgesics available to clinicians.

The location of the opioid μ, δ, and κ receptors and their endogenous ligands within the central nervous system provides valuable anatomic information regarding the sites of pain processing and mediation.[28,29] Receptors and ligands are found in areas that are thought to mediate the perception of pain, such as laminae I and II in the spinal cord, the spinal trigeminal nucleus, and the brain periaqueductal gray area. Areas involved in the modulation of affective behaviors (amygdala, thalamus, cortex, and locus caeruleus), motor control (globus pallidus and caudate putamen), and autonomic nervous system and neuroendocrine functions (medulla oblongata and median eminence) in response to pain likewise are rich in opioid receptors and endogenous peptides. The N/OFQ receptor is found in higher concentrations in the hippocampus and cortex and has been suggested to be involved with drug reward and reinforcement, in addition to learning and memory.

Morphine and related opioids seem to produce analgesia by inhibiting ascending pathways that carry pain information gathered from primary sensory neurons, in addition to activating descending pain control systems that normally operate through the ventromedial medulla down into the dorsal horn of the spinal cord.[30] Opioids acting in the preiaqueductal gray on μ receptors decrease GABA-ergic inhibition of the descending pathways through the ventromedial medulla.[31] Morphine is much more effective against sharp intermittent pain than dull continual pain. The analgesia produced does not usually affect the other sensations, and unconsciousness does not occur with appropriate analgesic doses. The administration of morphine to subjects not experiencing pain usually results in unpleasant feelings, including nausea, vomiting, and drowsiness.

MORPHINE PHARMACOLOGY

In addition to analgesia, morphine and most other opioids produce many characteristic responses centrally and peripherally.[32] Respiratory depression via μ receptor inhibtion of the brainstem respiratory control centers is common and may limit the dose of opioid that can be used. Rate and depth of respiration are depressed by opioids. The respiratory depression can be reversed rapidly by naloxone. Morphine also produces nausea and vomiting via stimulation of the chemotrigger zone in the area postrema, and miosis (constriction of the pupil) via stimulation of the parasympathetic nerves innervating the pupil. Both of these responses can be attributed partially to μ receptor activation. Additionally in the central nervous system, morphine increases prolactin release, decreases cough, and occasionally produces seizures. The seizures, which are more common with meperidine owing to one of its metabolites, usually respond better to naloxone than to conventional antiepileptic agents.

In the periphery, morphine and most other opioids produce histamine release, which causes skin flushing and a feeling of warmth. Hypotension, especially orthostatic hypotension, also can occur. In the gastrointestinal tract, especially the duodenum, opioids via μ and κ receptors increase overall resting tone and decrease propulsive movements.[33] Additionally, they often decrease intestinal, pancreatic, and biliary secretions. By way of centrally mediated and peripherally mediated mechanisms, opioids tend to be immunosuppressive. This effect is thought to be largely μ receptor mediated.

Morphine undergoes conjugation with glucuronic acid to form two major metabolites: morphine-3-glucuronide and morphine-6-glucuronide (Fig. 3).[34] Usually, conjugation of a parent compound leads to a more water-soluble metabolite that is inactive and excreted more easily via renal mechanisms. This is true for morphine-3-glucuronide, which is inactive and excreted readily by the kidneys and accounts for most of a given morphine dose. In the case of morphine-6-glucuronide, this compound has been found to be at least 100 times more potent than morphine in *in vitro* studies and *in vivo* as an analgesic when administered intracerebroventricularly to bypass the blood-brain barrier. Although more potent than morphine, the 6-glucuronide metabolite is much less able to enter the brain. The overall observed analgesic response to a given dose of morphine is probably due to a combination of the actions of the less potent, more easily central nervous system–penetrable morphine, in addition to that of the more potent, but less central nervous system–penetrable morphine-6-glucuronide metabolite. With long-term use of morphine, the 6-glucuronide metabolite has been shown to accumulate in tissues and may be more important than the parent morphine compound in producing analgesia and other effects.[35]

OPIOID STRUCTURE ACTIVITY RELATIONSHIPS

As is true for most alkaloids produced in nature, the naturally occurring morphine molecule synthesized by the poppy plant is enantiomerically pure. Although the ($-$) levorotatory enantiomer is the naturally occurring form, the ($+$) dextrorotatory compound has been synthesized but is inactive at all opioid receptors. There are five chiral centers in the morphine molecule: carbon numbers 5, 9, and 14 in the (R) configuration and carbon numbers 6 and 13 in the (S) configuration (Fig. 4). Minor structural changes to the basic morphine molecule can lead to dramatic changes in the pharmacodynamic (receptor affinity and intrinsic activity) and pharmacokinetic (oral absorption, distribution, metabolism, elimination) profiles of a newly synthesized compound. Most structural manipulations have centered around the number 3, 6, and 7 carbons of morphine and the tertiary nitrogen. Most substitutions of morphine's number 3 hydroxy group lead to significantly decreased analgesic activity. Replacing the

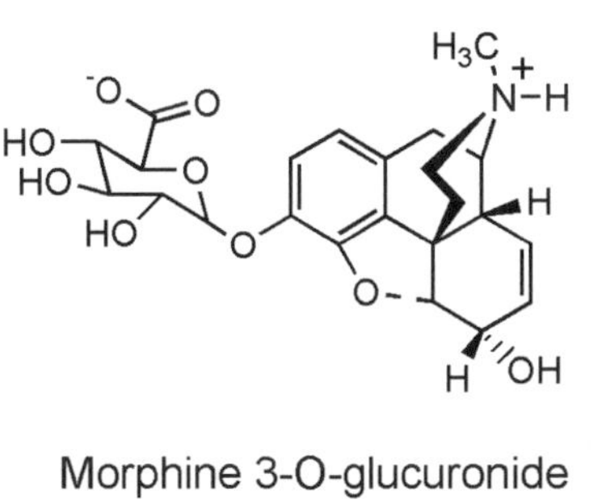

Morphine 3-O-glucuronide

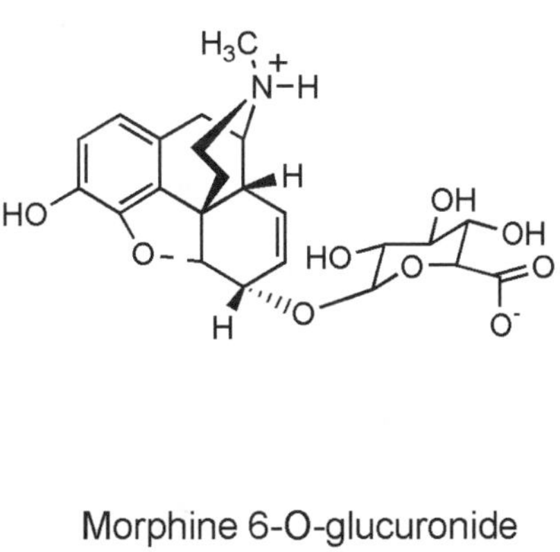

Morphine 6-O-glucuronide

Figure 3. Metabolites of morphine.

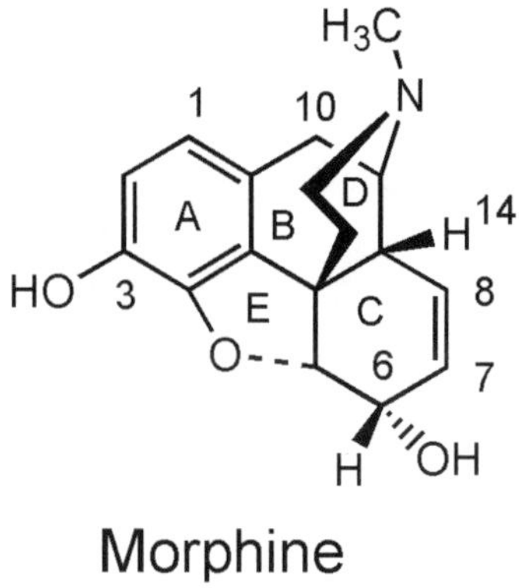

Morphine

Figure 4. Morphine structure with ring numbering.

number 6 hydroxy group with hydrogen increases activity. Reducing the double bond at numbers 7 and 8 significantly increases activity. The addition of bulky substituents at the tertiary nitrogen can produce a more potent agonist or, in some cases, a pure antagonist.

Specific morphine analogs of interest deserve mention (Fig. 5). Heroin is the 3,6-diacetyl derivative of morphine and is much more lipophilic than morphine. Although weaker than morphine at the μ receptor, the parent compound heroin produces a potent analgesic response as a result of its ease at crossing the blood-brain barrier and as a result of its conversion to the more potent deacetylated metabolites, 6-monoacetyl-morphine and morphine. Codeine, the 3-methoxy derivative of morphine, is converted by the cytochrome P-450 enzyme CYP2D6 to morphine. As such, codeine is less potent than morphine. Other useful morphine analogs include oxycodone, hydrocodone, oxymorphone, hydromorphone, levorphanol, and tramadol (Fig. 5). Tramadol has other activities, such as its ability to block norepinephrine and serotonin reuptake, and should not be used in patients receiving monoamine oxidase inhibitors.[36] These compounds are μ receptor agonists with differing potencies. Nalbuphine, butorphanol, and buprenorphine also are morphine analogs, but function as mixed agonists-antagonists. In opioid-naïve individuals, these agents produce analgesia; however, in opioid-dependent individuals, these agents typically precipitate withdrawal symptoms. Additionally, naloxone and naltrexone are pure receptor antagonists at all subtypes (Fig. 6). These compounds are chemically similar to morphine, having large substitutions at the tertiary nitrogen atom. These compounds are devoid of all agonist activity and precipitate withdrawal symptoms in individuals who are opioid-dependent.

A chemical class of compounds, the phenylpiperidines, includes the opioids meperidine, loperamide, and diphenoxylate (Fig. 5). The latter two opioids are used for their antidiarrheal properties because they lack central nervous system activity at normal therapeutic doses. Meperidine is metabolized to normeperidine, which has been implicated in this compound's ability to produce seizures. Additionally, meperidine should not be used in patients receiving monoamine oxidase inhibitors or dextromethorphan because of a dangerous serotoninergic potentiation. A chemically related compound is propoxyphene, which is about one half as potent as codeine and often is combined with aspirin to potentiate its action.

Pentazocine is an example of the chemical class of benzomorphans and is a mixed agonist/antagonist at μ receptors in addition to being a κ agonist (Fig. 7). The analgesic activity of

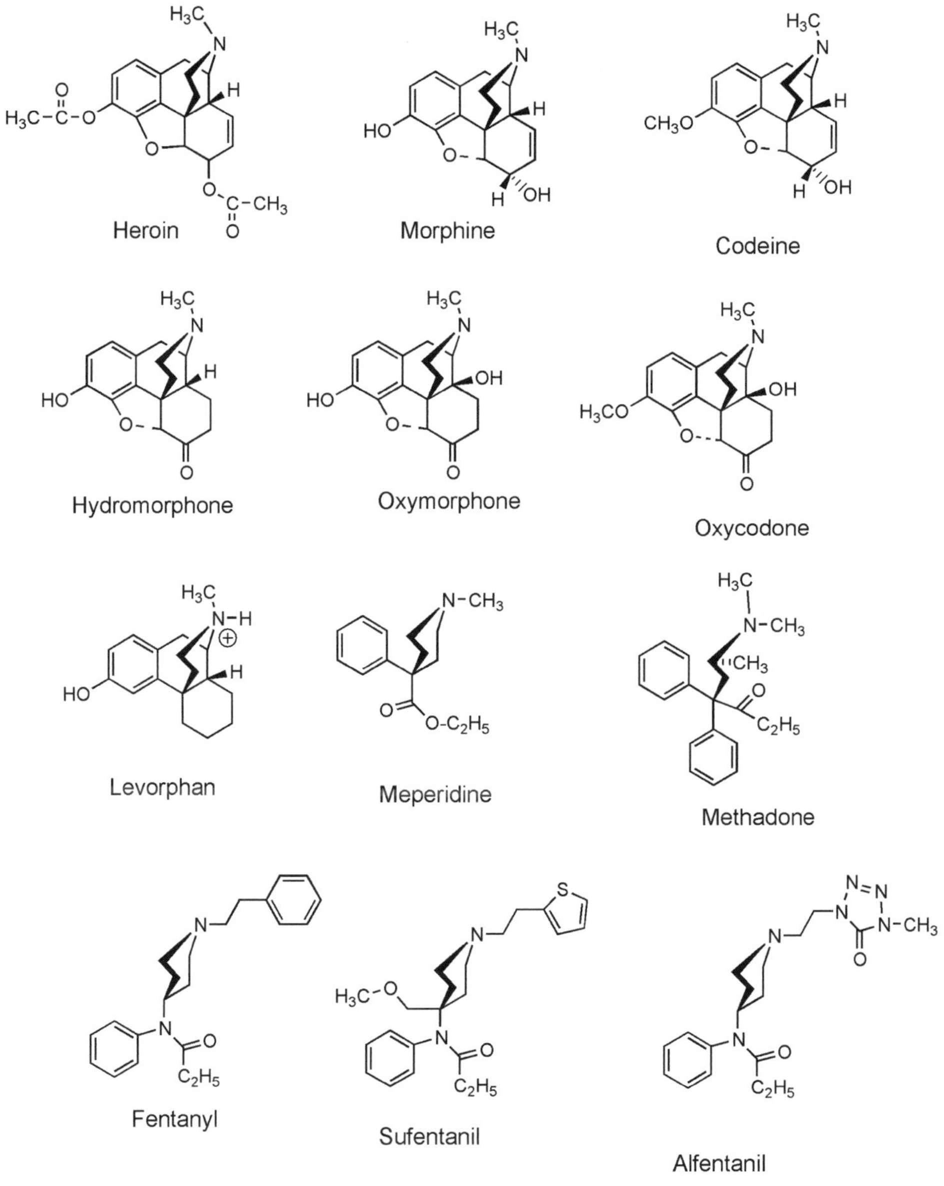

Figure 5. Mu opioid receptor agonists.

pentazocine is similar to that of morphine; however, abuse potential is significantly less than that of morphine.[37]

The propionanilides, which include fentanyl, sufentanil, and alfentanil, are extremely potent analgesics (Fig. 5). Largely because of their superior lipid solubility, sufentanil and fentanyl are 1,000 and 100 times as potent as morphine in producing analgesia.[38] These agents are μ agonists that produce the classic respiratory depression and most other typical adverse

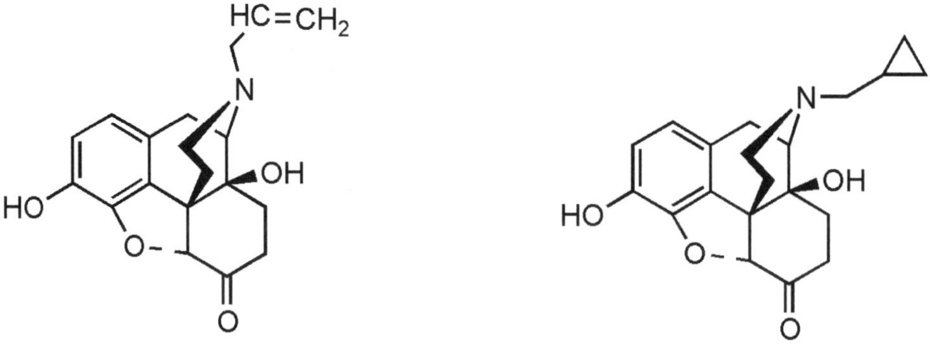

Naloxone   **Naltrexone**

Figure 6. Opioid Receptor antagonists.

opioid-like effects. These compounds do not produce histamine release, however, and are much less likely to cause hypotension. These agents are not substrates for the g-glycoprotein efflux system operating in the blood-brain barrier.

IDEAL OPIOID

The ideal opioid analgesic does not yet exist. Such a compound most likely would be highly selective for receptors that mediate analgesic actions of the opioids, whether supraspinal or spinal. Additionally the compound would be selective for receptors or areas of the brain and spinal cord that mediate pain, without acting at other sites that mediate the unwanted gastrointestinal, respiratory, and cardiovascular effects. The ideal agent would not be subject to adverse drug interactions, would act quickly, and would be able to be reversed quickly. Finally, the abuse potential and the ability to produce tolerance would be minimal. Medicinal chemists continue to synthesize new compounds, whether they be small-molecular-weight

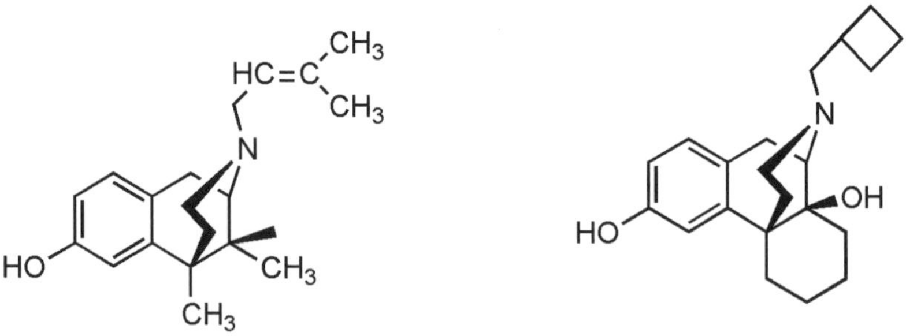

pentazocine   **butorphanol**

Figure 7. Mixed acting opioid agonist-antagonists.

organic molecules or peptides, in the hope of finding the ideal opioid analgesic compound. Until peptides can be delivered efficiently into the central nervous system, their therapeutic utility is unlikely. Additionally, because the neuronal wiring and receptors that mediate responses to pain and account for analgesia also are involved with other functions in the body, the likelihood of finding such an ideal agent seems remote. The currently available opioids are extremely valuable tools in the effective treatment of pain.

REFERENCES FOR ADDITIONAL READING

1. Huxtable RJ, Schwarz SKW: The isolation of morphine: First principles in science and ethics. Mol Interv 1:189–191, 2001.
2. Gustein HB, Akil H: Opioid analgesics. In Hardman JG, Limbird LE (eds): Goodman and Gilman's Pharmacological Basis of Therapeutics. 10th ed. New York, McGraw-Hill, 2001, pp 569–619.
3. Maher TJ, Johnson DJ: Receptors and drug action. In Foye WO, Williams DA, Lemke TL (ed): Principles of Medicinal Chemistry. 5th ed. Baltimore, Lippincott Williams & Wilkins, 2002, pp 86–99.
4. Fries DS: Opioid analgesics. In Foye WO, Williams DA, Lemke TL (eds): Principles of Medicinal Chemistry. 5th ed. Baltimore, Lippincott Williams & Wilkins, 2002, pp 453–479.
5. Wandel C, Kim R, Wood M, Wood A: Interaction of morphine, fentanyl, sufentanil, alfentanil, and loperamide with the efflux drug transporter p-glycoprotein. Anesthesiology 96:913–920, 2002.
6. Pert CB, Snyder SH: Opiate receptor: Demonstration in nervous tissue. Science 70:2243–2247, 1973.
7. Akil H, Owens C, Gutsein H, et al: Endogenous opioids: Overview and current issues. Drug Alcohol Depend 51:127–140, 1998.
8. Grossman A: Opioids and stress in man. J Endocrinol 119:377–382, 1988.
9. Pan ZZ, Hirakawa N, Fields HL: A cellular mechanism for the bidirectional pain-modulating actions of orphanin FQ/nociceptin. Neuron 26:515–522, 2000.
10. Donnerer J, Cardinale G, Coffey J, et al: Chemical characterization and regulation of endogenous morphine and codeine in the rat. J Pharmacol Exp Ther 242:583–587, 1987.
11. Weitz CJ, Faull KF, Goldstein A: Synthesis of the skeleton of the morphine molecule by mammalian liver. Nature 330:674–677, 1987.
12. Martin WR, Eades CG, Thompson JA, et al: The effects of morphine- and nalorphine-like drugs in non-dependent and morphine-dependent chronic spinal dog. J Pharmacol Exp Ther 197:517–532, 1976.
13. Zagon IS, McLaughlin PJ: Production and characterization of polyclonal and monoclonal antibodies to the zeta (ζ) opioid receptor. Brain Res 630:295–302, 1993.
14. Paul D, Bodnar RJ, Gistrak MA, Pasternak GW: Different μ receptor subtypes mediate spinal and supraspinal analgesia in mice. Eur J Pharmacol 168:307–314, 1989.
15. Schoffelmeer ANM, Rice KC, Jacobson AE, et al: μ-, δ- and κ-opioid receptor-mediated inhibition of neurotransmitter release and adenylate cyclase activity in rat brain slices: Studies with fentanyl isothiocyanate. Eur J Pharmacol 154:169–178, 1988.
16. McCleskey EW, Gould MS: Ion channels of nociception. Annu Rev Physiol 61:835–856, 1999.
17. Zadina JE, Hackler L, Ge LJ, Kastin AJ: A potent and selective endogenous agonist for the mu-opiate receptor. Nature 386:499–502, 1997.
18. Schwyzer R: Molecular mechanism of opioid receptor selection. Biochemistry 25:6335–6342, 1986.
19. Sofuoglu M, Portoghese PS, Takemori AE: Differential antagonism of δ opioid agonists by naltrindole and its benzofuran analog (NTB) in mice: Evidence for δ opioid receptor subtypes. J Pharmacol Exp Ther 257:676–680, 1991.
20. Negri L, Potenza RL, Corsi R, Melchiorri P: Evidence for two subtypes of delta opioid receptors in rat brain. Eur J Pharmacol 196:335–336, 1991.

21. Zaki PA, Bilsky EJ, Vanderah TW, et al: Opioid receptor types and subtypes: The δ receptor as a model. Ann Rev Pharmacol Toxicol 36:379–401, 1996.

22. Clark JA, Liu L, Price M, et al: Kappa opiate receptor multiplicity: Evidence for two U50,488-sensitive kappa 1 subtypes and a novel kappa 3 subtype. J Pharmacol Exp Ther 251:461–468, 1989.

23. Bertorelli R, Calo G, Ongini E, Regoli D: Nociceptin/orphanin FQ and its receptor: A potential target for drug discovery. Trends Pharmacol Sci 21:233–234, 2000.

24. Reisine T, Bell GI: Molecular biology of the opioid receptors. Trends Neurosci 16:506–510, 1993.

25. Jordan BA, Devi LA: G-protein-coupled receptor heterodimerization modulates receptor function. Nature 399:697–700, 1999.

26. Pei G, Kieffer BL, Lefkowitz RJ, Freedman NJ: Agonist-dependent phosphorylation of the mouse delta-opioid receptor: Involvement of G-protein-coupled receptor kinases but not protein kinase C. Mol Pharmacol 48:173–177, 1995.

27. Bohn LM, Lefkowitz RJ, Gainetdinov RR, et al: Enhanced morphine analgesia in mice lacking β-arrestin 2. Science 286:2495–2498, 1999.

28. Hiller JM, Zhang Y, Bing G, et al: Immunohistochemical localization of mu-opioid receptors in the rat brain using antibodies generated against a peptide sequence present in a purified mu-opioid binding protein. Neuroscience 62:829–841, 1994.

29. Ji RR, Zhang Q, Law PY, et al: Expression of mu-, delta- and kappa-opioid receptor-like immunoreactivities in rat dorsal root ganglia after carrageenin-induced inflammation. J Neurosci 15: 8156–8166, 1995.

30. Pasternak GW: Pharmacological mechanisms of opioids analgesics. Clin Neuropharmacol 16: 1–18, 1993.

31. Vaughan CW, Ingram SL, Connor MA, Christie MJ: How opioids inhibit GABA-mediated neurotransmission. Nature 390:611–614, 1997.

32. Martin WR: Pharmacology of opioids. Pharmacol Rev 35:283–323, 1983.

33. Manara L, Bianchetti A: The central and peripheral influences of opioids on gastrointestinal propulsion. Annu Rev Pharmacol Toxicol 25:249–273, 1985.

34. Christup LL: Morphine metabolites. Acta Anaesthesiol Scand 41:116–122, 1997.

35. Milne RW, Nation RL, Somogyi AA: The disposition of morphine and its 3- and 6-glucuronide metabolites in humans and animals, and the importance of the metabolites to the pharmacological effects of morphine. Drug Metab Rev 28:345–472, 1996.

36. Duthie DJ: Remifentanil and tramadol. Br J Anaesth 81:51–57, 1998.

37. Brogden RN, Speight TM, Avery GS: Pentazocine: A review of its pharmacological properties, therapeutic efficacy and dependence liability. Drugs 5:6–91, 1973.

38. Sanford T, Gutstein HB: Fentanyl, sufentanil and alfentanil: Comparative pharmacology. Clin Anesth Updates 6:1–20, 1995.

Chapter 9

Clinical Pharmacology of Opioids

Piotr K. Janicki, MD, PhD / Winston C. Parris, MD, FACPM

Opioid analgesics are well known for their ability to reduce the perception of pain without a loss of consciousness. They also are known for problems of tolerance, physical dependence, and potential for development of addiction after repeated administration.

Clinical pharmacology of currently available opioid analgesics is determined by two major factors: (1) pharmacokinetic properties of individual opioid analgesics and (2) their opioid receptor properties. What this means in clinical practice is that two opioids with the same opiate receptor binding pattern (e.g., μ opioid receptor agonists) might be clinically dissimilar because of the differences in their pharmacokinetics (i.e., bioavailability, distribution, half-life, and metabolic pattern). Opioids with apparently similar pharmacokinetics may produce different clinical effects because of the different pattern of the opiate receptor activation based on the interactions with different types of opiate receptors binding to the different receptor regions within one opiate receptor subtype. More recently, a third important factor was added: the genetic polymorphism in the opiate receptor gene and cytochrome P-450 isoform and uridine glucuronosyltransferase genes involved in the opioid metabolism. This genetic polymorphism seems to be responsible for most of the interindividual differences in the analgesic effectiveness of opioids and their side effects in humans.

RECEPTOR PROPERTIES OF OPIOID ANALGESICS

The opioid receptors belong to the large superclass of G protein–coupled receptors, which all possess the same general structure: an extracellular aminoterminal region, seven transmembrane domains, and an intracellular carboxyterminal tail structure. From the practical point of view, there seem to be three major opiate receptor subtypes, termed μ (the morphine receptor, MOR), κ (the ketocyclazocine receptor), and δ (the endorphin/enkephalin receptor). σ receptors first were described in 1976 as opiate receptors but later were determined to be a distinct class of receptors with two subtypes, σ_1 and σ_2. The observations of Mei and Pasternak[1] indicate an increasing importance of σ_1 receptors as a modulatory system influencing the analgesic activity of opioid drugs. From the currently used opioids, only pentazocine interacts with this type of receptor. The most well-known agonists and antagonists of classic receptors are summarized in Table 1. μ-receptor is a main molecular target for opioid analgesic activity and is subdivided into μ_1 and μ_2. μ_1 receptors predominate at the supraspinal level. In the dorsal horn of the spinal cord, morphine analgesia is mediated by μ_2 receptors. Other pharmacologic effects of opioids also are related to interaction with specific receptors. Respiratory depression is mediated by μ_2 receptors in the brain stem, whereas constipation is mediated by μ_2 receptors within the brain and in the intestinal plexus.[2]

TABLE 1

Agonists and Antagonists of Major Types of Opioid Receptor Subtypes

Drug	μ	δ	κ
Opioid peptides			
Enkephalins	Antagonist	Agonist	
β-Endorphin	Agonist	Agonist	
Dynorphin	Weak agonist		
Agonist			
Codeine	Weak agonist	Weak agonist	
Fentanyl, sufentanil, alfentanil, ramifentanil	Agonist		
Meperidine	Agonist		
Methadone	Agonist		
Morphine	Agonist	Weak agonist	
Agonist-antagonists			
Buprenorphine	Partial agonist		
Pentazocine	Antagonist or partial agonist		Agonist
Antagonist:			
Naloxone	Antagonist	Antagonist	Antagonist

Advances in genomic research encourage the search for pharmacogenetic causes of variability in individual responses to pain and opioid drugs. Studies using mice deficient in μ opioid receptor (MOR) showed that the μ receptor is crucial for the analgesic and respiratory depressant properties of morphine. Antisense probes targeting exon 1 of the MOR receptor gene blocked analgesia caused by morphine but not that by morphine-6-glucuronide (M6G), heroin, or 6-acetylmorphine, suggesting that these agents might be acting on a splice variant of the μ receptor.[3,4] Subsequent research using knockout mice with disruptions of either the first or second coding exons of MOR-1 provided further genetic evidence for a unique receptor site for M6G and heroin analgesia.[5] Several pure μ opiate receptor agonists (i.e., morphine and fentanyl), acting through the activation of the same μ receptor, may bind at different locations on the receptor. In this respect, it was shown that the minimal (one amino acid) mutation in the MOR produced different receptor activation patterns by fentanyl and morphine. These different patterns may explain partly the observation that patients with cancer-related pain refractory to morphine respond more adequately to fentanyl or sulfentanil.[6]

So far, the most prevalent single nucleotide mutation of the MOR gene is substitution of position A118 $\longrightarrow$ G. An analysis of blood samples from 100 white volunteers resulted in 77.2% frequency of the homozygous (A/A) MOR wild-type genotype; 21.8% of this population possessed the heterozygous (A/G) genotype, whereas only 1% was homozygous for the mutated MOR allele (G/G).[7] This alteration in the MOR gene produces alterations in the amino acid sequence (Asn40 $\longrightarrow$ Asp) localized in the extracellular N-terminal region of the MOR and results in the loss of a putative glycosylation site of the receptor. Loetsch et al[8] showed for the first time that in vivo effects of an opioid (M6) are affected by the A118G polymorphism in the MOR gene. These authors reported that the potency of M6G to constrict the pupils in humans was significantly lower in heterozygous carriers of the A118G polymorphism. An even lower potency of M6G to constrict pupils was observed in one homozygous A118G individual. In contrast, the constrictive effects of morphine on pupils were not affected significantly in carriers of the A118G polymorphism.

These observations indicate that the morphine metabolite M6G does not contribute to the acute central effects of morphine to any major extent; however it may contribute significantly to the morphine-like side effects with prolonged morphine administration in patients with impaired kidney function. Patients with the A118G polymorphism may have a lower risk for side effects of M6G. The differential activity of morphine and M6G in carriers with A118G polymorphism also may be explained by the fact that A118G-induced mutation in MOR, which is localized at the extracellular N-terminal of the receptor, affects the binding of large ligands such as β-endorphins or M6G, without changing the binding of smaller molecules such as morphine or enkephalins.[9] Genotyping of the human MOR gene has revealed several other single nucleotide polymorphisms that exist infrequently in the general population and give rise to alterations in the amino acid sequence of the human MOR (Table 2). For several of these mutations in the structure of MOR, substantial changes in the functionality of MOR were reported. Even if the definite proof of clinical significance of these MOR variants is still lacking, it is likely that carriers of the mutant alleles might display altered responses to opioid analgesics.[10,11]

Humans also differ from one another in MOR densities. Binding studies to postmortem brain samples and in vitro positron emission tomography radioligand analyses suggest 30% to 50% or larger ranges of individual human differences in MOR densities. Elucidation of the genetic bases for these differences in receptor expression would represent a substantial advance in understanding of individual differences in nociceptive behaviors and drug responses.[12]

TABLE 2

Summary of Partially Characterized Single Nucleotide Polymorphisms of the Human μ Opioid Receptor*

Allele Localization on Chromosome 10	MOR Localization	Reported Frequency	Effect on Opioid Binding to MOR	Effect on MOR Function	Confirmed Clinical Significance
Exon1 C17T	Ser4Arg				
Exon1	Ala6Val	0.1–1%			
Exon1 A118G	Asn40Asp	10–20%	Yes (M6G, endorphins)	No	Yes
Exon2 C440G	Ser147Lys				
Exon2 A→G	Asn152Asp		No	Low-density expression	
Exon3	Arg260His	0.1–1%			
Exon3 G→A	Arg265His	0.1–1%	No	Yes	
Exon3 T→C	Ser268Pro	0.1–1%	No	Yes	
Exon3 G820A	Asp274Asn				

*About 30 more single nucleotide polymorphism sites were reported in intron and untranslated fragments of MOR.

PHARMACOKINETICS OF OPIOIDS

Absorption and Routes of Administration

The speed of onset and duration of action for any opioid depend on the specific drug chosen and its formulation (tablet with immediate or slow release). Opioids are well absorbed after oral or rectal administration. Drugs absorbed from the gut are subject to first-pass metabolism in the liver, however, in addition to some degree of metabolism by enzymes localized in the intestinal wall, and should be given at higher doses than when given parenterally. The onset of opioid action is fastest after intravenous dosing because there is no delay in absorption. Opioid doses and frequency should be titrated to the patient's response and analgesic needs when changing the route of administration or the type of formulation.

The *oral route* is the preferred route of administration for chronic pain because it is the most convenient and cost-effective. Oral opioids are available in tablet, capsule, and liquid forms and in immediate-release and controlled-release formulations. Controlled-release tablets become immediately released when crushed and are not appropriate for patients who are unable to swallow whole tablets. When patients cannot take medications orally, other noninvasive routes, such as rectal or transdermal routes, should be tried. During intravenous and subcutaneous administration, local irritation of the skin or vein may occur. Some opioids (codeine, oxycodone) have a high oral-to-parenteral potency ratio because they are protected from conjugation by substitution on C3 aromatic hydroxyl residue. Parenteral routes should be used only when simpler, less demanding, and less costly methods are inappropriate or ineffective.

Intramuscular administration of drugs should be avoided because this route can be painful and inconvenient, and absorption is unreliable. Intravenous and subcutaneous administration are effective alternatives. Patients who may benefit from continuous infusions of opioids include patients with persistent nausea and vomiting; patients with severe dysphagia or swallowing disorders; patients with delirium, confusion, stupor, or other mental status changes that make oral administration contraindicated because of concerns about pulmonary aspiration in an unprotected airway; patients on high doses of oral medications necessitating numerous tablets; patients who experience undesirable side effects in relation to each dose of an *as-needed* medication; and patients who require rapid incremental doses of analgesia.

The benefits of opioid infusions, compared with those of intermittent as-needed doses by intramuscular or subcutaneous injection, include less pain on injection and improved effectiveness. The intravenous route provides the most rapid onset of analgesia, but the duration of analgesia after a bolus dose is shorter than with other routes.

A *continuous intravenous infusion* provides the most consistent level of analgesia and is accomplished easily for patients who obtain opioid analgesia during the perioperative period in the form of patient-controlled analgesia. If intravenous access is not available or desirable, continuous subcutaneous opioid infusion offers a practical alternative in the hospital and at home. The subcutaneous administration of opioids provides levels in blood comparable to those with intravenous doses; the intravenous dose recommendations can be used.

The *rectal route* may be used when patients have nausea or vomiting or are fasting either preoperatively or postoperatively. The rectal route is contraindicated if there are lesions of the anus or rectum because placement of the suppository would cause pain. When converting from the oral to the rectal route, the therapy should be started with the same amount as the oral dose and titrated as needed.

The *transdermal route* is an increasingly important route of administration. Transdermal administration bypasses gastrointestinal absorption. Fentanyl currently is the only opioid commercially available in a transdermal form (TDS-Fentanyl). Four patch sizes are available and provide delivery of fentanyl at 25, 50, 75, or 100 μg/hr; there is flexibility in drug dosing. Patients requiring larger doses should be switched to an equianalgesic dose of an oral or subcutaneously administered opioid. In contrast to intravenous fentanyl, the transdermal administration of fentanyl is not suitable for rapid dose titration. Transdermal fentanyl should be considered when patients have relatively constant pain with infrequent episodes of breakthrough pain, such that rapid increases or decreases in pain intensity are not anticipated. As with other long-acting analgesics, all patients should be provided with oral or parenteral rapidly acting, short-duration opioids to manage breakthrough pain. The most commonly reported side effects of transdermal fentanyl administration are nausea, mental clouding, and skin irritation.

The *transnasal route* is an alternative delivery method that may be useful when patients no longer are able to tolerate the oral route. Although several agents currently are being studied, the only commercially available formulation is the mixed agonist-antagonist drug butorphanol, which is taken up rapidly by the vascular nasal mucosa. The major indication for its use is acute headache.

In properly selected patients, intraspinal or intraventricular (*neuraxial route*) infusions of opioids have the advantage of producing profound analgesia without motor, sensory, or sympathetic blockade. The short-term use of epidural analgesia is appropriate for some types of anesthesia and surgery, including postoperative pain control. The long-term use of epidural opioids is indicated when systemically administered oral or parenteral analgesics do not achieve adequate pain relief without unacceptable sedation, respiratory depression, or other side effects.

Analgesics may be administered intraspinally when pain is not well controlled by oral, transdermal, subcutaneous, or intravenous routes because side effects such as confusion and nausea limit further dose escalation. Documentation of the failure of maximal doses of opioids and coanalgesics administered through other routes should precede consideration of intraspinal analgesia. Before implantation of a permanent device, screening should be done to ensure adequate response to spinal therapy. A trial of graded opioid doses administered percutaneously through an epidural catheter generally indicates whether intraspinal therapy is warranted.

As with systemic opioid administration, the dose range for intraspinal opioid therapy varies widely, depending on the level of pain and tolerance. Any agent delivered into the epidural or intrathecal space should be free of preservatives because many preservatives and antioxidants can produce neurotoxicity when used intraspinally. All patients treated with intraspinal drugs should have access to rescue medications (oral or parenteral) for periods of breakthrough pain or in the case of catheter or drug delivery system malfunction. The coadministration of systemic opioids (which generally is not recommended for postoperative pain management) is safe in most cancer patients because they are tolerant to the respiratory depressant effects of the drugs.

Preservative-free morphine (Duramorph) is the most commonly used intraspinal drug. Alternative opioids, such as hydromorphone, fentanyl, or sufentanil, have been used intraspinally to manage cancer pain and may be useful substitutes when the patient experiences side effects from morphine. Intraspinal morphine may produce the same side effects of nausea, mental clouding, and sedation as in oral, rectal, or parenteral dosing because epidural or subarachnoid morphine is absorbed into the circulation. Lipophilic opioids, such as fentanyl and sufentanil, have a more limited cerebrospinal fluid distribution, but these drugs also gain access to the blood and are delivered to the brain via the systemic circulation.

In some patients, it is possible to give relatively small doses of opioid spinally and produce pain relief, while avoiding the side effects that can limit prior oral or parenteral dosing. Patients with a high degree of tolerance to systemic opioids may require large doses of spinal opioids, however, which may negate the advantages of this targeted approach because side effects still may be prominent at high dosage levels.

Experience with *intraventricular* morphine administration is increasing steadily, and results with this route compare favorably with those with intraspinal administration, with more than 90% of patients in published series benefiting significantly. Most important, intraventricular morphine is beneficial for recalcitrant pain resulting from head and neck malignancies and tumors that affect the brachial plexus. Complications are rare, the most important being infection. Intraventricular morphine requires the placement of a ventricular catheter connected to a subcutaneous (e.g., Ommaya) reservoir for intermittent administration or an infusion pump for continuous administration.

Distribution

The intensity of the analgesic effects of opioids is the result of the number of receptors occupied by the opioid, which is directly proportional to the concentration of drugs in the tissue compartment containing those receptors (e.g., brain, spinal cord). The onset and duration of action are related to the rise and fall of the number of receptors occupied. The uptake of the drug by a tissue is determined by its rate of delivery and the capacity of the tissue to accumulate the drug. Highest concentrations in tissues are a function of perfusion, the concentration gradient between plasma and the tissue, and the permeability coefficient of the drug. For most opioids, skeletal muscle is the largest reservoir. For highly lipophilic opioids (e.g., fentanyl), there is also significant concentration in adipose tissue. Ionization of the drug is important because nonionized drugs cross membranes more easily. Amphoteric agents (possessing an acidic and basic group, e.g., morphine [phenolic hydroxyl at C_3]) display greatest difficulty for brain entry. Other substitutions at C_3 improve blood-brain barrier penetration (e.g., heroin). Neonates lack the blood-brain barrier. Placental opioid transfer (uses in obstetric analgesia) can result in depressed respiration in the newborn.

Metabolism

Opioids with hydroxyl groups likely are conjugated with glucuronic acid in the liver by the phase 1 reaction by forming the opioid glucuronides, which then are excreted by the kidneys. Most opioid glucuronides are pharmacologically inactive, with the notable exception of morphine glucuronides (see later), which produce several pharmacologic effects. The renal dysfuction may produce decreased clearance of pharmacologically active glucuronides with the subsequent exacerbated pharmacologic response of the parent compounds.

An important group of conjugation reactions are performed by the uridine 5'-diphosphate–glucuronosyltransferases (UGTs), and at least 10 different UGT isoforms have been identified. The UGTs are involved in the metabolism of many opioid analgesics. Isoform specificity for these substrates has not been fully characterized, however. UGT2B7 is the only UGT isoform for which ontogeny has been characterized *in vitro* and *in vivo*, using morphine as the probe drug. Genetic polymorphisms have been identified for the UGT family. The impact of these genetic differences on drug metabolism remains to be established, however, because of overlapping isoform specificity of the drugs studied and a lack of specific probe substrates to test the activity of individual UGT isoforms in relation to these gene mutations. An information gap exists regarding the developmental and genetic aspects of UGT regulation and its potential impact on therapy.[13]

Some natural opioids and semisynthetic derivatives (e.g., codeine, oxycodone, hydrocodone, and dihydrocodeine) are metabolized by cytochrome P-450 isoforms CYP2D6 to metabolites of increased activity (e.g., morphine, oxymorphone, hydromorphone, and dihydromorphine) and isoforms CYP3A4 to various inactive metabolites of methadone, fentanyl, sufentanil, and alfentanil. CYP2D6 and CYP3A4 are genetically polymorphic. An estimated 4% to 10% of whites lack CYP2D6 activity (poor metabolizers) because of inheritance of two nonfunctional alleles. Different activity of this system might be responsible for the high interindividual variability in the pharmacokinetics of some opioids and may play a role in the different rate of development of opiate dependence.

Oxidative metabolism is the primary route of phenylpiperidine opioids (fentanyl, sufentanil, alfentanil) metabolism to the variety of inactive metabolites. Piperidine N-dealkylation by polymorphically expressed CYP3A4 was found to be the predominant pathway of liver microsomal metabolism.

N-demethylation pathway is the minor pathway for most opioids. Accumulation of the demethylated meperidine metabolite normeperidine produces excitatory side effects, however (see later). Patients with decreased renal function or on high dosages display central nervous system excitatory effects (e.g., seizures, more likely in children). Ester-type opioids are hydrolyzed by tissue-nonspecific esterases (remifentanil) or plasma pseudocholinesterases in addition to liver carboxyesterases (heroin).

Excretion

Most polar metabolites of opioids are excreted by the kidneys with small amounts excreted unchanged. Glucuronide conjugates also are excreted in bile and may undergo enterohepatic circulation, which probably has minor clinical significance.

CLINICAL PHARMACOLOGY OF FREQUENTLY USED OPIOID ANALGESICS

For the clinical use of opioids in chronic pain management, it is useful to classify them as weak or strong, to be used for mild-to-moderate or moderate-to-severe pain, depending on their relative potency. Weak opioids (e.g., codeine, oxycodone, hydrocodone, propoxyphene, meperidine, pentazocine) are used for less severe pain. Their efficacy is limited by an increased incidence of side effects at higher doses (e.g., nausea and constipation with codeine, central nervous system excitation with propoxyphene, dysphoric effects with pentazocine). Strong opioids (morphine, hydromorphone, methadone, fentanyl, sufentanil, alfentanil, remifentanil) are indicated for more severe pain. They have a wide therapeutic range and no ceiling effect for analgesia: Higher doses produce an increasing level of analgesia. A summary of most commonly used opioid analgesics follows.

Weak Opioid Analgesics

Codeine is the prototype of the weak opioid analgesics. It has weak affinity to the μ opioid receptor and about 15% of the analgesic potency of morphine. The half-life of codeine is 2.5 to 3 hours. Codeine is metabolized predominantly by glucuronidation to codeine-6-glucuronide (C6G). Minor metabolic pathways include N-demethylation to norcodeine and O-demethylation to morphine.[14] The latter is catalyzed by the polymorphically expressed CYP2D6.[15] There is increasing evidence that the analgesic effect of codeine is mediated by its O-demethylated metabolite morphine[16] and the glucuronidated morphine metabolite M6G. In humans, the analgesic activity of C6G has not been reported; however, antinociceptive responses after intracerebroventricular administration were reported in rats.[17] Constipation and nausea are the major side effects of codeine. Doses of codeine greater than 65 mg are not appropriate because of the increasing side effects.

Dihydrocodeine (Synalgos-DC) is similar in many aspects to codeine and has a pharmacokinetic pattern similar to codeine. It was not clear previously whether the analgesic effect of dihydrocodeine, similar to codeine, was attributed to the drug itself or its metabolite, dihydromorphine (DHM). Most of dihydrocodeine is conjugated to inactive dihydrocodeine-6-glucuronide. Less than 10% of dihydrocodeine is metabolized by N-demethylation to nordihydrocodeine and O-demethylation to DHM, and this latter conversion is mediated by polymorphically expressed cytochrome P-450 CYP2D6 enzyme. DHM, which has a stronger affinity to μ opiate receptor than morphine itself, is conjugated further to the next active metabolite, DHM-6-glucuronide, and inactive DHM-3-glucuronide.[18] Studies of the relative contribution of dihydrocodeine and DHM to analgesia after dihydrocodein administration[19] indicate that polymorphic differences in dihydrocodeine metabolism to DHM have little or no effect on the analgesic effect.

Hydrocodone and oxycodone are codeine derivatives and because of high bioavailability (>50%) are available as oral formulations, mostly in combination with nonopioid analgesics (several hundreds of preparations on the US market alone). Oxycodone and hydrocodone in similar doses are equivalent to morphine in effectiveness after oral administration and have only about 25% of morphine's effectiveness after parenteral (not currently available on the market) administration. The half-lives of hydrocodone and oxydone are similar to codeine. They possess analgesic and antitussive activity. Both drugs undergo extensive hepatic conjugation and oxidative degradation to a variety of metabolites excreted mainly in urine.

The major metabolites of hydrocodone excreted into urine are conjugates of dihydrocodeine and nordihydrocodeine (both conjugated to approximately 65%). The O-demethylation to DHM conversion is mediated by polymorphically expressed cytochrome P-450 CYP2D6 enzyme; however, DHM is produced in minor amounts and is conjugated further in 85%. Traces of nordihydromorphine and hydrocodone were confirmed, and other metabolites of dihydrocodeine can be detected. Some of the hydrocodone metabolites (DHM, hydromorphone, dihydrocodeine) are pharmacologically active on the opioid receptors and may contribute in various degrees to analgesic activity of hydrocodone or produce unexpected side effects when their excretion is impaired (e.g., renal dysfunction).

Oxycodone undergoes oxidative hepatic metabolism and conjugation to inactive metabolites. Oxycodone is conjugated extensively (15% to 80% of the total dose) in the liver, and the minority undergoes demethylation and oxidation via multiple hepatic pathways into noroxycodone, oxymorphone, oxycodols, and their respective oxides. Only less than 10% of unchanged oxycodone is excreted in the urine. Oxymorphone, the active metabolite of oxycodone, is formed in a reaction catalyzed by CYP2D6, which is under polymorphic genetic control. The role of oxymorphone in the analgesic effect of oxycodone is not yet clear. Significant individual variation in oxycodone metabolism may account, however, for abnormal responses during treatment of chronic cancer pain.[20]

Oxycodone and hydrocodone have been considered weak analgesics because of their use in a fixed combination with acetaminophen and nonsteroidal antiinflammatory drugs. When oxycodone is used as a single oral agent, however, it has no ceiling effect for analgesia. Oxycodone seems to produce fewer side effects than morphine after oral administration. It is also available in immediate-release and controlled-release (OxyContin) oral formulations. Controlled-release oxycodone has the characteristics of an ideal opioid analgesic drug: short half-life, long duration of action, predictable pharmacokinetics, absence of clinically active metabolites, rapid onset of action, easy titration, no ceiling dose, minimal adverse effects, and minimal associated stigma.[21]

Meperidine is a relatively weak opioid μ agonist (10% efficacy of morphine) with significant anticholinergic and local anesthetic properties. The oral-to-parenteral ratio is 4:1. The anticholinergic properties of meperidine might be responsible for associated tachycardia, mydriasis, and clinically uncertain spasmolytic effects (e.g., decreased pressure in the biliary and urinary tracts). The half-life of meperidine is 3 hours. Meperidine is demethylated in the liver to normeperidine (half-life 15 to 30 hours), which has significant neurotoxic properties. Normeperidine is accumulated after long-term meperidine administration, particularly in patients with renal dysfunction, and may cause central nervous system excitatory effects, which may produce naloxone-irreversible multifocal myoclonus and grand-mal seizures. Short-term administration of meperidine has been associated with mild dysphoria. Meperidine must not be given to patients being treated with monoamine oxidase inhibitors because this combination may produce severe respiratory depression, hyperpyrexia, central nervous system excitation, delirium, and seizures. Meperidine use in the treatment of the treatment of acute and chronic pain has steadily declined in more recent years. In postanesthesia care units, meperidine is used frequently to treat postanesthestic shivering.

Propoxyphene (Darvon) is a synthetic analgesic that is structurally related to methadone and has opioid dose equipotency similar to codeine. The analgesic activity is confined to its d-steroisomer (dextropropoxyphene). It half-life is 6 to 12 hours, but the duration of effective analgesia is limited to 3 to 5 hours. Propoxyphene is demethylated in the liver to norpropoxyphene, which has a much longer half-life (30 to 60 hours) and is considered to have cardiac toxicity. Propoxyphene itself can produce seizures (naloxone-reversible) after overdose. Parenteral formulation of propoxyphene (not available on the U.S. market) is known to be extremely irritating for blood vessels and soft tissue. Propoxyphene does not offer any significant advantage over other weak opioids. In addition to being a μ receptor agonist, propoxyphene is a weak and noncompetitive N-methyl-D-aspartate (NMDA) receptor antagonist. The clinical significance of this fact is unknown (see discussion of methadone later).

Pentazocine (Talwin) is a semisynthetic derivative of the benzomorphinanes. In contrast to most currently used opioids, pentazocine interacts with κ-opioid receptors and σ receptors. These receptors' properties are responsible for the dysphoric and psychotomimetic effects of pentazocine. Because of weak antagonistic properties toward μ opioid receptor, pentazocine also is called a mixed opioid agonist-antagonist. Pentazocine is manufactured as the racemic (L/R, 50:50), but only L-isomer possesses analgesic activity. Pentazocine is well absorbed after oral administration. Given parenterally, the equianalgesic does of pentazocine is only two times higher than morphine. Increasing the dose to greater than 30 mg produces increasing dysphoria, however, with no increase in analgesia or respiratory depression. Pentazocine, in contrast to most other opioid analgesics, may cause tachycardia and hypertension after acute intravenous administration. The half-life of pentazocine is about 4 hours. Pentazocine is metabolized almost exclusively in the liver to inactive glucuronides and oxidation of the terminal methyl groups. Pentazocine is not indicated in the treatment of chronic pain. Intravenous pentazocine sometimes is used for acute pain control in patients with renal failure after anesthesia, secondary to its kidney-independent route of metabolism.

Tramadol (Ultram) is a synthetic analog of codeine that inhibits norepinephrine and serotonin reuptake and produces some central opiate receptor activity. Gillen et al[22] produced evidence that one of the metabolites of tramadol is responsible for μ opiate–derived analgesic effect. Tramadol is absorbed rapidly and extensively after oral doses and is metabolized in the liver. The metabolic pathway of tramadol involves O-demethylation to O-desmethyl tramadol, the active metabolite of tramadol, which is formed in a reaction catalyzed by CYP2D6, which is under polymorphic genetic control. There is one report of decreased tramadol effects on experimental pain in subjects that showed decreased metabolism of tramadol to its MOR active metabolite owing to a genetic decrease in CYP2D6 activity.[23] Tramadol also is metabolized by N-demethylation and nortramadol. In patients with moderate postoperative pain, intravenous tramadol is roughly equal in efficacy to meperidine or morphine; for severe acute pain, tramadol is less effective than morphine. After oral administration, tramadol equals in its analgesic potency codeine.[24]

Strong Opioid Analgesics

Morphine is a phenanthrene derivative and is the prototype μ receptor opioid agonist. All other opioids are compared with morphine when determining their relative analgesic potency. Morphine also is recommended by the World Health Organization as the drug of choice (first-line therapy) for the management of moderate-to-severe cancer pain. As with other strong opioid analgesics, there is no ceiling to the analgesic effect; however, side effects (particularly sedation and confusion) may intervene before optimal analgesia is achieved. The absorption of morphine after oral administration varies from 20% to 30%. Morphine is a relatively long-lasting opioid with analgesic effect lasting 4 to 5 hours, although its elimination half-life (2 hours) is less than that for shorter acting opioids (i.e., fentanyl). This discrepancy may be explained by the low solubility of morphine and its slower elimination from the brain compartment in relation to the plasma concentration, which also may be associated with its existence in an ionized state in the relatively acid brain compartment The relatively long analgesic activity of morphine also may be associated with the presence of the active morphine metabolites, which have half-lives of elimination longer than morphine itself.

The classic data concerning the pharmacologic effects of morphine and other opioids are confounded increasingly by evidence concerning the activity of their active metabolites. Morphine is considered to be an intermediate drug subject to pronounced presystemic elimination, and it is metabolized to several metabolites, most of them having some pharmacologic activity. Successive studies in the 1980s and 1990s determined the extraction pattern of morphine and its metabolites into urine. Approximately 2% to 8% of the dose typically is found in urine as unmetabolized morphine after oral or parenteral doses, whereas 50% to

80% of the dose administered by either route typically is recovered as glucuronide metabolites, mostly morphine-3-glucuronide (M3G) and M6G. Metabolic pathways of morphine involving its O-transmethylation to codeine, demethylation to normorphine, diglucuronidation to morphine-3,6-diglucuronide, conjugation to morphine-3-sulfate, and formation of morphine-ethereal-sulfate seem to have minor pharmacokinetic and pharmacologic significance. Morphine-3-sulfate and normorphine have been found in urine as minor metabolites, along with traces of other metabolites, but these have been more variable.

During oral or systemic administration of morphine in humans, glucuronidation (i.e., conjugation with glucuronic acid) at the phenolic and alcoholic hydroxyl groups at position 3 and 6 occurs to a large extent in the liver (Figure 1). UGT was identified as the enzyme responsible for production of glucuronides from morphine. UGT exists as a multigene family resulting in a range of isoenzymes, and at least 11 different forms of UGT have been identified. The functional heterogeneity also has been observed between the isoenzymes responsible for the glucuronidation of morphine in the 3- and 6-positions. The liver is the major site of metabolism of morphine, but evidence of extrahepatic glucuronidation has been reported. It was shown that the epithelium of the small and large intestine contributes with the liver to the formation of the active M6G; at the same time, the gastric, intestinal, and colonic epithelia are involved in the inactivation of morphine to M3G. Enterohepatic cycling of morphine has been described in different species, including humans. Glucuronides can be deconjugated to morphine by colonic flora after having been excreted via the bile to the gut lumen, and the parent compound subsequently can be reabsorbed.

The above-described metabolic pattern results in the formation of M3G and M6G. During long-term morphine administration, circulating concentrations of M3G and M6G markedly exceed those of morphine itself because hepatic metabolism converts approximately 70% of

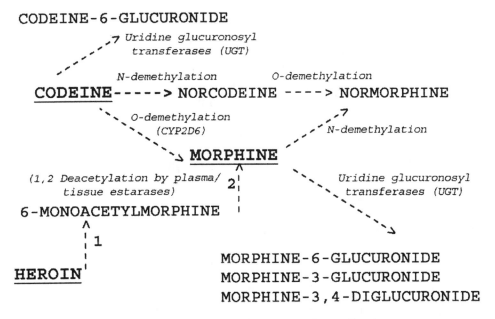

Figure 1. Metabolic pathways of codeine, morphine, and heroin.

morphine into M3G (60%) and M6G (10%). In adults, long-term oral administration of morphine produces variable plasma ratios of M3G to M6G, with reported mean ratios between 10:1 and 5:1. There also are marked ethnic differences in the morphine clearance; Chinese subjects were shown to metabolize morphine by glucuronidation (but not demethylation to normorphine) at much higher rates than white subjects.[25] These differences were associated with greater inhibitory effects produced by morphine in the latter group of subjects.[25]

Morphine glucuronide formation may be influenced by route of morphine administration. After a single intravenous dose of morphine, the molar ratio of M3G and M6G to morphine in plasma was significantly lower compared with oral morphine administration.[26] After oral administration of morphine in a single dose, M6G and M3G were found to be present at concentrations exceeding those achieved after rectal dosing of morphine.[27] These data suggest that rectal administration of morphine is associated with significant avoidance of hepatic biotransformation. Patients receiving morphine orally produced significantly greater amounts of M3G and M6G than patients receiving long-term parenteral morphine administration. In our own study involving terminal cancer patients, we found that some patients receiving morphine orally for prolonged periods had a significantly higher ratio of M3G and M6G to morphine in urine than patients receiving morphine systemically.[28]

Although the primary site of action of morphine is in the central nervous system, only small quantities of morphine cross the blood-brain barrier in adults. Compared with other more lipid-soluble opioids, such as codeine, heroin, and methadone, morphine crosses the blood-brain barrier at a considerably lower rate. Among opioids, morphine is relatively water soluble, which also would be expected in greater degrees for its glucuronide metabolites. The transfer half-life of M6G between plasma and effect site in the brain was consistently longer than that of morphine (6.4 hours and 2.8 hours).[29]

Both glucuronides of morphine are pharmacologically active. M6G has a relatively high affinity for the μ opioid receptors. The results of studies comparing the affinity of morphine and M6G with μ and δ opioid receptors indicate that M6G has fourfold lower affinity than morphine for the μ_2 receptor (i.e., mediating the respiratory depression and gastrointestinal effects of morphine) and for the total μ receptor, whereas there was no significant difference seen at the μ_1 and δ opioid receptors.

From all available knowledge, M6G was considered to be more potent than morphine, the reported relative potency ranging from a ratio of 2:1 to 650:1. In contrast to these data, the finding of Loetsch et al[29,30] indicates that by directly comparing central effects of morphine and M6G after short-term systemic administration, M6G was about 22 times less potent than morphine. Similarly, some reports revealed the lack of analgesic effects of M6G in studies that employed short-term M6G administration at dosages that produce M6G plasma concentrations comparable to those usually found after administration of analgesic morphine dosages.[30,31] M6G was shown clearly to be more potent than morphine when injected intrathecally to patients.[32] This discrepancy could be explained by the fact that the opioid effects attributed to M6G develop with a remarkable delay from the rise of M6G plasma concentrations caused by slow and incomplete transfer of M6G through the blood-brain barrier.

In contrast to M6G, M3G shows no affinity for the μ and δ-opioid receptors and is presumed to be devoid of analgesic activity.[33] Despite this apparent lack of activity, however, intracerebroventricular or intraperitoneal M3G has been reported to induce allodynia and hyperalgesia, and progressively higher doses of M3G produce behavioral excitation, myoclonus, and seizures.[34,35] These central excitatory effects of M3G may complicate the interpretation of behavioral measures of antinociception and interfere with the analgesic activity of morphine itself. The concentration of M3G in blood of patients taking morphine exceeds that of morphine approximately 20-fold, whereas the concentration of M6G is 2-fold higher than morphine. The analgesic effect of morphine is probably the result of complex interactions of the drug and its two main metabolites. The evidence for pharmacologic activity of M3G when administered indirectly (i.e., being blood borne) is much less convincing. In one of the few observations comparing the pharmacologic effects of different concentrations of morphine, M3G, and M6G in patients, Westerling et al[36] noted that M6G was four and eight times more potent than morphine in producing miosis and reduction of saliva production. The same pharmacokinetic/pharmacodynamic model indicated that intrinsic activities of M6G and morphine were similar for both effect parameters, whereas M3G was either inactive or opposed the effects of morphine and M6G.

Morphine glucuronides are eliminated from the body via urinary excretion. The slow elimination of glucuronides is important in patients with impaired renal function. The high plasma level of M6G was observed in patients with renal failure several days after termination of morphine treatment.[37] These patients might be expected to experience more metabolite-related side effects. These high levels of plasma M6G (without measurable plasma morphine concentrations) were accompanied by respiratory depression, sedation, and vomiting, which could be reversed by the opioid receptor antagonist naloxone. The most serious complications reported in patients with impaired renal function are encephalopathy and myoclonus.[38] It was shown that M6G-to-morphine ratio in these patients shows correlation with increased blood urea nitrogen or creatinine levels. There was a significant difference in the prevalence of myoclonus observed between patients receiving morphine via either the oral or parenteral route, with a threefold greater frequency in patients receiving oral morphine. These observations indicate cumulative properties of glucuronides in the body in the patients with high morphine dosage and impaired renal clearance.[39] In patients with renal failure, the retention of plasma M6G induces a progressive accumulation of this active metabolite in cerebrospinal fluid; this accumulation may explain the increased susceptibility to morphine in patients with renal failure.

Increasing numbers of cases reported in the literature describe situations in which chronic pain patients do not respond as expected to strong opioids.[40–42] These cases of nociceptive pain, not responsive to opioid narcotics, have become known as *paradoxical pain* or *overwhelming pain syndrome*. In the case of neurogenic pain, exemplified by postherpetic neuralgia, trigeminal neuralgia, painful diabetic neuropathy, reflex sympathetic dystrophy, and central (thalamic) pain, there is no direct nociceptive stimulation. The nociceptive impulses are generated as a result of neuronal dysfunction and do not follow classic pain pathways. Such pains are relatively resistant to the action of conventional analgesics, including opiates. Hyperalgesia, hyperesthesia, or other neuropathic pain syndromes unresponsive to even large doses of morphine in cancer patients sometimes may be accompanied by myoclonus.[43,44] Although only a few clinical descriptions of the relationship between hyperalgesia and myoclonus and high doses of morphine are available, experimental support from animal studies indicates that morphine, or its metabolites, plays a causative role for the observed behavioral syndrome. Nevertheless, the role of morphine metabolites as excitatory agents producing hyperalgesia and myoclonus remains an unresolved question in humans.

There is no apparent relationship between morphine and M6G concentrations in the plasma and cerebrospinal fluid and pain scores.[45,46] Although M6G is a potent analgesic itself, M3G could attenuate the opioid activity (including analgesia) of M6G in various experimental conditions. Patients' analgesic response to morphine seems to depend on their M3G-to-M6G ratio, with M6G being responsible for the analgesic effect. This ratio in plasma has been reported in several case reports of patients with malignant disease taking oral doses of slow-release morphine for long periods, and the ratio is usually in the 4.5:1 to 5:1 range. Goucke et al[47] reported that M3G-to-M6G ratios in 11 patients with morphine-resistant pain receiving long-term morphine therapy were similar to published values in patients with well-controlled pain. It is not known if interindividual differences in the metabolite ratios in patients are inherent or are induced by disease, by drugs per se, or by age. It is not known what the normal range of ratio is when morphine is given to opioid-naive subjects and what plasma concentrations of morphine and M6G are associated with effective analgesia. Pharmacokinetic studies indicate that with long-term dosing, plasma levels of M3G and M6G are higher than those of morphine itself.[48] The route of morphine administration also can influence the observed ratio of morphine and its metabolites. The concentration ratios of the active metabolite M6G to morphine and its inactive metabolite M3G are higher after prolonged oral morphine treatment than after systemic administration of morphine. Patients receiving morphine orally produced significantly greater amounts of its pharmacologically more active metabolite than patients receiving long-term systemic morphine treatment.

Several case reports describe the lack of analgesic effects of large and continuous doses of intrathecal morphine in patients with intractable pain in which the analysis of plasma and cerebrospinal fluid showed high levels of M3G but not M6G.[49,50] In one case, pain was relieved by intrathecal administration of M6G. The proposed explanation for the paradoxical pain produced a considerable amount of criticism, and the explanation of morphine resistance by the morphine metabolite is still highly controversial.[51,52]

So far, there are no systematic studies linking the M3G-to-M6G ratio in plasma during intrathecal morphine administration to the analgesic effectiveness of morphine. Little is known about the glucuronide metabolites and their concentration in cerebrospinal fluid and plasma after intrathecal morphine administration. It was reported that morphine metabolite concentrations were higher in plasma than in cerebrospinal fluid and that plasma-to-cerebrospinal fluid ratios for M6G and M3G were 1:0.08 and 4:1, suggesting that M6G penetrates the blood-brain barrier more easily than M3G.[53] In a different study in which morphine and M6G were measured in cerebrospinal fluid of cancer patients receiving long-term morphine treatment,[54] plasma contained approximately twice as much M6G as morphine, whereas cerebrospinal fluid contained only one fifth to one third as much. These data suggest that M6G in plasma is redistributed in cerebrospinal fluid, but to a far lesser extent than morphine. The metabolite concentrations observed in plasma of patients after intrathecal morphine administration most probably reflect hepatic biotransformation of free morphine in the plasma. Even if morphine glucuronidation has been shown in postmortem human brain tissue, the rate of glucuronidation in these tissue samples was low compared with that in liver. Some reports indicate, however, that morphine metabolites can be formed directly in vivo in cerebrospinal fluid after cerebroventricular administration of morphine.[55]

M3G was shown in plasma during long-term systemic and intraspinal administration of morphine in many clinical studies.[44] Although the properties of M3G in humans are unknown, M3G is a potent antagonist of some pharmacologic effects of M6G and morphine in rodents. The accumulation of M3G in the central nervous system may result in hyperalgesia, agitation, and myoclonus. The mechanism of this action is not known and might involve nonopioid receptor mechanisms. It also is possible that the abnormal metabolism of morphine, wherein large amounts of M3G are formed with little or no M6G, could produce higher than normal concentrations of M3G. The development of such abnormal metabolism is consistent with present knowledge of the nature and differential induction of the UGT enzyme,[56] which is responsible for the metabolism of morphine. If hyperalgesia, agitation, and myoclonus responses are due to a nonopioid receptor effect exerted by morphine or its metabolites, the use of non–UGT-metabolized opioids for patients requiring increasing doses of opioids or for patients not responding to long-term morphine treatment may be relevant and worthy of therapeutic monitoring. It was suggested that when faced with patients with paradoxical pain, physicians should consider the use of methadone instead of morphine because UGT do not metabolize methadone.

Diacetylmorphine (heroin, diamorphine) is semisynthetic lipid-soluble opioid analgesic prepared by diacetylating morphine. Heroin is extremely lipophilic and rapidly deacylated by three different esterases (pseudocholinesterase and nonspecific liver carboxylesterases hCE-1 and hCE-2) to active metabolites 6-monoacetyl-morphine (6-MAM) and morphine, which then undergo further metabolic changes described earlier for morphine.[57] Heroin does not have any demonstrated advantages over morphine in pain treatment and is not available on the U.S. pharmaceutical market (schedule I drug). The administration of heroin is a less efficient way of delivering morphine. Diamorphine is used currently in several European countries as the substitute pharmaceutical preparation to control heroin dependence.

Hydromorphone (Dilaudid) is a phenantrene-derivative structural analog of morphine and may be produced in the body by N-demethylation of hydrocodone. Hydromorphone is highly hydrophilic and has a strong affinity μ opioid receptor. When administered parenterally, 1.5 mg of hydromorphone is equivalent to 10 mg of morphine. The oral-to-parenteral ratio is 5:1, and the oral bioavailability of hydromorphone is about 30% to 40%. The duration of analgesic action of hydromorphone is similar to morphine (3 to 4 hours), and the metabolic pathways for its degradation are similar to morphine. After systemic administration, hydromorphone is metabolized primarily to hydromorphone-3-glucuronide (H3G), which, similar to the corresponding M3G, is not only devoid of analgesic activity but also evokes a range of dose-dependent excitatory behaviors, including allodynia, myoclonus, and seizures in animal models. The relative concentrations of H3G in cerebrospinal fluid and plasma in relation to other hydromorphone metabolites are unknown. The reported incidence of neuroexcitatory side effects (allodynia, myoclonus, seizures) in patients given large doses of hydromorphone (and morphine) has increased, however.[38] Cessation of hydromorphone (or morphine) or rotation to a structurally dissimilar opioid (from morphine/hydromorphone to methadone or fentanyl) usually results in a restoration of analgesia and resolution of the neuroexcitatory opioid side effects over a period of hours to days.

Methadone (Dolophine) is a synthetic, open-chain derivative μ opioid receptor agonist. In addition to its opioid receptor interactions, methadone is an antagonist of NMDA receptor. Methadone is a racemic mixture of two enantiomers (R/S, 50:50), and R-methadone accounts for most of its opioid effect. Methadone is equipotent to morphine after parenteral administration. The pharmacokinetics and pharmacodynamics of methadone are highly variable, which indicates the necessity of the individualized dose and interval titration. The oral bioavailability varies considerably in the range of 40% to 99%. Intestinal metabolism by cytochrome P-450 3A4 (CYP3A4) in the intestinal wall may contribute to the high variability in presystemic methadone inactivation.[58] The disposition of the active enantiomer, R-methadone, can be predicted in part by CYP3A4 activity and protein binding to α_1-AGP (ORM2), whereas S-methadone disposition is not well explained by the above-mentioned factors. Despite these differences, central nervous system effects were difficult to interpret on the basis of plasma R-methadone pharmacokinetics.[59]

The methadone plasma level decline follows the biexpotential model (2 to 3 hours of initial phase and 15 to 60 hours of terminal phase), which accounts for the discrepancy between moderate length (6 to 8 hours) of analgesic action and the tendency for drug accumulation with repeated dosing. Plasma protein binding and rate of hepatic extraction also influence the highly variable half-life. Methadone is metabolized by genetically expressed CYP3A4 in human liver and has no known active metabolites. It is sequentially N-demethylated to the inactive metabolites 2-ethylidene-1, 5-dimethyl-3, 3-diphenylpyrrolidine (EDDP) and 2-ethyl-5-methyl-3, 3-diphenylpyraline (EMDP). Because it is excreted almost exclusively in feces, methadone has been proposed as a safe and effective analgesic for patients with chronic renal failure. When urine pH is greater than 6.0, however, the remaining renal clearance of methadone is decreased significantly; older patients and patients with cancer also may have decreased clearance. The repeated use of methadone necessitates careful individual titration. In some patients with cancer, the long half-life of methadone offers the advantage of extending dosing intervals to 12 hours; however, further research is needed in this area.[60]

In vitro data showed that methadone and dextropropoxyphene, in addition to being opioid receptor agonists, are weak noncompetitive NMDA receptor antagonists. Clinical anecdotes suggest that the NMDA receptor antagonism of these opioids may play a significant role in the pharmacologic action of these compounds; however, no clinical studies have been conducted to support this issue. Much evidence points to the involvement of NMDA receptors in the development and maintainance of neuropathic pain. In neuropathic pain, a presumed opioid-insensitive component generally is involved, which apparently can be blocked by NMDA receptor antagonists. To obtain complete analgesia, however, a combination of an NMDA receptor antagonist and an opioid receptor agonist is needed. Ebert et al.[61] discussed evidence for the NMDA receptor antagonism of these compounds and its relevance for clinical pain treatment; an overview of structure-activity relationships for the relevant opioids as noncompetitive NMDA receptor antagonists was presented. They concluded that although the finding that some opioids are weak noncompetitive NMDA receptor antagonists in vitro has generated much attention among clinicians, no clinical studies have been conducted to evaluate the applicability of these compounds in the treatment of neuropathic pain conditions.

Because of its relatively weak drug abuse potential, methadone is used extensively for the opioid detoxification or maintenance programs. There are, however, many problems associated with methadone use. Among these is the obvious risk of substituting one addiction for another. Although methadone is safer to use and legal if taken in a clinic, an addiction to methadone is harder to break than one to heroin. If a patient decides after several months on methadone maintenance to discontinue it, the detoxification is generally longer and more uncomfortable. Use of methadone reduces cravings for heroin, but methadone maintenance, unless combined with counseling, does nothing to alleviate the social and emotional consequences of long-term use. Also, methadone's side effects can include orthostatic hypotension, nausea, insomnia, constipation, and allergic reactions.

Current trends toward outpatient surgery and closed-loop computer-controlled drug administration have created a demand for short-acting analgesic agents. Such agents not only produce rapid patient recovery after completion of the procedure, but also provide almost immediate intraoperative control over the analgesic state of the patient. The family of the phenylpiperidine opioid analgesics, which include the traditional agents fentanyl, alfentanil, and sufentanil and newly introduced ramifentanil provides the wide spectrum of intravenous analgesic opioids for controlled infusion during anesthesia and intensive care.

Fentanyl is the oldest synthetic phenylpiperidine-derivative opioid agonist that interacts primarily with μ receptors. Intravenous preparations of fentanyl are the most widely used opioids for intravenous analgesia in the settings of perioperative pain control. Fentanyl is about 80 times more potent than morphine. It is highly lipophilic and binds strongly to plasma proteins. Because of its stong lipophilic properties, fentanyl also is used for the transdermal and transmucosal routes of administration.

Fentanyl undergoes extensive metabolism in humans. Systemic elimination occurs primarily by hepatic metabolism. When administered as a lozenge for oral transmucosal absorption, swallowed fentanyl is subject to first-pass metabolism in the liver and possibly small intestine. Piperidine N-dealkylation to norfentanyl was found to be the predominant pathway of liver microsomal metabolism. Amide hydrolysis to despropionylfentanyl and alkyl hydroxylation to hydroxyfentanyl were comparatively minor pathways. Hydroxynorfentanyl was identified as a minor, secondary metabolite arising from N-dealkylation of hydroxyfentanyl. Microsomal norfentanyl formation was inhibited significantly by the cytochrome P-450 3A4 (CYP3A4) inhibitor troleandomycin and the CYP3A4 substrate and competitive inhibitor midazolam and was correlated significantly with CYP3A4 protein content and catalytic activity. Of six expressed human P450 isoforms (P450s 1A2, 2B6, 2C9, 2D6, 2E1, and 3A4), only CYP3A4 exhibited significant fentanyl dealkylation to norfentanyl. These results indicate the predominant role of CYP3A4 in the primary route of hepatic fentanyl metabolism. Human duodenal microsomes also catalyzed fentanyl metabolism to norfentanyl; the average rate was approximately half that of hepatic metabolism. Rates of duodenal norfentanyl formation were diminished by troleandomycin and midazolam and were correlated significantly with CYP3A4 activity, suggesting a prominent role for CYP3A4. These results show that human intestinal and liver microsomes catalyze fentanyl metabolism, and N-dealkylation by CYP3A4 is the predominant route in both organs. The fraction of fentanyl lozenge that is swallowed likely undergoes significant intestinal and hepatic first-pass metabolism. Intestinal and hepatic first-pass metabolism and systemic metabolism may be subject to individual variability in CYP3A4 expression and to drug interactions involving CYP3A4.[62]

The transdermal therapeutic system for fentanyl (Duragesic) delivers drug continuously to the systemic circulation for 72 hours. This route of administration may be indicated for patients with chronic pain who are unable to take opioids orally and do not require a rapid dose titration. The transdermal absorption of fentanyl is similar from chest, abdomen, or thigh. After application of the transdermal patch, the initial (first 4 hours) systemic absorption is low and increases steadily to reach steady-state within 12 to 24 hours from application. After removal of the transdermal patch, serum fentanyl concentration decreases about 50% in approximately 16 hours. These considerations translate clinically to a delay of several hours in the onset of analgesia after initial application and a persistence of analgesia and side effects long after removal of the transdermal system. The more recently available formulations of fentanyl for transmucosal administration (lozenges) were introduced for pediatric sedation in the preoperative setting and are characterized by relatively fast systemic absorption and limited duration of action.

Fentanyl is used widely via the epidural and intrathecal route, mostly in combination with different local anesthetics to provide neuraxial analgesia. After those routes of administration, because of the strong lipophilic properties, the spread of fentanyl throughout the epidural or intrathecal space is limited. In addition to the local spinal effects, a significant part of fentanyl is absorbed into the systemic circulation with subsequent pharmacologic effects on supraspinal sites.

Sufentanil (Sufenta) is about five times more potent than fentanyl. The pharmacokinetics of sufentanil are similar to fentanyl, and most pharmacokinetic properties of fentanyl can be applied to sufentanil. The slightly smaller volume of distribution for sufentanil and similar clearance (13 to 15 mL/min/kg) may account for the shorter elimination half-life of sufentanil compared with fentanyl (164 minutes versus 3.1 to 7.9 hours). As with fentanyl, sufentanil is metabolized rapidly and extensively in the liver, and CYP3A4 is responsible for sulfentanil N-dealkylation to norsufentanil.[63] Because of its lipophilic properties, protein binding, and the large volume distribution reflecting the strong tissue affinity of sufentanil, however, the slow release of sufentanil from muscle and fat keeps the plasma concentration relatively low and is the rate-limiting step in the elimination of sufentanil from the body. The similarities between fentanyl and sufentanil pharmacokinetics imply similar pharmacodynamic properties for both drugs, with sufentanil having a slightly more rapid onset of effect and a slightly shorter duration of action.

Alfentanil (Alfenta) is relatively lipid soluble but considerably less than fentanyl and sufentanil. The lower lipid solubility of alfentanil accounts for its small volume of distribution (about 25% of fentanyl and sufentanil). Rapid and almost complete hepatic metabolism of alfentanil results in only about 0.4% of alfentanil excreted unchanged in the urine. The clearance of alfentanil is approximately half of fentanyl and sufentanil. There is considerable unexplained variability in alfentanil pharmacokinetics, particularly systemic clearance. Alfentanil is metabolized extensively in vivo, and systemic clearance depends on hepatic biotransformation. CYP3A4 was shown to be the predominant P-450 isoform responsible for human liver microsomal alfentanil metabolism. This observation, combined with the known population variability in CYP3A4 activity, provides a mechanistic explanation for the interindividual variability in alfentanil disposition.[64] The greater decrease of alfentanil's volume of distribution relative to the decrease in its clearance results in a significantly shorter terminal elimination half-life. The terminal elimination half-life for alfentanil varies between 70 and 111 minutes and is shorter than for fentanyl and sufentanil. Alfentanil's small volume of distribution and short elimination half-life preclude significant accumulation of the drug in the body and render it a useful drug for continuous infusion and rapid titration.

Remifentanil (Ultiva) is the most potent μ receptor agonist from this series and in contrast to other opioids is characterized by the unique pharmacokinetic pattern resulting from its exclusive degradation by the plasma and tissue nonspecific esterases. Remifentanil is not a substrate for plasma pseudocholinesterase, and patients deficient in pseudocholinesterase or with atypical pseudocholinesterases expect to have normal duration of action. Remifentanil has ultrarapid onset of action and peak effect and short duration of action. The hydrolysis of ramifentanil at labile ester linkage results in the production of carboxylic acid metabolite, which represents the principal (>95%) of remifentanil. The carboxylic acid metabolite is essentially inactive and is excreted by the kidneys with an elimination half-life of approximately 90 minutes. Remifentanil is highly lipophilic (more than fentanyl and sufentanil) and has a much greater volume of distribution (about 100 mL/kg) compared with the aforementioned intravenous opioids. Because of its rapid distribution and metabolism in the plasma and tissue, blood concentrations of remifentanil decline 50% in 3 to 6 minutes after 1 minute or after prolonged continuous infusion and are completely independent (in contrast to any other opioid analgesic) of duration and magnitude of drug administration. The pharmacodynamic effects of remifentanil follow the measured blood concentrations, allowing direct control between dose, blood levels, and response. Because of its rapid onset and termination, the use of remifentanil may be associated with impaired ventilation through the muscle rigidity in patients who are not paralyzed at the beginning of high-dose infusion. Rapid termination of analgesic effects after infusion produces virtually no residual analgesia after termination of infusion so that the postoperative analgesia has to be provided by other, longer-acting opioids.

Drug Interactions With Opioid Analgesics

Widespread use of opioid analgesics in patients with all kinds of diseases opens a variety of possible interactions between analgesics and other drugs that might be administered concomitantly to the patient.[65] Many of these drug interactions are of little clinical importance. Some drug interactions have been reported to result in serious clinical problems, however. Drug interactions can predominantly affect the pharmacokinetics or the pharmacodynamics of the drug. Most important pharmacokinetic drug interactions occur at the level of drug metabolism or protein binding. Acceleration of methadone metabolism caused by CYP3A4 induction by antiretroviral drugs or rifampicin (rifampin) has caused methadone withdrawal symptoms. Lack of morphine formation from codeine produced by CYP2D6 inhibition by quinidine may result in an almost complete loss of the analgesic effects. Alterations of methadone protein binding caused by an inhibition of α_1-acid glycoprotein synthesis by alkylating substances are another possibility for predominantly pharmacokinetically based drug interactions during opioid treatment. Inhibition of P-glycoprotein by anticancer drugs could result in altered transmembrane transport of morphine, methadone, or fentanyl, although this has not been shown to be of clinical relevance. Synergistic effects of systemically administered opioids with spinally or topically delivered opioids or anesthetics have been reported frequently. The same is true for the opioid-sparing effects of co-administered nonopioid analgesics. Antidepressants, anticonvulsants, or α_2-adrenoreceptor agonists also have been shown to exert additive analgesic effects when administered together with an opioid. Inconsistent findings are reported, however, regarding the treatment of patients with opioid-induced nausea and sedation because coadministration of antiemetics either increased or decreased the respective adverse effects or revealed additional unwanted drug effects.

Opioid Tolerance, Dependence, and Addiction

Opioid tolerance and physical dependence are expected with long-term opioid treatment and should not be confused with psychological dependence (*addiction*), manifested as drug abuse behavior. Physical dependence on opioids is revealed when the opioid is discontinued abruptly or when opioid antagonist (naloxone, naltrexone) is administered and typically is manifested as anxiety, irritability, chills and hot flashes, joint pain, lacrimation, rhinorrhea, diaphoresis, nausea, vomiting, and abdominal cramps and diarrhea. For opioids with short half-lives (i.e., codeine, hydrocodone, morphine, hydromorphone), the onset of withdrawal symptoms can occur within 6 to 12 hours and peak at 24 to 72 hours after discontinuation. For opioids with long half-lives (i.e., methadone, levorphanol, transdermal fentanyl), the onset of the abstinence syndrome may be delayed for 24 hours or more after drug discontinuation and may be of milder intensity.

The appearance of the abstinence syndrome defines physical dependence on opioids, which may occur after just 2 weeks of opioid therapy but *does not imply psychological dependence or addiction.*

Most patients with cancer take opioids for more than 2 weeks, and only rarely do they exhibit the drug abuse behaviors and psychological dependence that characterize addiction. Pain often is treated inadequately because of reluctance about using opioid analgesics and fear that they will be abused. Although international and national expert groups have determined that opioid analgesics are essential for the relief of pain, little information has been available about the health consequences of the abuse of these drugs. In a retrospective study in this area, Joranson et al[66] evaluated the proportion of drug abuse related to opioid analgesics and the trends in medical use and abuse of five opioid analgesics used to treat severe pain—fentanyl, hydromorphone, meperidine, morphine, and oxycodone—in a nationally representative sample of hospital emergency department admissions resulting from drug abuse. They reported that from 1990 to 1996, there were increases in medical use of morphine (59%), fentanyl (1,168%), oxycodone (23%) and hydromorphone (19%) and a decrease in the medical use of meperidine (35%). During the same period, the total number of drug abuse mentions per year owing to opioid analgesics increased (only 6.6%), although the proportion of mentions for opioid abuse relative to total drug abuse mentions decreased from 5.1% to 3.8%. Reports of abuse decreased for meperidine (39%), oxycodone (29%), fentanyl (59%), and hydromorphone (15%) and increased for morphine (3%). The authors concluded that the trend of increasing medical use of opioid analgesics to treat pain does not seem to contribute to increases in the health consequences of opioid analgesic abuse.[66]

Patients with cancer occasionally require discontinuation or rapid decreases in doses of opioids when the cause of pain is eliminated effectively by antineoplastic treatments or pain perception is modified by neuroablative or neurolytic procedures. In such circumstances, the opioid abstinence syndrome can be avoided by withdrawal of the opioid on a schedule that provides half the prior daily dose for each of the first 2 days, then reduces the daily dose by 25% every 2 days thereafter until the total dose (in morphine equivalents) is 30 mg/d. The drug may be discontinued after 2 days on the 30 mg/d dose.

Tolerance to opioids is defined as the need to increase dose requirements over time to maintain pain relief. For most cancer patients, the first indication of tolerance is a decrease in the duration of analgesia for a given dose. Increasing dose requirements are correlated most consistently with progressive disease, which produces increased pain intensity. Patients with stable disease do not usually require increasing doses.

Suzuki et al[67] focused on the relationships between opioid receptor types and physical and psychological dependences. μ and δ, but not κ opioid receptor agonists produce physical dependence. From behavioral, biochemical, and molecular biologic studies, it is suggested so far that development of physical dependence on morphine results predominantly from an activation of μ_1 and μ_2 opioid receptors, which causes functional changes in protein G transporters, adenylate cyclase, protein kinases A and C, β-adrenoceptor, and NMDA receptor in the locus caeruleus. There have been significant advances in studies on psychic dependence. Activation of the mesolimbic dopamine system may lead to psychological dependence on opioids. μ and δ_1 opioid receptor agonists activate the mesolimbic dopamine system to induce a rewarding effect, whereas the rewarding effect of δ_2 opioid receptor agonists may be produced through a nondopaminergic system. There are complicated interactions among opioid receptor types. The activation of κ opioid receptor suppresses physical and psychic dependences on μ and δ opioid receptor agonists, but the activation of δ opioid receptor potentiates the dependence on μ opioid receptor agonists. The clinical use of morphine in patients with cancer pain would not lead to dependence, probably because of the balance of the opioid system coming from these interactions.

REFERENCES FOR ADDITIONAL READING

1. Mei and Pasternak J Pharmacol Exp Ther 2002, 300, 1070–4
2. Manfredi et al, In Cancer Pain Management, ed. Parris, WCV, Butterworth-Heinemann, 1997, 49–64
3. Rossi et al, FEBS Lett 1995, 369,192–6;
4. Rossi et al, Neurosci Lett 1996, 216, 1–4
5. Schuller et al, Nature Neurosci 1999, 2,151–6
6. Paix A et al, Pain 1995, 63, 263–9)
7. Groesch et al, Br J Clin Pharmacol 2001, 52, 711–714
8. Loetsch et al, Pharmacogenetics 2002, 12, 3–9
9. Hoellt, Pharmacogenetics 2002, 12, 1–2
10. Wang et al, J Biol Chem 2001, 276, 34624–30
11. Befort et al, J Biol Chem 2001, 276, 3130–7
12. Uhl et al, Proc Natl Acad Sci USA, 1999, 96, 7752–5
13. deWildt et al, Clin Pharmacokinet 1999, 36, 439–52
14. Yue et al, Br J Clin Pharmacol 1991, 31, 635–42
15. Yue et al, Br J Clin Pharmacol 1989, 28, 639–45
16. Eckhardt et al, Pain 1998, 76, 27–33
17. Srinivasan et al, Pharm Res 1996, 13, 296–300
18. Aderjan et al, Ther Drug Monitor 1996, 20, 561–9
19. Webb et al, Br J Clin Pharm 2000, 52, 35–43
20. Heiskanen et al, Acta Oncol 2000, 39, 941–7
21. Levy, Eur J Pain 2001, 5, 113–6
22. Gillen et al, Naunyn-Schmiedebergs Arch Pharmacol 2000, 362, 116–22
23. Poulsen et al, Eur J Clin Pharmacol 1996, 51,289–95
24. Lewis et al, Am J Health Syst Pharm 1997, 54, 643–52
25. Zhou et al, Clin Pharmacol Ther 1993, 54, 507–13
26. Osborne et al, Clin Pharmacol Ther 1990, 47, 12–9
27. Babul et al, Clin Pharmacol Ther 1993, 54, 286–92
28. Janicki et al, Eur J Chem Clin Biochem 1991, 29: 391–3
29. Loetsch et al, Anesthesiology 2001, 95, 1329–38
30. Loetsch et al, Anesthesiology 1997, 87, 1348–58
31. Motamed et al, Anesthesiology 2000, 92, 355–60
32. Grace et al, Anesth Analg 1996, 83, 1055–9
33. Hewett et al, Pain 1993, 53, 59–63
34. Gong et al, Pain 1992, 48, 249–55
35. Igawa et al, Br J Pharmacol 1993, 110, 257–62
36. Westerling et al, Ther Drug Monit 1995, 17, 287–301
37. Peterson et al, Eur J Clin Pharmacol 1990, 38, 121–4
38. Smith, Clin Exp Pharmacol Physiol 2000, 27, 524–8
39. Schneider et al, Br J Clin Pharmacol 1992, 34, 431–3
40. Arner et al, Pain 1988, 33, 11–23
41. Bowsher Br Med J 1993, 306: 473–4
42. Morley et al, Lancet 1992, 340, 1045
43. Sjogren et al, Pain 1993, 55, 93–7
44. Sjogren et al, Acta Anaesth Scand 1993, 37, 780–2
45. vanDongen et al, Br J Clin Pharmacol 1994, 38, 271–3
46. Somogyi et al, Clin Pharmacokinet 1993, 24, 413–20
47. Goucke et al, Pain 1994, 56, 145–9
48. Saewe in: Foley KM, Inturrisi CE, eds. Advances in pain research and therapy. New York: Raven Press, 1986, 45–4

49. Morley et al, Lancet 1992, 340, 1045
50. Parris et al, South Med J 1996, 417–9
51. Hardy, Br Med J 1993, 306, 793–4
52. Davis et al, Br Med J 1993, 306, 793
53. Hartley et al, Arch Dis Child 1993, 69, 55–8
54. Portenoy et al, Neurology 1991, 41, 1457–61
55. Sandouk et al, Eur J Drug Metab Pharmacokinet 1991, 3, 166–71
56. Lawrence et al, Biochem Pharmacol 1992, 43, 2335–40
57. Brzezinski et al, Drug Metab Disp 1997, 25, 1089–96
58. Oda et al, J Pharmacol Exp Ther 2001, 298, 1021–32
59. Boulton et al, Clin Pharmacol Ther 2001, 70, 48–57
60. Bruera et al, J Palliat Med 2002, 5, 127–38
61. Ebert et al, Biochem Pharmacol 1998,1, 553–9
62. Labroo et al, Drug Metab Dispos 1997, 25, 1072–80
63. Tateishi et al, Anesth Analg, 1996, 82, 167–172
64. Kharash et al, Anesthesiology 1997, 87, 36–50
65. Lotsch et al, Clin Pharmacokinet 2002, 41, 31–57
66. Joranson et al, JAMA 2000, 283, 1710–1714
67. Suzuki et al, Nippon Yakurigaku Zasshi, 1997, 109, 165–74

Chapter 10

Opioid Therapy in Chronic Non-Malignant Pain

Barth L. Wilsey, MD / Gagan Mahajan, MD / Scott M. Fishman, MD

Opioids are the gold standard of currently available analgesics, yet their use in the treatment of chronic non-malignant pain (CNMP) remains controversial.[1–3] Part of this controversy stems from an outdated or inaccurate understanding of appropriate use and risks of abuse or side effects. The decision to initiate opioid therapy in patients with CNMP should be based on a rationale for treatment with observable treatment endpoints and management of side effects.[4,5]

More than a century has passed since Florence Nightingale first resorted to opium injections to treat her chronic back pain.[6] To this day, there is still a scarcity of convincing scientific data to persuasively argue for or against long-term opioid therapy. The relative lack of evidenced-based medicine concerning opioid prescribing with no validated endpoints of analgesic therapy makes its role in clinical practice formidable. There are also challenges in measuring the positive and negative impact of treatment with opioids on the patient's quality of life.

Patients who use opioids for CNMP range from those using stable amounts of opioid with little variation to those whose requirements are seemingly never satisfied and whose dosages frequently escalate. But the prime motivator in the continuing controversy surrounding the use of opioids for CNMP derives from societal attitudes and beliefs. Resistance to chronic opioid therapy stems from social, medical, and legal stigmas. This chapter reviews these issues and discusses the major topics in the debate over opioid prescribing in the treatment of CNMP, including efficacy, toxicity, abuse potential, and the role of physical dependence and tolerance.

RATIONALE

Opioid therapy can be an integral part of a multidisciplinary approach to CNMP management. Often, one combines opioids with other modalities, including psychological treatment and physical rehabilitation. Simultaneously, interventional pain procedures and analgesics (antidepressants, anticonvulsants, nonsteroidal antiinflammatory drugs [NSAIDs], and opioids) may be prescribed. Much of the debate concerning the role of opioid therapy in CNMP management has centered on whether opioid therapy should be used as a first-line treatment. Should pain physicians withhold opioid therapy until other treatment options are exhausted? Although there is a lack of consensus on this important issue, opioid therapy tends to be used as a second-line treatment for CNMP for the following reasons:

- CNMP may respond to nonopioid pharmacological interventions such as NSAIDs for arthritic pain[7] and anticonvulsants or tricyclic antidepressants for neuropathic pain, such as postherpetic neuralgia.[8]

- At times, interventional pain management can be more effective in patients with certain types of CNMP (e.g., sympathetically maintained CRPS types I & II) than chronic drug management.
- Considering the noteworthy side effects and liability profiles of opioid treatment (see later), the risk-to-benefit ratio often demands that other options be employed before opioids.

Chronic opioid therapy should be considered in patients with CNMP when other interventions are not successful. Although the effectiveness of opioid therapy for certain types of CNMP remains controversial, there is no evidence suggesting that opioid therapy is contraindicated in circumstances in which it is not necessarily the first choice. Animal studies have shown a rightward shift of the opioid dose-response curve in experimental pain models related to nervous system injury,[9,10] suggesting that higher opioid doses may be required for patients suffering primarily from neuropathic pain or other forms of chronic severe pain. The limiting factor for opioid therapy in neuropathic pain treatment may be related to the development of significant side effects associated with the high doses of opioids needed rather than to the inherent tolerance found in these conditions. In instances in which tolerance is suspected, methadone may be the optimal choice, because its professed N-methyl-D-aspartate (NMDA) blocking action may reduce tolerance to opioids in patients with neuropathic pain.

In summary, a trial of opioid therapy should be considered when alternative analgesics, interventional pain procedures, and physical therapy are inadequate or inadvisable. Since antidepressants and anticonvulsants only provide 50% pain relief for only one out of three patients,[11] opioids are frequently used despite their narrow therapeutic window. Such use of opioids requires not only an comprehensive strategy that includes consideration of other potentially effective therapies that have less risk but also a clear sense of purpose and observable endpoints of treatment.

GUIDELINES

Because opioids are controlled substances with potential for abuse, they are often associated with stigma as well as regulation by the Drug Enforcement Administration and other state agencies. One of the major concerns of opioid prescribers is potential diversion through fraud, theft, forged prescriptions, or the illegal activities of unprincipled health professionals. Several national organizations, including the American Pain Society, have advanced guidelines for prescribing opioids to help with rational approaches to prescribing and avoiding potential adverse effects.[12] Guidelines often emphasize the importance of frequent monitoring to evaluate therapeutic effectiveness, including the patient's functional status.

ADMINISTRATION

The usual goal of effective opioid administration in patients with chronic pain is to provide constant, sustained analgesia over regular intervals.[13] This requires consideration of multiple factors. For instance, changing from one opioid to another requires knowledge of equianalgesic dosages. Since cross-tolerance between opioids may be incomplete, a patient who has become tolerant to one opioid drug can respond with effective analgesia to another opioid of less than equianalgesic dose. Pain in the tolerant patient can be a challenge because typical dosages for the opioid-naive patient do not apply. In these cases, careful titration is required.

Whether fixed dosing is better than PRN (*pro re nata*, "as needed") dosing is controversial, with each method having advantages for different situations. Fixed dosing allows consistent delivery for reaching the steady state, avoiding the high peak and low trough effect associated with on-demand dosing. It also prevents delays in delivery that can occur with on-demand schedules. However, opioids with longer half-lives may accumulate in fixed doses, and patients receiving their first exposure to opioids may require test dosing, which is most safely given on demand. Morphine and hydromorphone may take less than 24 hours to reach a steady state, whereas levorphanol or methadone can take up to a week. Employing conservative fixed dosing combined with PRN "rescue" dosing can be effective, particularly when there is a need to assess analgesia threshold.

Analgesic therapy with long-acting opioids offers convenient dose intervals that reach safe, effective steady-state levels.[14] Various controlled-release opioids are now available, including morphine (MS-Contin, Oramorph, Kadian), oxycodone (Oxycontin), and fentanyl (Duragesic Patch). Methadone and levorphanol are not formulated for sustained release but have intrinsically longer plasma half-lives than other typical opioids such as codeine, hydrocodone (Vicodin), oxycodone (Percocet), hydromorphone (Dilaudid), or morphine. The availability and ease of administration of orally administered opioids have made this route the most commonly employed. Many cancer patients, however, are unable to tolerate oral ingestion. Intravenous or subcutaneous infusion is commonly used in these cases, often with continuous dosing for constant effect. Infusion eliminates the first-pass effect and can be supplemented by "rescue" bolus doses. The subcutaneous route has several advantages; faster onset of analgesia compared with most oral preparations (although slower than intravenous), access that is usually uncomplicated (e.g., use in patients without intravenous access), and safer administration compared with the intramuscular route in patients with bleeding disorders or reduced muscle mass.

Many means of administering opioids are advantageous for patients with cancer[15] as well as patients undergoing surgery or other invasive or chemical therapies. Rectal suppositories are an alternative in patients unable to use parenteral or oral preparations. These are available containing morphine, hydromorphone, and oxymorphone. Sublingual, buccal, intranasal, and transdermal administration of opioids are also available. Fentanyl, an opioid with many times the potency of morphine, is offered as a transdermal patch with dosing every 3 days. It has the advantage of easy application in almost all patients with chronic severe pain but may be limited by skin sensitivity to the adhesive patch. Fentanyl is now also available as a rapid-onset transmucosal delivery product (Actiq). Epidural and intrathecal routes of opioid administration are also available, making opioids directly available to central regions densely populated with opioid receptors. This form of selective analgesia has the advantage of requiring small quantities of opioids, which predisposes to significantly fewer central and autonomic complications. This route is widely used in the postoperative and obstetric setting as well as for cancer patients.

Patient-controlled analgesia delivers intravenous or subcutaneous dosages of analgesic triggered by a button that is under the control of the patient. Ceilings can be placed on frequency and maximal dosage, and records of usage are easily maintained. Essentially, the patient titrates his or her own dosage delivered at individualized intervals according to the parameters set by the physician. Patient-controlled analgesia is widely used for treating postoperative pain and is finding broader use in cancer patients. A newer variant of this drug delivery system is patient-controlled epidural analgesia, which delivers epidural dosages of analgesic triggered by a button under the control of the patient.

TREATMENT ENDPOINTS

There are two critical issues related to treatment endpoints in opioid therapy for CNMP: (1) what should be considered a positive outcome of a trial of opioids and (2) when opioid therapy should be discontinued (or tapered) if the treatment is either effective or ineffective. Clinical studies in this area are limited.

Markers of benefit in patients treated with opioids for CNMP include subjective pain reduction and objective evidence of improvement of functional status and quality of life. However, psychological and social factors, as well as the status of coexistent disease, may influence pain perception, suffering, and entitlement and can alter the overall assessment.[16–18] Unfortunately, not all of these parameters will improve concomitantly and proportionately following the initiation of opioid therapy. It is well recognized that psychological factors may influence pain perception and that the reduction of pain from an opioid trial may not be as robust in a patient who has not adequately resolved other psychological amplifiers of pain perception. At the same time, pain reduction and improvement of functional status resulting from effective opioid analgesia may not be concordant with achievements occurring from psychological treatment. Determining treatment endpoints during an opioid trial may require flexibility in considering the many possible variations in efficacy and functional gain.

Pain reduction is always a subjective variable and as such can serve only as a single aspect of adequate chronic opioid therapy. Consider the patient who has daily pain rated 6 on a 1 to 10 pain severity scale, with significant disability associated with the pain. While opioid therapy may reduce subjective pain scores by only one point from 6 of 10 to 5 of 10, the treatment is clearly successful if there is evidence of increased function, such as return to work and improved ability to participate in physical rehabilitation. On the other hand, an opioid trial characterized by subjective reports of marked pain relief but no observable functional gains, and possibly even signs of functional loss such as voluntary unemployment, dysfunctional interpersonal relationships, or diminished physical activity, can be considered counterproductive. In cases in which function worsens, it is imperative to assess the possible contribution of opioid side effects, including sedation and cognitive impairment. In addition, signs of dysfunction always warrant consideration of, but do not confirm, possible addiction (see later). It is only with careful assessment that side effects can be recognized and managed, allowing chronic opioid therapy to be safe, with minimal adverse effects.

In addition to pain relief, restoration of function has become one of the primary treatment goals for the chronic pain patients on long-term opioid therapy. Unlike the patient with addiction whose level of function is impaired by substance use, the chronic pain patient's level of function should improve with adequate, judicious use of these medications. Patients with adequate analgesia should be expected to increase their function as a result of using opioids. It is optimal to collect collateral evidence of functional gains from family members or friends or from other caregivers such as psychologists or physical therapists. Increase in function can mean that the patient's quality of life has improved, as evidenced by enhanced activities of daily living, gains in employment, performance of household chores, and increased socializing and family activities. Decreased function in the chronic pain patient should raise suspicion that addiction may be a possible adverse consequence of opioid therapy. However, this is not the same as confirmation that addiction is responsible, as decreased function may be related to other factors beyond the patient's control, such as the opioid side effects of sedation or cognitive impairment. Deteriorating mental or physical health or a downward psychosocial spiral (loss of employment, legal difficulties, interpersonal or family difficulties) may necessitate additional support in the form of a multidisciplinary approach with referral to mental health providers.

Documenting improvement in function is a critical part of safe, well thought-out opioid management. For instance, documented evidence of improved function can go a long way toward mitigating concerns about addiction. Documenting functional endpoints of opioid therapy can provide a yardstick for improvement at the time of initiating opioid therapy and regular monitoring of these areas. As noted earlier, vigilance for recognizing decreased function is equally important, as this may be a sign of addiction. Many other formal indices can help monitor function in patients using chronic opioid therapy. For instance, visual analog scales for average pain levels or multidimensional scales that measure function and coping skills are often employed. Although questionnaires given to patients in pain clinics have previously attested to benefit vis-à-vis pain relief, documented gains in function following institution of opioids have been relatively uncommon.[19] However, there is some evidence that using opioids in combination with a psychological treatment regimen using behavioral interventions may improve a patient's functional level. Thus, a comprehensive treatment program using a multidisciplinary approach may offer the best chance of effective opioid therapy for CNMP.[20]

Another critical issue is when to discontinue opioid therapy if the treatment is deemed to be unsatisfactory. Determination of a treatment failure requires consideration of many possible contributing factors, including inadequate dose, inappropriate dosing schedule, improper drug delivery route, opioid-insensitive pain relating to the nature of the pain generator (e.g., neuropathic pain), involvement of unresolved contributors to pain such physical, psychological, and social disability, and development of side effects that limit dose escalation. Some patients appear resistant to one opioid and sensitive to another.[21]

How long effective opioid therapy should be continued remains a question with little science to guide decision-making and no clear consensus among practitioners. Pharmacological tolerance to opioids can develop during treatment (see later) and may necessitate an increase in dose to maintain the same therapeutic effect or rotation to an alternate opioid. Although some clinical studies have suggested a plateau of opioid dose requirement following an initial escalation, it is possible that progressive dose escalation may be required during prolonged opioid treatment. This implies that periodic opioid dose escalation may be necessary in some patients experiencing effective pain relief with opioid therapy. Clearly, decisions regarding the duration of effective opioid therapy should be made based on each patient's need, with full consideration of treatment efficacy relative to adverse effects as well as to the progression or regression of underlying pathologic condition. Once opioid therapy is started, it may not be possible to know how much pain would be present without opioid therapy unless opioids are discontinued (by slow controlled taper.)

CONSIDERATIONS FOR OPIOID SELECTION

Patients with moderate to severe chronic pain who have not improved with alternative non-opioid therapies should be assessed for potential benefit from opioid analgesics. Consideration should be given whether the patient is opiate naive. In those who are, an opiate trial can be given with a low-dose, short-acting opioid (SAO) such as propoxyphene, hydrocodone, or oxycodone. The rapid clearance and short half-life of SAOs should minimize toxic accumulation of the medication and thereby minimize risk of side effects. Just as with a long-acting opioid (LAO), SAOs should be taken at fixed-dosing intervals, as opposed to "as-needed," to avoid precipitation of anxiety and reinforcement of pain complaints and behaviors with additional analgesics. If a patient responds to the SAO and tolerates its side effects, he or she should be converted to an equianalgesic LAO dose if possible.

Although selection of any LAO largely appears to be empirical, a rational approach to prescribing can be aided by a careful review of the patient's medical history. Long considered the "gold standard" because it was the first LAO to market, of the relative hydrophilicity of sustained-release morphine formulations (MS Contin and Oramorph) actually makes it a less than ideal opioid. Because of the delay in transport across the blood-brain barrier, it has a slower onset of action compared with other opioids. Although its pharmacological activity is primarily due to the parent compound, morphine's analgesic effects can also be mitigated or perpetuated by two of its glucuronide metabolites. Morphine 3-glucuronide accounts for approximately 50% of the metabolites and causes generalized hyperalgesia, central nervous system irritability, and development of tolerance.[22] Morphine 6-glucuronide accounts for approximately 5% to 15% of metabolites and sustains the analgesia in addition to the side effects. Since morphine's elimination is dependent on hepatic mechanisms, it should be used with caution in cirrhotic patients. In addition, because it is excreted through the kidneys, the dose should be adjusted in patients with renal impairment to minimize the risk of adverse side effects associated with the aforementioned glucoronide metabolites.

In comparison to sustained-release morphine, sustained-release oxycodone (OxyContin) has a more sustained pharmacokinetic profile, which theoretically allows it to be solely administered on an every 12 hours dosing schedule. This, however, reflects a characteristic of the drug delivery system rather than a property of the drug itself. In spite of this, oxycodone does differ pharmacologically from morphine. On a milligram-for-milligram basis, oxycodone is more potent, has a quicker onset of analgesia, and has less plasma variation than morphine. Furthermore, oxycodone causes fewer side effects (hallucinations, dizziness, and pruritis). Thus, oxycodone may be advantageous in patients who are sensitive to the side effects of morphine and therefore have a narrower therapeutic window of analgesia. While it possesses some intrinsic analgesic properties via activation of the κ-opioid receptors, oxycodone is predominantly a prodrug metabolized by the cytochrome p450 2D6 enzyme into oxymorphone, a μ-opioid agonist. In the approximately 10% of the population with genetically low levels of this enzyme, higher than usual doses of oxycodone may be necessary to obtain pain relief. Analgesic efficacy may also be decreased in those who are concurrently taking medications known to inhibit the p450 2D6 enzyme. Therefore, careful dose adjustments must be made in those concurrently taking medications such as selective serotonin reuptake inhibitors, tricyclic antidepressants, or neuroleptics. Finally, because oxycodone is excreted by the kidneys, the dose should be adjusted in renal dysfunction.

Recently, there has been a tremendous resurgence of interest in methadone as an analgesic medication because of its NMDA receptor antagonistism, which theoretically complement its μ-opioid receptor agonist activity.[23,24] Numerous studies have demonstrated the involvement of NMDA receptor mechanisms in the development of opioid tolerance[25] and neuropathic pain.[26] Theoretically, then, methadone might mitigate opioid-induced tolerance, and methadone's potential advantage in treating neuropathic pain remains a compelling concept. The pharmacoeconomic benefit of methadone has also prompted reappraisal of this medication, since it is much less costly than other proprietary sustained-release opioids. Because its duration of effect is inherently long-acting (as opposed to being a sustained-release tablet like the other long-acting oral opioids), this is especially beneficial for patients with impaired gastrointestinal absorption secondary to "short-gut syndrome" or "dumping syndrome." Unlike the sustained-release oral opioids, methadone tablets can be broken in half or chewed. It is also available as an elixir, which is advantageous for patients with a gastrostomy feeding tube because the risk of clogging the tube with a crushed tablet is avoided. In addition, the elixir theoretically allows for a relatively more precise titration of methadone. This is advantageous in allowing one to minimize the potential for delayed-onset toxicity due to methadone's remarkable interindividual variability in metabolism. Because methadone is metabolized by the p450 family of enzymes, similar precautions as outlined for oxycodone (see earlier) must also be taken. Aside from possible drug interactions, methadone's efficacy can be influenced by gastric pH. Absorption of methadone will be higher, for example, in patients taking omeprazole. Changes in urinary pH can also influence renal excretion of methadone. Thus, polypharmacy or changes in either gastric or urinary pH increase the potential for toxic accumulation of methadone.

Originally formulated as part of a balanced anesthetic for use during surgical procedures, fentanyl is a lipophilic opioid with an inherently quicker onset of action than morphine. Its greater degree of potency compared with other opioids allows for the delivery of smaller quantities measured in micrograms per hour. Although considerd short acting, continuous absorption through the skin can provide sustained levels of analgesia. When applied as a transdermal patch in a single application, absorption for extended periods occurs, allowing for 3-day dosing with avoidance of the first-pass effect of the liver. Constipation and medication with laxatives may be reduced during fentanyl administration compared with orally administered opioids because of avoidance of passage of the opioid through the gastrointestinal tract. This lack of reliance upon gastrointestinal absorption provides the basis for recommending its use in patients with an inability to tolerate oral medications secondary to chronic nausea and vomiting, in those with impaired gastrointestinal absorption secondary to short-gut syndrome or dumping syndrome, and in those who are noncompliant with taking oral medications. Unlike the oral long-acting opioids, however, dose titration can sometimes be more challenging because of individual variations in transdermal absorption of the medication, fat stores, and muscle bulk. In addition, it can take up to 6 days before steady state is achieved after the dose is changed. Finally, the patch may be impractical for patients in whom it does not easily adhere to the skin, such as those who perspire excessively.

SIDE EFFECTS

The most common side effects of opioids are constipation, nausea, vomiting, sedation, urinary retention, pruritus, and respiratory depression. Any adverse effects from opioids may significantly limit therapy, and some can present life-threatening consequences. Fortunately, tolerance to most of the side effects occurs as time progresses. The exception to this general rule is opioid-induced constipation, which does not tend to resolve with time. Among the other opioid-related side effects, there are few predictors of which patients will experience which side effects or which particular opioids will produce them. It is sensible to expect side effects and whenever possible to take preventive action. Unfortunately, not all opioid-related side effects can be prevented. Thus, patients should be closely followed. The elderly are at particular risk, since they tend to be predisposed to some of these adverse effects. Effective management includes anticipation of side effects and use of preventative measures, such as laxatives for constipation. It is also necessary to choose the best medication with careful administration and to provide clear communication with the patient, family, and nurse to ensure prompt recognition and response to adverse effects.

Constipation

Constipation is the most predictable side effect of opioids. But unlike most others, tolerance does not develop. Thus, constipation can be expected throughout the duration of opioid administration. Constipation is such a reliable consequence that lack of constipation in a patient with normal gastrointestinal function may, in part, support concern that the opioid dose may be too low or even that opioids may be diverted. Preventative therapy with stool softeners and adequate fluid intake is a mainstay of opioid therapy and should be offered at the time opioids are started and continued throughout opioid treatment. Since opioids block intestinal motility, passive agents such as stool softeners and bulking agents such as bran or psyllium derivatives alone will be inadequate because opioid-related constipation require agents that directly stimulate gut motility. Thus, active stimulating laxatives are recommended over passive modalities. It is advisable to recommend a cathartic at the time of initiating opioid therapy. This might include senna tablets every day or twice a day or bisacodyl, either 5 mg PO at bedtime or 10 mg rectal suppository PRN at bedtime. Alternatively, one might employ cascara 4 to 12 ml at bedtime. Severe constipation may respond to oral administration of osmotic laxatives such as lactulose or an opioid antagonist such as naloxone. The latter maneuver exploits the extensive metabolism of naloxone after oral administration, which limits its systemic bioavailability. The exact dosing regimen of oral naloxone for constipation is uncertain. It is suggested that an initial oral dose of naloxone should not exceed 5 mg. In our institution, we start with 1.2 mg to 2.4 mg PO (3–6 small ampules) every 4 hours until the first bowel movement, or for five doses. If ineffective, another series with a higher dose (3–5 mg per dose) can be tried. Since nonopioid effects can contribute to constipation, naloxone will only reverse the opioid-induced effects and will not reverse nonopioid effects, such as anticholinergic side effects from tricyclic antidepressants. Thus, oral naloxone usually works only when the constipation is solely opioid-related.

There are other ways of counteracting opioid-induced constipation. For instance, there is some evidence that opioid products that are not delivered by an enteric route, such as transdermal fentanyl, may be less prone to inducing constipation as compared with equivalent oral morphine.[27] Alternatively, a drug whose side effect profile includes diarrhea can coexist well with constipating opioids. Misoprostol (Cytotec), used commonly to protect the gastric mucosa from NSAID toxicity, is often associated with diarrhea. Since it can reverse opioid-related constipation and protect the gastrointestinal mucosa, it is a compelling addition to combination therapy with opioids and NSAIDs. However, misoprostol must be avoided in pregnant patients owing to its potential to stimulate uterine contraction.

Nausea and Vomiting

Although nausea and vomiting are seen early in some cases of opioid therapy, severe protracted nausea and vomiting due solely to opioids are rare. Opioid-related nausea and vomiting are usually transient, with tolerance to this side effect developing in 2 to 3 days. One might elect the temporary addition of antiemetics, although there are other alternatives.

Since nausea and vomiting often become less significant within several days of initiating therapy with opioids, the alternative is a reduction of the opioid dose to the minimum that produces acceptable analgesia; this step alone may prove to be all that is necessary before resuming upward titration. Alternatively, a change in the route of administration may also alleviate symptoms (e.g., IV to PR). If these simple measures fail, it may be necessary to consider opioid rotation, which requires substituting one opioid agent for an another equianalgesic opioid. It is not clear why one opioid should produce nausea and vomiting in an individual patient while another does not, or why changing to a different opioid often reduces or eliminates emetic side effects. Patients with a history of severe nausea with previous opioid treatment may benefit from pretreatment with an antiemetic or avoidance of the previous offending opioids.

Opioid-induced nausea and vomiting are thought to result from activation within the brainstem area responsible for afferent input to the emetic center termed the medullary chemoreceptor trigger zone. Effective antiemetic agents include the antihistamines (e.g., hydroxyzine), serotonin antagonists (e.g., ondansetron), dopamine antagonists (e.g., droperidol, haloperidol, and metoclopramide) and anticholinergics (e.g., scopolamine). It is not clear which of these drug classes is most effective for opioid-induced nausea and vomiting, so the choice is usually made on an empirical basis. Opioid-related nausea may be related to orthostasis or ambulation, thus possibly involving vestibular dysfunction and thus possibly best resolved with antivestubular antiemetics (i.e., antihistamines). Since the single most effective antiemetic is not always predictable, an agent may be chosen for its secondary benefits, such as its promotility, sedation, an antipruritic effect, anxiolytsis, or antipsychotic properties. Of course, other causes of nausea and vomiting, not related to opioids, must be considered. These include chemotherapy (particularly with cisplatin), radiation therapy, metastases (particularly to brain and gastrointestinal tract), increased intracranial pressure, peptic ulcer disease, esophagitis, gastritis, electrolyte and acid-base imbalance, uremia, liver disease, infection, pregnancy, fear, and anxiety.

Sedation

Opioid-related sedation is common and can indicate either excess drug or even delirium. It is usually temporary, resolving over time as patients accommodate to a new opioid drug or new dose. Reducing the opioid dose to the minimal level required for adequate analgesia is the first step to managing significant sedation. In more acute and severe cases, opioid cessation and reversal with antagonists may be necessary. Sedation that occurs late in treatment may be related to accumulation of the opioid medication or its metabolites. In such a case, resolution may occur with increasing of the dose interval or changing to a different agent. Sometimes converting a patient from a long-acting opioid to a short-acting one is necessary to avoid sedation. Also, one should consider other causes of sedation, such as other drugs that affect the central nervous system, encephalopathy, and so on. For patients with waxing and waning levels of consciousness with altered mental status, the diagnosis of delirium should be entertained. Hospitalization may be necessary with discontinuation of opioids, as well as all other medications that can cause delirium, such as antihistamines, anticholinergics, and NSAIDs (among many others). For unremitting opioid-related sedation that is not related to altered mental status, stimulants such as dextroamphetamine can reduce sedation if other therapeutic options are not successful. Dextroamphetamine 2.5 to 5.0 mg can be administered in the morning and increased on a daily basis until a satisfactory level of stimulation occurs. If the resultant stimulation is effective but short lived, another dose at noon can be added. It is best to avoid administering stimulants later in the day to avoid insomnia the following night.

Pruritus

Oral opioid–induced pruritus is uncommon. It is somewhat more common in patients treated with intravenous or intramuscular opioids and relatively frequent in patients treated with intrathecal and epidural opioids. Such effects often vary with specific agent and dose. Parenteral opioid–induced pruritus is usually mild but can rarely be moderate to severe. Tolerance to opioid-induced pruritus usually occurs quickly. Such pruritus is often localized to the face or, less often, the perineum, but it can become generalized. The mechanism of opioid-induced pruritus is not well understood. Suggested hypotheses include μ-receptor stimulation, histamine release, local excitation of dorsal horn neurons, and central migration of spinal opioids to the brainstem.

Since pruritus may be an idiosyncratic response to a certain opioid, it may respond to a change in opioid agents. Small doses of naloxone that are inadequate for reversing analgesia can be effective for opioid-related pruritus: 0.5 to 1.0 μg/kg IV q10min prn or 10 to 40 ug IV per hour as a continuous infusion (and reduce if there is evidence of decreased analgesia). A new long-acting opioid antagonist, nalmefene, permits every 6 hours administration for pruritis (and nausea and vomiting) and therefore may be less problematic if pruritus is non-remitting and a continuous infusion is deemed logistically problematic. Antihistamines may also be effective. The antipruritic efficacy of antihistamine therapy may, in part, be related to sedation and therefore nonsedating antihistamines may be less effective than the sedating antihistamines. Small dosages of propofol (10 mg IV push q10min $\times$ 2–3 dosages) are also effective for controlling some cases of intractable pruritus due to spinal opioids. At low doses, adverse effects from propofol are minimal. It is recommended, however, that administration of this sedative hypnotic be confined to a monitored setting.

Respiratory Depression

Depressed respiration is obviously one of the most serious of the opioid side effects. Tolerance to opioid-induced respiratory depression usually develops early in the course of chronic therapy, so that with long-term therapy, respiratory depression is rarely a problem. Depressed respiratory drive may occur more rapidly when oral or intravenous opioids are combined with epidural or intrathecal opioids. Likewise, combining opioids with other sedating drugs can worsen the respiratory depressant effect of the opioid. Usually, the patient first manifests sedation as a promontory sign of respiratory depression. Unfortunately, this cannot be detected during the evening hours when the patient is "sleeping." Since the respiratory depression seen after administration of epidural and intrathecal opioids occurs 12 hours or so after injection, the sign of sedation may be lost during sleep and one has to rely on more subtle indices (e.g., shallow breathing). For this reason, it is advisable to use pulse oximetry in patients in whom clinical wisdom would indictate that increased surveillance is necessary (e.g., very young or elderly patients, patients with obesity or major thoracoabdominal surgery). Significant acute respiratory depression can be managed with the opiate receptor antagonist naloxone. The doses of naloxone for treating respiratory depression is

0.1 mg IV push repeated every 10 to 15 minutes as needed. Naloxone may provide a brisk response but also has a brief duration of action that can require frequent dosing or continuous intravenous administration. It is best to monitor such patients in an intensive care unit.

Particular care must be given to the rapid administration of naloxone in a patient who has had prolonged opioid exposure, since this can precipitate an aggressive and possibly dangerous withdrawal. In special cases, particularly in a patient predisposed to alveolar fluid collections (e.g., one with congestive heart failure or adult respiratory distress syndrome), reversal of opioid actions can induce pulmonary edema, possibly as a result of reversal of opioid-induced pulmonary vascular smooth muscle relaxation.

OPIOID TOLERANCE, PHYSICAL DEPENDENCE, AND ADDICTION

Pharmacological tolerance and physical dependence are pharmacological properties of a drug and are not synonymous with addiction. Both can develop following opioid treatment. However, sustained analgesia without the interplay of tolerance is common, and a patient may remain on a stable dose indefinitely. It is not clear how much opioid exposure is needed to induce tolerance or physical dependence.

Tolerance

Tolerance occurs when a fixed dose of opioid produces decreasing analgesia so that a dose increase is required to maintain a stable effect. Tolerance usually develops to most opioid side effects, even more commonly than it develops to analgesia. Compensating for decreased analgesic efficacy in a tolerant patient requires either changing the opioid or increasing the dose. A patient who has become tolerant to one opioid drug may respond with adequate analgesia to another. This phenomenon is referred to as "lack of cross tolerance" and comes into play when opioid rotation is used. Mechanisms underlying this clinical observation are not completely understood but may relate to the differential opioid receptor affinities of different opioid agonists. Equianalgesic dosages are not necessary in the opioid-tolerant patient. When a new opioid agent is started in a tolerant patient, a one half of the equianalgesic dose can be given and the dose titrated to effective analgesia. By taking advantage of lack of cross-tolerance, it is thus possible to reduce the total amount of (equianalgesic) opioid administered.

Recent studies have demonstrated the involvement of the NMDA receptor in mechanisms of opioid tolerance.[25,28] It may be beneficial to combine an NMDA receptor antagonists with an opioid to attenuate tolerance. Such agents include dextromethorphan, memantine, amantadine, and ketamine. Appropriate ratios for such combinations for tolerance reduction have yet to be determined. Since methadone has activity at both the opioid (agonist) and the NMDA (antagonist) receptors, opioid rotation to methadone may be beneficial in instances of opioid tolerance. However, precautions must be taken when changing to methadone from another opioid, since methadone may be more potent (mg/mg) in opioid-tolerants patients than in those who are opioid naive.[29–31]

Physical Dependence and Withdrawal

Physical dependence relates to the expression of a withdrawal syndrome upon sudden drug cessation. It may reflect a biochemical adaptation from chronic exposure to a drug. Thus, duration of opioid treatment is likely a significant factor contributing to the development of opioid-related physical dependence.

Fear of opioid dependence may lead to undertreatment. However, opioid withdrawal is rarely life threatening and usually occurs with a regular progression of symptoms. Withdrawal usually begins with increased irritability, restlessness, anxiety, insomnia, yawning, sweating, rhinorrhea, and lacrimation. If allowed to progress, there may be dilated pupils, gooseflesh, tremor, chills, anorexia, muscle cramps, nausea, vomiting, abdominal pain, agitation, fever, tachycardia, and other features of heightened sympathetic activity. Laboratory data may reveal leukocytosis, ketosis, metabolic acidosis/respiratory alkalosis, and electrolyte imbalance.

The withdrawal syndrome may be seen with sudden discontinuation of an opioid or administration of an opioid antagonist. However, abrupt discontinuation of shorter acting opioids such as morphine or hydromorphone is more likely to produce withdrawal symptoms than discontinuation of agents with longer plasma half-lives, such as methadone or transdermally administered fentanyl. Slow, systematic tapering of opioids at a rate of 15% to 20% every few days can usually prevent withdrawal. Slow weaning of bedtime doses may help avoid the sleep disturbances that are often associated with opioid cessation.

Signs of sympathetic hyperactivity can be treated with sympatholytics such as clonidine and beta-blockers. However, these agents can produce their own problems. For instance, clonidine may produce hypotension or sedation and its antiwithdrawal effects may be antagonized by tricyclic antidepressants. Although the addition of clonidine can effectively blunt objective findings of sympathetic hyperactivity, it remains controversial whether clonidine or other sympatholytics increase or mask subjective symptoms of withdrawal, such as anxiety, insomnia, and restlessness. Such treatment is often begun at dosages of 10 to 20 μg/kg/day in three divided doses with subsequent adjustments to reduce signs of withdrawal while limiting hypotension. Clonidine can be maintained for 4 days for short-acting opioids and 14 days for long-acting opioids. Tapering of clonidine can then occur over 4 to 6 days.

Opioid Addiction and Pseudoaddiction

Opioid addiction is a biopsychosocial disorder characterized by compulsive use of opioids resulting in physical, psychological, and social dysfunction to the user and continued use despite that dysfunction. Opioid addiction should be distinguished from pseudoaddiction, a phenomenon that mimics signs of addiction but results from undertreatment. Whereas addiction is marked by dysfunction with the use of the drug that stimulates the disease, pseudoaddiction resolves when the drug that the patient seeks is increased and the patient notes both pain relief and improved function. There has been increased interest in rapid opioid detoxification with intravenous naloxone and general anesthesia. Such treatment offers rapid effects but is of unproven long-term value.

SUMMARY

The use of opioids for the treatment of CNMP remains controversial, and there is no universally accepted consensus on whether, when, and how opioid therapy should be administered. Clinicians who choose to offer chronic opioid therapies must formulate rational and individualized regimens according to strategies such as those described in this chapter. Safe opioid therapy requires a program for ongoing close monitoring of pain relief and possible side effects. In addition, it is important to document observable treatment endpoints. Ideally, treatment endpoints should include functional improvement as verifiable objective signs. Experience dictates that improvements in functionality are more frequently encountered when a multidisciplinary team is employed. Together with a caring medical team, many individuals with intractable pain can be helped by the judicious application of medical and cognitive and behavioral treatments.

REFERENCES FOR ADDITIONAL READING

1. Portenoy RK: Opioid therapy for chronic nonmalignant pain: A review of the critical issues. J Pain Symptom Manage 11:203, 1996.
2. Robinson RC, Gatchel RJ, Polatin P, et al: Screening for problematic prescription opioid use. Clin J Pain 17:220, 2001.
3. Pappagallo M, Heinberg LJ: Ethical issues in the management of chronic nonmalignant pain. Semin Neurol 17:203, 1997.
4. Barkin RL, Barkin D: Pharmacologic management of acute and chronic pain: Focus on drug interactions and patient-specific pharmacotherapeutic selection. South Med J 94:756, 2001.
5. Society AP: Principles of analgesic use in the treatment of acute pain and chronic cancer pain. Clin Pharm 9:601, 1990.
6. Prest VQJ: Dear Miss Nightingale: A selection of Benjamin Jowett's Letters to Florence 1860–1893. Oxford University Press, New York: 1987.
7. Bertin P: Current use of analgesics for rheumatological pain. Eur J Pain 4(Suppl A):9, 2000.
8. Watson CP: The treatment of neuropathic pain: Antidepressants and opioids. Clin J Pain 16(2 Suppl):S49, 2000.
9. Ossipov MH, Lopez Y, Nichols ML, et al: Inhibition by spinal morphine of the tail-flick response is attenuated in rats with nerve ligation injury. Neurosci Lett 199:83, 1995.
10. Mao J, Price DD, Mayer DJ: Experimental mononeuropathy reduces the antinociceptive effects of morphine: Implications for common intracellular mechanisms involved in morphine tolerance and neuropathic pain. Pain 61:353, 1995.
11. McQuay H, Moore R: An Evidence-Based Resource for Pain Relief. Oxford University Press, Oxford, 1998.
12. http://www.ampainsoc.org/advocacy/opioids.htm.
13. Portenoy RK: Current pharmacotherapy of chronic pain. J Pain Symptom Manage 19(1 Suppl):S16, 2000.
14. Reder RF: Opioid formulations: Tailoring to the needs in chronic pain. Eur J Pain 5(Suppl A):109, 2001.
15. Mercadante S, Fulfaro F: Alternatives to oral opioids for cancer pain. Oncology (Huntingt) 13:215; discussion 226, 1999.
16. Dworkin RH, Hetzel RD, Banks SM: Toward a model of the pathogenesis of chronic pain. Semin Clin Neuropsychiatry 4:176, 1999.
17. Vlaeyen JW, Crombez G: Fear of movement/(re)injury, avoidance and pain disability in chronic low back pain patients. Man Ther 4:187, 1999.
18. Feldman SI, Downey G, Schaffer-Neitz R: Pain, negative mood, and perceived support in chronic pain patients: A daily diary study of people with reflex sympathetic dystrophy syndrome. J Consult Clin Psychol 67:776, 1999.
19. Moulin DE, Iezzi A, Amireh R, et al: Randomised trial of oral morphine for chronic non-cancer pain. Lancet 347:143, 1996.
20. Kroenke K, Swindle R: Cognitive-behavioral therapy for somatization and symptom syndromes: A critical review of controlled clinical trials. Psychother Psychosom 69:205, 2000.

21. Quang-Cantagrel ND, Wallace MS, Magnuson SK: Opioid substitution to improve the effectiveness of chronic noncancer pain control: A chart review. Anesth Analg 90:933, 2000.

22. Smith MT: Neuroexcitatory effects of morphine and hydromorphone: Evidence implicating the 3-glucuronide metabolites. Clin Exp Pharmacol Physiol 27:524, 2000.

23. Gagnon B, Bruera E: Differences in the ratios of morphine to methadone in patients with neuropathic pain versus non-neuropathic pain. J Pain Symptom Manage 18:120, 1999.

24. Sang CN: NMDA-receptor antagonists in neuropathic pain: Experimental methods to clinical trials. J Pain Symptom Manage 19(1 Suppl):S21, 2000.

25. Price DD, Mayer DJ, Mao J, Caruso FS: NMDA-receptor antagonists and opioid receptor interactions as related to analgesia and tolerance. J Pain Symptom Manage 19(1 Suppl):S7, 2000.

26. Parsons CG: NMDA receptors as targets for drug action in neuropathic pain. Eur J Pharmacol 429:71, 2001.

27. Allan L, Hays H, Jensen NH, et al: Randomised crossover trial of transdermal fentanyl and sustained release oral morphine for treating chronic non-cancer pain. BMJ 322:1154, 2001.

28. Bespalov AY, Zvartau EE, Beardsley PM: Opioid-NMDA receptor interactions may clarify conditioned (associative) components of opioid analgesic tolerance. Neurosci Biobehav Rev 25:343, 2001.

29. Oneschuk D, Bruera E: Respiratory depression during methadone rotation in a patient with advanced cancer. J Palliat Care 16:50, 2000.

30. Ripamonti C, De Conno F, Groff L, et al: Equianalgesic dose/ratio between methadone and other opioid agonists in cancer pain: Comparison of two clinical experiences. Ann Oncol 9:79, 1998.

31. Bruera E, Pereira J, Watanabe S, et al: Opioid rotation in patients with cancer pain: A retrospective comparison of dose ratios between methadone, hydromorphone, and morphine. Cancer 78:852, 1996.

Chapter 11

Opioids: Adverse Effects and Their Management

Jennifer A. Elliott, MD / Susan E. Opper, MD

Opiates have been a mainstay in the management of pain for centuries. They are among the most effective known analgesics. However, the use of opiates in clinical practice is not without risk of undesired effects. Many of the undesirable effects of these agents occur as a result of their binding to the very receptors that mediate analgesia. Among the adverse effects commonly seen after opioid analgesic administration are pruritus, nausea, constipation, urinary retention, sedation, and, most fear-inspiring, respiratory depression. Some adverse effects of particular opiates are related directly to their metabolism to other active molecules that may possess neuroexcitatory effects, may have greater analgesic potency than their parent compounds, or may act to antagonize the analgesic effects of their parent compounds. Less understood at the present time is the potential for opiates to alter such things as immune function. Other phenomena, such as tolerance, physical dependence, and addiction, may also occur in the setting of opioid administration. Clinicians often poorly understand the distinction among these entities, and apprehension about the potential for their development, as well as fear of interference by governmental regulatory agencies,[1] may result in avoidance of opiate prescribing. Opioid agonist-antagonist drugs are occasionally used in pain management applications because of the perception that there may be a lower incidence of significant adverse effects or a lower likelihood of addiction to these substances, which may not in fact be true. On the other hand, opioid antagonists may provide a useful role in the management of certain opioid-induced side effects without sacrificing analgesia. In this chapter, we explore some of these issues and provide information regarding management of opioid-induced side effects.

OPIOID RECEPTORS

Four major opiate receptor types have been described. These include three classical receptors, μ, δ, and κ, and the more recently discovered nociceptin/orphanin FQ (N/OFQ), the "orphan" opioid receptor. They are found in many locations, including the brain, spinal cord, and peripheral nervous system. Each receptor has its own unique localization and function. Various receptor subtypes have been proposed (e.g., $\mu 1,2$, $\delta 1,2$ and $\kappa 1$–4)[2] (Table 1). All four receptor types are G protein–coupled receptors. Activation of opioid receptors leads to inhibition of adenyl cyclase activity. Suppression of voltage-gated calcium currents and activation of inward potassium currents then ensue.

The μ receptor is the most clinically relevant of the opioid receptor types. Both spinal and supraspinal effects promote analgesia and affect mood. Respiratory depression, sedation, and gastrointestinal inhibition are troublesome adverse effects mediated through the μ receptor. Other μ effects include physical dependence and tolerance. $\mu 1$ receptor agonism leads to

TABLE 1

Opioid Receptor Subtypes and Their Physiological Activities

Receptor type	Subtype	Effects
Mu	μ1 μ2	Supraspinal analgesia Physical dependence Euphoria Sedation Respiratory depression Constipation Orthostatic hypotension Arteriolar/venous dilation
Delta	δ1,2	Spinal analgesia Euphoria Potentiates mu receptor analgesia
Kappa	κ1,2,3	Spinal analgesia Sedation Miosis Supraspinal analgesia (K3)

Data from Jackson and Lipman[3] and Lipman and Jackson[4]

analgesia. μ2 effects are more negative, with the occurrence of respiratory and gastrointestinal suppression.

δ Receptor agonists are potent analgesics in animals, but their role in humans is less defined. These receptors are associated with endogenous opioid peptides, particularly at the spinal level. There appear to many similarities between the μ and δ receptors and fewer similarities between these receptors and the κ receptor.

The κ receptor mediates analgesia and sedation but little respiratory depression. A role for the κ receptor in visceral pain control has been described. Mice deficient in κ receptors demonstrate dramatic increases in response to visceral pain.[5] However, the commercial development of analgesic κ receptor agonists has been limited by their psychomimetic effects and dysphoria, which occur particularly at higher doses.

The novel N/OFQ receptor was cloned in 1994. It was initially called opioid-receptor-like 1 and nicknamed the "orphan" opioid receptor.[6] No binding of classic endogenous opioid peptides has been demonstrated for this receptor. Instead, its endogenous ligand has been shown to be nociceptin. Supraspinally, nociceptin is antianalgesic, reversing morphine-induced analgesia. However, its spinal action appears to be potentiation of the analgesia of intrathecal morphine. The N/OFQ receptor has many complex effects on behavior and may play a role in opiate dependence and withdrawal.

OPIOID METABOLITES

The metabolic byproducts of opioid metabolism may contribute to the side effects realized with chronic opioid administration. Certain conditions may contribute to increased levels of the various metabolites, including choice of analgesic and route of administration. Other contributing factors include hepatic induction and renal compromise. Morphine metabolism via glucuronidation occurs predominantly in the liver, but the brain and kidney may also be sites where this occurs. Glucuronides are excreted in the bile and urine. These compounds are highly polar and would not be expected to cross the blood-brain barrier easily. However, recent studies have suggested that these compounds may exist in a folded form, with masking of the polar groups facilitating brain penetrance.[7] The central nervous system (CNS) concentration of these metabolites slowly increases with chronic administration.

The major metabolites of morphine are morphine-3-glucuronide (50%) and morphine-6-glucuronide (10%) (FIGURE 1). Morphine-6-glucuronide (M6G) has very potent analgesic effects, 45 to 800 times greater than morphine when placed intrathecally, despite very similar μ1 receptor affinity.[8] M6G has less affinity for μ2 receptors and at equianalgesic doses may cause less respiratory depression in humans than morphine. Other differences include M6G's longer duration of effect and slower onset of action as compared with morphine. The analgesic effect of morphine may be attributed more to the effects of M6G than the parent compound with chronic administration. Despite the initial enthusiasm regarding the drug's clinical use as an analgesic, human studies have been inconsistent in proving the analgesic efficacy of M6G. In addition, its slow transfer into the CNS makes this compound less than an ideal analgesic for systemic administration. M6G may show more promise with intrathecal use. The half-life of M6G is increased in the setting of renal failure. In the patient

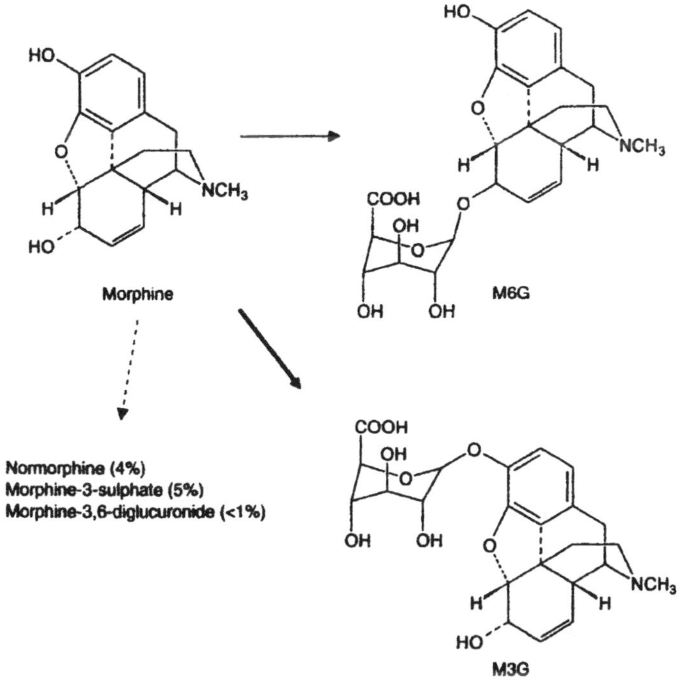

Figure 1. Major metabolites of morphine in humans The main metabolite is morphine-3-glucuronide (M3G). About 10% of morphine is metabolised to morphine-6-glucuronide (M6G). Other metabolites are normorphine, morphine sulphate and morphine-3,6-diglucuronide, probably with little clinical importance. (Reprinted with permission from Lotsch J, Geisslinger G: Morphine-6-glucuronide: An analgesic of the future? Clin Pharmacokinet 40:485, 2000.)

with normal renal function, adverse side effects from M6G are seldom seen, but if renal function is compromised, severe side effects such as unconsciousness and respiratory depression may be realized.

In contrast, morphine-3-glucuronide (M3G) is not an analgesic and shows little opioid receptor binding. M3G may actually antagonize morphine-associated analgesia and respiratory depression. Therefore, M3G may play a role in the development of tolerance. When morphine and M3G are administered together, behavioral excitation as well as allodynia and hyperesthesia have been reported. For example, rats demonstrated hyperactivity with increased exploring and grooming, shaking, and electroencephalographic (EEG) spiking with epileptiform discharges in a study in which they received high-dose morphine or M3G intracerebroventricularly.[9] Interestingly, these findings were exacerbated, rather than reversed, by the administration of opioid antagonists, lending support to a nonopioid receptor effect. M3G may be responsible for some of the adverse excitatory effects of morphine, such as myoclonus following high-dose or chronic morphine administration. Neuroexcitatory effects have also been seen after administration of large doses of hydromorphone and are attributed to hydromorphone-3-glucuronide (H3G) accumulation. The mechanism whereby M3G causes neuroexcitation is not known. Despite the fact that N-methyl-D-aspartate (NMDA) antagonism attenuates the excitatory effects of M3G, it does not appear that M3G has any affinity for NMDA receptors. Further, M3G appears to have no effect on the uptake or release of the excitatory amino acid glutamate.

In the setting of these adverse excitatory effects, it has been suggested that "opioid rotation" be undertaken, whereby a structurally dissimilar opiate such as methadone or fentanyl is substituted therapeutically for morphine or hydromorphone. This often leads to abatement of these neuroexcitatory effects with clearance of the M3G or H3G. In addition, changing from systemic to intracerebroventricular dosing will minimize M3G production, as hepatic glucuronidation is bypassed. Oral dosing leads to the greatest metabolite formation. Rectal dosing leads to significantly less hepatic transformation.[10]

Normeperidine is the major and sole active metabolite of meperidine. There may be significant accumulation of this compound in the setting of renal failure. Normeperidine has both analgesic (although less than that of meperidine) and neuroexcitatory effects. Seizures have occurred in renally compromised patients receiving meperidine, presumably due to normeperidine accumulation. Other signs and symptoms of CNS excitation due to normeperidine accumulation include delirium, restlessness, irritability, tremors, and myoclonus. These symptoms usually precede seizure activity. Normeperidine has a longer elimination half-life than meperidine (14–21 hours normally, but with renal compromise, it may be greater than 35 hours). Normeperidine accumulation may occur with large and frequent dosing. In addition, medications that induce hepatic enzymes may lead to enhanced hepatic production of normeperidine. These medications include chlorpromazine, phenytoin, and phenobarbital. Prior meperidine use may also cause hepatic enzyme induction and greater normeperidine formation. Opioid antagonists may actually worsen the neurotoxic effects of normeperidine. Use of naloxone may precipitate seizure activity. A better approach to treatment in this circumstance is to discontinue meperidine and use benzodiazepines or other anticonvulsants. Some authors have advocated that meperidine not be used for patient-controlled analgesia (PCA), particularly if high use is anticipated.

OPIOID AGONIST-ANTAGONISTS

The development of mixed agonist-antagonists occurred because of the desire to produce opioids with fewer addictive and respiratory depressant effects. These compounds do show a ceiling effect to respiratory depression, but, at the usual doses, the intensity of respiratory depression appears the same as with pure agonist medications. In addition, higher doses of the agonist-antagonist opioids have led to severe psychomimetic effects that are not reversible with naloxone. The agonist-antagonists also pose the risk of inducing withdrawal in the patient on chronic opiate therapy.

The agonist-antagonist group is a heterogeneous one, encompassing drugs that act both as agonists at the κ receptor and as antagonists at the μ receptor (the nalbuphine-like agents). Buprenorphine is unique, acting as a partial agonist at the μ receptor solely. The nalbuphine-like group includes pentazocine, butorphanol, and dezocine. All three of these drugs have lower abuse potential than the pure agonists, such as morphine. However, cases involving abuse and misuse have occurred. Table 2 gives equianalgesic doses for these agents compared with morphine.

Pentazocine was the first drug of this group to be widely used, and it is available in oral, rectal, and parenteral formulations. Adverse side effects including hallucinations, euphoria, and dysphoria have been reported in up to 20% of patients given pentazocine.[12] Potentially hazardous hemodynamic effects of this drug include increased pulmonary artery pressure and increased left ventricular work[13]; therefore, use of pentazocine is not recommended in the setting of coronary artery disease.

Butorphanol is an effective analgesic for labor pain and has been used via the epidural route for postoperative pain. However, significant respiratory depression of greater duration than from morphine has been reported with epidural administration of this agent.[14] No oral form of butorphanol is available, and there is a high incidence of drowsiness and sedation with this opioid. Nasal butorphanol has been used for the treatment of severe headaches.[15] Some concern regarding its abuse prompted its rescheduling to Schedule IV of the Controlled Substances Act.

Nalbuphine has shown less reliable analgesia when compared with morphine.[16] Fewer side effects of the excitatory nature are seen, and less constipation and nausea are experienced with nalbuphine as compared with morphine. However, inadequate analgesia limits its usefulness.

TABLE 2

Dosing of Opioid Agonist-Antagonists*

Drug	Dose (mg)
Pentazocine	30–60
Butorphanol	1–3
Nalbuphine	12
Dezocine	10
Buprenorphine	0.2–0.3
Meptazinol	100

*Equivalent analgesic doses, based on single parenteral doses relative to morphine 10 mg intramuscularly or subcutaneously (Reprinted with permission from Lippman M, Mok MS: Epidural butorphanol for the relief of postoperative pain. Anesth Analg 67:418,1988.)

Dezocine is equipotent to the analgesic effect of morphine, with a more rapid onset and shorter duration.[17] The incidence of adverse effects does not appear to be problematic, with fewer psychomimetic reactions and little nausea and vomiting. The analgesic effect of dezocine appears superior to that of butorphanol. The principal adverse effect of its use is drowsiness. No oral form is available; therefore, dezocine has not proved useful for chronic pain.

Buprenorphine is unique and may show the most promise of this class of opioids. A partial agonist with lower intrinsic activity than morphine, its action at the μ receptor exhibits a ceiling effect. The antinociceptive activity curve is actually bell-shaped, with increasing doses resulting in a paradoxical reduction in antinociception (FIGURE 2).[18] The oral formulation shows poor analgesia due to presystemic elimination. Buprenorphine has a long duration of analgesia, 6 to 9 hours, because of a slow dissociation from the receptor. Because of this high affinity, naloxone may not easily reverse respiratory depression caused by this agent. For this reason, buprenorphine is not recommended for labor analgesia. Respiratory stimulants, such as doxapram, may be more effective in reversing the respiratory depressant effects of buprenorphine. A sublingual form of buprenorphine is available, but its use in treating chronic pain is limited because of adverse side effects of dizziness, nausea, and drowsiness, as well as inadequate pain relief. However, constipation is much less of a problem.[19] Because of its long duration, lack of receptor antagonist effects, and absence of the effect of euphoria, buprenorphine may prove useful as an alternative to methadone in the treatment of heroin dependence. Currently, it is a therapeutic option for withdrawal in Australia and France.[20]

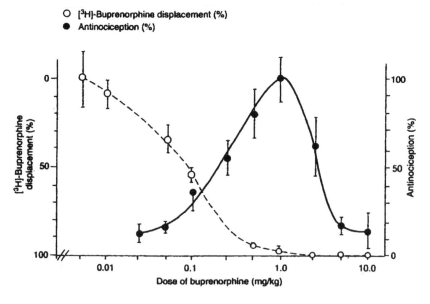

Figure 2. Dose-response curve for antinociception utilizing buprenorphine. (Reprinted with permission from Dum JE, Herg A: In vivo receptor binding of the opiate partial agonist, buprenorphine, correlated with its agonistic and antagonistic actions. Br J Pharmacol 74:627, 1981.)

COMMON OPIOID-INDUCED SIDE EFFECTS AND THEIR MANAGEMENT

Side effects induced by opioid administration can range from relatively minor annoyances such as itching to life-threatening respiratory depression. Common adverse effects in clinical practice include pruritis, nausea and vomiting, constipation, and sedation. These adverse effects may occasionally limit opioid administration when they become severe. Certainly, one of the most effective things that can be done to achieve decreased adverse effects of these agents is to reduce the opiate dose. There are several ways to effect dose reduction. The addition of adjuvants for pain control can be very helpful. Some of the most commonly employed adjuvants are non-steroidal anti-inflammatory drugs (NSAIDs), acetaminophen, α_2-agonists, local anesthetics, NMDA antagonists, and medications that are effective for neuropathic pain such as tricyclic antidepressants and anticonvulsants. Physical modalities such as transcutaneous electrical nerve stimulation may also be beneficial. As with any condition, the treatments selected must be tailored to the individual's particular pain problem and to his or her coexisting morbidities.

It is not uncommon for hospitalized patients receiving intermittent opiate boluses intravenously or intramuscularly to experience nausea and vomiting or sedation followed by inadequate analgesia several hours later. These patients may benefit from use of patient-controlled analgesia (PCA), which will allow for smaller doses at a greater frequency. PCA may help to limit the peak-and-trough effect of bolus dose administration and allow for more consistent blood concentrations that remain in the therapeutic range rather than at supratherapeutic (which often results in nausea and vomiting or other side effects) or subtherapeutic (resulting in inadequate analgesia) levels (FIGURE 3).[21] One may even find that

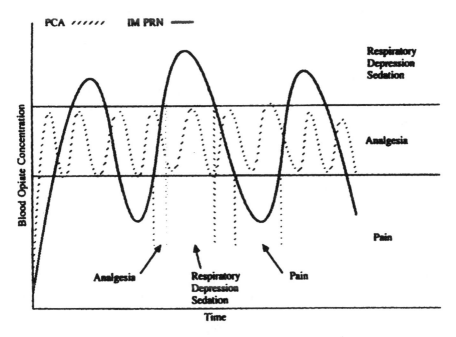

Figure 3. Comparison between intramuscular as-needed analgesia and patient-controlled analgesia. (Reprinted with permission from Ashburn M, Smith K: The management of postoperative pain. Surg Rounds 14:129, 1991.)

lower total doses of the opiate analgesic may be needed by this approach as opposed to the bolus dose approach, as the patient is better able to modulate the amount of medication needed to achieve the desired level of analgesia without side effects. Occasionally, when a patient cannot tolerate a particular opiate, switching to an alternate opiate may allow for improved tolerability.[22]

Other therapies, such as the use of opioid antagonists or agonist/antagonists, have been explored as a means of managing opioid-induced side effects. One of the primary applications of opioid antagonists seems to be in the management of opioid-associated constipation, which is discussed in detail later in this chapter. These agents have also been used in the treatment of other adverse effects of opioid therapy, however. One study compared the use of intravenous nalbuphine (a κ agonist/μ antagonist) 60 μg/kg/hr to naloxone (a pure opioid antagonist) 2 μg/kg/hr or placebo infusion in the management of side effects from epidurally administered morphine in 75 postoperative total abdominal hysterectomy patients. It was found that the incidence of nausea and vomiting and pruritis was highest in the placebo group, whereas the requirement for analgesic rescue was highest in the naloxone-treated group. The patients who received nalbuphine in conjunction with their epidural morphine therapy experienced fewer opioid-associated side effects and had a similar rescue analgesic usage pattern to that seen in the placebo-treated group. This suggests a potential role for systemic opioid agonist/antagonist therapy to manage anticipated adverse effects from epidurally administered opioids.[24]

Pruritus

It is not clear why itching occurs after opioid administration. Pruritus may occur with the use of both opiates that induce significant histamine release and those that do not and therefore is probably not completely related to this phenomenon. However, antihistaminics are often used for the treatment of this complaint, with some relief. Diphenhydramine is perhaps the most commonly used of these agents, but newer histamine-blocking agents are also employed. It has been postulated that itching may be a central effect induced by opioid binding in the medulla and spinal cord.[25] This may explain the higher incidence of itching seen after intraspinal opioid administration than with systemic administration.[26] Low doses of opioid antagonists (e.g., commonly 10–40 μg naloxone) are often used for rescue when itching becomes intolerable. This does not typically result in appreciable decreases in analgesia. Small doses of the anesthetic induction agent, propofol, have also been used in patients suffering opiate-induced pruritus[27] or nausea and vomiting,[28] particularly after intraspinal administration of the opioids, with some benefit.

Nausea and Vomiting

Nausea and vomiting are very common after opiate administration. These side effects appear to be related to stimulation of receptors in the chemoreceptor trigger zone in the medulla. A number of agents that act on receptors in the chemoreceptor trigger zone can be used to combat opioid-induced nausea and vomiting. These agents include $5HT_3$ receptor antagonists (e.g., ondansetron, dolasetron), dopamine receptor antagonists (e.g., metoclopramide, phenothiazines such as promethazine), muscarinic receptor antagonists (e.g., scopolamine), cannabinoid receptor agonists (e.g., dronabinol), and H_1 receptor antagonists (e.g., diphenhydramine).[29]

Sedation

Sedation may occur during opiate therapy, particularly when high-dose opiates are employed, as in the treatment of rapidly accelerating cancer-associated pain. It may also be seen in the postoperative period, when patients are in pain but still have some residual anesthetic that can accentuate the sedation seen after opioid administration. Several studies have evaluated the use of amphetamines as adjuncts to opiate therapy in these circumstances. In one study involving cancer pain patients, the use of methylphenidate was found to result in lower levels of sedation associated with opioid use. Additionally, patients receiving methylphenidate along with their opioids required fewer doses of opioid for breakthrough pain than those receiving placebo, suggesting enhanced analgesic potency of this combination as compared with opioids alone.[30] Another study in postoperative patients using a combination of morphine with dextroamphetamine versus placebo revealed that patients receiving combination opioid/amphetamine therapy had a lower incidence of sleepiness. Interestingly, the investigators also found that the addition of 10 mg of dextroamphetamine appeared to provide a degree of analgesia equivalent to that achieved with twice the actual morphine dose (e.g., administration of 6 mg of morphine with 10 mg dextroamphetamine appeared to result in the same degree of analgesia seen when 12 mg of morphine alone was given.)[31] Thus, amphetamines may not only act to combat the sedative side effects of opioid therapy but may also, in fact, enhance the analgesic effects of such treatment. Newer nonamphetamine stimulant agents, such as modafinil, are also available for treatment of opioid-associated sedation. It is unclear whether modafinil enhances the analgesic effects of opioid therapy.

Respiratory Depression

Respiratory depression is the most dreaded potential complication of opiate administration. Fear of this complication often results in underdosing, particularly by inexperienced practitioners dealing with opioid-tolerant individuals. Other signs of opioid toxicity, such as sedation, usually precede the onset of respiratory depression. Opioids reduce brainstem respiratory center responsiveness to CO_2 and thereby can depress respiratory drive. The respiratory pattern in opioid toxicity is typically that of a slowed respiratory rate, which may progress to frank apnea. In cases of significant opioid-induced respiratory depression, immediate treatment with an opiate antagonist is indicated. This typically would involve administration of naloxone, 0.4 to 2 mg every 2 minutes, up to 10 mg in 10 minutes.[32] Such therapy should be reserved only for cases of true emergencies related to opioid-induced respiratory depression, in which the individual's life is at risk. The use of naloxone may precipitate acute opioid withdrawal in individuals tolerant to opiates. It also will reverse the analgesia afforded by opiates, which can precipitate a pain crisis that is difficult to manage, as in the postoperative patient. In the patient with underlying cardiac disease, the resultant increases in heart rate and blood pressure can create acute coronary ischemia. Pulmonary edema can also occur after administration of naloxone.[33] It must also be remembered that the duration of action of most opiates will outlast the duration of a single bolus of naloxone, which may result in delayed onset of recurrent respiratory depression many hours later. This can have unfortunate consequences if not anticipated, and any patient at risk for such recurrent respiratory depression is probably best served by being placed in a monitored setting and being given a continuous naloxone infusion. In situations in which the degree of respiratory depression is mild, small aliquots of naloxone can be used judiciously such that the adverse effects associated with naloxone administration are avoided.

Constipation

Constipation is one side effect of opiate therapy that patients do not tend to develop a tolerance to over time. Traditionally, prevention and management of opiate-induced constipation has been with the use of stool softeners and with bulk and stimulant laxatives. Recent studies have been conducted to evaluate the usefulness of intravenous and oral opioid antagonist therapy for this common problem. The agents studied have included naloxone, methylnaltrexone, and ADL 8-2698, an investigational opioid antagonist. Naloxone given orally seems to reduce opioid-induced constipation. Typically, doses of 2 to 4 mg are given up to three times per day to start. In one study of patients on chronic opioid therapy who were given naloxone orally, investigators found that adequate laxation was achieved at a mean daily dose of 17.5 mg of naloxone. A small number of patients studied developed some signs and symptoms of opioid withdrawal during oral naloxone administration, typically at doses ranging from 6 to 20 mg. Twenty-two patients were initially enrolled in this study, with only one patient failing to complete the study due to severe symptoms of opioid withdrawal. Of the 17 patients who ultimately completed the study, 4 experienced mild to moderate symptoms of withdrawal.[34] Another study using oral naloxone versus placebo in nine patients on chronic opiate therapy found that while all the patients using oral naloxone had improvement of their constipation, several also experienced significant symptoms of opioid withdrawal and reversal of analgesia. The doses of naloxone used in this study ranged from 2 to 4 mg three times daily.[35] Both studies involved only a small population of subjects, but it appears that the results are somewhat discrepant with regard to the frequency of significant systemic opioid antagonist effects from administration of oral naloxone. However, it does appear from both studies that there is, in fact, some potential for this to occur.

Methylnaltrexone, a derivative of naltrexone, is another opioid antagonist that has been studied for management of opioid-induced constipation. It is a peripherally restricted opioid antagonist that does not cross the blood-brain barrier. A pilot study of four chronic methadone maintenance patients given intravenous methylnaltrexone for opioid-induced constipation revealed that all four subjects had a laxation response shortly after administration of the drug. One subject, who had received a dose of 0.45 mg/kg of methylnaltrexone, had to be withdrawn from the study because of protracted severe abdominal cramping following its administration. Another subject who received this same dose did not experience significant adverse effect after its administration. The other two subjects received lower doses of methylnaltrexone (up to 0.15 mg/kg), with laxation and no adverse affects. None of the subjects in the study exhibited evidence of opioid withdrawal.[36] Thus, methylnaltrexone offers potential promise in the management of opioid-associated constipation without risk of systemic opioid withdrawal.

Likewise, the investigational compound ADL 8-2698 may provide benefit for management of opioid-associated constipation without risk of reversal of systemic opioid effects. Like methylnaltrexone, ADL 8-2698 is a peripherally restricted opioid antagonist that does not cross the blood-brain barrier and is poorly absorbed after oral administration. Studies have been performed to evaluate the effects of ADL 8-2698 on gastrointestinal transit time in healthy volunteers given morphine. Fourteen subjects were given three combinations of drugs consisting of oral placebo/intravenous saline, oral placebo/intravenous morphine, and oral ADL 8-2698/intravenous morphine. It was found that morphine administration resulted in increases in gastrointestinal transit time, which were prevented by administration of ADL 8-2698. A second group of subjects undergoing molar extraction was employed to evaluate whether ADL 8-2598 administration diminishes the analgesic effects of morphine when these drugs are given concomitantly. Forty-five subjects were given combinations of oral ADL 8-2698 (4 mg)/intravenous morphine (0.15 mg/kg), oral placebo/intravenous morphine (0.15 mg/kg), or oral placebo/intravenous saline. It was found that the visual analog pain scores were higher in the group receiving intravenous saline than in the groups receiving morphine plus oral placebo or morphine plus oral ADL 8-2698. It appeared that there was no significant difference in visual analog pain scores among subjects in the groups receiving morphine with or without ADL 8-2698.[37] Further study of ADL 8-2698 in 78 patients undergoing partial colectomy or hysterectomy procedures suggests that this compound may provide benefit in the management of postoperative ileus, with earlier return of bowel function, and consequently reduced length of hospital stay versus patients receiving conventional postoperative care.[38,39] It therefore appears that future management of refractory severe opioid-associated gastrointestinal effects may be afforded with the use of methylnaltrexone and ADL 8-2698 without the risk of systemic opioid withdrawal or reversal of analgesia, which will undoubtedly enhance the quality of life of many individuals on chronic, and even acute, opioid therapy.

Immune Effects

A complex interaction exists between the nervous and immune systems. The central nervous system's effects on lymphoid tissue and immune cells modulate the immune system. In turn, immune cells play a role in endogenous opioid secretion. Activated memory-T lymphocytes secrete a variety of opioids, including β-endorphin, enkephalin, and small amounts of dynorphin. Peripheral opioid receptors in the tissues are up-regulated during inflammation. The secretion of localized analgesic opioids by the immune cells may act as a first line of analgesic defense.

Analgesia, or its lack thereof, may contribute to immune function. Several studies have highlighted the relationship between perioperative pain relief and improvement in immune function. Page and Ben-Eliyahu[40] demonstrated that cancer surgery performed without morphine analgesia led to increased retention of cancer cells and a greater number of metastases. Some cancer cells possess membrane receptors for opioids. Opioid agonists, including morphine and methadone, have been found to suppress the growth of lung cancer cells in vitro. Programmed cell death, or apoptosis, of human lung cancer cells was increased following opiate exposure.[41]

However, some controversy exists between the relationship of opiate analgesia and immune function. Recently introduced studies in both animals and humans have shown that morphine, particularly in high doses, may be immunosuppressive. It has been postulated that morphine may alter the resistance of an organism to infection. Various effects of opioids on immune cells include suppression of B lymphocyte antibody production and suppression of natural killer cell activity.[42] Opioids may play a detrimental role in combating infection. High doses of morphine (25 mg/kg) in rats led to increased death following *C. albicans* infection.[43] Although many studies have questioned whether chronic administration of morphine has any effect on immune function, Carpenter and colleagues[44] demonstrated that chronic administration of morphine in swine led to an increased incidence of herpes virus infection. In vitro studies have demonstrated that morphine does increase the rate of HIV-1 replication and modifies the host response to parasitic infections.[45]

The μ receptor appears to play a significant role in the adverse immunological effects of opioids. In one study, chronic morphine administration in wild-type mice led to lymphoid atrophy and decreased natural killer activity. However, in μ receptor–deficient mice, these effects were not observed. Interestingly, the central administration of the specific δ-receptor agonist DPDPE led to increased natural killer cell activity.[46] There appears to be a great deal of evidence for a central effect of opiates on immune function. A supraspinal rather than a spinal mechanism appears likely.

Other Adverse Effects of Opioid Administration

Some of the more common and more frightening adverse effects of opioid therapy have been described in detail, but a few other less common adverse effects deserve mention. Urinary retention is not a frequently observed consequence of systemic opioid administration, but it is seen with some regularity after epidural or intrathecal opioid administration, particularly in young men. This effect may persist for hours after dosing of the opioid and may be reversed with the use of naloxone.[47] Hearing loss has been reported with both licit and illicit use of opioids. In particular, heroin[48] and hydrocodone[49] abuse have been reported to result in the development of profound hearing loss, which may or may not be reversible in particular individuals. It must be emphasized that the cases of reported hearing loss associated with hydrocodone were in individuals using hydrocodone/acetaminophen in doses that exceeded the maximum recommended daily Tylenol consumption.

TOLERANCE, PHYSICAL DEPENDENCE, AND ADDICTION

Tolerance

Tolerance occurs with the use of many common drugs. It is defined as the reduction in response to a drug after repeated administration, resulting in the need for higher doses of the drug over time to produce effects previously achieved at lower doses.[50] Tolerance to various effects of a drug may occur after variable lengths of exposure to that drug. For example, tolerance to the euphoric effects of opiates may occur early in the course of their use, whereas it is known that the constipating effects of opiates tend to persist after long-term use of these drugs (i.e., there is little development of tolerance to these effects). Tolerance to other effects of opiate use, such as sedation, respiratory depression, and nausea and vomiting, tends to occur at an intermediate duration of exposure as compared with euphoria and constipation. As with these generally undesirable effects of opiate use, tolerance to the pain-relieving effects of opiates also occurs with time. Tolerance thus explains why habitual heroin users escalate their drug use over time. It also explains why some patients require dose escalation during the course of their pain treatment. In many chronic, stable pain states, however, the requirement for dose escalation may not be seen for extended periods of time. In patients with dynamic causes of pain, such as rapidly growing cancer, dose escalation may represent progression of the underlying disease process rather than the development of tolerance.

The development of tolerance may have several causes. Some drugs may induce an increase in the rate of their own metabolism via liver enzyme activation after repeated exposure, which is commonly seen with the use of drugs such as barbiturates. Exposure to other drugs over extended periods may result changes in receptor density or in signal transduction/receptor linked second messenger systems that cause decreased apparent effectiveness of the drug.[51] This is presumed to be the mechanism by which opioid tolerance develops. It is also thought that the development of tolerance to opioids may be associated with NMDA receptor activation, and that use of NMDA receptor antagonists in conjunction with opioid administration may delay or prohibit the development of tolerance.[52] Other agents such as nimodipine, a dihydropyridine calcium channel blocker, may also offer benefit in delaying the onset of opioid tolerance in certain individuals. The use of nimodipine 120 mg in daily divided doses was found to have efficacy in reducing opioid dose escalation and resulted in some decreases in opioid requirements in a study involving cancer pain patients.[53]

One phenomenon that has been seen in individuals exposed to opioids over time is that of hyperalgesia, or lowered threshold for painful stimulation. Investigators have found that the actions of opioids occur via G-protein linked receptors. It appears that two subtypes of these G-protein linked receptors exert the actions of opioid agonists (FIGURE 4). The clinical effects of antinociception afforded by opioid administration occur via activation of an inhibitory G-protein linked receptor. Activation of this receptor results in decreases in cyclic AMP production, with attendant alteration in K^+ and Ca^{2+} conductance. This in turn causes diminution in the action potential duration within the dorsal root ganglion and thereby causes decreased neurotransmitter release, resulting in clinical analgesic effects. At the same

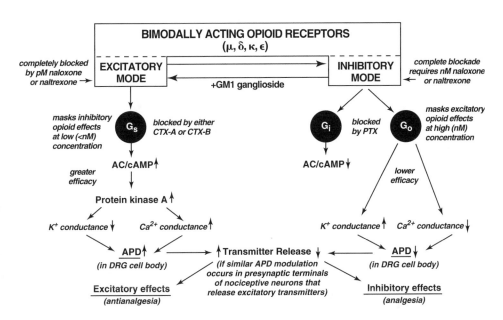

Figure 4. Stimulatory and inhibitor G-protein linked opioid receptors. AC = adenyl cyclase; cAMP = cyclic AMP; CTX = cholera toxin; PTX = pertussis toxin; APD = action potential duration; DRG = dorsal root ganglion; pM = picomolar; nM = nanomolar. (Reprinted with permission from Crain SM, Shen KF: GM1 ganglioside-induced modulation of opioid receptor-mediated functions. Ann NY Acad Sci 845:106, 1998.)

time, however, a stimulatory G-protein linked receptor is activated by the presence of opioid agonists. It is this receptor that appears to be responsible for the antianalgesic or hyperalgesic effects of opioid administration. This excitatory wing of the opioid receptor activation pathway is also thought to play a role in the development of tolerance/dependence seen during long-term opioid administration (FIGURE 5). The use of low doses of the opioid antagonists naloxone and naltrexone to block the activation of the excitatory opioid receptor has been evaluated. It appears that 1000-fold lower doses of these agents are required to block the function of the excitatory (antianalgesic) than the inhibitory (analgesic) pathway.[54] This mechanism may explain the finding that coadministration of low doses of an opioid antagonist with an opioid agonist enhances the analgesic potency of the opioid agonist, as noted in this study.

Cross-Tolerance

Cross-tolerance is another issue commonly encountered during the clinical use of opiates. Higher doses (as compared with those used in opioid-naive individuals) are often required in opioid-tolerant patients, even after switching from the opioid they have been chronically

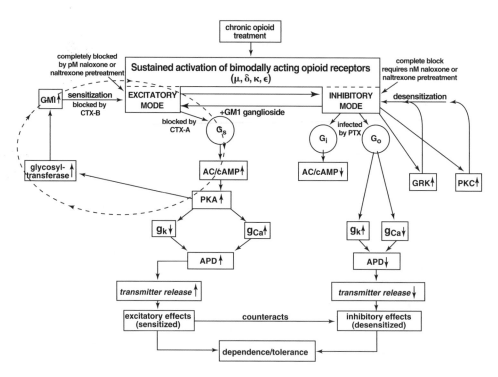

Figure 5. G-protein linked opioid receptors and the development of tolerance. AC = adenyl cyclase; cAMP = cyclic AMP; PKA = protein kinase A; GRK = G-protein-coupled receptor kinases; PKC = protein kinase C: CTX = cholera toxin; PTX = pertussis toxin; APD = action potential duration; g_{Ca} = calcium conductance; g_k = potassium conductance. (Reprinted with permission from Crain SM, Shen KF: Modulation of opioid analgesia, tolerance and dependence by GS-coupled GM1 ganglioside-regulated opioid receptor functions. Trends Pharmacol Sci 19:358, 1998.)

using to an alternate opioid formulation. Many practitioners believe that there may not be complete cross-tolerance among all opiates, and therefore most will factor in a dose reduction when converting a patient from one opiate to another.

Physical Dependence

Physical dependence is closely linked with the onset of tolerance. It is a normal consequence of repeated exposure to opiates over time, typically occurring after use of these agents for more than 1 week. Physical dependence is associated with the development of an abstinence or withdrawal syndrome upon abrupt drug discontinuation, rapid dose reduction, or drug antagonist administration. Withdrawal from opiates manifests with several recognizable symptoms, including mydriasis, tachycardia, sweating, restlessness, nausea and vomiting, dysphoria, yawning, and fever. It is not life-threatening and may manifest 6 to 12 hours after cessation of short-acting opiate preparations, or as long as 72 to 84 hours after discontinuation of long-acting preparations such as methadone.[51] Withdrawal can be managed by reintroducing an opiate, and the intensity of the withdrawal symptoms may be attenuated with the use of α_2-agonists such as clonidine.[55]

Addiction

Addiction, as defined by the Diagnostic and Statistical Manual of Mental Disorders (DSM-IV), is "a maladaptive pattern of substance use leading to clinically significant impairment or distress."[56] The American Society of Addiction Medicine further defines addiction in the setting of opioid therapy for pain management to include "adverse consequences associated with the use of opioids; loss of control over the use of opioids; and preoccupation with obtaining opioids, despite the presence of adequate analgesia."[57] This includes compulsive use, use despite harm, and craving. Behaviors that can be seen in the opioid addicted patient in the pain clinic include requests for early refills of opioid prescriptions, obtaining prescriptions from multiple sources, use of opioids from nonsanctioned sources (e.g., a relative's prescription, obtaining opioids on the street), and noncompliance with nonopioid components of therapy. An extensive list of behaviors, which may be more or less predictive of problematic drug use, has been established by Portenoy[58] (TABLE 3). The issue of addiction is often misunderstood by clinicians, as some practitioners mistakenly consider opioid tolerance or dependence to indicate addiction. However, as discussed earlier, tolerance and physical dependence are normal physiological responses to long-term opioid exposure, whereas addiction is an aberrant pattern of behavior involving compulsive and harmful drug use. Addiction in the pain patient population is reported to be quite rare,[59] yet fear of this problem often results in withholding of opioid therapy on the part of the physicians. Several screening tools may be used to help clinicians determine whether candidates for opioid maintenance are at risk for addictive behaviors. The Minnesota Multiaxial Personality Inventory (MMPI), which includes scales that may predict risk, and the Structured Clinical Interview for the DSM-IV are among the tools available for this purpose.[60] It may therefore be of value to request a psychological consultation prior to initiation of long-term opioid therapy to help establish whether treatment might be complicated by problems of addiction, although this approach is not foolproof. It also may be useful to set specific guidelines with patients selected for long-term opioid therapy, which

TABLE 3
Portenoy's Predictive Factors for Problematic Drug Use

Probably more predictive
  Selling prescription drugs
  Prescription forgery
  Stealing or "borrowing" drugs from others
  Injecting oral formulations
  Obtaining prescription drugs from nonmedical sources
  Concurrent abuse of alcohol or illicit drugs
  Multiple dose escalations or other noncompliance with therapy despite warnings
  Multiple episodes of prescription "loss"
  Repeatedly seeking prescriptions from other clinicians or emergency rooms without informing prescriber or after warning to desist
  Evidence of deterioration in the ability to function at work, in the family, or in social settings, that appears to be related to drug use
  Repeated resistance to changes in therapy despite clear evidence of adverse physical or psychological effects from the drug
Probably less predictive
  Aggressive complaining about the need for more drug
  Drug hoarding during periods of reduced symptoms
  Requesting specific drugs
  Openly acquiring similar drugs from other medical sources
  Unsanctioned dose escalation or other noncompliance with therapy on one or two occasions
  Unapproved use of the drug to treat other symptoms
  Reporting psychic effects not intended by the clinician
  Resistance to a change in therapy associated with "tolerable" adverse effects, with expressions of anxiety related to the return of severe symptoms

Reprinted with permission from Portenoy RK: Opioid therapy for chronic nonmalignant pain: A review of critical issues. J Pain Symptom Manage 11:203, 1996.

can be achieved through the use of an opioid "contract," listing parameters of behavior that will not be permitted during the course of opioid maintenance.

Pseudoaddiction

The term *pseudoaddiction* has been coined to describe specific behaviors, which resemble addictive behaviors, in individuals who experience inadequate pain management. This condition often manifests when inappropriate doses or dosing intervals are established, which may be particularly common in opioid-tolerant individuals. Pseudoaddiction evolves in a characteristic pattern. It arises when the patient has been offered inadequate analgesia and subsequently demands higher doses or more frequent dose administration. The patient may display overt pain behaviors in an effort to obtain additional analgesia. This is often followed by resistance to dose escalation on behalf of members of the health care team, who may interpret these behaviors as indicating addiction. It culminates in a crisis of mistrust, in which the patient feels angry and isolated, while members of the health care team feel frustrated and tend to avoid interaction with the patient.[61] The key difference between pseudoaddiction and true addiction is the resolution of "drug seeking" and overt pain behaviors in the former after adequate analgesia has been established. This issue is of particular importance in the cancer pain population, in which rapid dose escalation may be required to overcome the pain of a rapidly growing tumor. Care must be taken not to attribute dose escalation to addiction in such a setting.

CONCLUSION

Opioids have provided humankind with a means of controlling severe pain; however, their use is not without risk of significant adverse effects. More is becoming known about opioid receptor subtype function, and hopefully this information will help us develop opioid agonists with fewer unintended side effects and lower abuse liability in the future. For the time being, physicians who utilize opioids in the management of pain must be cognizant of the potential adverse effects these agents may produce, including pruritus, nausea and vomiting, sedation, constipation, and, most feared, respiratory depression. Additionally, opioid selection should be made with knowledge of the potential for metabolic byproducts of these agents to cause harm in certain patient populations. Lastly, a thorough understanding of the concepts of tolerance, physical dependence, and addiction and their differentiation from one another is necessary to avoid inappropriately withholding treatment from those patients who are in greatest need of alleviation from suffering.

REFERENCES FOR ADDITIONAL READING

1. Zenz M, Willweber-Strumpf A: Opiophobia and cancer pain in Europe. Lancet 341:1075, 1993.
2. Pasternak GW: Pharmacological mechanisms of opioid analgesics. Clin Neuropharmacol 16:1, 1993.
3. Jackson KC II, Lipman AG: Opioid analgesics. In: Tollison CD, Satterthwaite JR, Tollison JW, eds. Practical Pain Management, 3rd ed. Lippincott Williams & Wilkins, Philadelphia, 2002.
4. Lipman AG, Jackson KC: Opioids. In: Warfield C, Bajwa Z, eds. Principles and Practice of Pain Management, 2nd ed. New York: Mcgraw-Hill (to be published).
5. Black D, Trevethick M: The kappa opioid receptor is associated with the perception of visceral pain. Gut 43:312, 1998.
6. Darland T, Grandy DK: The orphanin FQ system: An emerging target for the management of pain? Br J Anaesth 81:29, 1998.
7. Carrupt P-A, Testa B, Bechalany A, et al: Morphine-6-glucuronide and morphine-3-glucuronide as molecular chameleons with unexpected lipophilicity. J Med Chem 34:1272, 1991.
8. Christup LL: Morphine metabolites. Acta Anaesthesiol Scand 41:116, 1997.
9. Labella FS, Pinsky C, Havlicek V: Morphine derivatives with diminished opiate receptor potency show enhanced central excitatory activity. Brain Res 172;263, 1979.
10. Babul N, Darke AC: Disposition of morphine and its glucuronide metabolites after oral and rectal administration: Evidence of route specificity. Clin Pharmacol Ther 54:286, 1993.
11. Mchugh GJ: Norpethidine accumulation and generalized seizure during pethidine patient-controlled analgesia. Anaesth Intensive Care 27:289, 1999.
12. Taylor M, Galloway DB, Petrie JC, et al: Psychomimetic effects of pentazocine and dihydrocodeine tartrate. BMJ 2:1198, 1978.
13. Alderman EL, Barry WH, Graham AF, Harrison DC: Haemodynamic effects of morphine and pentazocine differ in cardiac patients. N Engl J Med 287:623, 1972.
14. Lippman M, Mok MS: Epidural butorphanol for the relief of postoperative pain. Anesth Analg 67:418, 1988.
15. Bowdle TA, Galer BS: Agonist-antagonist and partial agonist opioids: Pharmacologic mechanisms and clinical application in the treatment of headache. Headache Q 4:322, 1993.
16. Brady MM, Furness G, Fee JPH: A comparison of the analgesic and sedative effects of nalbuphine and morphine following hip replacement. B J Anaesth 58:1332, 1986.
17. Hoskin PJ, Hanks GW: Opioid agonist-antagonist drugs in acute and chronic pain states. Drugs 41:326, 1991.
18. Bowdle TA: Adverse effects of opioid agonists and agonist-antagonists in anaesthesia. Drug Safety 19:173, 1998.

19. Adriaensen H, Mattelaer B, Van Meenen H: A long term clinical and pharmacokinetic assessment of sublingual buprenorphine in patients suffering from chronic pain. Acta Anaesthesiol Belg 1:33, 1985.

20. Wodak A, Hall WD: Buprenorphine: Better late than never. MJA 175:349, 2001.

21. Graves DA, Foster TS, Batenhorst RL, et al: Patient-controlled analgesia. Ann Intern Med 99:360, 1983.

22. Galer BS, Coyle N, Pasternak GW, Portenoy RK: Individual variability in the response to different opioids: Report of five cases. Pain 49:87, 1992.

23. Ashburn MA, Ready LB: Postoperative pain. In: Loeser J, ed. Bonica's Management of Pain, 3rd ed. Lippincott Williams & Wilkins, Philadelphia, 2001.

24. Wang JJ, Ho ST, Tzeng JI: Comparison of intravenous nalbuphine infusion versus naloxone in the prevention of epidural morphine-related side effects. Regional Anesth Pain Med 23:479, 1998.

25. Thomas DA, Williams GM, Iwata K, et al: Multiple effects of morphine on facial scratching in monkeys. Anesth Analg 77:933, 1993.

26. Ballantyne JC, Loach AB, Carr DB: Itching after epidural and spinal opiates. Pain 33:149, 1988.

27. Borgeat A, Wilder-Smith OHG, Saiah M, Rifat K: Subhypnotic doses of propofol relieve pruritis induced by epidural and intrathecal morphine. Anesthesiology 76:510, 1992.

28. Torn K, Tuominen P, Tarkkila P, Lindgren L: Effects of sub-hypnotic doses of propofol on the side effects of intrathecal morphine. Br J Anaesth 73:411, 1994.

29. Pasricha PJ: Prokinetic agents, antiemetic agents, and agents used in irritable bowel syndrome. In: Goodman and Gilman's Pharmacologic Basis of Therapeutics, 10th ed. McGraw-Hill, New York, 2001, pp 1021–1058.

30. Bruera E, Chadwick S, Brenneis C, et al: Methylphenidate associated with narcotics for the treatment of cancer pain. Cancer Treatment Rep 71:67, 1987.

31. Forrest WH, Brown BW, Brown CR, et al: Dextroamphetamine with morphine for the treatment of postoperative pain. N Engl J Med 296:712, 1977.

32. Hazinski MF, Cummins RO, Field JM, eds. Handbook of Emergency Cardiovascular Care for Healthcare Providers. American Heart Association, 2000.

33. Flacke JW, Flacke WE, Williams GD: Acute pulmonary edema following naloxone reversal of high-dose morphine anesthesia. Anesthesiology 47:376, 1977.

34. Meissner W, Schmidt U, Hartmann M, et al: Oral naloxone reverses opioid-associated constipation. Pain 84:105, 2000.

35. Liu M, Wittbrodt E: Low dose oral naloxone reverses opioid-induced constipation and analgesia. J Pain Sympt Manage 23:48, 2000.

36. Yuan CS, Foss JF, O'Connor M, et al: Effects of intravenous methylnaltrexone on opioid-induced gut motility and transit time changes in subjects receiving chronic methadone therapy: A pilot study. Pain 83:631, 1999.

37. Liu SS, Hodgson PS, Carpenter RL, Fricke JR: ADL 8-2698, A trans-3,4-dimethyl-4-(3-hydroxy-phenyl) piperidine, prevents gastrointestinal effects of intravenous morphine without affecting analgesia. Clin Pharmacol Therap 69:66, 2001.

38. Taguchi A, Sharma N, Saleem RM, et al: Selective postoperative inhibition of gastrointestinal opioid receptors. N Engl J Med 345:935, 2001.

39. Schmidt WK, Kehlet H, Pappagallo M, Foss J: ADL 8-2698: Profile of a novel GI-tract restricted mu opioid receptor antagonist. Symposium on "Recent Advances in the Treatment of Opioid Bowel Dysfunction and Postfunction Ileus," American Pain Society, April 21, 2001.

40. Page GG, Ben-Eliyahu S: The immune suppressive nature of pain. Semin Oncol Nursing 13:10, 1997.

41. Maneckjee R, Minna JD: Opioids induce while nicotine suppresses apoptosis in human lung cancer cells. Cell Growth Different 5:1033, 1994.

42. Mellon RD, Bayer BM: Evidence for central opioid receptors in the immunomodulatory effects of morphine: Review of potential mechanism(s) of action. J Neuroimmunol 83:19, 1998.

43. Tubaro E, Borelli G, Croce C, et al: Effect of morphine on resistance to infection. J Infect Dis 148: 656, 1983.

44. Carpenter GW, Garza HH Jr, Gebhardt BM, Carr DJ: Chronic morphine treatment suppresses CTL-mediated cytolysis, granulation, and cAMP responses to alloantigen. Brain Behav Immun 8:185, 1994.

45. Peterson PK, Gekker G, Schut R, et al: Enhancement of HIV-1 replication by opiates and cocaine: The cytokine connection. In: Friedman H, Klein TW, Specter S, eds. Advances in Experimental Medical Biology Plenum Press, New York, 1993, pp 181–188.

46. Gaveriaux-Ruff C, Matthes HWD, Peluso J, Kieffer BL: Abolition of morphine-immunosuppression in mice lacking the μ-opioid receptor gene. Proc Natl Acad Sci U S A 95:6326, 1998.

47. Chaney MA: Side effects of intrathecal and epidural opioids. Can J Anaesth 42:891, 1995.

48. Ishiyama A, Ishiyama G, Baloh RW, Evans CJ: Heroin-induced reversible profound deafness and vestibular dysfunction. Addiction 96:1363, 2001.

49. Oh AK, Ishiyama A, Baloh RW: Deafness associated with abuse of hydrocodone/acetaminophen. Neurology 54:2345, 2000.

50. Dorland's Illustrated Medical Dictionary, 27th ed. W.B. Saunders Company, Philadelphia, 1988.

51. O'Brien CP: Drug addiction and abuse, In: Goodman and Gilman's Pharmacologic Basis of Therapeutics, 10th ed. McGraw-Hill, New York, 2001, pp 621–642.

52. De Leon-Casasola O, Yarussi A: Pathophysiology of opioid tolerance and clinical approach to the opioid-tolerant patient. Cur Rev Pain 4:203, 2000.

53. Santillan R, Hurle MA, Armijo JA, et al: Nimodipine-enhanced opiate analgesia in cancer patients requiring dose escalation: A double-blind, placebo-controlled study. Pain 76:17, 1998.

54. Crain SM, Shen KF: Antagonists of excitatory opioid receptor functions enhance morphine's analgesic potency and attenuate opioid tolerance/dependence liability. Pain 84:121, 2000.

55. O'Brien CP: A range of research-based pharmacotherapies for addiction. Science 278:66, 1997.

56. American Psychiatric Association: Diagnostic and Statistical Manual of mental Disorders. 4th ed. American Psychiatric Association, Washington, D.C., 1994.

57. The American Society of Addiction Medicine: Public Policy Statement on Definitions Related to the Use of Opioids in Pain Treatment. www.asam.org 1997 (April).

58. Portenoy RK: Opioid therapy for chronic nonmalignant pain: A review of the critical issues. J Pain Sympt Manage 11:203, 1996.

59. Porter J, Jick H: Addiction rare in patients treated with narcotics. N Engl J Med 302:123, 1980.

60. Robinson RC, Gatchel RJ, Polatin P, et al: Screening for problematic prescription of opioid use. Clin J Pain 17:220, 2001.

61. Weissman DE, Haddox JD: Opioid pseudoaddiction: An iatrogenic syndrome. Pain 36:363, 1989.

Chapter 12

Opioid Tolerance and Dependence

Jianren Mao, MD, PhD / Lucy Chen, MD

Despite extensive efforts searching for new pharmacologic tools for pain treatment, opioids remain the most efficacious among the clinically available analgesic agents. The development of tolerance to and dependence on opioid analgesics presents practical challenges, however, for the use of opioids in the clinical setting.

DEFINITIONS

Opioid tolerance is a pharmacologic phenomenon.[1, 6] The development of pharmacologic tolerance after repeated use of opioids necessitates an increase in opioid dosage to maintain the equivalent analgesic effects.

Physical dependence is characterized by a constellation of clinical symptoms and signs on withdrawal (abstinence) from opioids after their prolonged use.[1, 6] Physical dependence on opioids should not be confused with addiction.

Addiction to opioids is a subset of substance abuse disorders characterized by compulsive use of opioids despite the resultant harm to the user and society.[1, 6] *Pseudoaddiction* may be seen in certain pain patients whose pain is inadequately controlled with opioid analgesics.

CLINICAL FEATURES OF OPIOID TOLERANCE AND DEPENDENCE

Pharmacologic tolerance is a real issue that is underlined by cellular and molecular mechanisms.[2, 7] Apparent tolerance to opioids is reflected by unexplained dose escalation during the course of opioid therapy. Not all increases in opioid use are attributable to the development of pharmacologic tolerance, however, and tolerance across subclasses of opioid drugs is often incomplete. Tolerance to side effects of opioids, such as constipation and respiratory depression, is often unreliable and occurs much later than tolerance to the analgesic effects.

Clinical manifestations of tolerance to opioids may be confounded by the disease progression and related psychological issues.[2, 7] Both conditions would lead to escalation of opioid use. Although clear clinical distinctions between true pharmacologic tolerance and increased opioid demand secondary to other factors may prove difficult, every effort should be made to investigate the underlying causes of increased opioid demand during the course of therapy. An increased pain state because of disease progression may be curtailed by appropriate adjunctive therapies, such as radiation therapy in cancer patients, rather than merely increasing the opioid dose. In general, opioid doses should not be increased simply based on changes in pain scores.

Physical dependence on opioids becomes clinically relevant only when withdrawal from opioids occurs.[2, 7] Withdrawal symptoms and signs include fatigue, yawning, increased anxiety, lacrimation, coryza, pupillary dilation, piloerection, diaphoresis, and increased sensitivity to pain. In more severe cases, tachycardia, abdominal cramping, diarrhea, nausea, vomiting, insomnia, and craving for opioids may follow. These symptoms and signs peak at about 48 to 72 hours after the initial withdrawal. The withdrawal process could be extremely uncomfortable and bothersome; rarely it becomes life-threatening. In patients receiving mixed opioid and benzodiazepine treatment, possible withdrawal from benzodiazepines always should be considered because life-threatening seizure may occur in such circumstances.

The opioid withdrawal phenomenon may be iatrogenic in many cases.[2, 7] Examples include (1) inappropriate dose conversion from one opioid to another or from one route of drug administration to another, (2) too large a decrease in an opioid dose during a tapering process, and (3) use of an opioid with mixed agonist-antagonist properties after prolonged opioid therapy.

MECHANISMS OF OPIOID TOLERANCE AND DEPENDENCE

Understanding mechanisms of opioid tolerance and dependence has been the focus of bench studies, and significant progress has been made.[2, 4, 5] Some important findings from investigations into the cellular and molecular mechanisms of opioid tolerance and dependence are as follows:

1. Three major subtypes of opioid receptors, μ, δ, and κ receptors, have been cloned. These receptors belong to a superfamily of G protein–coupled receptors. G protein activation serves as a coupling between opioid receptors and rectifying K^+ channels, leading to membrane hyperpolarization in most circumstances. Uncoupling G protein from opioid receptors has been implicated in the mechanisms of opioid tolerance.
2. There may be down-regulation of opioid receptors after prolonged exposure to opioid agonists. This down-regulation may be seen as changes in receptor density and affinity.
3. The cyclic adenosine monophosphate/protein kinase A system may be up-regulated during the development of opioid tolerance and may contribute to opioid withdrawal.
4. Activation of the N-methyl-D-aspartate (NMDA) receptor, a subgroup of excitatory glutamate receptors, has been implicated in the development of opioid tolerance and dependence. Among the three major opioid receptor subtypes, the role of NMDA receptors in μ opioid tolerance has been well established.
5. The NMDA receptor–mediated activation of intracellular cascades such as protein kinase C and nitric oxide may play a pivotal role in the development of opioid tolerance and dependence.
6. Opioid actions may be negatively modulated by cholecystokinin, an endogenous neuropeptide, in the central nervous system. In animal studies, morphine-6-glucuronide and morphine-3-glucuronide, two active morphine metabolites, potentiated and reduced the analgesic effects of μ opioid agonists.

An interesting observation has been made with regard to the relationship between opioid tolerance and neuropathic pain. Many studies have indicated similarities in the cellular and molecular mechanisms between opioid tolerance and neuropathic pain. Those findings may explain in part the reduced efficacy of opioid analgesics in treating neuropathic pain and a possible increase in pain sensitivity after prolonged exposure to opioid analgesics. These studies also raise the possibility that blockade of the NMDA receptor by using clinically available NMDA receptor antagonists may be beneficial for reducing pathologic pain and preventing opioid tolerance.

PREVENTING AND MANAGING OPIOID TOLERANCE AND DEPENDENCE

The experimental findings from bench studies and clinical observations provide several guidelines for preventing and managing opioid tolerance and dependence.[2–5, 7]

1. Withdrawal symptoms and signs may be minimized if the measured steps of opioid tapering are observed. In general, a 20% to 30% reduction of an opioid dose every 2 to 3 days until the discontinuation of opioid therapy would be sufficient to prevent withdrawal symptoms and signs.
2. In case of withdrawal, supportive measures should be taken to minimize the discomfort. In severe cases, clonidine has been used to treat withdrawal symptoms and signs. The mechanism of action of clonidine is unclear.
3. Because of incomplete cross-tolerance among subclasses of opioids, opioid rotation should be considered if a substantial increase in dose demand for one opioid is noted. The dose for a new opioid may be about 50% to 75% of the replaced one. The patient should be followed closely to ensure that an adequate dose conversion is made between two agents to avoid withdrawal symptoms and signs.
4. Although clinically available NMDA receptor antagonists are less potent and selective, several agents may be considered, including dextromethorphan, methadone, and ketamine. The combined use of opioids and NMDA receptor antagonists may increase opioid analgesic efficacy and retard the development of tolerance and dependence in the clinical setting.
5. Whenever possible, adjunctive medications, such as nonsteroidal antiinflammatory drugs, should be considered as part of the treatment regimen to reduce the total amount of opioid analgesics.
6. Laboratory studies indicated that the combination of an opioid and an ultra-low dose of an opioid receptor antagonist, such as naltrexone, may enhance opioid analgesic efficacy. Whether such treatment would reduce the development of tolerance is unknown.

SUMMARY

The presence of tolerance to and dependence on opioids should not discourage physicians from using opioids for pain management, particularly for cancer pain management. Many issues regarding tolerance and dependence may be minimized by the thoughtful formulation of an opioid treatment plan.

REFERENCES

1. American Academy of Pain Medicine (AAPM) and American Pain Society (APS): The use of opioids for the treatment of chronic pain: A consensus statement. Seattle, APS Press, 1997.

2. Bruera E, Pereira J: Neuropsychiatric toxicity of opioids. In: Jensen TS, et al (eds): Proceedings of the 8th World Congress on Pain. New York: IASP Press, pp 717–738.

3. Crain S, Shen KF: Antagonists of excitatory opioid receptor functions enhance morphine's analgesic potency and attenuate opioid tolerance/dependence liability. Pain 82:1–11, 1999.

4. Mao J: NMDA and opioid receptors: their interactions in antinociception, tolerance and neuroplasticity. Brain Res Rev 30:289–304, 1999.

5. Mao J, Piece DD, Mayer DJ: Mechanisms of hyperalgesia and morphine tolerance: A current view of their possible interactions. Pain 62:259–274, 1995.

6. O'Brience CP: Drug addiction and drug abuse. In: Hardman JG, et al (eds): Goodman and Gilman's Pharmacological Basis of Therapeutics. New York: McGraw-Hill, 1996, pp 557–577.

7. Reisine T, Pasternak G: Opioid analgesics and antagonists. In: Hardman JG, et al (eds): Goodman and Gilman's Pharmacological Basis of Therapeutics. New York: McGraw-Hill, 1996, pp 521–556.

Chapter 13

Treatment of Pain with Anticonvulsants: A Basic Science Approach

YiLi Zhou, MD, PhD / Salahadin Abdi, MD, PhD

Antiepileptic drugs (AEDs) have been used to treat seizures and pain syndromes. Carbamazepine (CBZ) has been a mainstay for treatment of trigeminal neuralgia. Gabapentin (GBP) is used widely for variety of pain conditions. Valproic acid has a potential to reduce the frequency of migraine attack. Newly released AED pregabalin and oxcarbazepine (OBZ) are derivatives of GBP and CBZ. These new derivatives may be more effective and pose fewer side effects than their elder generations. These medications can block sodium channels and calcium channels, facilitate opening of chloride channels, increase function of the γ-aminobutyric acid (GABA) system, and modulate multiple neurotransmitters. Other mechanisms are yet to be revealed. Animal studies of the effects of AEDs on chronic and acute pain have provided some scientific basis for using these agents for pain management.

CARBAMAZEPINE

CBZ acts mainly by decreasing repetitive firing of action potentials in depolarized neurons through blockade of voltage-dependent sodium channels.[5] In an *in vitro* study, CBZ and its derivative OBZ were found to interfere with adenosine receptor agonists 3H-L-phenylisopropyladenosine (A1) and 3H-N-ethylcarboxamidoadenosine (A2) to combine with adenosine receptors.[18] It is believed that the central nervous system effects of CBZ and OBZ are related partially to their interaction with A1 and A2 adenosine receptors.[31]

Microinjections of CBZ into the periaqueductal gray (PAG) matter suppress pain-related behavior in rats. This effect was blocked by pretreatment with bicuculline, a GABA receptor antagonist. CBZ may exert its central effect through the GABAergic systems in PAG.[17] The administration of CBZ also can elevate brain serotonin levels and pain threshold in rats.[34]

CBZ has been the treatment of choice for the management of trigeminal neuralgia. In a rat model of trigeminal neuropathic pain produced by a chronic constriction injury of the infraorbital branch, CBZ was effective in alleviating allodynia-like behavior.[23] Satoh and Foong[35] applied bradykinin solution to the tooth pulp of rabbits, which induced single neuronal intermittent paroxysmal activities in the subnucleus reticularis dorsalis and trigeminal subnucleus caudalis. Treatment with CBZ significantly suppressed such a paroxysmal response. Administration of CBZ also can block the increase of spontaneous activity in spinal cord neurons induced by spinal nerve ligation in rats.[7]

CBZ may have antinociceptive and antiinflammatory property. Mashimoto et al[32] found that a subcutaneous injection of CBZ decreased nociceptive pain behavior in rats as measured by the tail flick test. This antinociceptive property was blocked by caffeine, an adenosine A1/A2 receptor antagonist. It was suggested the antinociceptive effect of CBZ might be produced via an activation of the adenosine A1 receptors. Bianchi et al[4] reported CBZ can reduce hyperalgesia and edema induced by brewer's yeast injection in the rat hindpaw. They found CBZ reduced inflammatory exudate, prostaglandin E_2–like activity, and substance P concentrations in the exudates in a dose-dependent fashion.

OXCARBAZEPINE

OBZ is a keto derivative of CBZ. It can block sodium-dependent action potentials. OBZ has been released in the United States as a second-line treatment for partial seizure. Experience with trigeminal neuralgia patients showed that OBZ can be effective and has fewer adverse effects than CBZ.[12, 38]

Animal studies support the notion that OBZ could be a possible candidate for the treatment of trigeminal nerve pain. Kiguchi et al[29] recorded evoked potentials from the superficial layers of the caudal part of the trigeminal spinal tract nucleus in anesthetized rats. Electrical stimulation to the maxillary canine tooth pulp was used as a nociceptive stimulus. The P3 component of the evoked potentials, related to nociception, was suppressed significantly by intravenous injection of OBZ in a dose-dependent manner. Microinjections of MHD (an active metabolite of OBZ) into the recording site of the trigeminal spinal tract nucleus suppressed the P3 component. Given fewer adverse effects of OBZ than CBZ, it is worthwhile to investigate further whether OBZ could be a better choice for trigeminal neuralgia.

GABAPENTIN

GBP has a chemical structure similar to GABA. It seems not to act directly at the GABA-binding site in the central nervous system, however. The mechanism of action is still unclear. It may enhance the release or activity of GABA and seems to inhibit voltage-dependent sodium channels.

GBP can reduce mechanical allodynia in a neuropathic pain model in animals.[1, 13, 15] Field et al[15] studied static and dynamic allodynia in rats caused by injection of streptozocin. Static and dynamic allodynias were blocked by GBP and pregabalin is a dose-dependent manner, not by morphine or amitriptyline. It was suggested that GBP and pregabalin possess a superior antiallodynic profile than morphine and amitriptyline. Abdi et al[1] observed the effects of GBP on behavioral signs of mechanical allodynia produced by tight ligation of the left L5 and L6 spinal nerves in rats. GBP increased the threshold for mechanical allodynia 30 minutes after treatment, and the effect lasted for at least 1 hour. Electrophysiologic monitoring did not find that GBP influences the rate of continuing ectopic discharge of the injured afferent fibers, whereas this continuing discharge was suppressed by injection of lidocaine. It is believed that GBP increases the threshold of allodynia mainly through a central mechanism. Increased spontaneous activities of spinal neurons have been observed in partial spinal nerve ligation in rats. This increased spinal neuron activity can be blocked by GBP.[7] GBP may have an antinociceptive capacity through the peripheral mechanism.[6] Simultaneous microinjection of GBP and formalin into the hind paws of rats significantly reduced flinching and lifting and licking behavior, whereas microinjection of GBP into the contralateral hind paw did not. It was suggested that GBP might have a peripheral site of action.

An animal study showed that GBP and pregabalin can block hyperalgesia caused by thermal injury. Jun and Yaksh[28] induced hyperalgesia with a mild thermal injury to the hind paw of rats. Intrathecal injection of GBP produced a dose-dependent reversal of the hyperalgesia.

A similar reversal was observed after intrathecal delivery of pregabalin. The effects of intrathecal GBP and pregabalin were reversed by intrathecal D-serine. It is suggested that gabapentinoids can selectively modulate the facilitation of spinal nociceptive processing otherwise generated by persistent small afferent input induced by tissue injury.

GBP and pregabalin could be effective in the treatment of postoperative pain. Field et al[14] studied thermal hyperalgesia and tactile allodynia caused by an acute incision of the plantaris muscle of the hind paw in rats. A single subcutaneous dose of GBP or pregabalin, 1 hour before surgery, blocked the development of allodynia and hyperalgesia caused by surgical incision.

PREGABALIN

Similar to GBP, pregabalin is a 3-alkylated GABA analog. Pregabalin has been shown to be able to displace GBP from the its binding site, increase rate of GABA synthesis, increase GAD activity, alter nonsynaptic GABA release, bind to the $\alpha_2 \delta$ subunit with the possibility of reducing calcium influx into neurons, and reduce K^+ induced monoamine release in vitro.[15]

Animal studies found pregabalin can decrease mechanical allodynia induced by chronic constrictive injury of spinal nerves (Chung model),[13, 15] mechanical hyperalgesia caused by carrageenan,[16] and a mild thermal injury[27, 28] in rats. Pregabalin seems more effective than GBP at nonsedating doses.[27] Injection of pregabalin into the central nervous system resulted in a 20% to 30% reduction in joint swelling and prevented the development of heat hyperalgesia and spontaneous pain in a rat model of acute arthritis. The antihyperalgesic and antiinflammatory properties of pregabalin probably are mediated through a central neurogenic mechanism.[21] Pregabalin also may be able to reduce postoperative pain in animal models.[16] The effectiveness of pregabalin in treating human pain has not been investigated well yet.

LAMOTRIGINE

Lamotrigine is a broad-spectrum AED used for generalized, partial, and refractory seizures. Although it has shown efficacy for trigeminal neuralgia[37] and painful diabetic neuropathy,[11] it failed to show its effectiveness in human immunodeficiency virus painful neuropathy.[36] The proposed mechanism of lamotrigine is to block voltage-dependent sodium channels and inhibit glutamate and aspartate release.[36]

Nakamura-Craig and Follenfant[33] reported that lamotrigine could be used to treat neuronal sensitization and possibly inhibit the development of this sensitization. When lamotrigine (10 to 100 mg/kg) was administered orally before prostaglandin E_2 subplantar injection, it significantly decreased hyperalgesia in an animal model. It also inhibited the development of sustained hyperalgesia induced by multiple subplantar injections of prostaglandin E_2. Lamotrigine induced analgesia in a model of chronic hyperalgesia in streptozotocin-induced diabetic rats.

Hunter et al[22] compared the antinociceptive effect of lamotrigine and GBP in chronic constriction injury and spinal nerve ligation models. The investigators found that lamotrigine (10 to 100 mg/kg subcutaneously) and GBP (30 to 300 mg/kg intraperitoneally) reversed cold allodynia (chronic constriction injury model). Only GBP reversed tactile allodynia (spinal nerve ligation model), however. Christensen et al[8] compared the effect of lamotrigine and GBP on mechanical allodynia–like behavior in a rat model of trigeminal neuropathic pain induced by chronic constriction of infraorbital nerve. It was found that repeated (30 and 50 mg/kg) but not single (30 to 100 mg/kg) injections of intraperitoneal GBP partially alleviated the mechanical allodynia–like behavior, whereas single (5 to 100 mg/kg) and repeated (5 to 30 mg/kg) intraperitoneal injections of lamotrigine failed to reduce the mechanical allodynia–like behavior. GBP rather than lamotrigine may be a better therapeutic approach for the clinical management of some trigeminal neuropathic pain disorders

VALPROATE

Valproate has been used for migraine prophylaxis,[25] neuropathic pain,[19] and a variety of seizure disorders. This wide spectrum of activities is reflected by several different mechanisms of action. Valproate can enhance the GABAergic system by increasing the synthesis and blocking the degradation of GABA.[20, 26] Valproate seems to reduce the release of the excitatory amino acid γ-hydroxybutyric acid and to attenuate neuronal excitation induced by N-methyl-D-aspartate (NMDA)–type glutamate receptors. Valproate also exerts direct effects on excitable membranes.[30]

Valproate has been used for migraine prophylaxis. It may act through activation of GABA receptors to modulate the c-fos activity in trigeminal nociceptive neurons innervating the meninges. Cutrer and Moskowitz[9] tested the effect of valproate on c-fos activity in the trigeminal nucleus. Hartley guinea pigs were pretreated with valproate 30 minutes before activation of trigeminal afferent fibers by intracisternal injection of capsaicin. Valproate ($\geq$ 10 mg/kg intraperitoneally) reduced c-fos-labeled cell expression within the trigeminal nucleus caudalis (lamina I, II) by 52% ($P < 0.05$). This effect was blocked by bicuculline (GABA antagonist), suggesting the importance of GABA receptors. Evidence indicates that c-fos-related trigeminal nucleus hyperactivity is associated with migraine attacks. The suppressive effect of valproate on c-fos activity may account for its utility in migraine prophylaxis.

The clinical efficacy of valproate for neuropathic pain has not been established.[19] Animal studies failed to show any supportive evidence for this treatment. Yamashiro studied hyperactive neuronal discharges in the thalamic nuclei in a rat neuropathic pain model induced by a surgical lesion to C5 dorsal nerve root.[36a] Administration of phenytoin and diazepam reduced the hyperactive firing. No effect was seen with valproic acid.

Animal studies have not revealed an antinociceptive effect of sodium valproate. Aley and Kulkarni[2] compared the antinociceptive effect of sodium valproate with other GABA agonists and baclofen on radiant heat–induced nociception in mice. Sodium valproate failed to enhance the reaction time to radiant heat as other drugs did. Concomitant administration of any of these agents with morphine showed a potentiation of morphine-induced analgesia.

TOPIRAMATE

Anecdotal data show that topiramate may reduce migraine frequency[10] and treat refractory intercostal neuralgia.[3] It was approved by the Food and Drug Administration (FDA) as an adjunct treatment for partial and secondary generalized seizures. The mechanisms of action include blockade of sodium channels, enhancement of GABA inhibition, and attenuation of kainate-induced responses at glutamate receptors. Controlled studies in human pain-related disorders and animal study data are needed, however.

TIAGABINE

Tiagabine, a new AED, may have antinociceptive property via the GABA system. Ipponi et al[24] found that systemic administration of tiagabine, 30 mg/kg intaperitoneally, increased nearly twofold the extracellular GABA levels in rats and increased significantly the rat paw pressure nociceptive threshold in a time-correlated manner. Dose-related significant tiagabine-induced antinociception was observed at doses of 1 and 3 mg/kg intraperitoneally in the mouse hot plate and abdominal constriction tests. The tiagabine antinociception was antagonized completely by pretreatment with the selective GABA(B) receptor antagonist, CGP 35348 (3-aminopropyl-diethoxy-methyl-phosphinic acid), but not by naloxone. It is suggested that tiagabine causes antinociception as a result of raised endogenous GABA levels, which in turn activate GABA(B) receptors. Applications of tiagabine in human pain-related disorders are yet to be studied.

LEVETIRACETAM

Levetiracetam was released for partial seizures in 1999 in the United States. Its role in pain management has not been defined. It has a specific binding site confined to the synaptic plasma membranes of cells in the central nervous system.[24a] The mechanism of action is still unknown, however. Levetiracetam does not modulate inhibitory and excitatory neurotransmission, and it does not displace ligands from binding sites. It does not affect channel proteins. Levetiracetam has no effect on glutamate receptors, GABA transaminase, or glutaminate decarboxylase.

ZONISAMIDE

Zonisamide has been approved by the FDA as add-on therapy for the treatment of partial seizures. Its role in pain relief is being investigated. Zonisamide is able to block sodium channels and T-type calcium channels.[36a,36b] An animal study revealed zonisamide could scavenge hydroxyl radicals (OH) and inhibit nitric oxide synthase activity induced by NMDA in the rat hippocampus. Zonisamide may protect neurons from free radical damage and stabilization of neuronal membranes. It also can facilitate dopaminergic and serotoninergic neurotransmission and weakly inhibits carbonic anhydrase. Electrophysiologic studies showed zonisamide modulates descending excitatory and inhibitory mechanisms in the cat trigeminal complex.

CONCLUSION

The management of neuropathic pain continues to be a challenge to clinicians. Although there are numerous medications available, physicians face a dilemma when weighing their efficacies against side effects. Expanding clinical applications of AEDs in pain management provide a new hope, especially because of the few side effects the new AEDs, such as GBP, and pregabalin, and OBZ, have. Studies on the use of AEDs in animal models of experimental pain have yielded crucial information regarding the mechanisms of antinociceptive and antineuropathic properties of these medications. These studies may also help to identify newer generations of AEDs that have significant clinical efficacy with fewer side effects for the treatment of human pain. Future studies should focus on how to translate the basic science findings into clinical settings.

REFERENCES FOR ADDITIONAL READING

1. Abdi S, Lee DH, Chung JM: The anti-allodynic effects of amitriptyline, gabapentin, and lidocaine in a rat model of neuropathic pain. AnesthAnalg 87:1360–1366, 1998.
2. Aley KO, Kulkarni SK: GABAergic agents-induced antinociceptive effect in mice. Methods Find Exp Clin Pharmacol 11:597–601, 1989.
3. Bajwa ZH, Sami N, Warfield CA, Wootton J: Topiramate relieves refractory intercostal neuralgia. Neurology 1917, 1999.
4. Bianchi M, Rossoni G, Sacerdote P, et al. Carbamazepine exerts anti-inflammatory effects in the rat. Eur J Pharmacol 294:71–74, 1995.
5. Brodie MJ, Ditcher MA: Antiepileptic drugs. N Engl J Med 334:168–175, 1996.
6. Carlton SM, Zhou S: Attenuation of formalin-induced nociceptive behaviors following local peripheral injection of gabapentin. Pain 76:201–207, 1998.
7. Chapman V, Suzuki R, Chamarette HL, et al: Effects of systemic carbamazepine and gabapentin on spinal neuronal responses in spinal nerve ligated rats. Pain 75:261–272, 1998.
8. Christensen D, Gautron M, Guilbaud G, Kayser V: Effect of gabapentin and lamotrigine on mechanical allodynia-like behavior in a rat model of trigeminal neuropathic pain. Pain 93:147–153, 2001.
9. Cutrer FM, Moskowitz MA: Wolff Award 1996. The actions of valproate and neurosteroids in a model of trigeminal pain. Headache 36:579–585, 1998.
10. Dodick DW, Capobianco DJ: Treatment and management of cluster headache. Curr Pain Headache Rep 5:83–91, 2001.
11. Eisenberg E, Lurie Y, Braker C, et al: Lamotrigine reduces painful diabetic neuropathy: A randomized, controlled study. Neurology 57:505–509, 2001.
12. Farago F: Trigeminal neuralgia: Its treatment with two new carbamazepine analogues. Eur Neurol 26:73–83, 1987.
13. Field, J, Bramwell S, Hughes J, Singh L: Detection of static and dynamic components of mechanical allodynia in rat models of neuropathic pain: Are they signaled by distinct primary sensory neurons? Pain 83:303–311, 1999.
14. Field MJ, Holloman EF, McCleary S, et al: Evaluation of gabapentin and S-(+)-3-isobutylgaba in a rat model of postoperative pain. J Pharmacol Exp Ther 282:1242–1246, 1997.
15. Field MJ, McCleary S, Hughes J, Singh L: Gabapentin and pregabalin, but not morphine and amitriptyline, block both static and dynamic components of mechanical allodynia induced by streptozocin in the rat. Pain 80:392–398, 1999.
16. Field MJ, Oles RJ, Lewis AS, et al: Gabapentin and S-(+)-3-isobutylgaba represent a novel class of selective antihyperalgesic agents. Br J Pharmacol 121:1513–1522, 1997.
17. Foong FW, Satoh M: The periaqueductal gray is the site of the antinociceptive action of carbamazepine as related to bradykinin-induced trigeminal pain. Br J Pharmacol 83:493–497, 1984.
18. Fujiwara Y, Sato M, Otsuki S: Interaction of carbamazepine and other drugs with adenosine (A1 and A2) receptors. Psychopharmacology (Berl) 90:332–335, 1986.
19. Hardy JR, Rees EA, Gwilliam B, et al: A phase II study to establish the efficacy and toxicity of sodium valproate in patients with cancer-related neuropathic pain. J Pain Symptom Manage 21: 204–209, 2001.
20. Hitchcock E, Teixeira M: Anticonvulsant activation of pain-suppressive systems. Appl Neurophysiol 45:582–593, 1982.
21. Houghton AK, Lu Y, Westlund KN: S-(+)-3-isobutylgaba and its stereoisomer reduces the amount of inflammation and hyperalgesia in an acute arthritis model in the rat. J Pharmacol Exp Ther 285:533–538, 1998.

22. Hunter JC, Gogas KR, Hedley LR, et al: The effect of novel anti-epileptic drugs in rat experimental models of acute and chronic pain. EurJPharmacol 254:153–160, 1997.

23. Idanpaan-Heikkila JJ, Guilbaud G: Pharmacological studies on a rat model of trigeminal neuropathic pain: Baclofen, but not carbamazepine, morphine or tricyclic antidepressants, attenuates the allodynia-like behavior. Pain 79:281–290, 1999.

24. Ipponi A, Lamberti C, Medica A, et al: Tiagabine antinociception in rodents depends on GABA(B) receptor activation: Parallel antinociception testing and medial thalamus GABA microdialysis. Eur J Pharmacol 368:205–211, 1999.

24a. Jain KK: An assessment of levetiracetam as an anti-epileptic drug. Expert Opin Investig Drugs 9(7): 1611–1624, 2000.

25. Jensen R, Brinck T, Olesen J: Sodium valproate has a prophylactic effect in migraine without aura: A triple-blind, placebo-controlled crossover study. Neurology 44:647–651, 1994.

26. Johannessen CU: Mechanisms of action of valproate: A commentary. Neurochem Int 37:103–110, 2000.

27. Jones DL, Sorkin LS: Systemic gabapentin and S(+)-3-isobutyl-gamma-aminobutyric acid block secondary hyperalgesia. Brain Res 810:93–99, 1998.

28. Jun JH, Yaksh TL: The effect of intrathecal gabapentin and 3-isobutyl gamma-aminobutyric acid on the hyperalgesia observed after thermal injury in the rat. AnesthAnalg 86:348–354, 1998.

29. Kiguchi S, Ichikawa K, Kojima M: Suppressive effects of oxcarbazepine on tooth pulp-evoked potentials recorded at the trigeminal spinal tract nucleus in cats. Clin Exp Pharmacol Physiol 28:169–175, 2001.

30. Loscher W: Valproate: A reappraisal of its pharmacodynamic properties and mechanisms of action. Prog Neurobiol 58:31–59, 1999.

31. Marangos PJ, Post RM, Patel J, et al: Specific and potent interactions of carbamazepine with brain adenosine receptors. Eur J Pharmacol 1983; 93:172–182, 1983.

32. Mashimoto S, Ushijima I, Suetsugi M, et al: Stress-dependent antinociceptive effects of carbamazepine: A study in stressed and nonstressed rats. Prog Neuropsychopharmacol Biol Psychiatry 28:159–168, 1998.

33. Nakamura-Craig M, Follenfant RL: Effect of lamotrigine in the acute and chronic hyperalgesia induced by PGE2 and in the chronic hyperalgesia in rats with streptozotocin-induced diabetes. Pain 63:33–37, 1995.

33a. Oommen KJ, Mathews SC: Zonisamide: A new antiepileptic drug. Clin Neuropharmacol 2(4): 192–200, 1999.

34. Pinelli A, Trivulzio S, Tomasoni L: Effects of carbamazepine treatment on pain threshold values and brain serotonin levels in rats. Pharmacology 54:113–117, 1997.

35. Satoh M, Foong FW: A mechanism of carbamazepine-analgesia as shown by bradykinin-induced trigeminal pain. Brain Res Bull 10:407–409, 1983.

36. Simpson DM, Olney R, McArthur JC, et al: A placebo-controlled trial of lamotrigine for painful HIV-associated neuropathy. Neurology 54:2115–2119, 2000.

36a. Suzuki S, Kawakami K, Nishimura S, et al: Zonisamide blocks T-type calcium channel in cultured neurons of rat cerebral cortex. Epilepsy Res 12(1):21–27, 1992.

36b. Yamashiro K, Iwayama K, Kurihara M, et al: Neurones with epileptiform discharge in the central nervous system and chronic pain. Experimental and clinical investigations. Acta Neurochir Suppl (Wien) 52:130–132, 1991.

37. Zakrzewska JM, Chaudry Z, Nurmikko TJ, et al: Lamotrigine in refractory trigeminal neuralgia: Results from a double-blind placebo controlled cross-over trial. Pain 73:223–230, 1997.

38. Zakrzewska JM, Patsalos PN: Oxcarbazepine: A new drug in the management of intractable trigeminal neuralgia. J Neurol Neurosurg Psychiatry 52:472–476, 1989.

Chapter 14

Anticonvulsant Drugs in the Treatment of Chronic Pain States

John P.R. Loughrey, MB, BCh, MRCPI, FCARCSI / Howard S. Smith, MD

The popular classification of pain into nociceptive, in which somatic or visceral tissue sustains an insult, and neuropathic continues to be of some clinical value from a treatment perspective. Nociceptive pain generally responds better to antiinflammatory and opioid medication. Neuropathic pain is defined as pain due to dysfunction of the nervous system in the absence of ongoing neural tissue damage. The elucidation of the role of the central nervous system in chronic pain states, together with the relative success and lack of toxicity of the newer generation drugs has resulted in an increase in anticonvulsant prescribing in the United States. Recent reviews have established the anticonvulsant drugs as among the first-line agents in the treatment of neuropathic pain.[1-4] However, the clinical evidence-base for widespread use of these agents has been slow to emerge. The difficulty with randomized trials of agents to treat neuropathic pain is that it represents such a wide range of clinical entities. Thus, most randomized controlled trials of these agents focus on the classic neuropathic pain disorders with well-defined causes or clinical presentations such as post-herpetic neuralgia (PHN), painful diabetic neuropathy (PDN), and trigeminal neuralgia (TN). This chapter reviews the basic mechanism of action, pharmacology, and clinical utility of the more commonly used agents from this category in the management of chronic neuropathic pain.

NEUROPATHIC PAIN

The property of the nervous system in adapting to an external insult or stimulus at a cellular level is known as *neuroplasticity*. This appears to play a key role in the development and continuation of chronic pain syndromes. Neuropathic symptoms include spontaneous burning, shooting pains, hyperalgesia, and paradoxical sensory loss. Nonpainful stimuli often evoke painful responses (allodynia), and repetitive stimuli lead to an increase in pain. These latter symptoms may represent peripheral sensitization, in which nociceptors have a reduced threshold for stimuli. An increase in sodium channel density has been observed following peripheral nerve injury.[1,5] Neuromas can generate ectopic electrical impulses at the regenerating tips in the damaged primary nociceptive afferents at various levels in the nervous system from the dorsal root ganglia to demyelinated regions of a root or nerve.[6] Ectopic neuronal activity may be due to a change in voltage-sensitive pain specific Na^+ channels. The peripheral and central neuronal hyperexitability observed partially explains the mechanism of symptom alleviation by the membrane-stabilizing properties of the anticonvulsant drugs.[7]

Neuropathic symptoms encompass disorders of varying etiology but with similar clinical phenomena. Physicians encountering chronic pain problems should realize the potential for central and peripheral sensitization phenomena mixed with ongoing nociceptive pain states, and that a combination of pain-sustaining mechanisms probably exists in many pain disorders. It is therefore easy to justify a trial of anticonvulsant medications as part of a treatment algorithm in the treatment of many resistant chronic pain problems.

MECHANISMS OF ACTION

The improved understanding of the pathophysiology of the both central and peripheral neuropathic pain disorders has helped to shed light on the mechanisms of action of drugs used to treat these disorders, in addition to identifying agents for study in the future (TABLE 1).

Sodium channels are found in all nerve cells and are primarily involved in nerve impulse transmission. Nine or more different subtypes of sodium channels are known, which may be divided into tetrodotoxin (TTX) sensitive or resistant. In models of epilepsy, the anticonvulsant Na^+ channel blocking agents alter primary and transmission neurons, acting as membane stabilizers that alter the threshold for firing in neural tissue. The biochemical similarity between neuropathic pain and epilepsy provides a logical explanation for the clinical efficacy of these agents. A TTX-resistant Na^+ channel subtype, PN3, which is located in the dorsal root ganglion, may have specific importance in pain transmission.[8] The identification of more specific targets will lead to drugs with fewer of the side effects related to generalized Na^+-channel blockade.

Alteration of not only Na^+ but also Ca^{2+}, γ-aminobutyric acid (GABA), substance P, and N-methyl-D-aspartate (NMDA) systems in neuropathic pain models also partially explains the mechanism of action of other anticonvulsants (see TABLE 1). These other non-Na^+ channel-blocking mechanisms are proposed to also have an effect on central or peripheral sensitized neurons via direct or indirect augmentation of central nervous system inhibitory pathways (increasing GABA activity), or reduction in release of excitatory amino acids such as glutamate.

ANTIEPILEPTIC DRUGS

A comparison of the various AEDs is made in the following paragraphs. Although there exists a growing number of antiepileptic rugs (AEDs) and clinical use of AEDs for amelioration of neuropathic pain is increasing, the number of randomized trials of AEDs for pain relief is limited. Four AEDs that have been studied in randomized clinical trials for providing pain relief in neuropathic pain states include carbamazepine, gabapentin, lamotrigine, and phenytoin. The results of studies with carbamazepine and gabapentin have been favorable, but conflicting results exist with phenytoin and lamotrigine.[34]

TABLE 1

Proposed mechanism of action of drugs in clinical use

Proposed Mechanism of Action	Drug
GABA enhancement	Gabapentin, topiramate, valproic acid
NA$^+$ current blockade	Carbamazepine, oxcarbazepine, phenytoin, lamotrigine, sodium valproate
Ca^{2+} current blockade	Gabapentin, oxcarbazepine
Reduced excitatory amino acid	Phenytoin, topiramate, lamotrigine
Anti-inflammatory effect	Gabapentin, lamotrigine

There is certain no consensus when it comes to the clinical use of epileptic drugs in the treatment of neuropathic pain. Criticisms of some of the gabapentin data[99] include-that stable doses of tricyclic antidepressants and/or opioids were continued. In one of the eight-week trials[17] patients in the gabapentin group reported a reduction of the daily pain scores (on a 0–10 scale) from 6.3 to 4.2, as compared with a half-point reduction (from 6.5 to 6.0) in the placebo group.[17] However, the patients with a 4.2 pain score would still have been eligible to participate in the study, so it is difficult to assess just how clinically significant this decrement was for these patients. Mao and Chen, in 2000, concluded that more data are needed before any notions can be supported that gabapentin should be considered as a first-line treatment for neuropathic pain with better efficacy, fewer side effects, and a favorable cost/efficiency ratio.[99]

Although AEDs continue to be used frequently for neuropathic and sometimes other types of pains, mystery still surrounds some of their basic mechanisms of action. For example, in the normal state, it appears that gabapentin does not directly interact with the NMDA receptor. It is conceivable, however, that gabapentin affects NMDA receptor-mediated currents in the presence of protein kinase C, which is evolved from inflammation. This seems to be plastic, depending on baseline phosphorylation state.[100] In spite of uncertainties in the basic science and clinical analgesic applications of AEDs, many more AEDs seem to be under development. Other carbamazepine derivatives—10-acetoxy—10/1—dihydro—5H—dibenz[b,f]azepine—5—carboxamide (BIA2–093) and 10,11—dihydro-10-hydroxyimino-5H-dibenz[b,f]azepine—5-carboxamide (BIA 2–024), recently developed by BIAL[101]—may hold promise in the future if it can be demonstrated that they exhibit improved efficacy, fewer side effects (better risks/benefit ratio) and more favourable cost-effectiveness.

A comparison on the various AEDs is made in the following paragraph. NNT (stands for "number needed to treat") is the number of patients who need to be treated to obtain one patient with more than 50% pain relief. It is a commonly used tool to compare the efficacy of individual treatments.

Gabapentin (Neurontin)

A structural analogue of GABA (hence its name), this agent is considered by many practitioners to be the first-line drug for treatment of PHN and PDN because of its tolerability and efficacy, which has been confirmed in well-designed randomized controlled trials. It does not actually act at the GABA receptor but does cause an increase in global GABA activity. GABA is one of the primary neurotransmitter inhibtors, along with glycine.

Prior to 1993, there were six major drugs available in the United States for the treatment of patients with epilepsy. These included phenobarbitol, phenytoin, carbamazepine, primidone, valproic acid/sodium valproate, and ethosuximide. Gabapentin was introduced into clinical practice in 1993 as an adjunctive agent for partial seizures in adults but is now established mainly as a successful drug in the management of neuropathic pain.[9–11] The mode of action as an anticonvulsant is incompletely understood. Evidence exists for an action on Ca^{2+} via the binding protein associated with a subunit of the Ca^{2+} channel (α-2-δ subtype),[12] probably an N-type Ca^{2+} channel, with both peripheral and central effects and a partial effect on the high-frequency firing of sodium-dependent action potentials. Inflammation may actually alter receptor complex subunits (e.g., phosphorylating/dephosphorylating), thereby modulating receptor functions and interactions. In animal models of carrageenan-induced inflammatory pain, gabapentin has been shown to have an antinociceptive effect,[13] which may partly explain the clinical success with this drug as an adjunctive agent outside the classic chronic neuropathic pain disease states. An effect on mood in patients with bipolar disorder may partially explain the success in some patients with neuropathic pain and significant psychopathology.

Gabapentin, 1-(aminomethyl)cyclohexaneacetic acid, is a bitter-tasting crystalline substance with a molecular weight of about 171. It is available in 100 mg capsules, 300 mg capsules, 400 mg capsules, 600 mg tablets, and 800 mg tablets, and in an oral solution 250 mg/5 mL. It has an amino-acid like structure and exists as a zwitterion at physiologic pH. It is transported by the L-system amino acid transporter, similar to L-leucine and L-valine. Bioavailability is roughly 60% and time to maximum plasma concentration is 2 to 3 hours. If possible, antacids should be taken more than 2 hours before or more than 2 hours after gabapentin ingestion, so as to maximize bioavailability. The elimination half-life is generally considered to be 9 hours but may range from 4 to 22 hours.[14] The drug is excreted renally, and in 11 anuric patient given a single oral dose of 400 mg gabapentin, the half-life was 132 hours on nonhemodialysis day and 3.8 hours during dialysis.[15]

The gabapentin dose should be reduced in renal dysfunction. The manufacturer recommends the following dosing:

Creatinine clearance	Gabapentin dose
< 60 mL/min	400 mg PO tid
30–60 mL/min	300 mg PO tid
1.5–30 mL/min	300 mg PO qd
< 15 mL/min	300 mg PO qod

A maintenance dose of 200 to 300 mg is recommended following each 4 hours of hemodialysis as a significant amount of drug is removed during dialysis. The drug is absorbed by a saturable pump dependent mechanism, so more frequent dosing intervals will lead to higher blood levels, particularly at high doses. With a range of 300 to 3600 mg/day in three or four divided doses, a reasonable mean efficacious dose is 1800 mg/day, although some clinicians have used more than 6 g/day. Dose increases are usually made every 4 days, but some clinicians titrate faster without significant problems. The NNT for PHN and PDN in well-designed studies has been found to be 3.2 and 3.7, respectively.[16,17] It is excreted without undergoing hepatic metabolism and has a very favorable side effect profile comprising somnolence, fatigue, poor concentration, anorexia, nausea, ataxia, dizziness, rash, purpuric lesions, peripheral edema, stuttering, anxiety, parathesias, arthralgias, twitching, tremor, abnormal vision, and headache, which result in discontinuation of the drug in about 13% of patients.

Gabapentin has emerged as a first-line anticonvulsant for the treatment of neuropathic pain based mostly on a favorable side effect profile as compared with other anticonvulsants. There now exist four large randomized trials of gabapentin for amelioration of neuropathic pain.[16–19] Backonja and associates[16] performed a randomized double-blind placebo-controlled, 8-week trial of gabapentin for the symptomatic treatment of painful diabetic neuropathy. Eighty-four patients were in the gabapentin group with 70 (83%) completing the study, and 81 patients were in the placebo group with 65 (80%) completing the study. The gabapentin group's mean daily pain scores went from 6.4 to 3.9 (P < .001) versus the placebo group's, which went from 6.5 to 5.1. There was also statistically significant improvement in the gabapentin group in sleep interference scores, Short-McGill Pain Questionnaire scores, Patient

Global Impression of change, and clinical Global Impression of changes as well as various measures on the Short Form-36 quality of life questionnaire scores and the Profile of Mood States values. The most common side effects were in the gabapentin group and included dizziness, somnolence, and confusion.

Rowbotham and colleagues conducted a multicenter, randomized, double blind, placebo-controlled, parallel dosing, 8-week trial of gabapentin for the treatment of post-herpetic neuralgia. The first phase of the study involved a 4-week titration period to a maximum dosage of 3600 mg/d. One hundred thirteen patients were in the gabapentin group with 89 (78.8%) completing the study, and 116 patients received placebo with 95 (81.9%) completing the study. The gabapentin group had a significant reduction in average daily pain score from 6.3 to 4.2 points, as compared with a change from 6.5 to 6.0 in the placebo group (P < .01). Somnolence, dizziness, ataxia, and peripheral edema were more frequent in the gabapentin group.

Rice and associates[18] conducted a randomized, placebo-controlled, 7-week study that confirmed that gabapentin is effective and well tolerated for the treatment of post-herpetic neuralgia. One hundred eleven patients were randomized to placebo, 115 to gabapentin 1800 mg/day, and 108 to gabapentin 2400 mg/d. The final difference in pain in the treated groups versus the placebo group was 18.8% for the 1800 mg dose (P < .01) and 18.7% for the 2400 mg dose (P < .01). Sleep interference diaries revealed similar improvements in sleep for both gabapentin groups (P < .01). Overall, gabapentin was well tolerated, with the most common side effects being dizziness and somnolence.

Serpell and coworkers[19] conducted a double-blind, randomized, placebo-controlled, 8-week study to evaluate the efficacy and safety of gabapentin doses up to 2400 mg/d in patients with neuropathic pain. The study took a novel approach by using inclusion criteria based on specific pain symptoms. The study included patients with diverse neuropathic pain syndromes, with at least two of the following: allodynia, burning pain, shooting pain, or hyperethenia. One hundred fifty-two patients were randomized to receive placebo and 153 patients were randomized to received gabapentin. The average daily pain diary score was compared from the final week to baseline values. The score decreased by 1.5 (21%) in the gabapentin group and by 1.0 (14%) in the placebo group (P = .048, rank-based ANCOVA). Gabapentin cay be started at a dose of 300 mg orally at night on day 1, increased to 300 mg orally twice a day on day 2, and increased to 300 mg orally three times a day on day 3. Patients may begin to experience efficacy (i.e., analgesia) within a week. The dose should be titrated as appropriate but may be doubled to 1800 mg/d by week 2, increased to 2400 mg/d by week 3, and increased to 3600 mg/d or greater if necessary or appropriate by week 4. Roughly 80% of patients tolerate gabapentin and the above titration schedule.[16–19]

Carbamazepine (Tegretol)

The analgesic properties of carbamazepine in patients with TN were published first in 1962. Chemically related to the tricyclic andidepressants, this drug decreases sodium and potassium conductance, and its primary mechanism of action on neuropathic pain is thought to be Na^+-channel blockade. Like most of the anticonvulsants, owing to the frequency-dependent nature of blockade of ionic conductance, it suppresses the spontaneously firing A delta and C fibers involved in hyperexitability states and not the normally conducting motor and touch nerve fibers.

Four randomized, double-blinded, crossover trials have been published that confirm the superiority of carbamazepine to placebo in treating TN.[20–23] With a NNT of 2.6 for this disorder,[24] carbamazepine remains the treatment of choice with responses usually observed after 5 to 14 days in as many as 89% of patients. It also appears efficacious in treating PDN. It has not been found to be as successful in treating PHN and central pain.

Carbamazepine, 5-carbamoyl-5-H-dibenzo(b,f)azepine, is a tricyclic compound containing an azeping ring with a double bond, two benzene rings, and one amide group with a molecular weight of about 236.[25] The peak plasma concentration generally occurs about 4 to 8 hours (infrequently up to 26 hours) after oral administration. The steady-state half-life in situation of chronic dosing ranges from about 10 to 20 hours, and bioavailability is approximately 75% to 85%.[26] The protein-bound fraction of carbamazeine is roughly 75% but varies with changes in serum alpha L-acid glycoprotein.[27,28] Carbamazepine is predominantly biotransformed via epoxidation (about 40%), hydroxylation (about 25%), glucuronidation (about 15%) and sulfuration (about 5%).[26] Carbamazepine is predominantly metabolized via cytochrome p450 3A4 to carbamazepine–10, 11-epoxide (a metabolite with equipotent anticonvulsant activity in animal models), which has a somewhat shorter half-life than its parent compound. Metabolism is almost complete with its major metabolite, carbamazepine-epoxide, being hydrolyzed to yield trans-10,11,dihydroxy-carbamazepine.[26] Carbamazepine induces its own metabolism (autoinduction), which may result in increased clearance, shortened serum half-life, and decreased serum levels after multiple repeated dosing.[29]

Carbamazepine may significantly interact with multiple medications (especially antiepileptic drugs). The Physicians Desk Reference (PDR) has a black-box warning regarding a very low incidence of aplastic anemia and agranulocytosis. Titration of the daily dose is usually in increments of 100 mg/week, from 200 mg/day to a median effective dose of 600 to 900 m/day in two divided doses. Rarely should doses exceed 1200 mg/day. It causes gastrointestinal side effects, in addition to the less common agranulocytosis, aplastic anemia (1 in 15,000 exposed), and hyponatremia (via antidiuretic hormone secretion) necessitating slow titration and occasional blood sampling. Dizziness and somnolence are the most common side effects and necessitate withdrawal from clinical trials of up to 11% of patients. Rash may lead to erythema multiforme or Stevens-Johnson syndrome.

Four double-blind trials have compared patients treated with carbamazepine to active control subjects. Vilming and coworkers[30] found it superior to tizanidine for the treatment of TN. Lindstrom and Lindblom[31] found equal efficacy with tocainide for TN. Lechin[32] found it less effective than pimozide for TN, but pimozide had a high frequency of adverse effects (83%). Gomez-Perez[33] found equal efficacy with nortriptyline and fluphenazine for painful diabetic neuropathy. Overall, the NNT for carbamazepine treatment of painful and was 3.3.[34]

Oxcarbazepine (Trileptal)

Oxcarbazepine (10,11-dihydro-10-oxo-5H-debenz(b,f)azepine-5-carboxanide) is an analogue of carbamazepine with a keto group at the 10 carbon position. Oxcarbazepine is roughly 50% protein bound in the plasma. Oxcarbazepine is a prodrug for 10-hydroxy-oxcarbazepine, the active metabolite of which has a half-life of about 8 to 10 hours. This monohydroxy derivative is generally excreted either unchanged in the urine or as a glucuronide conjugate. The dose should be at least cut by half if the patient has significant renal insufficiency.

Oxcarbazepine appears to have fewer drug interactions than carbamazepine, as well as less binding to serum proteins, linear pharmacokinetics, and no clinically significant hepatic autoinduction.[35]

The most frequent adverse effects experienced include dizziness and vertigo, weight gain and edema, gastrointestinal symptoms, fatigue, and allergic-type reactions. Cross-allergy to carbamazepine occurs in about 25% of patients and may be severe.[36]

Severe blood dyscrasias have not been reported, although isolated drops of white blood cell count below 3000 have occurred. Asymptomatic mild hyponatremia (especially in the elderly) may not be uncommon, but treatment of emergent hyponatremia (serum sodium < 125 mEg/L) occurred in 3% of patients.[37] Routine serum sodium monitoring is not necessary but should be used if individual clinical factors warrant this.[38] Precautions should be followed, with women using hormonal contraception methods due to enzyme induction interactions.[38]

Oxcarbazepine produces a blockade of voltage-sensitive sodium channels leading to stabilization of hyperexcitable neuronal membranes, inhibition of repetitive neuronal firing, and diminution of propagation of synaptic impulses.[39]

Oxcarbazepine is available as 150 mg, 300 mg, and 600 mg film-coated tablets as well as in oral suspension at 60 mg/mL.

The mechanism of action seems to involve both by both Na^+ and Ca^{2+} channel blockade, however, as with carbamazepine, most data suggest that the mechanism of action of these compounds is predominantly due to sodium channel inhibition. Several studies have reported on its efficacy in the treatment of TN as front-line therapy and in patients who did not respond to carbamazepine as well as other neuropathic conditions, thus proposing a niche role for this drug in treatment plans for neuropathic pain and perhaps radiculopathic pain as well.[40–42] Doses of 150 mg/day slowly titrated by 150 mg to 300 mg per week up to 1800 mg as appropriate in two divided doses are generally well tolerated. Patients should also be switched from carbamazepine to oxcarbazepine slowly, avoiding "overnight switching."

Savk and associates[43] reported on a small number of patients with notalgia paresthetica, a sensory neuropathy that generally presents with pruritis on the back, who responded reasonably well to oxcarbazepine.

Phenytoin (Dilantin, Epanutin)

Phenytoin was the first anticonvulsant to be reported, in 1942, to have efficacy in the treatment of neuropathic pain of TN.[44] Despite this, few randomized controlled trials exist on the analgesic efficacy of the drug, with a probable NNT for PDN reported to be in the range of other existing anticonvulsants.[24] Three randomized clinical trials exist of analgesic effectiveness in various neuropathic pain conditions, two for diabetic neuropathy[45,46] and one for various neuropathies.[47] Although results were somewhat conflicting for diabetic neuropathy, overall the NNT was calculated to be 2.1.[34] It blocks $Na+$ channels and at high concentrations may inhibit presynaptic glutamate release. Phenytoin is a weak acid with limited aqueous solubility. Enteral administration yields slow variable and sometimes partial absorption. Peak concentration in plasma may occur as early as 3 hours or as late as 12 hours following single-dose administration. Phenytoin is about 90% protein bound (albumin) and is biotransformed mainly via the hepatic endoplasma reticulum. Although multiple metabolites exist, the major metabolite (60–70%) is a parahydroxyphenyl derivative and is inactive. Up to a plasma concentration of 10 μg/mL, elimination is via first-order kinetics (plasma half-life, roughly 6–24 hours). At higher concentrations, dose-dependent elimination predominates (plasma half-life, roughly 20–60 hours).

Phenytoin is available as 30 mg, 50 mg, and 100 mg tablets, as 300 mg extended-release kapseals, and as a liquid concentration 125 mg/1.5 mL and 50 mg/1 mL. Daily doses of 300 mg/day are usual and can be taken at once. Ataxia, nystagamus, and slurred speech may occur in 10% of patients. Gingival hyperplasia, facial hair thickening, a narrow therapeutic window, and interaction with other drugs requiring serum level monitoring remain probable reasons for its relative nonpopularity.

Topiramate (Topamax)

Topiramate, 2,3:4,5–bis-O-(1-methylethylident)-beta-D-fructopyranose sulfamate, is a sulfonamide relative (a sulfamate–substituted monosaccharide) that exists as a white crystalline power with a bitter taste. Topiramate is most soluble in alkaline solutions (pH 9–10). Many mechanisms have been postulated to explain its mechanism of action, including blocking voltage-dependent sodium channels, potentiating the inhibitory action of GABA transmission, and blocking the excitatory action of the D-amino-3-hydroxy-5-methyl-4-isoxazole-propionic acid subtype of glutamate receptor.[48] Although topiramate may inhibit carbonic anhydrase, this does not appear to contribute significantly to its mechanism of action. Topiramate also may selectively attenuate nicotine-induced increases in monoamine releases, although whether this action is any clinical significance if speculative.[49] Topiramate is well absorbed after oral administration, with serum protein binding being less than 15%.[48] The half-life is 18 to 24 hours and clearance is predominantly via the kidneys with a small hepatic component.[48]

Topiramate is available as 15 mg, 25 mg, 100 mg, and 200 mg tablets as well as in gelatin capsules with "sprinkles" (small white spheres) in doses of 15 mg and 25 mg. The usual starting dose is 25 to 30 mg at night, which can be increased slowly over 8 weeks as appropriate to 400 mg/day in two divided doses. Gradual initiation of topiramate therapy may significantly improve patient compliance.[50] The side effect profile includes fatigue, anorexia, weight loss, asthenia, dizziness, tremor, headaches, cognitive dysfunction, and urolithiasis (1.5% due to carbonic anhydrase inhibitor activity).[51] The weight loss recorded has been up to 7% of body weight and seems to peak at 15 to 18 months of therapy.[48,52]

Although dose-ranging studies did not reveal a high incidence of cognitive dysfunction, Rosenfeld and colleagues[52] reported cognitive side effects in 83% of 18 patients taking 400 mg/day.[52] Topiramate has also been anecdotally reported to alleviate various neuropathic pain states (including painful diabetic neuropathy), intercostal neuralgia, and trigeminal neuralgia.[53–55]

Lamotrigine (Lamictal)

Lamotrigine, like gabapentin, was introduced for adjunctive treatment of partial seizures. Early animal data indicated that it was promising as an analgesic, and evidence is accumulating for a role in the treatment of neuropathic pain.[56–58] It is a phenyltriazine derivative that blocks voltage dependent Na^+ channels and inhibits release of the excitatory transmitters, glutamate, and aspartate. Zakrzewska and coworkers[59] has shown it to be superior to placebo in the treatment of TN, although a daily dose of 200 mg/day was ineffective at controlling neuropathic symptoms in various neuropathic pain conditions in one trial.[60] Lamotrigine is available as 100 mg, 150 mg, and 200 mg tablets. The starting dose is 25 to 50 mg/day increasing slowly as appropriate in small increments every 14 days to 200 to 500 mg/day in two divided doses. Up to 10% of patients develop a rash, which can rarely progress into Stevens-Johnson Syndrome (3/1000) or toxic epidermal necrolysis (PDR black box warning) and somnolence can occur. Other side effects may include dizziness, nausea, constipation, ataxia, and diplophia. Long-term use of lamotrigine can lead to accumulation and binding to melanin–rich tissues in the body (especially the eyes), leading to visual blurriness. The optimal doses in neuropathic pain disorders are not known. Peak plasma levels following oral administration occur within 1 to 4 hours and interactions can occur with the other anticonvulsants due to moderate protein binding (55%) and drug metabolism. The coadministration of phenytoin or barbiturates shortens the half-life of lamotrigine through enzyme induction. The metabolism of lamotrigine is decreased with valproic acid and doses, if it is used concurrently, should not exceed 150 mg/day. Lamotrigine can cause increased plasma carbamazepine levels, producing clinical toxicity. Lamotrigine may also have analgesic efficacy in central post-stroke pain[61] as well as HIV polyneuropathy.[62]

Valproic Acid and Divalproex Sodium (Depakote)

Valproate (2-propylpentanoic acid) is a broad-spectrum anticonvulsant originally used as an organic solvent. Valproic acid is a highly protein bound, branched-chain fatty acid that undergoes beta-oxidation and easily penetrates the blood-brain barrier. Divalproex sodium is a stable coordinated complex of equal quantities of sodium valproate and valproic acid. Its mechanism of action seems to be multifactorial and may include increasing GABA levels by inhibiting enzymes involved in its degradation (eg GABA transaminase [probably not a major contribution in therapeutic doses] and succinic semialdehyde dehydrogenase) and/or increasing GABA synthesis (facilitation of synthesis via glutamatic acid dehydrogenase [GAD]); selectively enhancing post-synaptic GABA responses; direct effect of valproic acid on neuronal membranes voltage dependent sodium channels, calcium dependent potassium currents, and/or T-type calcium currents; and reduction of excitatory transmission by excitatory amino acids (e.g., aspartate), although there is no convincing direct evidence to support this.[63]

Valproic acid is roughly 80% to 95% bound to plasma proteins, rapidly absorbed throughout the intestine, and highly bioavailable (ingestion of food may significantly slow the onset of peak levels after oral administration). The half-life is roughly about 15 hours (range, 6–16 hours). Valproic acid is available in the United States, as 250 mg capsules, as the sodium salt in tablets (125 mg to 250 mg), as the sodium salt (sodium valproate) in syrup (250 mg/5 mL), as enteric–coated and delayed-release tablets of sodium divalproex (125 mg, 250 mg, 500 mg), and as a particulate presentation (sprinkles). The starting dose of valproic acid usually is 250 mg per day, and the dose can be slowly titrated upward as appropriate to about 1200 mg/day, generally given in two divided doses. Valproic acid has a PDR black box warning for hepatotoxicity, teratogenicity, and pancreatitis.

Valproic acid has multiple drug interactions and idiosyncratic, dose-related, as well as hypersensitivity significant adverse reactions requiring monitoring of blood tests. Side effects include gastrointestinal upset, nausea, vomiting, weight gain, tremor, rash, CNS depression, hair loss, pancreatitis, and severe hepatic and hematological toxicity. The most common clinical use for valproic acid appears to be for migraine headaches.[64–71] It has also been used for chronic daily headaches.[72] In early trials of patients with trigeminal neuralgia who received valproic acid, 50% experienced relief, whereas 37% of patients with lacinating pain due to various causes experienced relief.[73] Sodium valproate has also been studied in patients with cancer-related neuropathic pain.[74]

Clonazepam (Klonopin)

Although structurally related to and considered to belong to the benzodiazepine family of drugs, the antiepileptic mechanism of action of clonazepam is thought to involve potentiation of inhibitory GABA neurotransmission. Clonazepan, a GABA-B agonist-like bacelofen (and therefore in general they should not be used concurrently), is 81% to 98% absorbed following oral administration, with peak plasma levels occurring in 1 to 4 hours.[75] It is highly bound to plasma proteins (86%) and is highly lipid soluble.[75] Clonazepan has a long elimination half-life of roughly 18 to 36 hours (single-dose studies, 18.7–39 hours, and multiple-dose studies, 31–42 hours) and does not seem to have significant hepatic enzyme induction issues.[75] It is metabolized predominantly by reduction of the nitro groups, yielding inactive 7-amino derivatives.[75] Conjugated metabolites are excreted in the urine.[75] Clonazepan is available as 0.5 mg (scored), 1 mg, and 2 mg tablets. Commencing at 0.5 mg at night and increasing slowly up to 4 mg/day as appropriate, some success has been achieved with this dose in treating the cranial neuralgias, including glossopharyngeal neuralgia and cluster headache.[76,77] The reduction in pain scores achieved with clonazepam may also be due to the known effects on anxiety and muscle spasticity. Sedation is the main side effect, but liver enzyme elevations and blood dyscrasias should be monitored from time to time. Drowsiness, dizziness, and fatigue are also not uncommon.

Pregabalin

Pregabalin, like gabapentin, is a GABA analog, but without direct agonist effect at the receptor. Earlier animal work demonstrated potential efficacy in neuropathic pain models,[78] but a question over the safety of the agent arising from animal studies has halted progress on trials of the efficacy of pregabalin on neuropathic pain.[79]

Tiagabine

Tiagabine is derived from nipecotic acid and inhibits the uptake of GABA presynaptically. The antinociceptive effect is abolished by pretreatment with GABA-B receptor antagonists in animal models.[80] Tiagabine increases GABA levels in the brain.[81] Tiagabine has a bioavailability of roughly 90% and a serum half-life of about 7 hours and is approximately 95% protein bound. Its half-life may be shortened to 2 to 3 hours when it is administered concurrently with enzyme-inducing AEDs. It is metabolised via the cytochrome p-450 system (mostly 3A) by carbon oxidation of the thiopetene ring, followed by conjugation with glucorinic acid. Tiagabine is available in 2 mg, 4 mg, 12 mg, 16 mg, and 20 mg tablets. The starting dose is 4 mg orally at night and may be increased slowly as appropriate by 4 mg each week. Although it is usually given three times a day, clinicians have used two to four doses per day, and adult maintenance doses for epilepsy range between 32 to 56 mg/d. As with all AEDs, no dose range or therapeutic blood concentration exists for analgesic effects.

Felbamate

Felbamate is a dicarbamate that can inhibit NMDA-evoked potentials. Imamura and Bennett,[82] in a neurobiological study in rats, demonstrated that felbamate reduced mechanoallodynia/hyperalgesia as well as thermal hyperalgesia. This agent continues to be the most effective analgesic AED in their rat models for induced neuroapathy pain. (Unfortunately, due to potential side effects it is not used as an analgesic.) Felbamate's theraputic efficacy in the laboratory may be due to its multiple mechanisms of action, which include inhibition of NMDA and AMPA/kainate receptors, potentiating GABA receptor–mediated chloride channels, and inhibiting spontaneous discharges from voltage-dependent sodium channels. It has been reported to be effective in cases with refractory trigeminal neuralgia at doses of 400 to 800 mg tid.[83] Because of the potential for bone marrow and liver toxicity, its current use in the clinical arena is only in patients with refractory epilepsy.

Levetiracetam (Keppra)

Levetiracetam, a pyrrolidone (2-oxopyrrolidine) family derivative, although developed as a cognitive enhancing agent, possesses antiepileptic in addition to anxiolytic features. It may act via an unknown binding site in the brain.[84] Biochemical evidence exists for an effect on several neurochemical transmission systems, including the dopaminergic and glutamate pathways. It does appear to have a GABA-mediated effect, although it does not have significant affinity for GABA receptors.[85] The inhibition of higher voltage activated calcium currents may contribute somewhat to its mechanism of action. Lukyanetz and colleagues[86] published data suggesting that levetiracetam selectively inhinits N-type calcium channels. It is used as adjunctive therapy for partial seizures and is potentially useful in treating photosensitive epilepsy. Levetiracetan is available in 250 mg, 500 mg and 750 mg tablets. The recommended starting dose is 1000 mg/day in two divided doses, increasing slowly over a month to 2000 mg/day as appropriate. It is absorbed rapidly and almost completely with peak levels reached within an hour after administration. The half-life is about 8 hours, and it is largely unbound to plasma proteins, with 66% renally excreted in the unchanged form. The remainder is transformed to inactive form by hydrolysis of the acetamide group. Side effects include nausea, ataxia, headache, dizziness, asthenia, and sedation or somnolence. Reports of the coding term "infection" (common cold, upper respiratory infection) were not preceded by low neutrophil counts and probably were due to selection of adverse event coding terms.[87] Concurrent use of levetiracetam and carbamazepine should be monitored closely, as there seems to be a potential pharmaceodynamic interaction (i.e., serum drug levels are unaffected), leading to symptoms of carbamazepine toxicity.[88]

Vigabatrin

Vigabatrin selectively and irreversibly inhibits the aminotransferase enzyme that catabolizes GABA (GABA-T). It has antinociceptive properties in animal models of neuropathic pain[89] but has not been approved in the United States because of reports of retinal toxicity. Vigabatrin irreversibly inactivates GABA-T (pyridoxal form) by interacting with the pyridoxal phosphate cofactor to form a Schiff base at the active site of GABA–T. A proton from the

Schiff base irreversibly binds to a nucleophilic acid at the GABA-T active site which blocks other substrates.[90] Vigabatrin may possibly induce psychiatric syndromes.

Zonisamide (Zonegran)

Zonisamide is a sulfonamide drug that is used for adjunctive therapy for partial seizures. Zonisamide (1,2-benzisoxazole-3-methane sulfonamide) blocks sodium channels and reduces low voltage-dependent T-type calcium currents, stabilizing neuronal membranes and suppressing neuronal hypersynchronization.[91] Zonisamide may also inhibit nitric oxide synthase activity induced by NMDA receptor complex activation, which could contribute to analgesic effects in neuropathic pain.[92] It appears to bind to the GABA receptor and may facilitate dopaminergic and serotonergic neurotransmission. Additionally, it possesses carbonic anhydrase inhibitor activity (although this probably does not contribute to its mechanism of action)[93] and exhibits in vivo antioxidant properties, scavenging free radicals.[94] Zonisamide is available in a 100 mg capsule. The starting dose is 100 mg orally at night and may be increased slowly as appropriate: 100 mg per week to 400 mg/d. In the elderly, because of the long half-life, dosing can be started at 100 mg orally every third day, then changed to 100 mg every other day and then to 100 mg every night. A capsule with 50 mg is planned for the future.

Zonisamide is contraindicated in patients with hypersensitivity to sulfonamides. Due to its carbonic anyhydrase inhibiting activity, it may potentially lead to the development of renal calculi. A report exists of the possible induction of a systemic lupus erythematosus–like syndrome by zonisamide[95] as well as its potentially leading to renal tubular acidosis.[96] These cases resolved after discontinuation of the drug.[95,96]

Zonisamide is 40% to 50% protein bound, metabolized by the liver by biotransformation (reduction cleavage of the benzisoxazole ring by the cytochrome p450 system), and excreted by the kidneys with a plasma half-life of 63 hours. Drug interactions have been noted with carbamazepine and phenytoin. Anorexia, somnolence, dizziness, ataxia, fatigue, and nystagamus are known side effects.[91]

Stiripentol

Stiripentol is an α-ethylene alcohol derivative with anticonvulsant activity but an unknown mechanism of action. Stiripentol does inhibit GABA uptake and GABA-transaminase.[97] This agent is not currently clinically available in the United State.

Clobazam (Mystan)

Clobazam is an AED that is a 1, 5-benzodiazepine with nitrogen atoms in the 1 and 5 positions of the heterocyclic ring and a different pharmacological profile from that of 1,4-benzodiazepines.[98] Although clobazam has a lower affinity for the benzodiazepine receptor than 1,4-benzodiazepines, it appears to possess selectivity for the omega-2 receptor (anticonvulsant activity) compared with the omega-1 receptor (e.g., sedation).[98] It therefore also may have somewhat less association with dependency problems than 1,4-benzodiazepines. This agent is not currently available clinically in the United States.

TREATMENT STRATEGIES

Gabapentin and carbamazepine are the first choice drugs for patients with chronic pain disorders with a neuropathic pain component. Owing to its superior safety profile and lack of drug interactions, gabapentin is the most commonly prescribed anticonvulsant in the United States for chronic pain. For TN, carbamazepine retains an excellent record of efficacy, and most physicians consider it to be a first-line drug (TABLE 2). Second-line agents include oxcarbazepine and phenytoin for TN, valproic acid for migraine prophylaxis, and clonazepam for other cranial neuralgias. Lamotrigine and topiramate do not have a sufficient evidence-base for widespread use, but knowledge of their mechanisms of action suggests a role for these in patients who do not respond to first-line agents. The combination of agents with differing mechanisms of action, such as gabapentin and topiramate, may also have a role in resistant pain disorders.

CLINICAL PEARLS

1. The key to patient tolerability of the anticonvulsants as therapy in chronic pain states is slow titration to the intended dose, because a significant number of patients have intolerance of even the newer agents. The clinician should be familiar with the pharmacokinetic differences of the various AEDs (TABLE 3).
2. Outside of the classic neuropathic pain disorders, trials of these agents can be used as adjunctive therapy, but the greatest clinical success will continue to be with TN, PHN,

TABLE 2

Treatment Strategies with Anticonvulsants for Neuropathic Pain Disorders

Pain disorder	First Line	Second Line	Third Line
Painful diabetic neuropathy	Gabapentin	Topiramate Oxcarbazepine Zonisamide	Phenytoin
Trigeminal neuralgia	Carbamazepine	Gabapentin Oxcarbazepine	Phenytoin Topiramate Lamotrigine
Post-herpetic neuralgia	Gabapentin	Carbamazepine Oxcarbazepine Topiramate	Valproate Lamotrigine
Migraine	Valproate	Gabapentin Levetiractem	Tiagabine Topiramate
Cranial neuralgias	Carbamazepine	Gabapentin Oxcarbazepine	Phenytoin Lamotrigine
Central Pain	Carbamazepine	Gabapentin Oxcarbazepine Zonisamide Topiramate	Phenytoin Lamotrigine Valproate Clonazepam
Neuropathy/Radiculopathy	Gabapentin	Oxcarbazepine Topiramate Zonisamide	Valproate Tiagabine

TABLE 3

Pharmacological Properties of Antiepileptic Drugs

Antiepileptic Drug	Clinical Adult Dose Analgesic Range (mg/d)	Protein Binding (%)	Half-life (hr)	Excretion (Metabolic)	Usual Adult Analgesic Dosing Regimen
Carbamazepine	200–800	75	10–20	Hepatic	Carbatrol or Tegretol–XR, bid; tid, other forms
Gabapentin	900–3600	<10	5–9	Renal	tid
Oxcarbazepine	300–1800	50	9 (8–10)	Renal	bid
Phenytoin	300–600	90	Varies with concentration 12–36	Mostly hepatic/renal	qhs
Topiramate	50–400	15	18–30	Mostly renal/hepatic	bid
Lamotrigine	50–300	55	24 (15–30)	Hepatic glucoronide conjugation	bid
Valproate	500–1200	Concentration dependent 90	15 (6–16)	Liver	Valproicacid, tid; divalproexsodium, bid
Clorazepam	0.5–4	85	23 (20–40)	Liver	qhs
Tiagabine	12–44	95	5–10	Mostly hepatic/renal	tid
Zonisamide	100–400	40	60 (25–60)	Hepatorenal	qhs
Levetiracetam	1000–2000	<10	7 (6–8)	Mostly renal/hepatic	bid
Clobazam	10–40	85	18	Hepatic	qhs
Stiripentol	1500–3000	99	4–12	Hepatic	bid

and PDN. Because the optimal doses of the newer agents for many pain disorders are undefined, individually titrating to efficacy or the limit of side effects is a useful exercise.

3. Because some of these agents have separate and distinct mechanisms of action, combining two different drugs may lead to success in managing chronic neuropathic pain.

CONCLUSION

Anticonvulsant drugs are effective in treating neuropathic pain disorders. As the knowledge of the central mechanisms underlying pain increases and evidence gathers for the efficacy of the anticonvulsants outside the classic neuropathic pain states, including acute pain,[102] we may see the development of new treatment approaches in which anticonvulsants play a wider role. The success of drugs that do not act primarily by Na^+ channel blockade, such as gabapentin, has led to a surge in interest in developing other analgesic agents that may target neuropathic pain. Developing a multimodal approach in treatment strategies for chronic neuropathic pain with the anticonvulsants requires a working knowledge of the proposed mechanism of action of each, in addition to potential interactions and side effect profiles of each agent.

REFERENCES

1. Woolf CJ, Mannion RJ: Neuropathic pain: Aetiology, symptoms, mechanisms, and management. Lancet 353:1959, 1999.
2. Backonja MM: Anticonvulsants (antineuropathics) for neuropathic pain syndromes. Clin J Pain 16 (2 Suppl):S67, 2000.
3. MacPherson RD: The pharmacological basis of contemporary pain management. Pharmacol Ther 88:163, 2000.
4. Ross EL: The evolving role of antiepileptic drugs in treating neuropathic pain. Neurology 55(5 (Suppl 1)):S41, discussion S54, 2000.
5. Devor M: Neuropathic pain and injured nerve. Br Med Bull 47:619, 1991.
6. Burchiel KJ: Carbamazepine inhibits spontaneous activity in experimental neuromas. Exp Neurol 102:249, 1988.
7. Tanelian DL, Brose WG: Neuropathic pain can be relieved by drugs that are use-dependent sodium channel blockers: Lidocaine, carbamazepine, and mexiletine. Anesthesiology 74:949, 1991.
8. Sangameswaran L, Delgado SF, Fish LM, et al: Structure and function of a novel voltage-gated tetrodotoxin-resistant sodium channel specific to sensory neurons. J Bio Chem 27:5953, 1996.
9. Laird MA, Gidal BE: Use of gabapentin in the treatment of neuropathic pain. Ann Pharmacother 34:802, 2000.
10. Herranz JL: [Current data on gabapentin]. Rev Neurol 30 Suppl 1:S125, 2000.
11. Tremont-Lukats IW, Megeff C, Backonja MM: Anticonvulsants for neuropathic pain syndromes: Mechanisms of action and place in therapy. Drugs 60:1029, 2000.
12. Gee NS, Brown JP, Dissanayake VU, et al: The novel anticonvulsant drug, gabapentin (Neurontin) binds to the alpha-2-delta subunit of the calcium channel. J Bio Chem 271:5776, 1996.
13. Stanfa LC, Singh L, Williams RG, Dickenson AH: Gabapentin, ineffective in normal rats, markedly reduces C-fibre evoked responses after inflammation. Neuroreport 8:587, 1997.
14. Comstock TJ, Sica DA, Bockbrader HN, et al: Gabapentin pharmacokinetics in subjects with various degrees of renal function [abstract]. J Clin Pharmacol 30:862, 1990.
15. Halstenson CE, Keane WF, Tuerck D, et al: Disposition of gabapentin (GAB) in hemodialysis (HD) patients [abstract]. J Clin Pharmacol 32:751, 1992.
16. Backonja MM, Beydoun A, Edwards KR, et al: Gabapentin for the symptomatic treatment of painful neuropathy in patients with diabetes mellitus. A randomised controlled trial. JAMA 280:1831, 1998.
17. Rowbotham M, Harden N, Stacey B, et al: Gabapentin for the treatment of postherpetic neuralgia: A randomized controlled trial. JAMA 280:1837, 1998.
18. Rice ASC, Maton S: Postherptic Neuralgia Study Group: Gabapentin in post herpetic neuralgia: A randomised, double blind, placebo-controlled study. Pain 94:215, 2001.
19. Serpell MG, and the Neuropathic Pain Study Group: Gabapentin in neuropathic pain syndromes: A randomised, double blind, placebo-controlled trial. Data on file at Pfizer.
20. Killian JM, Fromm GH: Carbamazepine in the treatment of neuralgia. Arch Neurol. 19:129, 1968.
21. Rockliff BW, Davis EH: Controlled sequential trials of carbmazepine in trigeminal neuralgia. Arch Neurol 15:129, 1966.
22. Campbell FG, Graham JG, Zikha KJ: Clinical trial of carbamazepine (Tegretol) in trigeminal neuralgia. J Neurosurg Neurol Psych 29:265, 1966.
23. Nicol C: A four year double blind randomized study of tegretol in facial pain. Headache 9:54, 1969.
24. McQuay H, Carroll D, Jadad AR, et al: Anticonvulsant drugs for management of pain: A systematic review. BMJ 311:1047, 1995.
25. Gagneux AR: The chemistry of carbamazepine. In: Birkmeyer E, ed. Epileptic seizures—Behaviour—Pain. Birkmeyer, Vienna, Austria, 1976, pp 120–126.
26. Faigle JW, Feldman KF: Pharmacokinetic data of carbamazepine and its major metabolites in man.

In: Schneider H, Janz D, Gardner-Thorpe C, Meinardi H, Shervin AL, eds. Clincal Pharmacology of Antiepileptic Drugs. Springer-Verlag, Berlin, 1975, pp 159–165.

27. Hooper WD, Dubetz JK, Brohner F, et al: Plasma protein binding of carbamazepine. Clin Pharmacol Ther 17:433, 1978.

28. Baruzzi A, Contin M, Perucca E, et al: Altered serum protein binding of carbamazepine in disease states associated with an increased alpha 1–acid glycoprotein concentration. Eur J Clin Pharmacol 31:85, 1986.

29. Bertilsson L, Hojer B, Tybring G, et al: Autoinduction of carbamazepine metabolism in children examined by a stable isotope technique. Clin Pharmacol Ther 27:83, 1980.

30. Vilming ST, Lyberg T, Latastex: Tizanidine in the management of trigeminal neuralgia. Cephalgia 6:181, 1986.

31. Lindstrom P, Lindblom U: The analgesic effect of tocainide in trigeminal neuralgia. Pain 28:45, 1987.

32. Lechin F, van der Dijs B, Lechin ME, et al: Pimozide therapy for trigeminal neuralgia. Arch Neurol 46:960, 1989.

33. Gomez-Perez FJ, Choza R, Rios JM, et al: Nortriptyline–fluphenazine vs. carbamazepine in the symptomatic treatment of diabetic neuropathy. Arch Med Res 27:525, 1996.

34. Backonja M: Anticonvutsants and antiarrhythmics in the treatment of neuropathic pain syndromes In: Hansson PT, Field HL, Hill RG, Marchettini P, eds. Neuropathic Pain: Pathophysiology and Treatment Progress in Pain Research and Management, Vol 21. IASP Press, Seattle, 2001.

35. Pendlebury SC, Moses DK, Eadie MJ. Hyponatremia during oxcarbazepine therapy. Hum Toxicol 8:337, 1989.

36. Dam M: Practical aspects of ox carbazepine treatment. Epilepsia 35(suppl 3):S23, 1994.

37. Glauser TA: Oxcarbazepine in the treatment of epilepsy. Pharmacotherapy 21:904, 2001.

38. Smith PE: The UK Oxcarbazepine Advisory Board Clinical recommendations of oxcarbazepine. Seizure 10:87, 2001.

39. McLean NJ, Schmutz M, Wamil AW, et al: Oxcarbazepine: Mechanisms of action. Epilepsia 35 (suppl 3):55, 1994.

40. Beydoun A, Kutluay E: Oxcarbazepine. Expert Opin Pharmacother 3:59, 2002.

41. Farago F: Trigeminal neuralgia: Its treatment with two new carbamazepine analogues. Eur Neurol 26:73, 1987.

42. Zakrzewska JM, Patsalos PN: Oxcarbazepine: A new drug in the management of intractable trigeminal neuralgia. J Neurol Neurosurg Psychiatry 52:472, 1989.

43. Savk E, Bolukbasi O, Akyol, et al: Open pilot study treatment on oxcarbazepine for the treatment of notalgia paresthetica. J Am Acad Dermatol 45:630, 2001.

44. Bergouignan M: Cures heureuses de nevralgies faciales essentielles par diphenyl-hydantoinate de soude. Rev Laryngol Otol Rhinol 63:34, 1942.

45. Saudek CD, Werns S, Reidenberg MM: Phenytoin in the treatment of diabetic symmetrical polyneuropathy. Clin Pharmacol Ther 22:196, 1977.

46. Chadda VS, Mathur M: Double-blind study of the effects of diphenylhydantoin sodium in diabetic neuropathy. J Assoc Physician India 26:403, 1978.

47. McCleane GJ: Intravenous infusion of phenytoin relieves neuropathic pain: A randomized, double-blinded placebo-controlled, crossover study. Anesth Analg 89:985, 1999.

48. Ben-Nemachem E: Potential antiepileptic drugs: Topiramate. In: Levy RH, Mattson RH, Meldrum BS, eds. Antiepileptic Drugs, 4th ed. Raven Press, New York, 1995, pp 1063–1069.

49. Schiffer WK, Gerasimov MR, Marstellar DA, et al: Topiramate selectively attenuates nicotine induced increases in monoamine release. Synapse 42:196, 2001.

50. Biton V, Edwards KR, Montouris GD, et al: Topiramate titration and tolerability. Ann Pharmacother 35:173, 2001.

51. Privitera M, Fincham R, Penry J, et al: Topiramate placebo-controlled dose-ranging trial in refractory partial epilepsy using 600-, 800-, and 1000-mg daily dosages. Topiramate YE study Group. Neurology 46:1678, 1996.

52. Rosenfeld WE, Holmes GB, Hunt TL, et al: Topiramate: Effective dosing enhances potential for success [abstract]. Epilepsia 33(suppl 3):118, 1992.
53. Edwards K, Glantz MJ, Button J, et al: Efficacy and safety of topiramate in the treatment of painful diabetic neuropathy: A double-blind, placebo-controlled study. Neurology 54(S3):A81, 2000.
54. Bajwa ZZH, Sami N, Warfield CA, et al: Topiramate relieves refractory intercostal neuralgia. Neurology 52:1917, 1999.
55. Zvartau-Hind M, Din MU, Gilani A, et al: Topiramate relieves refractory trigeminal neuralgia in MS patients. Neurology 55:1587, 2000.
56. McCleane GJ: Lamotrigine in the management of neuropathic pain: A review of the literature. Clin J Pain 16:321, 2000.
57. Devulder J, De Laat M: Lamotrigine in the treatment of chronic refractory neuropathic pain. J Pain Symptom Manage 19:398, 2000.
58. di Vadi PP, Hamann W: The use of lamotrigine in neuropathic pain. Anaesthesia 53:808, 1998.
59. McCleane G: 200 mg daily of lamotrigine has no analgesic effect in neuropathic pain: A randomised, double-blind, placebo controlled trial. Pain 83:105, 1999.
60. Zakrzewska JM, Chaudhry Z, Nurmikko TJ, et al: Lamotrigine (Lamictal) in refractory trigeminal neuralgia: results from a double blind placebo controlled crossover trial. Pain 74:223, 1997.
61. Vestergaard K, Anderssen G, Gottruptt, et al: Lamotrigine for central poststroke pain: A randomised controlled trial. Neurology 56:184, 2001.
62. Simpson DM, Olney R, McArthur JC, et al: A placebo-controlled trial of lamotrigine for painful HIV-associated neuropathy. Neurology 54:2115, 2000.
63. Johannessen CU: Mechanisms of action of valproate: A commentatory. Neurochem Int 37:103, 2000.
64. Gallagher RM, Mueller LL, Freitag FG: Divalproex sodium in the treatment of migraine and cluster headache. J Am Osteopath Assoc 102:92, 2002.
65. Norton J: Use of intravenous valproate sodium in status migraine. Headache 40:755, 2000.
66. Rothrock JF: Clinical studies of valproate for migraine prophylaxis. Cephalalgia 17:81, 1997.
67. Rothrock JF, Kelly NM, Brody ML, et al: A differential response to treatment with divalproex sodium in patients with intractable headache. Cephalalgia 14:241, 1994.
68. Silberstein SD: Divalproex sodium in headache: Literature review and clinical guidelines. Headache 36:547, 1996.
69. Silberstein SD, Wilmore LJ: Divalproex sodium: Migraine treatment and monitoring. Headache 36;239, 1996.
70. Silberstein SD, Collins SD: Safety of divalproex sodium in migraine prophylaxis: An open-label, long-term study. Long-Term Safety of Depakote in Headache Prophylaxis Study Group. Headache 39:633, 1999.
71. Mathew NT, Saper JR, Silberstein SD, et al: Migraine prophylaxis with divalproex. Arch Neurol 52:281, 1995.
72. Freitag FG, Diamond S, Diamond ML, et al: Divalproex in the long-term treatment of chronic daily headache. Headache 41:271, 2001.
73. Swerdlow M, Cundill JG: Anticonvulsant drugs used in the treatment of lacinating pain: A comparison. Anaesthesia 36:1129, 1981.
74. Hardy JR, Rees EA, Gwilliam B, et al: A phase II study to establish the efficacy and toxicity of sodium valproate in patients with cancer-related neuropathic pain. J Pain Symptom Manage 21:204, 2001.
75. Sata S: Benzodiazepines, clonazepam. In Levy RH, Mattson RH, Meldrum BS, eds. Antiepileptic Drugs, 4th ed. Raven Press, New York, 1995, pp 725–734.
76. Caccia MR: Clonazepam in facial neuralgia and cluster headache: Clinical and electrophysiological study. Eur Neurol 13:560, 1975.
77. Smirne S, Scarlato G: Clonazepam in cranial neuralgias. Med J Aust 1:93, 1977.
78. Field MJ, McCleary S, Hughes J, Singh L: Gabapentin and pregabalin, but not morphine and amitripty-

line, block both static and dynamic components of mechanical allodynia induced by streptozocin in the rat. Pain 80:391, 1999.

79. Selak I:Pregabalin (Pfizer). Curr Opin Investig Drugs 2:828, 2001.

80. Ipponi A, Lamberti C, Medica A, et al: Tiagabine antinociception in rodents depends on GABA(B) receptor activation: Parallel antinociception testing and medial thalamus GABA microdialysis. Eur J Pharmacol 368:205, 1999.

81. During M, Mattson R, Scheyer R, et al: The effect of tiagabine on extracellular GABA levels in the human hippocampus [abstract]. Epilepsia 33(suppl 3):83, 1992.

82. Imamura Y, Bennett GJ: Felbamate relieves several abnormal pain sensations in rats with an experimental peripheral neuropathy. J Pharmacol Exp Ther 275:177, 1995.

83. Cheshire WP: Felbamate relieved trigeminal neuralgia. Clin J Pain 11:139, 1995.

84. Noyer M, Gillard M, Matagne A, et al: The novel antiepileptic drug levetiracetam (ucbL059) appears to act via a specific binding site in CNS membranes. Eur J Pharmacol 286:137, 1995.

85. Sills GJ, Leach JP, Fraser CM, et al: Neurochemical studies with the novel anticonvulsant levetiracetam in mouse brain. Eur J Pharmacol 325:35–40, 1997.

86. Lukyanetz EA, Shkryl VM, Lostyuk PG: Selective blockade of N-type calcium channels by levetiracetam. Epilepsia 43:9, 2002.

87. French J, Edrick P, Cramer JA: A systematic review of the safety profile of levetiracetam: A new antiepileptic drug. Epilepsy Res 47:77, 2001.

88. Sisodiya SM, Sander JW, Patsalos PN: Carbamazepine toxicity during combination therapy with levetiracetam: A pharmacodynamic interaction. Epilepsy Res 48:217, 2002.

89. Alves ND, de Castro-Costa CM, de Carvalho AM, et al: Possible analgesic effect of vigabatrin in animal experimental chronic neuropathic pain. Arq Neuropsiquiatr 57:916, 1999.

90. Jung MJ, Lippert B, Metcalf BW, et al: Gamma–vinyl–GABA (4-amino-hexenoic acid) a selective irreversible inhibitor of GABA-T: Effects on brain GABA metabolism in mice. J Neurochem 29:797, 1977.

91. Peters DH, Sorkin EM: Zonisamide: A review of its pharmacodynamic and pharmacokinetic properties, and therapeutic potential in epilepsy. Drugs 45:760, 1993.

92. Noda Y, Mori A, Packer L: Zonisamide inhibits nitric oxide synthase activity induced by N-methyl-D-aspartate and buthionine sulfoximine in the rat hippocampus. Res Commun Mol Pathol Pharmacol 105:23, 1999.

93. Masuda Y, Noguchi H, Karasawa T: Evidence against a significant implication of carbonic anhydrase inhibitory activity of zonisamide in its anticonvulsive effects. Arzneimittelforschung 44:267, 1994.

94. Mori A, Noda Y, Packer L: The anticonvulsant zonisamide scavenges free radicals. Epilepsy Res 30:153, 1998.

95. Mutoh, Hidaka Y, Hirose Y, et al: Possible induction of systemic lupus erythematosus by zonisamide. Pediatr Neurol 25:340, 2001.

96. Inoue T, Kira R, Kaku Y, et al: Renal tubular acidosis associated with zonisamide therapy. Epilepsia 41:1642, 2000.

97. Poisson M, Huguet F, Savattier A, et al: A new type of anticonvulsant, stirpentol. Pharmacological profile and neurochemical study. Arzenmittelforschung 34:199, 1984.

98. Nakajima H: A pharmacological profile of clobazam (Mystan), a new antiepileptic drug. Nippon Yakurigaku Zasshi. 118:117, 2001.

99. Mao J, Chen LL: Gabapentin in pain management. Anesth Analg 91:680, 2000.

100. Gu Y, Huang LY: Gabapentin actions on N-methyl-D-aspartate receptor channels are protein kinase C-dependent. Pain 93:85, 2001.

101. Ambrosio AF, Soares-Da-Silva P, Carvalho CM, et al: Mechanisms of action of carbamazepine and its derivatives, oxcarbazepine, BIA 2–093, and BIA 2–024. Neurochem Res 27:121, 2002.

102. Bonicalzi B, Canavero S, Cerruti F, et al: Lamotrigine reduces total postoperative analgesic requirement: A randomized double-blind placebo-controlled pilot study. Surgery 122:567, 1997.

Chapter 15

Antiepileptic Drugs and Pain

Gary McCleane, MD

Almost 60 years ago, it was suggested that the antiepileptic drug (AED) phenytoin could have an analgesic effect in the treatment of neuropathic pain.[1] Since then, this suggestion has been transformed into a conviction that the broad range of drugs with an anticonvulsant effect also possess analgesic effects when used to treat neuropathic pain.[2,3] Indeed, with some of the newer AEDs, greater quantities of them are used to treat neuropathic pain than are used to treat epilepsy.[4]

Given the similar pathophysiological origins of epilepsy and neuropathic pain, that is, aberrant neural function with ectopic discharge, it should be of little surprise that agents that are effective for one condition can be equally effective for the other. Conversely, the temptation to a pharmaceutical company to establish an analgesic effect of an AED that has failed to demonstrate a superior anticonvulsant effect than its rivals is likely to provide the pain clinician with a drug that fails to have a greater analgesic effect than its rivals as well.

Although AEDs possess analgesic effects, they differ from what one might consider more conventional analgesics. With the use of opioids or nonsteroidal antiinflammatory drugs (NSAIDs) there is, usually, marginal benefit to be obtained by changing from one drug in that class to another, given that these drugs are unified by a mode of action (in the case of opioids, largely effect on opioid receptors). In contrast, AEDs are unified by a therapeutic effect (decrease in seizure frequency, analgesia) rather than a mode of action (TABLE 1).

The knowledge of these differing modes of actions have important clinical implications. Although there may be little rationale for changing from one opioid to another in the face of lack of therapeutic effect, there is every reason for changing from one AED to another when confronted with therapeutic failure, as each new AED tried targets a different receptor or neurotransmitter. Even in the case of phenytoin and carbamazepine, which share a common sodium channel-blocking effect, it is possible that different sodium channels are targeted by each agent. Again, this potential use of a variety of AEDs is suggested by the epilepsy experience, in which change in AED or the use of a combination of AEDs is common practice and finds its foundation in vast clinical experience as well as scientific knowledge.

TABLE 1

Putative Mode of Action of Antiepileptic Drugs

Antiepileptic drug	Mode of action
Phenytoin	Sodium channel blockade[5]
Carbamazepine	Sodium channel blockade[6]
Clonazepam	γ-Aminobutyric agonist
Gabapentin	Action on $\alpha\,\delta$-2 subunit of calcium channel[7]
Lamotrigine	Decrease glutamate release[8] and action on voltage gated cation channels[9]
Harkoseride	Action of strychnine-sensitive glycine channel

CHOICE OF ANTIEPILEPTIC DRUG

Clearly, no single AED will produce analgesia in all subjects with neuropathic pain who take it. As previously discussed, there must be a willingness to change agent if analgesia is not apparent. As yet, we have no clear indication of which AED has the most chance of producing analgesia in any of the etiological conditions that produce neuropathic pain, nor do we really know which AED has the most profound effect on the primary symptoms and signs of neuropathic pain (numbness, burning, paresthesia/dysesthesia, shooting/lancinating pain, and allodynia) as well as overall perception of pain. There is a perception that AEDs have the most effect on the shooting component of neuropathic pain, but this feeling is based on anecdotes rather than evidence from clinical studies. The absence of an animal model for shooting or lancinating pain or indeed burning or paresthesia or dysesthesia hinders our proper understanding of individual AEDs' potential effects. Therefore, choice is determined by a judgment of the potential analgesic benefit from use balanced against the risk of side effects. Although the extent of potential analgesia produced by different AEDs is broadly similar, side effects differ widely. In most cases, treatment palliates rather than cures the pain in question, and treatment and consequent side effects are likely to be long term.

Broadly speaking, the newer AEDs such as gabapentin and lamotrigine have less effect on cognitive function than carbamazepine and phenytoin.[10,11] Gabapentin can produce somnolence[12] (a side effect that can be used if a greater proportion of the daily dose is given at night in a subject who has insomnia), whereas lamotrigine can cause insomnia. A wide variety of side effects are possible with any individual AED. It would be inappropriate to list all the side effects of AEDs, as these are recorded in the product literature, but rather to mention in passing those that are of particular importance. Unfortunately, while we have knowledge of which AED can have an analgesic effect and which is associated with potential side effects, we have no way of predicting which patient will derive analgesia or suffer side effects when a particular AED is used.

The issue of potential side effects is of particular importance when the source of the neuropathic pain is a condition that has multiorgan consequences. For example, in the subject with painful diabetic neuropathy, renal impairment may be present, and this must be considered when choosing the most appropriate AED. Liver enzyme induction is associated with the older AEDs particularly, and this again needs consideration in subjects already taking medication for other puroposes. With a few notable exceptions, the use of AEDs in the treatment of neuropathic pain is outside the approved use of the drugs in question, with the exception of carbamazepine and gabapentin.

Another feature of AED use that requires further elucidation is their role in preventing flareups of neuropathic pain, particularly as the severity of neuropathic pain often fluctuates widely. In the case of the more toxic AEDs, patients may be content to take a large dose of that agent and suffer the accompanying side effects during a flare-up of their pain but be more reluctant to take a dose that may have a prophylactic effect during a more settled phase of their condition.

SPECIFIC ANTIEPILEPTIC DRUGS

Phenytoin

Despite being one of the first AEDs to have an analgesic effect attributed to it, the use of phenytoin in subjects with neuropathic pain is not widespread. The early case report evidence has been substantiated by randomized controlled trials (RCTs),[13,14] but its use is compromised by tachyphylaxis.

Clonazepam

Case report evidence suggests that clonazepam may have a useful effect in treatment of the shooting pain associated with phantom limb pain.[19] Somnolence is a predominant effect, and with this drug's long half-life, daytime sedation may complicate use. As it belongs to the benzodiazepine group of drugs, anxiolysis and muscle relaxation may also be produced by its use, and this combination of properties may, in some patients, prove useful.

Carbamazepine

Carbamazepine remains perhaps the most widely used in AED in the treatment of pain. Early case reports now almost 40 years old[15,16] suggest analgesia when used in subjects with trigeminal neuralgia; these findings have subsequently been verified by RCTs[17,18] and vast clinical experience. The analgesic effect is not specific for trigeminal neuralgia and can be observed in patients with any neuropathic pain condition.

Sodium Valproate

Although associated with fewer side effects than carbamazepine, evidence of an analgesic effect is less robust and based on case reports. Caution is advised when using sodium valproate in females of childbearing age in view of the so-called "fetal valproate syndrome."

Gabapentin

Despite the name of this agent, it exerts its effect on α δ-2 subunits of a calcium channel[20] rather than influencing γ-aminobutyric acid (GABA) mediated transmission. Its effect on glutamate release may be implicated in its anti-allodynic action.[21]

Gabapentin is the only therapeutic agent possessing a license for use in the broad spectrum of conditions that produce neuropathic pain. Rapid dose escalation can reduce the duration of troublesome side effects. Its use in a wide range of conditions, from post-herpetic neuralgia[22] and painful diabetic neuropathy[23] to other neuropathic pain conditions,[24-28] is now verified. Interestingly, substantial evidence from animal pain models suggest that gabapentin can also have an antinociceptive effect in cases of nonneuropathic pain.[29-33] This effect has been confirmed, in human subjects although the analgesic effect is less pronounced than that observed in subjects with neuropathic pain.[34,35] Dose escalation up to 2400 mg daily (in selected cases, 3600 mg) may be required to achieve maximal effect.

Lamotrigine

Again, a strong body of evidence points to lamotrigine's possessing analgesic as well as anticonvulsant effects.[36-41] Perhaps the major side effect limiting rapid titration to a therapeutic dose is skin rash. The incidence of this is undoubtedly reduced by a more gradual increase of dose.

An issue surrounding all AEDs is the dose at which effect is maximal. With lamotrigine, it has been shown that a dose of 200 mg daily has no analgesic effect,[42] suggesting that higher doses need to be attained for the effect earlier mentioned to be achieved. In practice, patients may be placed on lamotrigine 50 mg daily, with the dose being increased by 50 mg daily on a weekly basis to 300 mg a day. Higher doses may be used, but, if no effect is observed at 300 mg a day, further increases are unlikely to produce analgesia. In view of the relatively long half-life of lamotrigine, once-daily dosing may be appropriate.

Case report evidence suggests that lamotrigine may reduce the symptoms of complex regional pain syndrome (type 1), with the sudomotor changes seen in this condition being alleviated along with pain and allodynia.[37] If this effect can be verified, it may provide a welcome alternative to the conventional, more invasive modes of treatment such as sympathetic blockade.

An interesting feature of lamotrigine is its potential neuroprotective effect, which has been demonstrated in several animal studies.[43,44] The human clinical relevance of this has yet to be defined, but an obvious attraction exists with use of an agent that not only reduces the symptoms associated with the nerve injury but may also diminish the extent of subsequent neural dysfunction.

Topiramate

It has been suggested that topiramate possesses analgesic properties when used for neuropathic pain.

Experimental Antiepileptic Drugs

Work proceeds with several novel AEDs. Information is beginning to emerge confirming an analgesic effect with pregabalin. Initial clinical experience with another AED, SPM 927 (Harkoseride), shows very encouraging results. This agent has an effect on strychnine-sensitive glycine channels, has an anticonvulsant effect, and has recently completed an open-label led trial in resistant neuropathic pain.[45] In this study, 6 of 25 subjects with previously resistant neuropathic pain (resistant being defined as lack of response to currently available AEDs, tricyclic antidepressants, opioids, and NSAIDs) derived significant analgesia from its use and continue to do so 1 year after commencing therapy. In some subjects, relief was total and tolerance to its analgesic effect has not yet become apparent.

Parenteral Antiepileptic Drugs

So far, this discussion has been centered on oral AEDs. There may be circumstances in which the oral route is unavailable or a rapid effect is required, and in these circumstances, parenteral use of an AED may be more appropriate. The evidence confirming parenteral efficacy of AEDs is surprisingly sparse. Phenytoin, known to produce analgesia when used orally, also has an analgesic effect when used intravenously.[46] Phenytoin has a pH of 11, and therefore extravasation after intravenous injection can lead to skin necrosis. Fosphenytoin, a water-soluble ester prodrug of phenytoin, has a neutral pH and consequently the danger of spillage into the tissues around the vein are minimal.

Because phenytoin and fosphenytoin are not milligram-for-milligram equivalent, to avoid inappropriate dosing fosphenytoin is measured in "phenytoin equivalent" (PE) units, with 1 mg phenytoin being therapeutically equal to 1 PE of fosphenytoin.

When used intramuscularly[47] and intravenously[48,49] analgesia can be seen. In the case of both intramuscular and intravenous use, it seems that subjects either derive benefit or do not. When benefit is observed, it is marked. This feature seems to be uniform for all AEDs. For example, in a randomized trial (crossover design), 48 subjects received a single intramuscular injection of 500 PE fosphenytoin and placebo on differing occasions. In the first 48 hours after injection, average pain scores fell from 7.49 to 6.75 on a 0 to 10 linear visual analogue scale (P = .01), a fall of 0.74. Although such a fall was statistically significant, it would not be particularly impressive from a clinical perspective. However, when the results from subjects who noted relief were compared with results from those who felt no relief, a differing outcome was seen: of the 28 who derived no relief, pain scores increased by 0.46 (P = .05), whereas in the 20 who obtained relief, pain scores fell by 2.42 (P < .001), a much more impressive fall.

The intramuscular dose of fosphenytoin is 500 PE and the immediate side effect of intramuscular injection is a short-lived but often intense burning sensation at the injection site. When used intravenously, 1500 PE can be infused over 24 hours. Side effects are common and often marked, but the analgesia produced often significantly outlives the half-life of the drug, with relief lasting weeks or even months not being unusual after a single 24-hour infusion.[50]

In view of the significant potential for side effects with intravenous infusion of fosphenytoin, it should not be used as a first-line treatment but rather as option for the subject with resistant pain.

It could be argued that, since both phenytoin/fosphenytoin and lidocaine/mexiletine are sodium channel blockers, lidocaine/mexiletine could be used in preference to phenytoin/fosphenytoin. However, from a clinical perspective, phenytoin/fosphenytoin can produce analgesia even when lidocaine/mexiletine has failed to do so, suggesting that they may be active at differing sodium channel receptors.

CONCLUSION

Antiepileptic drugs undoubtedly have an analgesic effect in some but not all subjects with neuropathic pain. If an individual AED, used in appropriate dose, fails to produce analgesia, there is logic for a similar trial with an alternative AED. In general, the newer AEDs may have more acceptable side effect profiles than the original members of this group, but as treatment is liable to be long term, thought must be given to the long- as well as short-term consequences of their use. When the oral route of administration is not available, the parenteral formulation of the drugs for which it is available has a similar efficacy to their oral derivatives.

REFERENCES FOR ADDITIONAL READING

1. Bergouignan M: Cures heureuses de nevralgies faciales essentielles par le diphenyldantoinate de soude. Rev Laryngol Otol Rhinol 63:41, 1942.

2. McQuay H, Carroll D, Jadad AR, et al: Anticonvulsant drugs for management of pain: A systematic review. BMJ 311:1047, 1995.

3. Kingery WS: A critical review of controlled clinical trials for peripheral neuropathic pain and complex regional pain syndromes. Pain 73:123, 1997.

4. McCleane GJ: Anticonvulsants: Epilepsy or pain. Pain Clinic 13: 87, 2001.

5. Wakamoti M, Kaneda M, Oyama Y, Akaike N: Effects of chlordiazepoxide, chlorpromazine, diazepam, diphenylhydantoin, flunitrazepam and haloperidol on the voltage-dependent sodium current of isolated mammalian brain neurones. Brain Res 494:374, 1989.

6. Schwarz J, Grigat G: Phenytoin and carbamazepine: potential and frequency dependent block of Na currents in mammalian myelinated nerve fibres. Epilepsia 30:286, 1989.

7. Gee NS, Brown JP, Dissanayake VU, et al: The novel anticonvulsant drug, gabapentin (Neurontin), binds to the alpha 2 delta subunit of a calcium channel. J Biol Chem 271:5568, 1996.

8. Cunningham MO, Jones RS: The anticonvulsant, lamotrigine decreases spontaneous glutamate release but increases spontaneous GABA release in the rat entorhinal cortex in vivo. Neuropharmacology 39:2139, 2000.

9. Lees G, Leach MJ: Studies on the mechanism of action of the novel anticonvulsant lamotrigine (Lamictal) using primary neuroglial cultures from rat cortex. Brain Res 612:190, 1993.

10. Cohen AF, Ashby L, Crowley D, et al: Lamotrigine (BW430C), a potential anticonvulsant: Effects on the central nervous system in comparison with phenytoin and diazepam. Br J Clin Pharmacol 20:619, 1985.

11. Cohen AF, Hamilton MJ, Peck AW, Yuen WC: Lamotrigine and carbamazepine: A comparison on psychomotor performance. Br J Clin Pharmacol 98:704, 1986.

12. Martin R, Meador K, Turrentine L, et al: Comparative cognitive effects of carbamazepine and gabapentin in healthy senior adults. Epilepsia 42:764, 2001.

13. Braham J, Saia A: Phenytoin in the treatment of trigeminal and other neuralgias. Lancet 2:892, 1960.

14. Chadda VS, Mathur MS: Double blind study of the effects of diphenylhydantoin sodium on diabetic neuropathy. J Assoc Physicians India 26:403, 1978.

15. Blom S: Trigeminal neuralgia: Its treatment with a novel anticonvulsant drug. Lancet 1:839, 1962.

16. Blom S: Tic douloureux treated with new anticonvulsant: Experiences with G32883. Arch Neurol 9:285, 1963.

17. Campbell FG, Graham JG, Zilkha KJ: Clinical trial of carbazepine (Tegretol) in trigeminal neuralgia. J Neurol Neurosurg Psychiat 29:265, 1966.

18. Rull J, Quibrera R, Gonzalez-Millan H, Lozano-Castenada O: Symptomatic treatment of peripheral diabetic neuropathy with carbamazepine: Double blind crossover study. Diabetologia 5:215, 1969.

19. Bartusch SL, Sanders BJ, D'Alessio JG, Jernigan JR: Clonazepam for the treatment of lancinating phantom limb pain. Clin J Pain 12:59, 1996.

20. Gee NS, Brown JP, Dissanayake VU, et al: The novel anticonvulsant drug, gabapentin (Neurontin), binds to the alpha delta 2 sub unit of a calcium channel. J Biol Chem 271:5768, 1996.

21. Maneuf YP, Hughes J, McKnight AT: Gabapentin inhibits the substance P facilitated K^+ evoked release of [^{3}H] glutamate from rat caudal trigeminal nucleus slices. Pain 93:191, 2001.

22. Rowbotham M, Harden N, Stacey B, et al: Gabapentin for the treatment of postherpetic neuralgia: A randomized controlled trial. JAMA 280:1837, 1998.

23. Backonja M, Beydoun A, Edwards KR, et al: Gabapentin for the symptomatic treatment of painful neuropathy in patients with diabetes mellitus. JAMA 280:1831, 1998.

24. Mellick G, Mellick LB: Reflex sympathetic dystrophy treated with gabapentin. Arch Phys Med Rehabil 78:98, 1997.

25. Houtchens MK, Richert JR, Sami A, Rose JW: Open label gabapentin treatment for pain in multiple sclerosis. Multiple Sclerosis 3:250, 1997.

26. Sist TC, Filladora VA, Miner M, Lema M: Experience with gabapentin for neuropathic pain in the head and neck: Report of 10 cases. Region Anesth 22:473, 1997.

27. McGraw T, Stacey BR: Gabapentin for treatment of neuropathic pain in a 12 year old girl. Clin J Pain 14:354, 1998.
28. Samkoff LM, Daras M, Tuchman AJ, Koppell BS: Amelioration of refractory dysesthetic limb pain in multiple sclerosis by gabapentin. Neurology 49:304, 1997.
29. Carlton SM, Zhou S: Attenuation of formalin-induced nociceptive behaviors following local peripheral injection of gabapentin. Pain 76:201, 1998.
30. Jun JH, Yaksh TL: The effect of intrathecal gabapentin and 3-isobutyl gamma amino butyric acid on the hyperalgesia observed after thermal injury in the rat. Anesth Analg 86:348, 1998.
31. Hunter JC, Gogas KR, Medley LR, et al: The effect of novel anti-epileptic drugs in rat experimental models of acute and chronic pain. Eur J Pharmacol 324:153, 1997.
32. Stanfa LC, Singh L, Williams RG, Dickenson AH: Gabapentin, ineffective in normal rats, markedly reduces C-fibre evoked responses after inflammation. Neuro Rep 8:587, 1997.
33. Shimoyama N, Shimoyama M, Davis AM, et al: Spinal gabapentin in antinociceptive in the rat formalin test. Neurosci Lett 222:65, 1997.
34. McCleane GJ: Gabapentin reduces chronic benign nociceptive pain: A double blind, placebo controlled crossover study. Pain Clin 12:81, 2000.
35. Werner MU, Perkins FM, Holte K, et al: Effects of gabapentin in acute inflammatory pain in humans. Reg Anesth Pain Med 26:322, 2001.
36. Zakrzewska JM, Chaudhry Z, Nurmikko TJ, et al: Lamotrigine (Lamictal) in refractory trigeminal neuralgia: Results from a double-blind placebo controlled crossover trial. Pain 73:223, 1997.
37. McCleane GJ: The symptoms of complex regional pain syndrome type 1 alleviated with lamotrigine: A report of 8 cases. J Pain 1:171, 2000.
38. Eisenberg E, Alon N, Daoud D, Yarnitsky D: Lamotrigine in the treatment of painful diabetic neuropathy. Eur J Neurol 5:167, 1998.
39. McCleane GJ: Lamotrigine in the management of neuropathic pain: A review of the literature. Clin J Pain 16:321, 2000.
40. Sotelo JC, Isanta MR, Felip M, Gimeno EB: Use of lamotrigine in a first line treatment for dysesthetic neuropathic pain. Analgesia 5:61, 2000.
41. Leandri M, Lunardi G, Inglese M, et al: Lamotrigine in trigeminal neuralgia secondary to multiple sclerosis. J Neurol 247:556, 2000.
42. McCleane GJ: 200 mg daily of lamotrigine has no analgesic effect in neuropathic pain: A randomised, double-blind placebo controlled trial. Pain 83:105, 1999.
43. Shauib A, Mahmood RH, Wishart T, et al: Neuroprotective effects of lamotrigine in global ischaemia in gerbils: A histological, in vivo micro dialysis and behavioral study. Brain Res 702:199, 1995.
44. Wiard RP, Dickerson MC, Beek O, et al: Neuroprotective properties of the novel anti epileptic lamotrigine in a gerbil model of global cerebral ischaemia. Stroke 26:466, 1995.
45. McCleane GJ: The anticonvulsant SPM 927 has an analgesic effect in human neuropathic pain. In Press.
46. McCleane GJ: Intravenous infusion of phenytoin relieves neuropathic pain: A randomized, double blind, placebo controlled crossover study. Anesth Analg 89:985, 1999.
47. McCleane GJ: Intramuscular fosphenytoin reduces neuropathic pain: A randomized, double-blind, placebo controlled, crossover study. Analgesia 4:479, 1999.
48. McCleane GJ: Intravenous fosphenytoin relieves chronic neuropathic pain: A double blind, placebo controlled, crossover trial. Analgesia 5:45, 2000.
49. Cheshire WP: Fosphenytoin: An intravenous option for the management of acute trigeminal neuralgia crisis. J Pain Sympt Manage 21:506, 2001.
50. McCleane GJ: Intravenous infusion of fosphenytoin produces prolonged pain relief: A case report. J Pain 3:156, 2002.

Chapter 16

α_2-Agonists (Bench)

Jennifer A. Elliott, MD / Howard S. Smith, MD

α_2-Agonists have been used for many years in the management of hypertensive disorders. Only in the relatively recent past has their role expanded to include applications in anesthesia and pain management. New α_2-agonists that may offer advantages over currently available agents are undergoing testing in animal models. Also, scientists have been able to characterize how α_2-receptors function and which receptor subtypes seem to be involved in α_2-agonist–mediated antinociception. As more has become understood about α_2-receptor subtype function, some investigators have begun to work on developing subtype-specific α_2-agonists to maximize therapeutic benefit and minimize side effects. This chapter briefly reviews what is known about α_2-receptor function and α_2-receptor subtypes. Information gleaned from preclinical studies of currently available and future α_2-agonists in animal models of pain states is presented.

The α_2-adrenoreceptor is a single polypeptide chain glycoprotein that belongs to the superfamily of receptors that incorporate seven transmembrane spanning domains. The cytoplasmic side is coupled to a guanine nucleotide binding protein (G protein), which generally facilitates intracellular second-messenger signaling cascades (usually via effector enzymes or interactions with ion channels).

There are three subtypes of α_2-adrenoreceptors: α_2A, α_2B, and α_2C (which share about three-quarters of similar amino acid residue identity). They occur at both presynaptic and postsynaptic locations. Agents that agonize the α_2-adrenergic receptor have traditionally been grouped into three major classes:

- Phenylethylamines (e.g., α-methyl norepinephrine)
- Imidazolines (e.g., clonidine, tizanidine, dexmedetomidine)
- Oxaloazepines (e.g., azepexole).

Clonidine is a selective α_2-agonist with an affinity ratio of 200:1 (α_2/α_1), which has been considered by some to be a partial agonist. Dexmedetomidine is a full, superselective α_2-agonist (an order of magnitude more selective than clonidine).[1]

The imidazolines also bind to the imidazoline receptors (e.g., I_1, and I_2). Although these receptors appear not to play a major role in providing analgesia, it is conceivable that they contribute to analgesia indirectly via interactions with cannabinoid (CB_1) receptors or α_2-receptors, or both.[2]

α_2-RECEPTORS

α_2-Receptors are known to function via a G protein–linked mechanism. Activation of these receptors results in many responses, including inhibition of cyclic adenosine monophosphate (cAMP) formation and the opening of K^+ channels. As K^+ leaves the affected cells, hyperpolarization occurs, which causes decreased impulse transmission in the activated nerve fibers. Decreased calcium conductance, which occurs via voltage-gated calcium channels, also seems to result in diminished neurotransmitter release from the activated neurons. Release of transmitters such as substance P may be attenuated.[3–5]

Although multifactorial and extremely complex, there appear to be five major potential mechanisms to explain the analgesia produced via α_2-adrenergic receptors (FIGURE 1).[6]

1. α_2-Adrenergic agonists can reduce sympathetic outflow by a direct effect on preganglionic outflow at the spinal level[7] as well as indirectly by diminishing free norepinephrine levels via effects on adrenal secretion.[8] These effects would seem to be intuitively beneficial in pain states in which the sympathetic nervous system is playing a significant proalgesic role.

2. α_2-Adrenergic receptors appear to play a role in the inhibition of transmitter release from primary afferent neurons,[9] probably via effects on a pertussis toxin-sensitive G protein ($G_{i/o}$).[10] Activation of this subunit could potentially lead to the opening of neighboring voltage-gated potassium channels[11] or G protein–coupled inwardly rectifying potassium (GIRK) channels.[12]

3. Additionally, the activation of the $G_{i/o}$ subunit via the α_2-adrenergic receptor diminishes the opening of voltage-gated N-type channels.[13] This would also lead to a dampening effect on transmitter release. The G protein interaction with N-type voltage-gated calcium channels results in a significant slowing of calcium conductance and a shift in the voltage dependence of these channels to more positive potentials (i.e., more po-

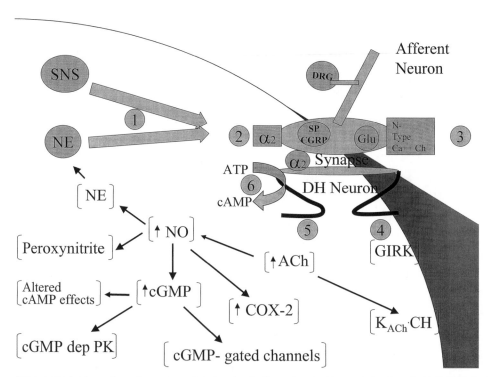

Figure 1. Mechanisms of α_2-adrenergic mediated analgesia. (Reproduced with permission from Smith H, Elliott J: Alpha$_2$ receptors and agonists in pain management. Curr Opin Anesthesiol 14:513–518, 2001.)

larization is needed to open channels).[14] This appears to be due to a shift in the channel gating mode from high probability of opening to low and medium probability of opening (i.e., "willing" mode to "reluctant" mode).[15, 16] Therefore, α_2-adrenoreceptor agonists may be synergistic with ziconotide or baclofen.

4. α_2-Adrenergic receptors may inhibit dorsal horn neurons by hyperpolarization secondary to potassium flux stimulation of G protein ($G_{i/o}$)–coupled inwardly rectifying potassium (GIRK) channels.[12, 17–19] It is conceivable that α_2-adrenergic receptors may be coupled to ion channels or adenyl cyclase,[14, 20] also producing antinoceptive effects.

5. Stimulation of α_2-adrenergic spinal receptors increases acetylcholine concentrations in the dorsal horn[21] and cerebrospinal fluid.[22] Increases in acetylcholine and resultant cholinergic receptor activation lead to increased in nitric oxide (NO) synthesis.[23, 24] Increased NO may contribute to various effects, including a potential positive feedback on norepinephrine release.[25] Also, NO may play a key part in the regulation of an inducible form of cyclooxygenase (COX-2) activity.[26] NO decomposes into other nitrogen oxides, such as nitrite (NO_2) and nitrate (NO_3) and may rapidly react with superoxide in vivo to yield peroxy nitrate (ONOO) [$NO + O_2^- \rightarrow ONOO$].[27] High concentrations of peroxynitrite may have significant deleterious effects (e.g., cytotoxicity).

6. Activation of $G_{i/o}$ by alpha$_2$-agonists binding to alpha$_2$-adrenoreceptors inhibits adenylate cyclase and thereby inhibits cyclic adenosine monophosphate (cAMP) formation.

It seems that different G protein α subunits may be involved in mediating the antinociceptive effects of clonidine and morphine. When oligodeoxynucleotides were directed against $G_{Z\alpha}$ in mice, researchers found that the antinociceptive effects of clonidine were diminished, whereas those of morphine were not. These two agents maintained a synergistic relationship despite the reduced antinociceptive effects of clonidine. Similarly, oligodeoxynucleotides were directed against the $G_{0\alpha}$ subunit, resulting in decreased antinociceptive effects of clonidine and morphine, but the synergism between these agents was preserved.[28] It seems that the antinociceptive effects of clonidine and morphine are mediated through different G protein α subunits, but synergy between these agents does not depend on activation of a single G protein α subunit.

Just as different G protein α subunits have been identified, subtypes of the α_2 receptor have been classified. Three receptor subtypes have been characterized: α_{2A}, α_{2B}, and α_{2C} adrenoceptors (see Table 1). Study of these receptor subtypes revealed that each may have a role in the development of neuropathic pain and antinociception. The distribution of α_2-receptor subtypes in rat and human dorsal root ganglia has been evaluated. In the rat, α_{2C} receptors constitute most of the α_2-receptors present in the dorsal root ganglia, whereas α_{2B}-receptors represent only a small percentage of the total α_2-receptor population.[29] In humans, it seems that most α_2-receptors present in dorsal horn cell bodies are α_{2A} and α_{2B} subtype receptors. α_{2B} and α_{2C} receptors constitute greater than 95% of α_2-receptors present in human dorsal root ganglia, each accounting for approximately 50% of the total α_2-receptor population.[30]

The effectiveness of α_2-agonists when given epidurally or systemically has been evaluated in rats. It was found that the degree of spinal antinociception of these agents correlated with their binding affinity for spinal cord α_2-receptors regardless of the route of administration (systemic versus epidural). Three α_2-agonists—clonidine, tizanidine, and dexmedetomidine—were used in this study. The antinociceptive potency of each agent was greater when given epidurally compared with systemic administration, and epidural administration was noted to result in a fivefold increase in the antinociceptive efficacy of these agents compared

TABLE 1

Features of α_2-Adrenergic Receptor Subtypes

	α_{2A}	α_{2B}	α_{2C}
Receptor Features			
Second messenger	Inhibitory G-protein	Inhibitory G-protein	Inhibitory G-protein
Transmembrane domains	7	7	7
Number of amino acids	450	450	461
Pharmacology			
AGONISTS			
Dexmedetomidine	+++	++	+
Clonidine	+++	++	+
UK 14304	+++	+	+
Oxmetazoline	+++	0	+
Tizanidine	+++		
ANTAGONISTS			
WB4101	+++	+	+
Antipamezole	+++	+++	+++
Idazoxan	++	++	++
Yohimbine	++	+++	+++
Prazosin	0	++	++
Imiloxan	0	++	++

Reproduced with permission from Childers MK: How alpha₂-adrenergic agonists relieve pain. In: Childers MK, ed. Use of Alpha₂-Adrenergic Agonists in Pain Management. Academic Information Systems, Columbia, MO, 2001, pages 13–27.

with systemic administration. The most potent antinociception was provided by dexmedetomidine, whereas the least was seen with tizanidine.[31]

To help determine which receptor subtypes may be involved in the development of sympathetically mediated pain, a mouse model was employed.[32] Populations of mice deficient in functional α_{2A}-receptors and normal mice that were subjected to chemical sympathectomy were used in this experiment. These mouse populations and normal control mice underwent tibial nerve sectioning. When the mice were observed for evidence of the development of mechanical and thermal hyperalgesia, it was found that mice lacking functional α_{2A}-receptors and mice that had had sympathectomy developed mechanical but not thermal hyperalgesia. The normal control mice developed mechanical and thermal hyperalgesia. This experiment suggests that intact sympathetic fibers and functional α_{2A}-receptors play a role in the development of thermal hyperalgesia because the mice lacking either component did not develop heat-associated hyperalgesia. It also seems to indicate independent mechanisms for the development of thermal and mechanical hyperalgesia because these same mice did show evidence of mechanical hyperalgesia. To evaluate whether the hyperalgesic behavior of these mice could be reversed by the administration of α_2-agonists, dexmedetomidine was given to the animals. (Dexmedetomidine created a dose-dependent decrease in the hyperalgesia exhibited by the control mice but did not reduce hyperalgesia in the α_{2A} receptor deficient mice, suggesting that the α_{2A}-receptor mediates the antihyperalgesic effects of α_2-agonists.)

Another study using α_{2A}-receptor–deficient mice was done to evaluate whether the α_{2A}-receptor subtype is responsible for mediating synergy between α_2-agonists and opioids. In a test of thermal nociception, morphine-associated antinociception was not affected by the lack of functional α_{2A}-receptors; however, administration of a nonspecific α_2-agonist to these mutant mice did not result in any observable antinociceptive effect. Normal mice displayed evidence of opioid–α$_2$-agonist synergy when these agents were administered together, but the mutant mice did not. In a test of substance P–associated behavior, it seemed that intraspinal morphine potency was decreased in the mutant mice compared with normal mice. The authors postulated this decrease was due to diminished potentiation of morphine effects by endogenous norepinephrine resulting from defective α$_{2A}$-receptors.[33]

Although these findings suggest that α$_2$-agonist antinociception is exerted via the α$_{2A}$-receptor, this may not be true in all cases. See the section on moxonidine for further explanation.

SPECIFIC α$_2$-AGONISTS

Clonidine

In pain management, clonidine is the most widely used of the currently available α$_2$-agonists. Some of the more recent animal research involving clonidine in models of pain has centered on the antinociceptive effects of intrathecal clonidine combined with various other agents in rats. One of the agents studied in combination with clonidine was epibatidine, a nicotinic acetylcholine receptor agonist. It was found that although epibatidine itself seemed to have little or no intrinsic antinociceptive effect when used in formalin-tested rats, the combination of epibatidine and clonidine exerted a greater than additive degree of antinociception. This finding indicates a synergistic relationship between these agents, and the researchers noted a sixfold leftward shift of the dose-response curve for the combination therapy compared with clonidine alone.[34] Another agent that has been studied in conjunction with clonidine is gabapentin. A rat model revealed a synergistic antinociceptive relationship between these agents when they were administered intrathecally.[35] A third study examined the interaction between clonidine and glutamate (N-methyl-D-aspartate [NMDA]/AMPA) receptor antagonists when given intrathecally. Synergism was noted when clonidine was administered with an NMDA or an AMPA receptor antagonist in rats.[36] Likewise, synergy between the α$_2$-agonist dexmedetomidine and the NMDA receptor antagonist ketamine was shown in another rat study in which these agents were administered intrathecally.[37]

Dexmedetomidine

Dexmedetomidine has an activity ratio of α$_2$-receptors to α$_1$-receptors of 1600:1 and seems to be more potent at binding α$_2$-receptors than clonidine.[38] An animal study using dexmedetomidine and another α$_2$-agonist, ST-91, evaluated whether these two agents exert their clinical effects via different α$_2$-receptor subtypes.[39] When these agents were used together in a rat model, supraadditive antinociceptive effects were seen. As mentioned previously, it seems that dexmedetomidine exerts its clinical effects through the α$_{2A}$-receptor, whereas ST-91 is thought to target primarily α$_{2C}$-receptors. The supraadditive antinociceptive activity of combined administration of dexmedetomidine and ST-91 seems to confirm that these agents exert their effects via separate receptor subtypes. If this is the case, the possibility of using combination α$_2$-agonist therapy to provide synergistic antinociception may arise in the future. This combination therapy may provide benefit in enhancing analgesia with lower doses of each α$_2$-agonist, which may allow for a decreased incidence of undesirable side effects.

An additional study involving the use of dexmedetomidine in a rat model of nerve injury revealed enhanced analgesic potency of this agent in this setting. There is a potential future role for dexmedetomidine in peripheral neuropathic pain states.[40]

To evaluate the pharmacokinetics and pharmacodynamics of dexmedetomidine given intrathecally, epidurally, and intravenously, Eisenach et al[5] used a sheep model. The same dose of dexmedetomidine was given by each route. When dexmedetomidine was given by the epidural route, 22% was absorbed into the intrathecal space, whereas there was no evidence of increased cerebrospinal fluid concentrations when it was administered intravenously. Cerebrospinal fluid levels of dexmedetomidine 10 minutes after administration were similar in animals that had received the drug either intrathecally or epidurally. The animals that received either intrathecal or epidural dexmedetomidine also displayed decreased mean arterial pressures after administration of the drug, whereas animals receiving intravenous doses did not. These blood pressure effects were more rapid and more pronounced after intrathecal administration when compared with epidural administration of dexmedetomidine. These data seem to indicate that the hypotensive effect of dexmedetomidine is due to activation of spinal α_2-receptors. Eisenach et al[5] concluded, based on these data, that it is likely epidural administration of dexmedetomidine in humans would result in analgesia and hypotension.[41] Although no published data are currently available regarding use of intraspinal dexmedetomidine in humans, it seems that intraspinal use may be limited by hypotension, which is also noted with intraspinal clonidine administration.

Tizanidine

Tizanidine has been evaluated in animal models of postoperative pain and neuropathic pain. Rats were used to determine the effectiveness of tizanidine in these circumstances. Although some improvement in mechanical allodynia was noted in the postoperative rat model, the degree of improvement was not deemed significant. One particular drawback noted during the administration of tizanidine, especially at the higher doses that might be needed to create significant antinociceptive benefit in postoperative pain, is sedation. The authors of this study believed there may be potential benefit in postoperative pain if tizanidine were given via the intraspinal route.[42] When used in a rat model of mononeuropathy, paw withdrawal latency increased after administration of tizanidine, with complete reversal of thermal hyperalgesia in animals receiving 1 to 2 mg/kg of tizanidine on days 4, 5, and 6 after nerve injury. As in the postoperative pain model, higher doses of tizanidine (e.g., 2 mg/kg), which were required for complete reversal of thermal hyperalgesia, were associated with decreased motor activity in the rats, a sign of sedation. At doses less than 2 mg/kg, no significant effect on motor activity was noted. This study suggests a role for the use of tizanidine in some neuropathic pain states.[43]

Moxonidine

Moxonidine currently is undergoing testing in animal models and is not yet available for clinical use in humans. In formalin-tested rats, moxonidine and morphine were found to be equipotent in reducing formalin-induced behavior,[44] but clonidine was found to be more potent than either of these agents. Moxonidine may have an advantage over clonidine, however, with regard to side effects, such as sedation, which often limit the use of clonidine.

Several studies were done in mice to evaluate for synergism between intrathecally administered moxonidine and several opioid receptor agonists. One model involved intrathecal use of morphine, deltorphin II, and DAMGO with moxonidine to determine whether these agents have synergistic antinociceptive effects in inhibiting substance P–associated pain behavior. When moxonidine was given with morphine (a nonselective opioid agonist) and deltorphin II (a δ selective opioid agonist), a synergistic relationship was observed. When moxonidine was given with DAMGO (a μ selective opioid receptor agonist), the antinociceptive effects were subadditive, indicating an antagonistic relationship.[45] The study authors suggested that moxonidine acts at a different α_2-receptor subtype than clonidine because clonidine has been found to synergize with DAMGO in other studies. The findings of this study imply a potential role for intrathecal combination therapy using morphine and moxonidine to provide synergism in the management of pain in humans. The synergistic relationship between intrathecally administered moxonidine and morphine also was noted in another study done on nerve-injured mice,[46] suggesting the potential usefulness of this combination in the management of neuropathic pain states.

Radolmidine

Radolmidine, similar to moxonidine, is undergoing testing in animals but has not been administered to humans. In a rat model, radolmidine was compared directly with dexmedetomidine for effectiveness in acute and chronic pain states. Each agent was administered intrathecally at varying doses. It was found that dexmedetomidine and radolmidine are equipotent in antinociceptive effects. It also was noted that rat locomotor activity was much more significantly decreased in the animals that received dexmedetomidine than in those that were given radolmidine, suggesting lower levels of sedation associated with radolmidine versus dexmedetomidine. This is likely due to the decreased capacity of radolmidine to cross the blood-brain barrier when compared with dexmedetomidine.[47] Based on the pharmacokinetic properties of radolmidine, it also seems that intraspinal administration of this agent may be required to exert significant clinical antinociceptive activity and that its effects are more spatially restricted than those of other α_2-agonists.[48] If the information obtained from rat studies can be extrapolated to humans, radolmidine may prove to be the optimal intraspinal α_2-agonist in the future, given its apparently superior side-effect profile. Systemic administration of this agent may not provide the same degree of benefit, however, significantly restricting its range of application.

CONCLUSION

Many advances have been made in the understanding of the α_2-receptor and agonists of its actions. Study of new and evolving α_2-agonists in animal models has furthered efforts to create optimal analgesic combination therapy. In the coming years, if much of the information obtained from these animal studies can be extrapolated to humans, we may have many more options available for pain management. On the horizon may be combination therapies using a variety of α_2-agonists with gabapentin, NMDA receptor antagonists, and acetylcholine receptor agonists. Patients may be able to derive benefit from such therapies as a result of the antinociceptive synergism provided by these combinations, along with overall decreases in required doses of the individual drugs and likely diminished incidence of undesirable side effects. Likewise, newer α_2-agonists with more receptor subtype–specific properties may provide greater antinociceptive efficacy compared with traditional agents, also with a lesser likelihood of prohibitive side effects. The information derived from bench study of the α_2 agonists suggests significant promise for the future of clinical α_2 agonist therapy in pain management.

REFERENCES FOR ADDITIONAL READING

1. Scheinin H, Virtanen R, MacDonald E, et al: Medetomidine—a novel α_2-adrenoreceptor agonist: A review of its pharmacodynamic effects. Prog Neuropsychopharmacol Biol Psychiatry 13:635, 1989.

2. Gothert M, Bruss M, Bonisch H, et al: Presynaptic imidazoline receptors: New developments in characterization and classification. Ann NY Acad Sci 881:171–184, 1999.

3. Docherty JR: Subtypes of functional alpha$_1$ and alpha$_2$ adrenoceptors. Eur J Pharmacol 361:1–15, 1998.

4. Khan ZP, Ferguson CN, Jones RM: Alpha$_2$ and imidazoline receptor agonists. Anesthesia 54:146–165, 1999.

5. Childers MK: How alpha$_2$ adrenergic agonists relieve pain. In: Childers MK, ed. Use of Alpha$_2$ Adrenergic Agonists in Pain Management. Academic Information Systems, Columbia, MO, 2001, pages 13–27.

6. Smith H, Elliott J: Alpha$_2$ receptors and agonists in pain management. Curr Opin Anesthesiol 14:513–518, 2001.

7. Eisenach JC, Tong C: Site of hemodynamic effects of intrathecal α_2-adrenergic agonists. Anesthesiology 74:766–771, 1991.

8. Gaumann DM, Yaksh TL, Tycee GM: Effects of intrathecal morphine, clonidine, and midazolam on the somatosympathoadrenal reflex response in halothane-anesthetized cats. Anesthesiology 73:425–432, 1990.

9. Go VLW, Yaksh TL: Release of substance P from the cat spinal cord. J Physiol 391:141–167, 1987.

10. Holz GG, Kream RM, Spiefel A, Dunlap K: G proteins couple alpha-adrenergic and GABA-B receptors to inhibition of peptide secretion from peripheral sensory neurons. J Neurosci 9:657–666, 1989.

11. Lledo PM, Homburger V, Bockaert J, Vincent JD: Differential F protein-medicated coupling of D2 dopamine receptors to $K+$ and Ca^{2+} currents in rate anterior pituitary cells. Neuron 8:455–463, 1992.

12. Shen K-Z, North RA, Surprenan TA: Potassium channels opened by noradrenaline and other transmitters in excised membrane patches of guinea-pig submucosa/neurones. J Physiol 445:581–599, 1992.

13. Kleuss C, Hescheler J, Ewel C, et al: Assignment of G-protein subtypes to specific receptors inducing inhibition of calcium currents. Nature 353:43–48, 1991.

14. Pollo A, Lovallo M, Shere E, et al: Voltage-dependent noradrenergic modulation of omega-conotoxin-sensitive Ca channels in human neuroblastome IMR32 cells. Pflugers Arch 422:75–83, 1992.

15. Delcour AH, Tsien RW: Altered prevalence of gating modes in neurotransmitter inhibition of N-type calcium channels. Science 259:980–984, 1993.

16. Bean BP: Neurotransmitter inhibition of neuronal calcium currents by changes in channel voltage dependence. Nature 340:153–156, 1989.

17. Jeftinija S, Korade Z: Mechanism of inhibitory action of enkephalins, norepinephrine, $(-)$ − Baclofen and somatostatin in the spinal dorsal horn: An in vitro study. In: Bond MR, Charlton JE, Woolf CJ, eds. Proceedings of the VIth World Congress on Pain. Elsevier Science, Amsterdam, 1991, pages 151–158.

18. Kuno Y, Reuveny E, Slesinger PA, et al: Primary structure and functional expression of a rat G-protein-coupled muscarinic potassium channel [see comments]. 1993;364:802–806, 1993.

19. North RA: Opioid receptor types and membrane ion channels. Trends Neursci 9:114–177, 1986.
20. Uhlen S, Wikberh JES: α₂-Adrenoceptors medicate inhibition of cyclic AMP production in the spinal cord after stimulation of cyclic AMP with forskolin but not after stimulation with capsaicin or vasoactive intestinal peptide. J Neurochem 52:761–767, 1989.
21. Clinch W, Tong C, Eisenach JC: Intrathecal alpha 2-adrenergic agonists stimulate acetycholine and norepinephrine release from the spinal cord dorsal horn in sheep: An in vivo microdialysis study. Anesthesiology 87:110–116, 1997.
22. Detweiler DJ, Eisenach JC, Tong C, et al: A cholinergic interaction in alpha-2 adrenoceptor-mediated antinociception in sheep. J Pharmacol Exp Ther 265:536–542, 1993.
23. Zhuo M, Meller ST, Gebhart GF: Endogenous nitric oxide is required for tonic cholinergic inhibition of spinal mechanical transmission. Pain 54:71–78, 1993.
24. Iwamoto EI, Marion L: Pharmacologic evidence that spinal muscarinic analgesia mediated by an L-arginine/nitric oxide/cyclic GMP cascade in rats. J Pharmacol Exp Ther 269:699–708, 1994.
25. Xu Z, Tong C, Pan H-L, et al: Intravenous morphine increases release of nitric oxide from spinal cord by α-adrenergic and cholinergic mechanism. J Neurophysiol 78:2072–2078; 1997.
26. Salvemini D, Misko TP, Masferrer JL, et al: Nitric oxide activates cyclooxygenase enzymes. Proc Natl Acad Aci U S A 90:7240–7244, 1993.
27. Beckman JS, Beckman TW, Chen J, et al: Apparent hydroxyl radical production by peroxynitrite: Implication for endothelial injury from nitric oxide and superoxide. Proc Natl Acad Sci 87:1620–1624, 1990.
28. Karim F, Roerig SC: Differential effects of antisense oligodeoxynucleotides directed against Gz alpha and Go alpha on antinociception produced by spinal opioid and alpha2 adrenergic receptor agonists. Pain 87:181–191, 2000.
29. Shi TJ, Serhan UW, Leslie F, Hockfelt T: Distribution and regulations of alpha2-adrenoceptors in rat dorsal root ganglia. Pain 84:319–330, 2000.
30. Ongioco RRS, Richardson CD, Rudner XL, et al: Alpha2-adrenergic receptors in human dorsal root ganglia: Predominance of alpha2b and alpha 2c subtype mRNAs. Anesthesiology 92:968–976, 2000.
31. Asano TA, Dohi S, Ohta S, et al: Antinociception by epidural and systemic alphax-adrenoceptor agonists and their binding affinity in rat spinal cord and brain. Anesth Analg 90:400–407, 2000.
32. Kingery WS, Guo TZ, Davies MF, et al: The alpha2 adrenoceptor and the sympathetic postganglionic neuron contribute to the development of neuropathic heat hyperalgesia in mice. Pain 85:345–358, 2000.
33. Stone LS, MacMillan LB, Kitto KF, et al: The alpha2a adrenergic receptor subtype mediates spinal analgesia evoked by alpha2 agonists and is necessary for spinal adrenergic-opioid synergy. J Neurosci 17:7157–7165, 1997.
34. Hama AT, Lloyd GK, Menzaghi F: The antinociceptive effect of intrathecal administration of epibatidine with clonidine or neostigmine in the formalin test in rats. Pain 91:131–138, 2001.
35. Cheng JK, Pan HL, Eisenach JC: Antiallodynic effect of intrathecal gabapentin and its interaction with clonidine in a rat model of postoperative pain. Anesthesiology 92:1126–1131, 2000.
36. Nishiuama T, Gyermek L, Lee C, et al: The analgesic interaction between intrathecal clonidine and glutamate receptor antagonists on thermal and formalin induced pain in rats. Anesth Analg 92:725–732, 2001.
37. Joo G, Horvath G, Klimscha W, et al: The effects of ketamine and its enantiomers on the morphine- or dexmedetomidine-induced antinociception after intrathecal administration in rats. Anesthesiology 93:231–241, 2000.
38. Kambiyashi T, Maze M: Clinical uses of alpha2-adrenergic agonists. Anesthesiology 93:1345–1349, 2000.
39. Graham BA, Hammond DL, Proudfit HK: Synergistic interactions between two alpha2 adrenoceptor agonists, dexmedetomidine and ST-91, in two substrains of Sprague-Dawley rats. Pain 85:135–143, 2000.

40. Poree LR, Guo TZ, Kingery WS, Maze M: The analgesic potency of dexmedetomidine is enhanced after nerve injury: A possible role for peripheral alpha2-adrenoceptors. Anesthes Analg 87:941–948, 1998.

41. Eisenach JC, Shafer SL, Bucklin BA, et al: Pharmacokinetics and pharmacodynamics of intraspinal dexmedetomidine in sheep. Anesthesiology 80:1349–1359, 1994.

42. Hord AH, Denson DD, Azevedo MI: Systemic tizanidine hydrochloride (Zanaflex) partially decreases experimental postoperative pain in rats. Anesth Analg 93:1307–1309, 2001.

43. Hord AH, Chalfoun AG, Denson DD, Azevedo MI: Systemic tizanidine hydrochloride (Zanaflex) relieves thermal hyperalgesia in rats with an experimental mononeuropathy. Anesth Analg 93:1310–1315, 2001.

44. Shannon HE, Lutz EA: Effects of the I1 imidazoline/alpha2-adrenergic receptor agonist moxonidine in comparison with clonidine in the formalin test in rats. Pain 85:161–167, 2000.

45. Fairbanks CA, Posthumus IJ, Kitto KF, et al: Moxonidine, a selective imidazoline/alpha2 adrenergic receptor agonist, synergizes with morphine and deltorphine II to inhibit substance P-induced behavior in mice. Pain 84:13–20, 2000.

46. Fairbanks CA, Nguyen HO, Grocholski BM, Wilcox GL: Moxonidine, a selective imidazoline/alpha2 adrenergic receptor agonist, produces spinal synergistic antihyperalgesia with morphine in nerve injured mice. Anesthesiology 93:765–773, 2000.

47. Xu M, Kontinen VK, Kalso E: Effects of radolmidine, a novel alpha2-adrenergic agonist compared with dexmedetomidine in different pain models in the rat. Anesthesiology 93:473–481, 2000.

48. Pertovaara A, Wei H: Attenuation of ascending nociceptive signals to the rostroventromedial medulla induced by a novel alpha2-adrenoceptor agonist, MPV-2426, following intrathecal application in neuropathic rats. Anesthesiology 92:1082–1092, 2000.

Chapter 17

α_2-Agonists (Bedside)

Jennifer A. Elliott, MD/Howard S. Smith, MD

α_2-Agonists have gained wider application in the field of pain management in the past few decades. These agents have proved useful in the treatment of a variety of painful conditions, including cancer pain, acute postoperative pain, neuropathic pain, chronic headaches, and myofascial pain/spasticity. Neuraxial administration of α_2-agonists in conjunction with opioids and local anesthetics has provided analgesic synergy, thereby allowing for lower opioid and local anesthetic doses and fewer associated side effects. Newer α_2-agonists have recently become available and have further expanded the role of α_2-agonists in anesthesia and pain management.

Clonidine, the oldest of the available α_2-agonists, has been used for a wide variety of painful conditions and is available for systemic and neuraxial delivery. Tizanidine has been used in the management of painful conditions involving spasticity and has undergone evaluation for use in other painful syndromes with apparent promise. Dexmedetomidine is currently available as an agent for use in intensive care unit (ICU) sedation. It appears that it may also provide benefit in other settings, such as the perioperative period, as it has analgesic and sedative properties yet also appears to have little effect on the respiratory system when compared with conventional sedatives and narcotics.

CLONIDINE

Clonidine is available for use in pain management applications in oral, transdermal, and epidural/intrathecal preparations. It is the most widely used of the currently available α_2-agonists for pain management applications. A large volume of literature exists regarding the use of clonidine for a range of pain syndromes, including cancer pain, complex regional pain syndrome, post-herpetic neuralgia, peripheral neuropathy, chronic headaches, and many others. In addition, clonidine has been used in conjunction with opioids and local anesthetics in a number of settings, including nerve blocks and epidural infusions for perioperative regional anesthesia and for management of intractable pain from cancer and other conditions.

Pharmacology and Metabolism

Clonidine is typically administered via the oral or transdermal route. It may also be used in epidural or intrathecal infusions. When administered orally, plasma levels of clonidine peak in 3 to 5 hours. Its half-life is approximately 12 to 16 hours. With the transdermal patch, it may take 2 days to achieve peak plasma concentrations. Duraclon, the form of clonidine used for neuraxial administration, reaches a peak plasma level approximately 19 minutes after administration. Nearly 50% of the absorbed dose of clonidine is hepatically metabolized, while

40% to 60% of the drug is eliminated unchanged in the urine within 24 hours. It does not appear that dose adjustment is necessary in patients with renal or hepatic insufficiency.[1–3]

Recommended starting doses of clonidine are 0.1 mg orally twice daily, 0.1 mg (daily dose) transdermal patch changed weekly, or 30 μg per hour by epidural infusion. Maximum recommended doses are 2.4 mg per day orally and 0.6 mg (daily dose) transdermal patch changed weekly. Bolus doses of epidural clonidine of 700 μg or more have been given; however, little information is available regarding continuous infusions of more than 40 μg per hour of Duraclon.[1–3]

Precautions and Adverse Effects

It is advised that caution be used in certain patients in whom treatment with clonidine is being considered. Owing to the antihypertensive properties of clonidine, it is suggested that patients with significant coronary insufficiency, a recent myocardial infarction, cerebrovascular disease, or chronic renal failure be closely monitored for evidence of adverse effects during institution of clonidine therapy. Caution should also be exercised when using clonidine in the elderly, as elderly individuals may poorly tolerate orthostatic hypotension, should it occur. Patients receiving concurrent treatment with calcium channel blockers, digitalis, or β-blockers may occasionally experience bradycardia or atrioventricular block with the initiation of clonidine therapy. Symptomatic bradycardia due to clonidine administration is typically responsive to atropine. Depression may occur during clonidine therapy, and therefore caution should be exercised when starting clonidine in individuals with a history of clinical depression. Clonidine is considered a category C drug when used during pregnancy. The use of Duraclon (neuraxial clonidine) is generally not recommended for pain management in obstetric, postpartum, or perioperative patients due to the risk of undesired hemodynamic effects such as hypotension or bradycardia.[1–3]

Commonly reported adverse effects from the use of clonidine preparations include hypotension, orthostasis, bradycardia, dry mouth, nausea, sedation, dizziness, confusion, and fever. Abrupt discontinuation of clonidine, regardless of its route of administration, can result in a withdrawal syndrome characterized by severe hypertension. The incidence of this seems to be higher in patients receiving β-blockers in conjunction with clonidine therapy. Other symptoms of withdrawal may include nervousness, tremor, agitation, and headache. The emergence of rebound hypertension during clonidine withdrawal is a potentially dangerous event that may result in hypertensive encephalopathy, cerebrovascular accident, or even death. Should such elevations in blood pressure become evident, it is recommended that clonidine therapy be reinstituted, or that an infusion of phentolamine be started. The best way to decrease the likelihood of withdrawal is to gradually decrease the dose of clonidine over 2 to 4 days prior to discontinuation.[1–3] It is interesting to note that rebound hypertension may occur in the absence of preexisting hypertension and has been observed even after abrupt discontinuation of epidurally administered clonidine.[4]

Clinical Studies Using Clonidine

The volume of clinical studies on the efficacy of clonidine for use in pain management is extensive. Only a limited number of these studies are described in detail in this chapter. The scope of painful conditions for which clonidine has been used is wide and includes postoperative pain, cancer-associated pain, painful neuropathies, post-herpetic neuralgia, headaches, labor pain, complex regional pain syndrome, restless leg syndrome, orofacial pain, and tourniquet pain, to name a few.

Oral clonidine has been used with success in the treatment of pain related to post-herpetic neuralgia. One study compared oral clonidine 0.2 mg to codeine 120 mg, ibuprofen 800 mg, or placebo for analgesic effectiveness in postherpetic neuralgia. Forty patients completed this study, which involved administration of single doses of each agent to be evaluated to each of the study subjects. Clonidine was the only agent that provided significant relief of pain in the population studied. It was noted that significant sedation and dizziness occurred fairly frequently with clonidine administration, which might make the use of clonidine in the elderly, who are most often afflicted with post-herpetic neuralgia, problematic.[5]

Oral clonidine has also been assessed as an adjunct for postoperative pain management. Although not all studies indicate the efficacy of clonidine for postoperative pain, many studies have shown decreased postoperative opioid analgesic use after the perioperative administration of clonidine. One such study was conducted in patients undergoing knee surgery (total knee replacement or hemiarthroplasty). Thirty-nine patients completed this study. These subjects received clonidine 5 μg/kg or placebo orally 90 minutes preoperatively and again 12 and 24 hours following this initial dose. All patients received general anesthesia with fairly standard doses of thiopental, fentanyl, and vecuronium for their surgeries. Postoperatively, patient-controlled analgesia (PCA) morphine was used for pain control, starting in the post-anesthesia care unit (PACU). It was found that the total usage of PCA morphine was lower in the clonidine-treated group than in the placebo group throughout the study period, with 37% less morphine used by the patients in the clonidine group compared with the placebo group at 36 hours postoperatively. It was also observed that fewer patients in the clonidine group experienced nausea or vomiting during this period compared with those in the placebo group, which may have been due to lower opioid consumption in the clonidine-treated group.[6]

Oral clonidine has been used in conjunction with epidural morphine for postoperative pain control. A study performed in patients undergoing total abdominal hysterectomy evaluated the effectiveness of oral clonidine administered preoperatively in conjunction with epidural morphine for the management of postoperative pain. Fifty-six women completed this study and were randomized into three treatment groups. The first group received oral clonidine 5 μg/kg 90 minutes preoperatively along with epidural morphine, 2 mg, administered prior to the induction of general anesthesia. The second group received oral placebo along with epidural morphine, 2 mg, preoperatively. The last group received oral clonidine 5 μg/kg and no epidural morphine preoperatively. All of these patients underwent general anesthesia and received epidural local anesthetic for their surgeries. PCA morphine was initiated postoperatively for pain control. It was found that the patients who received oral clonidine alone used PCA earlier than the other groups. Those patients receiving oral placebo and epidural morphine or oral clonidine and epidural morphine used similar amounts of morphine in the early postoperative period. As the patients progressed into their first postoperative day, the patients who had received clonidine along with epidural morphine were noted to consume less morphine than both of the other groups. This finding suggests that the use of clonidine orally prior to surgery may help to prolong the effects of epidurally administered morphine, thereby decreasing postoperative opioid requirements.[7]

Transdermal clonidine has been used in the management of several pain syndromes. It was evaluated for use as a prophylactic agent in the treatment of migraines in one study. Thirty patients were given clonidine 0.2 mg/day patches as well as matching placebo patches in this double-blind crossover study. During treatment with transdermal clonidine, 19 patients reported subjective improvement in headache measures such as headache frequency, severity, and duration. It was also noted that the use of schedule II narcotic rescue analgesics was significantly reduced during clonidine therapy. When this study was completed, 18 of the 19 clonidine responders elected to continue treatment with clonidine for their headaches.[8]

Several studies have demonstrated efficacy of epidurally administered clonidine as an analgesic. One such study was conducted in 19 healthy volunteers, in which the analgesic, respiratory, and hemodynamic effects of epidural clonidine were compared with intravenous alfentanil. Nine of the volunteers received epidural clonidine, while the other 10 subjects received intravenous alfentanil at three graded bolus/infusion rates. When performing ice immersion testing, it was found that alfentanil produced analgesia that varied with its plasma concentration. Subjects receiving epidural clonidine noted decreased pain perception in their feet, but not their hands, after ice immersion. This suggests that the analgesic activity of clonidine is mediated spinally, given the regional difference in pain perception between upper and lower extremities after lumbar epidural clonidine administration. Side effects observed in the clonidine-treated subjects included primarily profound sedation but also some hypotension and bradycardia. Alfentanil, on the other hand, produced respiratory depression at rest that was not seen after clonidine administration.[9]

Cancer pain has been successfully managed through the use of epidural clonidine. In a group of 85 patients with intractable cancer pain despite the use of escalating doses of opioids, epidural clonidine was compared to placebo for analgesic efficacy. All of the patients enrolled were taking morphine (or another opioid analgesic at equivalent doses) at doses of greater than 100 mg orally or intravenously, or more than 20 mg epidurally per day, or were intolerant of opioid-associated side effects which limited such dose escalation. These patients were given patient-controlled epidural morphine as a rescue agent during the trial. Patients received either clonidine 30 μg/hr or saline epidurally during the study period. In patients completing the study, clonidine was more effective than placebo, with 45% of patients experiencing subjective pain relief or using less epidural morphine in the clonidine group, as compared with 21% in the placebo group. It was also found that patients with neuropathic components to their pain (i.e., burning or shooting pain in a dermatomal or peripheral nerve distribution), who typically consumed more opioid analgesics than patients without neuropathic pain, derived even greater benefit from epidural clonidine than those without neuropathic pain. In this group, 56% of the patients had improvement in their pain during treatment with clonidine, as opposed to 5% during use of placebo. The most significant side effects noted during this study were hypotension and bradycardia. Overall, it appeared that epidural clonidine was effective in the management of cancer-associated pain, particularly that which had a neuropathic element.[10]

Refractory reflex sympathetic dystrophy (RSD) (complex regional pain syndrome I) has also been managed with epidural clonidine. A study involving 26 patients with severe RSD was performed to assess the usefulness of epidural clonidine for this condition. Patients received placebo, 300 μg, and 700 μg of epidural clonidine during the study. Those individuals who appeared to respond positively to the administration of epidural clonidine were then allowed to continue with epidural clonidine infusions at 10 to 50 μg/hr, if desired. During the bolus clonidine trial, visual analog pain scores were significantly reduced after the administration of 300 μg or 700 μg of clonidine, but not with placebo. Both doses of clonidine produced hypotension, bradycardia, and sedation, but the sedation was more profound with the 700 µg dose. Nineteen patients elected to proceed on to the continuous epidural clonidine infusion trial. These patients received epidural clonidine for a mean of 43 days at a mean rate of 32 µg/hr with continued pain relief. Thus, epidural clonidine appeared to provide relief in some patients with RSD after both acute and chronic administration.[11]

As with oral clonidine, use of epidural clonidine as an adjunct to postoperative opioid analgesia has been evaluated. Ninety-one patients were enrolled in a study in which either epidural morphine or a combination of epidural morphine and epidural clonidine was used for postoperative pain control. These patients all underwent major abdominal surgery under general anesthesia. At the end of surgery, all subjects received 2 mg of epidural morphine. The patients were followed for a period of 72 hours after surgery. During this time, they were all given continuous infusions of epidural morphine, with 6 mg/24 hours delivered on day 1, 4 mg/24 hours delivered on day 2, and 2 mg/24 hours delivered on day 3. The clonidine-treated group also received an infusion of epidural clonidine at 450 µg/24 hours on all 3 days. Rescue analgesia was provided in the form of 2 mg boluses of epidural morphine and 50 mg boluses of intravenous meperidine. The use of rescue analgesics was no different between the groups for the first 4 hours of the study, but after this, the clonidine-treated patients consistently used fewer doses of rescue opioid analgesics than did the patients receiving epidural morphine alone. The total number of epidural morphine rescue doses during the 72-hour period was 33 doses (66 mg) in the clonidine-treated group versus 68 doses (136 mg) in the epidural morphine–only group. Likewise, use of intravenous meperidine was 18 doses (900 mg) in 72 hours in the clonidine-receiving patients, compared with 30 doses (1500 mg) in 72 hours in the patients receiving epidural morphine alone. This study therefore indicated an opioid-sparing effect of epidural clonidine in patients who had undergone abdominal surgery.[12]

TIZANIDINE

Tizanidine has been used in the management of painful conditions involving spasticity. It is also becoming popular as a component of treatment in patients with myofascial pain, headache syndromes, and localized pain processes such as acute low back pain. It may also be effective for other conditions such as trigeminal neuralgia and may provide gastroprotective effects when used in conjunction with nonsteroidal antiinflammatory drugs in the management of pain.

Pharmacology and Metabolism

After administration of oral tizanidine, peak serum levels occur within 1 to 5 hours, depending on the dose given. Its elimination half-life is 4 to 8 hours, and it is hepatically metabolized with only a small fraction of the delivered dose excreted unchanged in the urine. It has been noted that in the presence of significant renal impairment, tizanidine clearance may be reduced by 50% or more, and therefore lower doses are recommended in this setting if the use of tizanidine is elected. It has also been observed that in women taking oral contraceptives, the clearance of tizanidine may be reduced by 50% as well, again necessitating a reduction in dose. Use of tizanidine in patients with hepatic impairment should be undertaken only with extreme caution, as there is a small potential for hepatic injury during tizanidine therapy. Tizanidine is a category C drug when used in pregnant patients. When used in the management of spasticity, the initial recommended dose of tizanidine is 4 mg, with subsequent increases in dosage by 2 to 4 mg at a time until satisfactory relief of spasticity is achieved. In the management of tension headaches, the usual starting dose of tizanidine is 2 mg three times daily, which may be increased to 4 to 6 mg three times daily as tolerated over the period of several weeks. Typically, tizanidine is administered in three divided doses per day. The maximum recommended daily dose of tizanidine is 36 mg. Thus far, little is known about the long-term effects of exposure to single doses of 6 to 16 mg or to daily doses of 24 to 36 mg.[13, 14]

Adverse Effects

The most commonly reported adverse events associated with the use of tizanidine are dry mouth, somnolence, asthenia, dizziness, hypotension, and bradycardia. Sedation may occur in a significant number of patients receiving tizanidine and has been reported to be severe in 10% of patients given the drug during clinical studies. This effect appears to be dose related. Hypotension also appears to be dose related and has been reported to occasionally be associated with bradycardia, orthostasis, dizziness, and, rarely, syncope. Perhaps the most worrisome potential adverse effect of tizanidine administration is hepatic injury. It was noted that approximately 5% of patients receiving tizanidine in clinical trials experienced elevations in aminotransferase levels to greater than three times the upper limit of normal during therapy. This effect typically resolved with the withdrawal of tizanidine. Most patients were asymptomatic, and these cases were picked up via surveillance with liver function test panels. A small number of patients receiving treatment with tizanidine may experience symptoms, such as nausea and vomiting, anorexia, abdominal pain, or jaundice, that suggest liver dysfunction. Three deaths due to hepatic failure in individuals taking this drug have been reported since tizanidine was released for use. In two cases, other potentially hepatotoxic agents were used concomitantly with tizanidine. In one individual who died of fulminant hepatic failure, no cause for the liver failure could be found aside from a reaction to tizanidine. The manufacturer of tizanidine therefore recommends that aminotransferase levels be measured at baseline, and at 1, 3, and 6 months when patients are placed on tizanidine. Patients on tizanidine for long periods may require additional intermittent surveillance beyond 6 months.[13, 14]

Clinical Studies Utilizing Tizanidine

A study in six healthy volunteers was conducted to evaluate the sedative and hemodynamic effects of tizanidine, as well as to determine which dose of tizanidine is equipotent to 150 μg of clonidine in creating these effects. Three doses of tizanidine in the amounts of 4, 8, and 12 mg and one dose each of clonidine 150 μg and placebo were administered to each subject during the study. When evaluating the sedative effects of the drugs, the most significant sedation was experienced after administration of 150 μg of clonidine. The most commonly reported side effect, dry mouth, was also most pronounced with the 150 μg dose of clonidine. Blood pressure declined with administration of both clonidine and tizanidine, and the degree of decline in blood pressure was similar when either 150 μg of clonidine or 12 mg of tizanidine was given. The investigators concluded that the sedative and hemodynamic effects of 12 mg of tizanidine are similar to those of 150 μg of clonidine, although of shorter duration.[15]

Several studies have been performed to evaluate the efficacy of tizanidine in the treatment of tension type, cluster, and chronic daily headaches. In one study of patients with chronic daily headaches, 39 patients received treatment with tizanidine for a period of 12 weeks. The maximum daily amount of tizanidine used was 18 mg, in divided doses. Ultimately, 77% of the patients completed the 12-week treatment period. Of the nine patients failing to complete the study, only three discontinued use of tizanidine due to side effects they considered to be mild to moderate in nature. These adverse effects included somnolence, dry mouth, hyperkinesis, and constipation. All of the patients who went on to complete the study reported decreased frequency, severity, and duration of their headaches, as well as decreased reliance on rescue analgesics. All of these measures showed significant improvement by the conclusion of the treatment period.[16]

A second study on the use of tizanidine in the treatment of chronic tension-type headaches involved 45 female patients. Of those patients initially enrolled in the study, 37 went on to complete it. Only two patients withdrew from the study because of side effects from tizanidine, namely drowsiness and dry mouth. During the study, patients received both tizanidine and placebo. The initial dose of tizanidine employed was 2 mg three times daily, which was gradually titrated up to 6 mg three times daily in patients who failed to respond to lower doses. Investigators found that during tizanidine therapy, patients recorded lower pain scores, used rescue analgesia less frequently, and had more headache-free days than when they were given placebo.[17]

Yet another study using tizanidine in the management of chronic headaches revealed that patients with a variety of headache types respond to this treatment favorably. The study subjects were recruited from a population of more than 350 patients being treated at a headache clinic. The authors reported on 222 patients who achieved improvement in their headaches during the study period. It appeared that 72 patients were still in the titration phase of the study when these results were published. It was noted that 55 patients had dropped out of the study after enrollment, with only 16 of these drop-outs being related to side effects. Patients with chronic tension-type headaches and chronic daily headaches reported a decline in the frequency of their headaches (by an average of 78%) and a decrease in the severity of their headaches (by an average of 50%). Those patients who also had a history of migraines additionally noted a decrease in the frequency and severity of their migraines. The average daily dose of tizanidine used during the course of this study was 26 mg.[18]

In a small study involving a group of five cluster headache patients treated with tizanidine, four patients noted some improvement with doses of 12 to 24 mg daily. Three of these patients discontinued other medications they had been using for their headaches during tizanidine therapy and reported no further cluster headache attacks during the period of follow-up (ranging from 8–12 weeks). Another patient had a reduction in frequency, intensity, and duration of attacks, while the remaining subject noted no improvement during treatment with tizanidine. These findings suggest that therapy with tizanidine may be beneficial in some patients suffering from cluster headaches.[19]

Aside from use in the management of headache disorders, use of tizanidine in the treatment of other painful syndromes such as acute low back pain, neuropathic pain, and trigeminal neuralgia has been explored. In a study conducted in patients with acute low back pain, 105 patients used either tizanidine 4 mg three times daily along with ibuprofen 400 mg three times daily or placebo three times daily with ibuprofen 400 mg three times daily. These patients were followed for a period of 7 days. Although patients in both groups had improvement in their back pain over this period, the patients in the group receiving tizanidine as part of their treatment saw improvement in their symptoms earlier, particularly with regard to pain at rest or at night, and in those with significant sciatica. Interestingly, it was also noted that patients in the group treated with tizanidine/ibuprofen had fewer gastrointestinal complaints, such as abdominal pain and indigestion, as compared with the patients taking placebo/ibuprofen.[20]

This finding of decreased gastrointestinal irritation when tizanidine is combined with a nonsteroidal antiinflammatory drug as compared with the use of a nonsteroidal antiinflammatory drug alone was also observed in patients receiving tizanidine/diclofenac for painful muscle spasm–related syndromes. In this study, 405 patients from 12 centers in six countries were initially enrolled, with 361 of these patients being available for assessment at the end of the 8-day study period. The patients received treatment with either tizanidine 2 mg twice daily plus diclofenac 50 mg twice daily or placebo twice daily plus diclofenac 50 mg twice daily for a period of 7 days. Investigators found that patients receiving the combination of tizanidine and diclofenac had a greater degree of improvement in measures of their pain than did those receiving placebo/diclofenac. They also found that significantly fewer patients in the tizanidine/diclofenac group reported adverse gastrointestinal symptoms than those in the placebo/diclofenac group. These results suggest synergism between the nonsteroidal antiinflammatory drugs and tizanidine in the treatment of some painful conditions, with the added benefit of fewer nonsteroidal antiinflammatory drug–associated gastrointestinal side effects when these agents are used together.[21]

An open-label study has been conducted on the use of tizanidine in patients with neuropathic pain. Twenty-two patients completed an 8-week trial period during which they received tizanidine titrated up to a maximum of 36 mg daily. At the conclusion of the 8-week titration period, two subjects reported complete relief of their pain, while 68% of the patients overall reported improvement in their symptoms. The mean dose of tizanidine used during the study was 23 mg per day.[22]

The effectiveness of tizanidine in treating patients with refractory trigeminal neuralgia has also been evaluated. Ten patients completed a single-crossover double-blind study using tizanidine and placebo. The doses of tizanidine used during this study were 6 to 12 mg daily. Eight of these 10 individuals noted significantly fewer paroxysms of trigeminal neuralgia while on tizanidine. After completion of the study, six subjects elected to continue therapy with tizanidine; however, all had recurrence of trigeminal neuralgia within 1 to 3 months. Thus, while tizanidine appears to be effective for the treatment of trigeminal neuralgia paroxysms, the benefit seemed to be of limited duration in this study. Further study may be necessary to determine whether any long-term benefit in the treatment of trigeminal neuralgia could be afforded through the use of tizanidine.[23]

Tizanidine may actually be able to modify some of the pathophysiological alterations seemingly associated with certain medical conditions. Russell and associates,[24] using an 8-week open-label study, demonstrated that tizanidine therapy for fibromyalgia syndrome led to a statistically significant drop in cerebrospinal fluid substance P levels, which correlated with improvement in various parameters of clinical outcome.

Tizanidine may also possess clinical utility for patients who are being "weaned" from high-dose opioid therapy, for patients with sleep disturbances (especially with initiation of sleep), and for patients with restless leg syndrome or periodic limb movement disorder.[25]

DEXMEDETOMIDINE

Dexmedetomidine has been approved for use in short term (<24 hours) sedation in the ICU, particularly in conjunction with mechanical ventilation. It also may provide some benefit in the management of postoperative pain and as an adjunct to general anesthesia.

Pharmacology and Metabolism

Dexmedetomidine has a distribution half-life of approximately 6 minutes and a terminal elimination half-life of approximately 2 hours. α_2 Selectivity is maintained with slow intravenous infusions of low to medium doses (10–300 µg/kg), whereas with rapid intravenous infusions or the use of high doses (>1000 µg/kg), both α_1 and α_2 activity occurs. This may account for some episodes of acute hypertension noted during dexmedetomidine infusion. No significant respiratory depression or oxygen desaturation has been noted when infusions in the range of 0.2 to 0.7 µg/kg/hr have been given. Dexmedetomidine is nearly completely metabolized via glucuronidation and the cytochrome p450 pathway, with very little excretion of unchanged dexmedetomidine in the urine and feces. Although the pharmacokinetics of dexmedetomidine do not appear to be altered by age, a higher incidence of bradycardia and hypotension has been noted in patients older than 65 years of age as compared with younger subjects, suggesting the potential need for dose reduction in the elderly population. Dose reductions are also recommended in the presence of significant hepatic insufficiency due to decreased rates of drug clearance (by nearly 50% versus healthy individuals in patients with severe hepatic impairment). Although the pharmacokinetics of dexmedetomidine do not appear to be significantly altered by the presence of renal insufficiency, it is unclear whether the elimination of dexmedetomidine metabolites is delayed in this setting, and therefore a dose reduction may also be necessary in these individuals. Dexmedetomidine has not undergone significant study in pregnant women and is considered a category C drug for use in pregnancy. The recommended loading dose for dexmedetomidine is 1 µg/kg given over 10 minutes, followed by a maintenance continuous infusion of 0.2 to 0.7 µg/kg/hr. It is not indicated for use for periods of greater than 24 hours.[26, 27]

Adverse Effects

Significant bradycardias and even sinus arrests have been reported during administration of dexmedetomidine, particularly with bolusing or with rapid infusion. These episodes have appeared to be responsive to anticholinergics (e.g., glycopyrrolate, atropine). Caution is advised when using dexmedetomidine in individuals with such conditions as heart block, severe ventricular dysfunction, hypovolemia, diabetes mellitus, and chronic hypertension, given the potential for exaggerated hypotension or bradycardia under these circumstances. Other adverse events that have been reported with the use of dexmedetomidine include hypertension or hypotension, nausea and vomiting, fever, hypoxia, tachycardia, and anemia. Owing to its pharmacological similarity to clonidine, there may be potential for the development of an abrupt clonidine-like withdrawal syndrome if dexmedetomidine is abruptly discontinued. It is unclear how significant this effect might be given the recommended short length of use of this agent. It has been observed that patients who receive doses above the recommended range of 0.2 to 0.7 µg/kg/hr may experience first-degree atrioventricular block or second-degree heart block. One individual who was given a bolus of undiluted dexmedetomidine suffered cardiac arrest but was successfully resuscitated.[26]

Clinical Studies Using Dexmedetomidine

The effects of increasing concentrations of dexmedetomidine have been studied in human volunteers. It was found that progressive increases in dexmedetomidine resulted in significant sedation, to the point of unconsciousness. Despite the presence of sedation, recall-recognition remained intact during administration of lower doses of dexmedetomidine. It was also observed that meaningful analgesia was present throughout the infusion period. Cold pressor testing was used to assess levels of analgesia during the infusion. Those subjects who remained conscious during the infusion of dexmedetomidine reported lowering of visual analog pain scores as the dexmedetomidine dosage was progressively increased. Other subjects rendered unconscious failed to respond to this form of stimulation (i.e., there was no grimacing, nor was there hemodynamic response to this painful stimulation). Some subjects had to be withdrawn from the study prior to achieving unconsciousness due to decreases in cardiac output or heart rate, increases in pulmonary artery pressures, changes in acid-base status, or agitation that investigators believed were significant enough to warrant termination of the dexmedetomidine infusion. Even at high doses during which unconsciousness was achieved, dexmedetomidine did not appear to cause any significant respiratory dysfunction.[28]

Several other studies have been conducted to evaluate the applications and side effects of dexmedetomidine in humans. When dexmedetomidine has been used as an adjunct to surgery, it has been shown to decrease requirements for anesthetics such as thiopental, isoflurane, and fentanyl in several settings.[29–32] It has also been noted to attenuate increases in blood pressure and heart rate related to laryngoscopy and tracheal intubation and to decrease intraocular pressure in ophthalmological surgery patients.[31, 32] In intubated ICU patients, the use of bolus dose dexmedetomidine (1 µg/kg) followed by continuous infusion maintenance (0.2–0.7 µg/kg/hr) resulted in decreased requirements for supplemental sedation with midazolam and analgesia with morphine (decreased by 80% and 50%, respectively, compared with patients receiving placebo infusion). The most prominent adverse effects during the dexmedetomidine infusion were significant hypotension or bradycardia, resulting in a decision to terminate infusion in a small number of patients.[33]

The analgesic properties of dexmedetomidine have been studied in both healthy volunteers and in patients undergoing laparoscopic tubal ligation. In five healthy volunteers, ischemic pain induced by use of a sphygmomanometer cuff inflated to 300 mm Hg for 2 minutes was less in subjects receiving either dexmedetomidine or fentanyl as compared with placebo. The most significant adverse effects seen during dexmedetomidine administration, as with the previously mentioned studies, were hypotension and bradycardia (for which atropine was given in two subjects).[34] In women undergoing laparoscopic tubal ligation, dexmedetomidine (0.2 µg/kg or 0.4 µg/kg) was compared with oxycodone (60 µg/kg) and diclofenac (250 µg/kg) for analgesic effects. Those patients receiving either diclofenac or the lower dose of dexmedetomidine required rescue with morphine earlier than those patients receiving either the higher dose of dexmedetomidine or oxycodone. Several doses of dexmedetomidine (0.4 μg/kg) were required to achieve the same reduction in visual analog pain scores as with a single dose of oxycodone. However, only 33% of patients in either the oxycodone group or the dexmedetomidine (0.4 μg/kg) group required further analgesic supplementation with morphine, as compared with 83% of the patients in the diclofenac group. The most significant adverse events seen after dexmedetomidine administration were significant sedation and bradycardia requiring treatment with atropine.[35]

As further information accumulates regarding the use of dexmedetomidine in the ICU, operating room, and postoperative settings, it seems this drug may well gain wider use. Its apparent analgesic sparing effects, its lack of significant respiratory depressant effects, and its lack of significant effect on recall-recognition at low doses distinguish this agent from most traditional sedatives and analgesics. These properties may help to define a niche for the use of dexmedetomidine in situations in which the use of other currently available sedatives and analgesics is undesirable.

CONCLUSION

α_2-Agonists have become a valuable addition to the pain management armamentarium in recent years. Clonidine, the most widely studied of the α_2-agonists, has proved to be efficacious in a wide variety of settings and may provide benefit in many circumstances due to its opioid-sparing effects. Clonidine has been used in the treatment of many painful conditions and has been delivered orally, transdermally, and neuraxially. Tizanidine has been successfully applied in the management of myofascial pain syndromes, headaches, and neuropathic pain and also has become an agent of choice in the treatment of painful spasticity. Dexmedetomidine is currently being used to provide sedation in the ICU but has potential for broader use in anesthesia and pain management. α_2-Agonists are generally well tolerated and will likely remain components of pain treatment for years to come.

REFERENCES FOR ADDITIONAL READING

1. Product Information: Catapres, Clonidine HCL. Boehringer Ingelheim, Ridgefield, Conn, 1996.
2. Product Information: Duraclon, Clonidine Hydrochloride Injection. Roxane Laboratories, Columbus, Ohio, 1/2000.
3. Drugdex Editorial Staff: Drugdex Drug Evaluations: Clonidine. Micromedex ® Healthcare Series Vol. 112, exp. 6/2002. Micromedex Thomson Healthcare,
4. Fitzgibbon DR, Rapp SE, Butler SH, et al. Rebound hypertension and acute withdrawal associated with discontinuation of an infusion of epidural clonidine. Anesthesiology 84:729–731, 1996.
5. Max MB, Schafer SC, Culnane M, et al: Association of pain relief with drug side effects in postherpetic neuralgia: A single-dose study of clonidine, codeine, ibuprofen, and placebo. Clin Pharmacol Ther 43:363–371, 1988.
6. Park J, Kolesar R, Beattie S: Oral clonidine reduces postoperative PCA morphine requirements. Can J Anaesth 43:900–906, 1996.
7. Goyagi T, Tanaka M, Nishikawa T: Oral clonidine premedication enhances postoperative analgesia by epidural morphine. Anesth Analg 89:1487–1491, 1999.
8. Bredfeldt RC, Sutherland JE, Kruse JE: Efficacy of transdermal clonidine for headache prophylaxis and reduction of narcotic use in migraine patients. J Fam Pract 29:153–158, 1989.
9. Eisenach J, Detweiler D, Hood D: Hemodynamic and analgesic actions of epidurally administered clonidine. Anesthesiology 78:277–287, 1993.

10. Eisenach JC, DuPen S, Dubois M, et al: The Epidural Clonidine Study Group: Epidural clonidine analgesia for intractable cancer pain. Pain 61:391–399, 1995.

11. Rauck RL, Eisenach JC, Jackson K, et al: Epidural clonidine treatment for refractory reflex sympathetic dystrophy. Anesthesiology 79:1163–1169, 1993.

12. Motsch J, Graber E, Ludwig K: Addition of clonidine enhances postoperative analgesia from epidural morphine: A double-blind study. Anesthesiology 73:1067–1073, 1990.

13. Product Information: Zanaflex, Tizanidine Hydrochloride. Athena Neurosciences, San Francisco, Calif, 4/2000.

14. Bunch C, Drugdex Editorial Staff: Drugdex Drug Evaluations: Tizanidine. Micromedex® Healthcare Series Vol 112, 3/2001. Micromedex Thomson Healthcare.

15. Miettinen TJ, Kanto JH, Salonen MA, Scheinin M: The sedative and sympatholytic effects of oral tizanidine in healthy volunteers. Anesth Analg 82:817–820, 1996.

16. Saper JR, Winner PK, Lake AE III: An open-label dose-titration study of the efficacy and tolerability of tizanidine hydrochloride tablets in the prophylaxis of chronic daily headache. Headache 41:357–368, 2001.

17. Fogelholm R, Murros K: Tizanidine in chronic tension-type headache: A placebo controlled double-blind cross-over study. Headache 32:509–513, 1992.

18. Krusz JC, Belanger J, Mills C: Tizanidine: A novel effective agent for the treatment of chronic headaches. Headache Q 11:41–45, 2000.

19. D'Alessandro R: Tizanidine for chronic cluster headache. Arch Neurol 53:1093, 1996.

20. Berry H, Hutchinson DR: Tizanidine and Ibuprofen in acute low-back pain: Results of a double-blind multicentre study in general practice. J Int Med Res 16:83–91, 1998.

21. Sirdalud Ternelin Asia-Pacific Study Group: Efficacy and gastroprotective effects of tizanidine plus diclofenac versus placebo plus diclofenac in patients with painful muscle spasms. Curr Ther Res 59:13–22, 1998.

22. Semenchuk MR, Sherman S: Effectiveness of tizanidine in neuropathic pain: An open-label study. J Pain 1:285–292, 2000.

23. Fromm GH, Aumentado D, Terrence CF: A clinical and experimental investigation of the effects of tizanidine in trigeminal neuralgia. Pain 53:265–271, 1993.

24. Russell I, Michalek J, Xiao Y, et al: Cerebrospinal fluid (CSF) substance P (SP) in fibromyalgia syndrome (FMS) is reduced by tizanidine therapy [abstract]. J Pain (Suppl) 3:15, 2002.

25. Smith HS, Barton AE: Tizanidine in the management of spasticity and musculoskeletal complaints in the palliative care population. Am J Hospice Pall Care 17:50–58, 2000.

26. Product Information: Precedex, Dexmedetomidine hydrochloride injection. Abbott Laboratories, Chicago, Ill, 2/2001.

27. Drugdex Editorial Staff: Drugdex Drug Evaluations: Dexmedetomidine. Micromedex ® Healthcare Series Vol. 112, exp. 6/2002. Micromedex Thomson Healthcare.

28. Ebert TJ, Hall JE, Barney JA, et al: The effects of increasing plasma concentrations of dexmedetomidine in humans. Anesthesiology 93:382–394, 2000.

29. Aantaa R, Kanto J, Scheinin M, et al: Dexmedetomidine, an alpha$_2$-adrenoceptor agonist, reduces anesthetic requirements for patients undergoing minor gynecologic surgery. Anesthesiology 73:230–235, 1990.

30. Aho M, Lehtinen AM, Erkola O, et al: The effect of intravenously administered dexmedetomidine on perioperative hemodynamics and isoflurane requirements in patients undergoing abdominal hysterectomy. Anesthesiology 74:997–1002, 1991.

31. Jaakola ML, Melkkila TA, Kanto J, et al: Dexmedetomidine reduces intraocular pressure, intubation responses and anesthetic requirements in patients undergoing ophthalmologic surgery. Br J Anaesth 68:570–575, 1992.

32. Scheinin B, Lindgren L, Randell T, et al: Dexmedetomidine Attenuates Sympathoadrenal responses to tracheal intubation and reduces the need for thiopentone and peroperative fentanyl. Br J Anaesth 68:126–131, 1992.

33. Venn RM, Bradshaw CJ, Spencer R, et al: Preliminary UK experience of dexmedetomidine, a novel agent for postoperative sedation in the intensive care unit. Anaesthesia 54:1136–1142, 1999.

34. Jaakola MJ, Salonen M, Lehtinen R, Scheinin H: The analgesic action of dexmedetomidine—a novel alpha$_2$-adrenoceptor agonist—in healthy volunteers. Pain 46:281–285, 1991.

35. Aho MS, Erkola OA, Scheinin H, et al: Effect of intravenously administered dexmedetomidine on pain after laparoscopic tubal ligation. Anesth Analg 73:112–118, 1991.

Chapter 18

Antidepressants: Basic Mechanisms and Pharmacology

Dan V. Iosifescu, MD / Jonathan E. Alpert, MD, PhD / Maurizio Fava, MD

Antidepressants are a heterogeneous group of pharmacological compounds with common therapeutic effects. These compounds have been used successfully in the treatment of major depressive disorder, anxiety disorders, and a variety of other conditions, including chronic pain.

We present in Chapter 19 a discussion of individual classes of antidepressants and their clinical use in depression and chronic pain. We focus in this chapter on the clinical pharmacology of antidepressants and the mechanisms of antidepressant drug action.

CLINICAL PHARMACOLOGY OF ANTIDEPRESSANTS

Elimination Half-Life and Blood Levels of Antidepressants

The elimination half-lives of several antidepressants are presented in Table 1. These data refer only to the parent compound; active metabolites can significantly prolong the half-life of antidepressants. For example, fluoxetine's active metabolite norfluoxetine has a half-life of 7 to 15 days.

Compounds with a half-life between 17 and 36 hours can be given once per day and maintain steady-state levels. Drugs with shorter half-lives have to be administered several times per day or once per day in extended-release formulations. Fluoxetine, which has a half-life of 4 days (87 hours) and a longer half-life (7–15 days) for its metabolite is available in a weekly formulation for maintenance therapy.[1]

There is a large individual variability in the blood levels obtained with a fixed dose of an antidepressant, due to individual variability in the activity of hepatic drug-metabolizing enzymes.[2] A relationship between blood levels and clinical response has been established only for tricyclic antidepressants.[3] For tricyclic antidepressants, blood level monitoring is also required to avoid toxicity. For other antidepressant agents, monitoring of blood levels can be used to avoid toxicity and for direct clinical decisions in using very high doses, but this is not part of routine care.[4]

The Effects of Antidepressants on Neurotransmitter Receptors and Transporters

The precise mechanisms by which antidepressant drugs exert their therapeutic effects on depression, anxiety, and pain are still unknown. Much is known, however, about the immediate interactions of antidepressant drugs with monoamine neurotransmitter transporters and receptors in the human brain.

TABLE 1

Elimination Half-Lives of Antidepressants

Antidepressant	Elimination Half-Live (hr)
Paroxetine	21
Fluoxetine	87
Sertraline	26
Fluvoxamine	19
Citalopram	35
Clomipramine	23
Imipramine	28
Amitriptyline	21
Desipramine	21
Amoxapine	8
Doxepin	17
Venlafaxine	3.6
Reboxetine	13
Nefazodone	3
Mirtazapine	30
Bupropion	12

Data from Richelson E: Pharmacology of antidepressants. Mayo Clin Proc 76:511–527, 2001.

The majority of antidepressants block the reuptake of neurotransmitters from presynaptic neurons. This is especially true for newer antidepressants, such as the specific serotonin reuptake inhibitors (SSRIs). Many antidepressants also directly block the post-synaptic neurotransmitter receptors. As seen in Table 2, the affinity of antidepressants for monoamine neurotransmitter transporters and receptors can be measured precisely.

The relationship between clinical efficacy and antidepressant receptor affinities is not well established. There is, however, a direct relationship between transporter and receptor affinities and the adverse effects of antidepressants. Antidepressants that inhibit the serotonin reuptake transporter (e.g., paroxetine, clomipramine, sertraline, fluoxetine) may induce gastrointestinal side effects (diarrhea, gastrointestinal upset), jitteriness, and sexual dysfunction. Antidepressants that inhibit the norepinephrine transporter (e.g., desipramine, reboxetine, amoxapine, doxepin) may induce tremors, tachycardia, diaphoresis, and hypertension as possible side effects. Blockade of the histamine H_1 receptor (e.g., mirtazapine, doxepin, amitriptyline) is related to sedation and weight gain. Antidepressants blocking the dopamine D_2 receptor (e.g., amoxapine) may induce extrapyramidal movement abnormalities and elevated prolactin levels as possible side effects. Blockade of the cholinergic muscarinic receptor (e.g., amitriptyline, clomipramine, imipramine) is related to blurred vision, dry mouth, constipation, urinary retention, tachycardia, and memory impairment. Antidepressants blocking the α_1-adrenoreceptors (e.g., doxepin, trazodone, nefazodone, amitriptyline, clomipramine) may induce postural hypotension, dizziness, and reflex tachycardia as possible side effects.

The antidepressant effects on neurotransmitter transporters and receptors occur within hours from the ingestion of the first dose. Adverse effects from antidepressants have similar rapid onset; there appears to be a close relationship between the specific synaptic effects of antidepressants and the side effects they engender. However, the clinical effects of antidepressants on mood as well as pain usually begin 2 to 4 weeks after the onset of treatment,

TABLE 2

Antidepressant Blockade of Monoamine Transporters and Receptors in the Human Brain*

Anti-depressant	Serotonin Transporter Inhibition	Norepi-nephrine Transporter Inhibition	Selectivity of Sero-tonin/ Norepi-nephrine Uptake Blockade	Dopa-mine Trans-porter Inhibition	α_1-Adreno-receptor Blockade	Dopamine D_2 Re-ceptor Blockade	Hista-mine H_1 Re-ceptor Blockade	Muscarinic Receptor Blockade	Serotonin 5-HT2A Receptor Blockade
Paroxetine	800	2.5	320	0.2	0.029	0.0031	0.0045	0.93	0.0053
Fluoxetine	120	0.41	300	0.028	0.017	0.0083	0.016	0.05	0.48
Sertraline	340	0.24	1400	4	0.27	0.0094	0.0041	0.16	0.01
Fluvoxamine	45	0.077	580	0.011	0.013	0	0.00092	0.0042	0.018
Citalopram	90	0.025	3500	0.0036	0.053	0	0.21	0.045	0.042
Clomipramine	360	2.7	140	0.045	2.6	0.53	3.2	2.7	3.7
Imipramine	70	2.7	27	0.012	1.1	0.05	9.1	1.1	1.2
Amitriptyline	23	2.9	8	0.031	3.7	0.1	91	5.6	3.4
Desipramine	5.7	120	0.05	0.031	0.77	0.0303	0.91	0.5	0.36
Amoxapine	1.7	6.2	0.27	0.023	2	5.6	4	0.1	97
Doxepin	1.5	3.4	0.43	0.0082	4.2	0.042	420	1.2	4
Venlafaxine	11	0.094	120	0.011	0	0	0	0	0
Reboxetine	1.7	14	0.12		0.0084	0.025	0.32	0.015	0.016
Nefazodone	0.5	0.28	2	0.28	3.9	0.11	4.7	0.0091	30
Mirtazapine	0.001	0.021	0.05	0.001	0.02	0.01	700	0.15	6.1
Bupropion	0.011	0.0019	5.8	0.19	0.022	0		0.015	0.0021	0.0011

*Potency (affinity) data are expressed as the inverse of the equilibrium dissociation constant K_d, multiplied by 10^{-7}.

Data from Richelson E: Pharmacology of antidepressants. Mayo Clin Proc 76:511–527, 2001.

and the full clinical benefit generally requires 4 to 6 weeks of treatment.[5] No antidepressant appears to have an onset of action significantly faster than the others. Several theories have tried to account for this delayed effect of clinical efficacy (see Theories on the Mechanisms of Antidepressant Drug Action).

THEORIES ON THE MECHANISMS OF ANTIDEPRESSANT DRUG ACTION

The earliest theory on the mechanism of action of antidepressants was the *monoamine hypothesis*. This hypothesis postulated that antidepressants' role is to correct a deficit of monoamine neurotransmitters, particularly serotonin (5-hydroxytriptamine; 5-HT) and norepinephrine.

The support for the monoamine hypothesis came from several observations. The locus coeruleus, a small retropontine nucleus that is the major source of the brain's adrenergic innervation, and the serotonin neurons originating in the brainstem raphe nuclei have modulatory roles, regulating global functions such as arousal, vigilance, attention, mood, and appetite. Certain drugs, such as reserpine, which deplete the monoamine neurotransmitters, induce a clinical state indistinguishable from depression, thus providing an animal model for the disease. Also, antidepressants such as monoamine oxidase inhibitors and tricyclic antidepressants (TCAs) increased by different mechanisms the amounts of monoamine neurotransmitters, resulting in clinical relief from depression. Such observations suggested that the action of antidepressant drugs is mediated through increasing noradrenergic or serotoninergic neurotransmission, thus compensating for a postulated initial deficit.

In its most simplistic form, this proved to be an inadequate theory on the biology of depression and the mechanisms of antidepressant drug action. There is a lack of evidence to prove that depression is characterized by diminished levels of noradrenergic or serotoninergic neurotransmission. Moreover, the effect of most antidepressants in raising the levels of neurotransmitters occurs very fast, in a matter of hours, while the latency for onset of clinical benefit is typically 2 to 4 weeks, and for the full clinical effect, 6 to 8 weeks.[5]

Given the limitations of the monoamine hypothesis, alternative explanations have been sought. Subsequent studies have shown that tricyclic antidepressants down-regulate β_1-adrenergic receptors over a period of 2 to 3 weeks, consistent with the occurrence of the therapeutic effect. Other studies have shown variable effects of antidepressants and electroconvulsive shock therapy on brain serotonin ($5\text{-}HT_2$) receptors. These findings have led to the *neurotransmitter receptor hypothesis*, postulating that antidepressants address preexisting abnormalities of receptors involved in neurotransmission. There is no clear evidence, however, demonstrating the link between modulation of neurotransmitter receptors and therapeutic effects on mood disorders or chronic pain. Changes in receptor numbers are currently seen as correlates of long-term administration, rather than a therapeutic mechanism.

Given the delayed onset of clinical effects, slow-onset changes in the nervous system have been sought to explain the mechanism of action of antidepressant drugs. According to the *hypothesis of neuronal gene expression*, antidepressant agents help correct a deficit of signal transduction in the post-synaptic neuron, despite normal levels of monoamines and post-synaptic receptors. The immediate action of antidepressant drugs is to raise the levels of monoamine neurotransmitters in the synaptic cleft. This process induces compensatory changes in the post-synaptic neuron, changes that ultimately involve activation of genes and protein synthesis. The changes in gene expression occur over several weeks, consistent with the time interval until the onset of antidepressant clinical.[6]

One candidate gene in this process is the gene for brain-derived neurotrophic factor (BDNF). BDNF has an important role in maintaining the viability of neurons. It enhances the growth and metabolism of several neuronal systems and serves as a neurotransmitter modulator. The gene for BDNF is down-regulated in conditions of stress and possibly in depression.[7] Infusing BDNF in the brains of depression-model animals leads to recovery of behavioral deficits. Administering antidepressants to animals enhances BDNF gene expression, thus reversing the effect of chronic stress.[8]

THEORIES ON THE MECHANISM OF ANTIDEPRESSANT DRUG ACTION IN CHRONIC PAIN

There is a large amount of clinical experience in using TCAs in the treatment of chronic pain, with TCAs appearing to have greater analgesic efficacy than SSRIs.[9-12] Antidepressants (especially TCAs) have been shown to be effective in a variety of conditions associated with chronic pain, even in the absence of major depression. Several mechanisms may be involved in this effect. TCAs inhibit norepinephrine and serotonin reuptake; this may enhance the activity of neuronal network implicated in the diffuse noxious inhibitory controls.[13]

Also, TCAs have an N-methyl-D-aspartate antagonist-like effect, which could relieve neuropathic pain by inhibiting neuronal hyperexcitability.[14] Inhibition of sodium channels explains both the proarrhythmic effects of TCAs and the membrane stabilization of peripheral and central neurons with a role in neuropathic pain.

In a review of the literature of antidepressants in chronic pain, Sindrup and Jensen[14] conclude that tricyclics with both norepinephrine and serotonin inhibition (e.g., amitriptyline) are more effective than noradrenergic tricyclic antidepressants (e.g., desipramine) in providing pain relief. The conclusion would be that pain control requires a combination of serotonergic and noradrenergic inhibition. This is consistent with data indicating that both serotonin and norepinephrine exert analgesic effects via descending pain pathways.[15–17] This finding may also explain the increased efficacy of TCAs, compared with selective serotonin reuptake inhibitors, in providing pain relief, as reported by some studies.[18] It can also explain the recently reported success of duloxetine, a dual serotonin-norepinephrine reuptake inhibitor (SNRIs), in treating both depression and painful physical symptoms among depressed patients,[19] and of venlafaxine, another SNRI, in treating neuropathic pain.[20] Mirtazapine, a histamine H1 receptor blocker, was also reported recently as efficacious in pain syndromes in cancer patients.[21]

MECHANISMS OF ACTION FOR NOVEL AGENTS WITH PUTATIVE ANTIDEPRESSANT EFFICACY

The Role of Cytokines and the Immune System

For a long time, researchers have noted the increased prevalence of depression among subjects with severe medical illness. One possible explanation involves the cytokines, nonantibody proteins released by cells on contact with antigens. Cytokines act as intercellular messengers, and levels of cytokines are increased in a variety of medical illnesses that involve activation of the immune system. Examples of such diseases include autoimmune diseases, stroke, trauma, cancer, and neurodegenerative diseases. Further observations have shown that the administration of cytokines such as interleukin-2, tumor necrosis factor, or interferon-α may induce depressive symptoms.[22] The decreased production of cytokines has a further impact on cortisol production and on the hypothalamic-pituitary-adrenal axis. Also, antidepressants have been shown to reduce the immune response and suppress cytokine production.[23] However, we do not yet know whether suppression of cytokine production represents a mechanism of action of antidepressants in depression associated with medical illness, or that it has any relevance to the antinociceptive effects of antidepressants.

The Neurokinin System and Substance P

Another class of peptides, the neurokinins, have been implicated in the pathology of both depression and pain. Neurokinins are secreted by brain cells and serve as neurotransmitters. The best known neurokin is substance P, which is released by neurons in response to inflammation. Substance P is associated with the pain response in neurogenic pain. Also, substance P is present in the spinal pain pathways and plays a role in the transmission of pain sensation at the level of the central nervous system.

Substance P antagonists have been researched for potential benefits in pain control. This led to the observation that symptoms of depression improved in patients with migraine (while the pain did not improve). It is possible that substance P and other related neurokinins act as neurotransmitters in brain circuits involved in mood regulation; these peptides are present in the amygdala and other brain areas involved in controlling emotional responses. This may be the mechanism of action for substance P antagonists in treating depression. Antagonists to the three major neurokinins (substance P, neurokinin A, and neurokinin B) are currently studied as potential antidepressants and antianxiety agents.[24] No definite results have been obtained yet, but this appears as a promising new avenue of pharmacological research in depression.

Further work elucidating the role of substance P in mood regulation may help explain the increased incidence of depression in patients with chronic pain and the efficacy of antidepressant drugs as pain medications.

NATURAL REMEDIES USED AS ANTIDEPRESSANTS

Natural remedies have been used for centuries and have become even more popular in the past decades. There are, however, limited data on the true efficacy or the mechanism of action of these substances.

Omega 3 Fatty Acids

Indirect evidence shows that populations with increased dietary intake of omega 3 fatty acids have a lower prevalence of depression. The rates of depression in North America are 10-fold greater than in Taiwan, while the dietary intake of omega 3 fatty acids in Taiwan is 200 mg higher than in the United States. Deficits of omega 3 fatty acids have been shown in the serum and cerebrospinal fluid of depressed subjects. In preliminary studies, adding omega 3 fatty acids to the diet has been correlated with the resolution of depression symptoms.[25]

The mechanism of action of omega 3 fatty acids in depression may be related to the known effect of reducing the inflammatory response and lowering cytokine levels. Other actions of omega 3 fatty acids that may have an antidepressant effect are the relaxation of brain microvasculature through α_2-adrenergic receptors (shown in vitro) and the stabilization of protein kinase C (similar to the mechanism of lithium).

St. John's Wort

The extract of St. John's wort (Hypericum perforatum) is used in Europe to treat mild and moderate depression. Several clinical trials have shown comparable efficacy with very low doses of TCAs. Hypericin is the presumed active compound among the many polycyclic phenols in St. John's wort.[26] Hypericin does not cross the blood-brain barrier but may act by inhibiting cytokine production, especially interleukins 1 and 6. Hypericin is also a weak reuptake inhibitor for several neurotransmitters (serotonin, norepinephrine, and dopamine).

Although two recent studies have questioned the efficacy of St. John's wort compared with SSRIs and placebo,[27, 28] these two US studies were rather inconclusive due to low assay sensitivity or study design issues (lack of an active comparator). Therefore, the issue concerning the efficacy of St. John's wort is still unresolved, and other large studies are underway for both major and minor depressive disorders.

S-Adenosyl Methionine

S-adenyl methionine (SAMe) is an important component for the brain cell metabolism, serving as the most important methyl donor in brain cells. SAMe activity depends on the levels of folate and vitamin B_{12}. Several studies have shown the antidepressant properties of SAMe to be superior to those of placebo and comparable to those of tricyclic antidepressants.[29] When SAMe is administered in conjunction with low doses of tricyclic antidepressants, patients may experience a faster onset of the antidepressant effect and fewer side effects.[26] Similar studies on the adjuvant role of SAMe when added to SSRIs are lacking. The precise mechanism of action for the putative antidepressant effects of SAMe is unknown.[30]

REFERENCES FOR ADDITIONAL READING

1. Burke WJ, Heindricks SE, McArthur-Miller D, et al: Weekly dosing of fluoxetine for the continuation treatment phase of major depression: Results for a placebo-controlled, randomized clinical trial. J Clin Psychopharmacol 20:423–427, 2000.
2. Lundmark J, Reis M, Bengtson F: Therapeutic drug monitoring of sertraline: Variability factors as displayed in the clinical setting. Ther Drug Monit 22:446–454, 2000.
3. Task Force on the Use of Laboratory Tests in Psychiatry: Tricyclic antidepressant-blood level measurements and clinical outcome: An APA Task Force report. Am J Psychiatry 142:155–162, 1985.
4. Burke MJ, Preskorn SH: Therapeutic drug monitoring of antidepressants: Cost implications and relevance to clinical practice. Clin Pharmacokinet 37:147–165, 1999.
5. Fava M, Davidson KG: Definition and epidemiology of treatment-resistant depression. Psychiatr Clin North Am 19:179–200, 1996.
6. Rangel YM, Kariko K, Harris VA, et al: Dose-dependent induction of mRNAs encoding brain-derived neurotrophic factor and heat-shock protein-72 after cortical spreading depression in the rat. Brain Res Mol Brain Res 88:103–112, 2001.
7. Reid IC, Stewart CA: How antidepressants work: New perspectives on the pathophysiology of depressive disorder. Br J Psychiatry; 178:299–303, 2001.
8. Russo-Neustadt A, Ha T, Ramirez R, Kesslak JP: Physical activity-antidepressant treatment combination: Impact on brain-derived neurotrophic factor and behavior in an animal model. Behav Brain Res 120:87–95, 2001.
9. Ansari A: The efficacy of newer antidepressants in the treatment of chronic pain: A review of current literature. Harvard Rev Psychiatry 7:257–277, 2000.
10. Collins SL, Moore RA, McQuay HJ, Whiffen P: Antidepressant and anticonvulsants for diabetic neuropathy and post-herptic neuralgia: A quantitative systematic review. J Pain Sympt Manage 20:449–458, 2000.
11. Lynch M: Antidepressants as analgesics: A review of randomized controlled trials. J Psychiatry Neurosci 26:30–36, 2001.
12. Sindrup SH, Jensen TS: Efficacy of pharmacological treatments of neuropthic pain: An update and effect related to mechanism of drug action. Pain 83:389–400, 1999.
13. Fields HL, Basbaum AI: Endogenous pain control mechanisms. In Wall PD, Melzak R, eds. Textbook of Pain. Churchill Livingstone, London, 1984, pages 142–152.
14. Sindrup SH, Jensen TS: Antidepressants in the treatment of neuropathic pain. In Hanson PT, Fields HL, Hill RG, Marchettini P, eds. Neuropathic Pain: Pathophysiology and Treatment, Progress in Pain Research and Management, Vol. 21. IASP Press, Seattle, 2001, pages 169–183.
15. Jones SL: Descending noradrenergic influences on pain. Prog Brain Res 88:381–394, 1991.
16. Richardson BP: Serotonin and nociception. Ann N Y Acad Sci 600:511–519, 1990.
17. Willis WD, Westlund KN: Neuroanatomy of the pain system and the pathways that modulate pain. J Clin Neurophysiol 14:2–31, 1997.

18. Max MB, Lynch SA, Muir J, et al: Effects of desipramine, amitriptyline, and fluoxetine on pain in diabetic neuropathy. N Engl J Med 326:1250–1256, 1992.

19. Detke MJ, Lu Y, Goldstein DJ, et al: Duloxetine, 60 mg/day, for major depressive disorder: A randomized double-blind placebo-controlled trial. J Clin Psychiatr 63:308–315, 2002.

20. Tasmuth T, Hartel B, Kalso E: Venlafaxine in neuropathic pain following treatment of breast cancer. Eur J Pain 6:17–24, 2002.

21. Theobald DE, Kirsh KL, Holtsclaw E, et al: An open-label, crossover trial of mirtazapine (15 and 30 mg) in cancer patients with pain and other distressing symptoms. J Pain Sympt Manage 23: 442–447, 2002.

22. Meyers CA: Mood and cognitive disorders in cancer patients receiving cytokine therapy. In: Danzer R, Wollman EE, Yirmiya R, eds. Cytokines, stress and depression. Kluwer Academic/Plenum Publishers, New York, 1999, pages 75–81.

23. Danzer R, Wollman E, Vitkovic L, Yirmiya R: Cytokines and depression: Fortuitous or causative association. Mol Psychiatry 4:328–332, 1999.

24. Haddjeri N, Blier P: Sustained blockade of neurokinin-1 receptors enhances serotonin neurotransmission. Biol Psychiatry 50:191–199, 2001.

25. Mischoulon D, Fava M: Docosahexanoic acid and omega-3 fatty acids in depression. Psychiatr Clin North Am 23:785–794, 2000.

26. Mischoulon D: Herbal remedies for mental illness. Psychiatr Clin North Am 6:1–19, 1999.

27. Shelton RC, Keller MB, Gelenberg A, et al: Effectiveness of St. John's wort in major depression: A randomized controlled trial. JAMA 285:1978–1986, 2001.

28. Hypericum Depression Study Group: Effect of Hypericum perforatum (St. John's wort) in major depressive disorder: A randomized controlled trial. JAMA 287:1807–1814, 2002.

29. Spillmann M, Fava M: S-adenosylmethionine (Ademetionine) in psychiatric disorders: Historical perspective and current status. CNS Drugs 6:416–425, 1996.

30. Alpert JE, Mischoulon D. One-carbon metabolism and the treatment of depression: Roles of S-adenosyl methionine (SAMe) and folic acid. In Natural Medication for Psychiatric Disorders (Mischoulon D, Rosenbaum JF, editors). Lippincott, Williams & Wilkins, Philadelphia, 2002.

Chapter 19

Antidepressants: Clinical Management

Dan V. Iosifescu, MD / Jonathan E. Alpert, MD, PhD / Maurizio Fava, MD

Antidepressants are effective treatment for major depression. In a survey of multiple antidepressants, 50% to 71% of depressed patients fully recovered when an adequate dose of any antidepressant is used for an adequate amount of time (at least 6 weeks). Of those who did not fully recover, 12% to 15% showed some improvement; whereas 19% to 34% failed to improve.[1]

Antidepressants also have broad efficacy for a range of conditions other than depression, particularly anxiety disorders (e.g., panic disorder, generalized anxiety disorder, social anxiety disorder, post-traumatic stress disorder, and obsessive-compulsive disorder), eating disorders, attention deficit hyperactivity disorders, premenstrual dysphoric disorder, and chronic pain.

A commonly used classification of antidepressant medications is as follows:

1. Selective serotonin reuptake inhibitors (SSRIs)
2. Cyclic antidepressants, including the tricyclic antidepressants (TCAs)
3. Monoamine oxidase inhibitors (MAOIs)
4. The miscellaneous category of "atypical antidepressants"

CLASSES OF ANTIDEPRESSANT MEDICATIONS

Selective Serotonin Reuptake Inhibitors

The advantages of SSRIs include a favorable side-effect profile, a broad spectrum of efficacy for comorbid disorders, a low potential for abuse and dependence, safety in overdose, and single daily dosing. A once-weekly formulation of fluoxetine is also now available.

The disadvantages of SSRIs include increased anxiety or "jitteriness" on initial dosing, side-effects such as sexual dysfunction, particularly anorgasmia and delayed ejaculation, headaches, gastrointestinal symptoms (nausea, diarrhea), agitation, insomnia, and drug-drug interactions by inhibiting the activity of cytochrome p450 isoenzymes. In rare cases, a serotonin syndrome can also occur when SSRIs are combined with monoamine oxidase inhibitors or with relatively serotoninergic agents (see Drug Interactions for more detail).

Mechanism of Action. Serotoninergic blockade at neuronal synaptic clefts occurs within hours of initiation of SSRI treatment. However, the typical time to response in patients with depression for all antidepressant medications, including the SSRIs, is 3 to 6 weeks; therefore, serotonin reuptake inhibition alone cannot account for antidepressant efficacy. It is likely that serotonin reuptake inhibition is at the origin of a chain of intracellular second-messenger systems that promote gene regulation, which in turn are ultimately responsible for the antidepressant actions of these medications (see Chapter 18 for more details).

Side Effects. All currently available SSRIs appear to be equally efficacious for depression; they differ primarily in their side effects, their half-lives, and their drug interactions. Some side effects are more common with some SSRIs than with others; however, one patient may find a particular SSRI sedating, while another might find the same SSRI activating.

The most common side effects of all the SSRIs are nausea (which tends to be worst during early treatment), reduced appetite, weight loss or gain, excessive sweating, headache, insomnia, jitteriness, sedation, dizziness, and sexual dysfunction, including decreased libido, delayed ejaculation, impotence, and anorgasmia. Other side effects include rash, dry mouth, and prolonged bleeding time (although this is usually variable and not clinically significant).

For reasons of tolerability and their benign side-effect profile, the SSRIs have become the first-line treatment for depressive disorder spectrum illnesses, ranging from dysthymia to severe major depression.

Half-Life. Half-lives vary greatly among the SSRIs. Although an antidepressant's half-life is not relevant to its treatment efficacy or its onset of action, it may be significant in terms of its side effects, its interactions with other agents, and its discontinuation-emergent symptoms. Medications with shorter half-lives may be useful when abrupt discontinuation is desired due to intolerable side effects or to medication interactions, but medications with shorter half-lives are more likely to cause the discontinuation-emergent symptoms (e.g., tachycardia, flu-like symptoms, dizziness, myalgias, anxiety, irritability, worsening of mood, jitteriness, and nausea). An SSRI with a longer half-life is more likely to "self-taper" and may be beneficial for a patient who is apt to miss occasional dosages.

Dosing. Given the fact that SSRIs have the potential to cause initial restlessness, insomnia, and increased anxiety, the starting doses should be low in patients who are particularly sensitive to somatic sensations (e.g., paroxetine 10 mg/day, sertraline 25 mg/day, fluvoxamine 25 mg/day, fluoxetine 10 mg/day, citalopram 10 mg/day). However, such patients may require at least average doses of SSRIs in order to achieve a response (e.g., paroxetine 40 mg/day, sertraline 100–150 mg/day, fluvoxamine 150–200 mg/day, fluoxetine 20–40 mg/day, and citalopram 20–40 mg/day).

Although dose-response curves have not been definitively established for the SSRIs, some patients who do not respond at a lower dose may benefit by having their dosage increased. SSRIs are hepatically metabolized and renally excreted; therefore, lower dosages may be required in hepatically compromised patients, and this is also true to a lesser degree in patients with renal failure.

Table 1 gives the recommended dosages of a number of commonly prescribed antidepressant drugs.

Drug Interactions. With the exception perhaps of citalopram, SSRIs may inhibit cytochrome p450 isoenzymes, potentially causing substrate levels to rise, or reducing conversion of a substrate (e.g., codeine) into its active form (see Drug Interactions for more detail).

TABLE 1

Recommended Dosage of Most Commonly Prescribed Antidepressant Medications

Drug	Sedative potency	Anticholin-ergic potency	Orthostatic Hypo-tension	Daily dose range (mg)	Initial dose (mg/day)	Dosing schedule	Half-life (h)
Selective Serotonin Reuptake Inhibitors							
Paroxetine (Paxil)	L	L	VL	10–50	10	qd	21
Sertraline (Zoloft)	VL	VL	VL	25–200	25	qd	26
Fluvoxamine (Luvox)	VL	VL	VL	50–300	25	qd	19
Fluoxetine (Prozac)	VL	VL	VL	10–80	10	qd	87
Citalopram (Celexa)	L	VL	VL	20–60	10	qd	35
Tricyclic Antidepressants							
Amitriptyline (Elavil)	H	VH	H	75–300	10–25	qd–bid	21
Amoxapine (Asendin)	L	M	M	75–300	10–25	qd–bid	8
Clomipramine (Anafranil)	H	H	H	75–250	12.5–25	qd–bid	23
Desipramine (Norpramin)	L	M	M	75–300	10–25	qd–bid	21
Doxepin (Sinequan)	H	H	M	75–300	10–25	qd–bid	17
Imipramine (Tofranil)	M	H	H	75–300	10–25	qd–bid	28
Maprotiline (Ludiomil)	M	L	M	75–225	10–25	qd–bid	43
Nortriptyline (Pamelor)	M	M	L	40–150	12.5–25	qd–bid	30
Protriptyline (Vivactil)	L	H	L	15–60	5–10	qd–bid	74
Trimipramine (Surmontil)	H	M	M	75–300	10–25	qd–bid	24
Monoamine Oxidase Inhibitors							
Phenelzine (Nardil)	L	VL	H	45–90	15	tid	3
Tranylcypromine (Parnate)	—	VL	H	30–60	10	bid	3
Atypical Antidepressants							
Venlafaxine (Effexor XR)	L	VL	—	75–225	37.5	qd	3.6
Nefazadone (Serzone)	M	VL	M	300–600	50	bid	3
Bupropion (Wellbutrin)	VL	VL	VL	200–400	75–100	bid	12
Mirtazapine (Remeron)	H	VL	VL	30–45	15	qd	30
Trazodone (Desyrel)	H	VL	H	150–400	50	qd	7.5

H, high; L, low; M, medium; VL, very low.
Modified from Arana GW, Rosenbaum IF: Handbook of Psychiatric Drug Therapy. Lippincott Williams & Wilkins, Philadelphia, 2000.

Tricyclic Antidepressants

Cyclic antidepressants have been in use for nearly 50 years and are generally as effective as SSRIs for depression. However, they have a more problematic side-effect profile and may be lethal in overdose. The term tricyclic signifies a shared chemical structure with two joined benzene rings.

Advantages of TCAs include their lower cost (when compared with SSRIs), the fact that they are well studied, and that they can be administered once a day. TCAs can be efficacious in SSRI nonresponders. Some evidence favors the use of TCAs in patients with severe melancholic depression.[2] In addition, TCAs have a more established track record than SSRIs in treating a variety of chronic pain conditions, including neuropathies, fibromyalgia, and migraine.[3, 4]

Disadvantages of TCAs include a wide range of adverse effects, including anticholinergic effects, orthostatic hypotension, effects on the cardiac conduction system, weight gain, sedation, sexual dysfunction, restlessness, "jitteriness," heightened anxiety on initial dosing, and cardiotoxicity in overdose. The combined direct and indirect cost of care with TCAs may be higher than with SSRIs because of the need for more frequent visits and for monitoring of serum levels and the electrocardiogram.[5]

Cyclic Antidepressant Categories. The TCAs can be divided into tertiary amines and their demethylated secondary amine derivatives. In addition, maprotiline (Ludiomil) is classified as a tetracyclic.

The tertiary amine TCAs include the following:

- amitriptyline (Elavil)
- imipramine (Tofranil)
- trimipramine (Surmontil)
- clomipramine (Anafranil)
- doxepin (Sinequan)

The secondary amine TCAs include the following:

- nortriptyline (Pamelor)
- desipramine (Norpramin)
- protriptyline (Vivactil)
- amoxapine (Asendin)

Categorization of Side Effects. Anticholinergic Effects. Anticholinergic side effects result from the affinity of TCAs for muscarinic cholinergic receptors. Anticholinergic symptoms include dry mouth, blurred vision, constipation, urinary hesitancy, tachycardia, and ejaculatory difficulties. Secondary amine TCAs tend to cause fewer anticholinergic effects than tertiary amine TCAs.

Antihistaminergic Effects. Antihistaminergic side effects results from histaminergic H_1 receptor blockade. Common side effects include sedation, carbohydrate craving, and weight gain. Weigh gain with TCAs can be substantial, averaging 1 to 3 lbs per month of treatment. Secondary amine TCAs tend to cause less sedation than tertiary amine TCAs.

α_1**-Adrenergic Receptor Blockade.** Orthostatic hypotension results from α_1-adrenergic receptor antagonism. Nortriptyline is generally thought to be less likely to cause orthostatic hypotension than tertiary amine TCAs.

Cardiac Effects. Cardiac toxicity may occur in susceptible individuals and following TCA overdose; the TCAs should be avoided in patients with bifascicular heart block, left bundle branch block, or a prolonged QT interval, because they may slow conduction through the atrioventricular node. TCAs have quinidine-like effects on cardiac conduction and are classified as class I antiarrhythmics. TCAs must be used with great caution with other drugs from this class, including quinidine, procainamide, and disopyramide. Baseline and follow-up electrocardiograms should be monitored, especially in older patients or those with cardiac conduction disorders, as well as in pediatric patients. TCAs can cause severe orthostatic hypotension in patients with congestive heart failure due to α_1-receptor blockade.

Dosage. Treatment should be initiated with lower doses (e.g., 10 mg/day for imipramine) in sensitive patients, to minimize the "activation syndrome" (restlessness, "jitteriness," palpitations, increased anxiety) noted upon initiation of treatment. Typical antidepressant doses are 100 to 300 mg/day for imipramine. The adverse effect profile of TCAs accounts for the high drop-out rate (30–70%) in published studies.

Toxicity. Tricyclic antidepressants have a low threshold for toxicity; overdose of even a 1-week supply may be lethal. Due to the lethality after overdose, it may be safer to treat acutely suicidal depressed patients with non-TCA antidepressants or to prescribe limited quantities of TCAs.

Manifestations of anticholinergic toxicity may including dilated pupils, blurred vision, dry skin, hyperpyrexia, ileus, urinary retention, confusion, delirium, and seizures. Additionally, arrhythmias, hypotension, and coma may develop. Although TCAs are highly plasma-bound and are not removed by hemodialysis, they are metabolized by hepatic microsomal enzymes. Patients who have overdosed on TCAs may require alkalinization of their serum, pressors, or ventilatory support to maintain survival.[6]

The TCAs should be avoided in patients with narrow angle glaucoma and prostatic hypertrophy, as symptoms related to these conditions may worsen because of anticholinergic effects. TCAs are also contraindicated with MAOIs (see Drug Interactions below).

Blood Levels. The relationship between serum levels and response is unclear, although most evidence points to a target level of at least 125 to 150 ng/mL (imipramine and desipramine levels). In general, TCAs have a linear relationship between increasing levels and effectiveness; some researchers have suggested that with nortriptyline there may be a U-shaped curve, with decreasing efficacy at blood levels above therapeutic range (50–150 ng/mL), although the evidence for such a view is not fully convincing, and some patients may benefit from higher levels. Blood levels may be useful in establishing compliance, higher than usual dose requirements (as in chronic smokers), or toxicity due to overdose or drug interactions.

Monoamine Oxidase Inhibitors

Monoamine oxidase (MAO) is found on the outer membrane of cellular mitochondria, where it catabolizes intracellular monoamines, including the central nervous system monoamines: dopamine, norepinephrine, serotonin, and tyramine. In the gastrointestinal tract and the liver, MAO catabolizes dietary pressor amines, such as dopamine, tyramine, tryptamine, and phenylethylamine. The currently available MAO inhibitors (MAOIs), such as phenelzine (Nardil), tranylcypromine (Parnate), and isocarboxazid (Marplan), are active on both MAO A and MAO B, thus increasing synaptic monoamine concentrations. Phenelzine, tranylcypromine, and isocarboxazid are relatively irreversible blockers of MAO activity, which takes about 14 days to regenerate after MAOI discontinuation. The anti-parkinsonian agent selegiline (Eldepryl), is a more selective MAO-B inhibitor, particularly at low doses (≤15 mg/day). It is also used for antidepressant properties, although higher doses are often required, and those doses are associated with lesser selectivity.

Advantages of MAOIs include their proven efficacy for the treatment of unipolar major depression. In "atypical" depression (characterized by mood reactivity plus hypersomnia, hyperphagia, extreme fatigue when depressed, and/or rejection sensitivity), MAOIs appear to be more effective than the TCAs.[7, 8] The MAOIs are often used in individuals with treatment-resistant depression, after successive treatment failures with more recent antidepressants. In addition, MAOIs have broad efficacy for anxiety disorders, including panic disorder and social anxiety disorder.

Disadvantages of MAOIs include their adverse effects profile (orthostatic hypotension, weight gain, and sexual dysfunction), particularly the need for dietary restrictions (to prevent hypertensive crisis), potentially fatal drug interactions (due to the interaction with sympathomimetic drugs or serotonergic drugs), and toxicity in overdose.

Side Effects. The most common side effects include postural hypotension, insomnia, agitation, sedation, impotence, delayed ejaculation, and anorgasmia. Others include weight change, dry mouth, constipation, and urinary hesitancy. Peripheral neuropathies have been reported and may be avoided by concomitant therapy with vitamin B_6.

Toxic Interactions. When patients on MAOIs ingest dietary amines, rather than being catabolized in the intestines and the liver, they are taken up in sympathetic nerve terminals and may cause the release of endogenous catecholamines with a resulting adrenergic crises. This is characterized by hypertension, hyperpyrexia, and other adrenergic symptoms such as tachycardia, tremulousness, and cardiac arrhythmias. The amine most commonly associated with these symptoms is tyramine, but others, such as phenylethylalamine and dopamine, may be involved.

Dietary Interactions. Dietary amines can be avoided by adherence to dietary restrictions and avoidance of tyramine-containing foods. The diet must be strictly followed. Patients must be instructed to avoid all matured or aged cheese, fermented or dried meats such as pepperoni and salami, fava and broad bean *pods* (not the beans themselves), tap beers, marmite yeast extract, sauerkraut, soy sauce, and other soy products such as tofu and tempe. All meats and cheese must be fresh and must have been stored and refrigerated or frozen properly. Up to two bottles of beer or glasses of wine may be consumed safely; this restriction includes nonalcoholic beers.[9]

Since endogenous MAO activity does not return to baseline immediately upon MAOI discontinuation, 2 weeks should transpire before after MAOI discontinuation before the diet is discontinued and a contraindicated medication is begun.

Dosage. Owing to the danger associated with consumption of tyramine-containing foods or sympathomimetic agents while taking a MAOI, with drug interactions, and with toxicity in overdose, MAOIs are usually reserved for patients with depression and anxiety that remain symptomatic after treatment with safer and better tolerated agents. Optimal doses for phenelzine range between 45 and 90 mg/day, whereas doses of tranylcypromine and isocarboxazid generally range between 30 and 60 mg/day. For selegiline, optimal doses range between 10 and 30 mg/day.

Medical Interactions. The MAOIs are contraindicated in patients with pheochromocytoma, congestive heart failure, and hepatic disease.

Atypical Antidepressants

The atypical antidepressants reflect a miscellaneous class of antidepressants, with varying mechanisms of action that differ from those of the SSRIs, TCAs, and MAOIs.

Bupropion (Wellbutrin, Wellbutrin SR). The mechanism of action of bupropion has not been fully elucidated, although it appears to block the reuptake of both dopamine and norepinephrine. Therefore, bupropion has sympathomimetic, stimulant-like effects. It is metabolized in the liver. Effective doses range between 200 and 400 mg/day (maximum, 450 mg/day); the starting dose is 75 mg every morning (or 100 mg every morning with the sustained release preparation, Wellbutrin SR). Common side effects include agitation, insomnia, weight loss, dry mouth, headache, constipation, and tremor. It has been noted to cause seizures, at a rate of 4 per 1000 subjects in its immediate release form. Its sustained-release (SR) form is associated with a somewhat lower seizure risk, comparable to that of the SSRIs. However, the risk of seizure markedly increases at doses greater than 450 mg/day and greater than 200 mg/dose. Bupropion may be more likely to induce seizures in patients with bulimia nervosa and histories of head trauma. It is generally safe in overdose, although fatalities have been reported. Bupropion is generally safe for patients with cardiac disease, although it may participate in drug interactions. It rarely induces sexual dysfunction and can even be beneficial as an adjunct in SSRI-induced sexual dysfunction. Its use is contraindicated with the MAOIs.

Mirtazapine (Remeron). Mirtazapine is an antagonist at inhibitory α_2-adrenergic auto- and heteroreceptors, leading to increased release of both serotonin and norepinephrine at the synaptic level. It is also a relatively potent histaminergic H_1 receptor antagonist. Effective doses range between 30 and 45 mg/day (maximum, 60 mg/day); the starting dose is 15 mg at bedtime. Common side effects include somnolence, weight gain, dizziness, dry mouth, constipation and orthostatic hypotension. Due to blockade of $5\text{-}HT_2$ and $5\text{-}HT_3$ receptors, mirtazapine may reduce SSRI-related sexual dysfunction and nausea when administered concomitantly.

Trazodone (Desyrel). Trazodone inhibits serotonin uptake, blocks serotonin $5\text{-}HT_2$ receptors, and may act as a serotonin agonist through an active metabolite. It is also an antagonist of α_1-adrenergic receptors. The metabolism is hepatic. Usual effective doses are 300 to 600 mg/day, usually given at bedtime. Trazodone is less lethal in overdose than the TCAs, although slightly more lethal than the SSRIs. The most common side effects are sedation, orthostatic hypotension, and headache. Priapism is a rare but serious side effect that requires immediate medical attention. Trazodone may induce arrhythmias in patients with preexisting heart disease. Trazodone is most commonly used at low doses (50–100 mg at bedtime) as an adjunctive medication for insomnia, owing to its sedating properties.

Nefazodone (Serzone). Nefazodone is chemically related to trazodone, with serotonin $5\text{-}HT_2$ blockade but with less α_1-blockade and fewer side effects. It is less likely to cause sexual dysfunction than SSRIs or TCAs and is less anticholinergic and histaminergic. The metabolism is hepatic. Nefazodone is effective in treating depression at doses between 200 and 600 mg/day.

Common side effects include somnolence, dizziness, dry mouth, nausea, constipation, headache, and amblyopia and blurred vision. Nefazodone is contraindicated with MAOIs. Nefazodone has been associated with rare but fatal hepatotoxicity.

Venlafaxine (Effexor, Effexor XR). Venlafaxine has a dual mechanism of action (serotonin and norepinephrine reuptake inhibitor, at doses greater than 150 mg/day; it is generally equivalent to an SSRI at lower doses). It is generally efficacious at doses between 75 and 375 mg/day; with a starting dose of 37.5 to 75 mg/day, typically in its extended release (XR) formulation.

The side effects of venlafaxine are similar to those of the SSRIs: nausea, insomnia, sedation, sexual dysfunction, and dizziness. Five to 7% of patients experience an increase in baseline diastolic blood pressure (especially at higher doses). Venlafaxine use is contraindicated with MAOIs.

Psychostimulants. Although the psychostimulants dextroamphetamine (Dexedrine), methylphenidate (Ritalin), and pemoline (Cylert) have not shown clear benefit in the long-term treatment of depression, they are frequently beneficial in apathetic geriatric patients, subjects with depression and comorbid attention deficit hyperactivity disorder, and as adjunctive medication in the treatment of refractory depression. Because of their potential for abuse, psychostimulants should be used cautiously in subjects with prior history of drug abuse or dependence. Side effects include insomnia, tremors, appetite change, palpitations, blurred vision, dry mouth, constipation, and dizziness. Arrhythmias and tachycardia have also been reported. Pemoline has been associated with hepatic toxicity. Newer formulations of amphetamine salts (Adderall) and methylphenidate (Concerta) offer the advantage of once-daily dosing and potentially less variability in drug blood levels throughout the day.

DRUG INTERACTIONS

Drug-drug interactions represent alterations in drug plasma levels, tissue concentrations, and drug effects associated with the use of two or more agents (prescribed, illicit, or over-the-counter) in close temporal proximity (including recent as well as concurrent use). The most important drug-drug interactions involving antidepressants are related to MAOIs. All other antidepressants may be involved in significant drug-drug interactions via the interactions with the cytochrome p450 isoenzymes or with post-synaptic receptors.

Drug-Drug Interactions with Monoamine Oxidase Inhibitors

Avoidance of toxic drug-drug interactions with MAOIs is critical. The concomitant use with MAOIs of serotonergic medications—serotonergic TCAs such as clomipramine, SSRIs, and venlafaxine—may result in the serotonin syndrome. The serotonin syndrome is characterized by an acute onset of at least three of the following 10 symptoms, coincident with the addition of or an increased dose of the serotoninergic agent: mental status changes, hyperreflexia, diaphoresis, agitation, tremor, diarrhea, myoclonus, fever, dyscoordination, and shivering. In its severe form, serotonin syndrome may include hyperthermia, coma, convulsions, and death. Other possible causes have to be ruled out (e.g., no recent neuroleptic addition or dose change).

The concomitant administration of MAOIs with certain narcotic analgesics can also result in a serotonin syndrome. This is most commonly seen with meperidine (Demerol), which has intrinsic serotoninergic properties. Codeine and morphine appear safer, although they may be potentiated by MAOIs. Other narcotics with serotoninergic properties (e.g., tramadol [Ultram]), as well as serotoninergic antimigraine agents including sumatriptan (Imitrex) have rarely caused problems but should be used with caution.

The MAOIs must be used with caution in patients with diabetes (due to possible potentiation of oral hypoglycemics and worsened hypoglycemia). It has been sugessted that low-dose MAOIs may increase sensitivity to insulin and that high-dose MAOIs may increase insulin resistance, but further studies are needed.

Sympathomimetics, both prescribed and over-the-counter, and relatively potent norepinephrine reuptake inhibitors such as TCAs may precipitate hypertensive crises when combined with MAOIs. Sympathomimetics are most commonly found in nasal decongestants (such as pseudoephedrine, ephedrine, and oxymetazoline [Afrin nasal spray]) and also include amphetamines and cocaine. Toxicity may also occur when the over-the-counter cough-suppressant dextromethorphan is used in the setting of an MAOI. The hypertensive crisis is characterized by sudden severe headache and nausea and may lead to stroke, pulmonary edema, and cardiac arrhythmias.

Prior to beginning an MAOI after discontinuation of a contraindicated antidepressant, the necessary drug-free time varies depending on the half-life of the previous antidepressant. At least five half-lives of the contraindicated medication must pass, with 2 weeks required after paroxetine and 5 weeks required after the use of fluoxetine. Conversely, at least 2 weeks must elapse between discontinuing an MAOI and starting a contraindicated agent. Under certain circumstances, MAOIs have been cautiously combined with certain TCAs and psychostimulants. However, this should be attempted only under the guidance of an experienced practitioner.

Drug-Drug Interactions Involving the Cytochrome p450 Isoenzymes

Cytochrome p450 isoenzymes, including the isoenzymes 1A2, 2C, 2D6, 3A3/4, are located on microsomal membranes throughout the body. Their mechanism of metabolism is best known in the liver and bowel wall, where they oxidatively metabolize medications as well as prostaglandins, fatty acids, and steroids. Alteration in function of these isoenzymes may cause clinically significant pharmacokinetic drug-drug interactions, via changes in drug levels (Table 2).

CYP450 2D6 inhibition by several antidepressants (fluoxetine, paroxetine, sertraline, and bupropion) may lead to increased levels of TCAs, β-blockers, antiarrhythmics, and several narcotic analgesics (codeine, hydroxycodone, oxycodone, tramadol, and dextromethorphan), which are all substrates for this enzyme. Also a potential consequence is inhibition of the conversion of codeine to its active form (morphine), with subsequent reduction of its efficacy.

CYP450 3A4 inhibition by nefazodone and fluvoxamine has potential consequences in increased levels of numerous commonly prescribed substrates, including carbamazepine, cyclosporine, alprazolam, midazolam, zolpidem, zaleplon, calcium channel blockers, statins, sildenafil, oral contraceptives, and pimozide (arrhythmia risk). By interacting with cisapride or pimozide, CYP450 3A4 inhibitors may lead to QT prolongation and torsades de pointes.

TABLE 2

Antidepressant Inhibition of Cytochrome p450 Isoenzymes

Drug	1A2	2C	2D6	3A
Selective Serotonin Reuptake Inhibitors				
Fluoxetine (Prozac)	0	++	++++(++++)	+(++)
Sertraline (Zoloft)	0	+(+)	+	+(+)
Paroxetine (Paxil)	0	0	+++	0
Fluvoxamine (Luvox)	++++	++	0	+++
Citalopram (Celexa)	0	0	+	0
Venlafaxine (Effexor XR)	0	0	(+)	0
Atypical Antidepressants				
Nefazadone (Serzone)	0	0	0	++++
Bupropion (Wellbutrin)	0	0	++++	0
Mirtazapine (Remeron)	0	0	0	0
St. John's Wort	0	0	0	—?

(), metabolite effect

—, suspected induction rather than inhibition

From Devane CL, Nemeroff CB: 2000 Guide to psychotropic drug interactions. Primary Psychiatry 7:X, 2000.

CYP450 1A2 inhibition by fluvoxamine may lead to toxicity on clozapine, theophylline, and other 1A2 substrates

CYP450 2C inhibition by fluoxetine, fluvoxamine, sertraline, tranylcypromine, ketoconazole, and fluconazole has a potential for increased levels of anticoagulant (warfarin) and diazepam.

For a more detailed list of inhibitors and substrates for the cytochrome P-450 isoenzymes, see TABLE 3.

MANAGEMENT OF COMMON SIDE EFFECTS

Although newer antidepressants tend to be better tolerated than the TCAs and the MAOIs, a series of side effects related to antidepressant use may interfere with the patient's compliance with treatment. Side effects may be understood in terms of the effects of antidepressants on specific receptors and transporters (see Chapter 18). Informing the patient of potential side effects and discussing options for their treatment can have a positive impact on the patient's compliance with the antidepressant therapy. Attempting to lower the dose of antidepressant, switching the time of administration or dividing the doses, and using pharmacological antidotes have been useful strategies in the management of significant side effects. For intolerable side effects, switching to another medication may prove necessary, but has to be weighed against potential loss of clinical efficacy.[10]

Cardiovascular Side Effects

Orthostatic hypotension, more common with the MAOIs, TCAs, and trazodone, is potentially more dangerous in the elderly. For those individuals, an SSRI or another agent with

TABLE 3

Inhibitors and Substrates for the Cytochrome p450 Isoenzymes

Isoenzyme	Substrates	Inhibitors	Inducers
2D6	TCAs, β-blockers, antiarrhytmics (mexiletine, flecainide, propafenone, encainide), diltiazem, nifedipine, nisoldipine, codeine, hydroxycodone, oxycodon, tramadol, odansetron, phenothiazines, risperidone, dextromethorphan, mCPP	Fluoxetine, paroxetine, sertraline, bupropion, phenothiazines, cocaine, methadone, yohimbine, quinidine, protease inhibitors, antimalarials, cimetidine, lansoprazole, antifungal (terbinafine)	?
3A	Pimozide, alprazolam, midazolam, zolpidem, zapelon, buspirone, carbamazepine, tertiary TCAs, quetiapine, clozapine, ziprasadone, haloperidol, cisapride, ergotamines, alfentanil, fentanyl, methadone, sildenafil, H_1 blockers, sibutramine, montelukast, oral contraceptive pills, testosterone, Ca^{++} channel blockers, cyclosporine, tacrolimus, HMG-CoA reductase inhibitors, amiodarone, propafenone, quinidine, antiretrovirals	Nefazodone, fluvoxamine, fluoxetine, sertraline, antifungals, macrolide antibiotics, antiretrovirals, quinupristin/dalfopristin, calcium channel blockers, grapefruit juice, cimetidine	Carbamazepine, pheytoin, oxcarbazepine, phenobarbital, ritonavir (chronic), efavirenz (also inhibitor), rifampin, ? St. John's wort
1A2	Clozapine, olanzapine, haloperidol, tertiary TCAs, tacrine, theophylline, aminophylline, caffeine, R-warfarin, cyclobenzaprine, propafenone, acetaminophen, phenacetin, pro-carcinogens	Fluvoxamine, fluorquinolones (ciprofloxacin, norfloxacin and others), cimetidine, antiarrhythmics (mexiletine, propafenone), zafirlukast	Omeprazole, cigarette smoking, charred meats (arylhydrocarbons), cruciferous vegetables (e.g., brussel sprouts).
2C subfamily	Diazepam, tertiary TCAs, pheytoin, THC, S-warfarin, nonsteroidal anti-inflammatory drugs, celecoxib, piroxicam, dapsone, propranolol, mephenytoin, THC, tolbutamide, glyburide, glipizide, rosiglitazone, tamoxifen, angiotensin II blockers (losartan, valsartan)	Fluoxetine, fluvoxamine, sertraline, tranylcypromine, omeprazole, valproate, isoniazid, ketoconazole, fluconazole, ritonavir, sulfaphenazole, ticlopidine, zafirlukast, fluvastatin, cimetidine	Rifampin, phenobarbital, carbamazepine

TCA, tricyclic antidepressant.
Modified from Alpert JE: Drug interactions in psychopharmacology. In: Stern TA, Herman JB, eds: Psychiatry: Update and Board Preparation. McGraw-Hill, New York, 2000, pages 381–390; DeVane CL, Nemeroff CB: 2000 Guide to psychotropic drug interactions. Primary Psychiatry 7:X, 2000; Eveshefsky L: Drug interactions of antidepressants. Psychiatr Ann 26:342–350, 1996; Greenblatt DJ, von Moltke LL, Harmantz JS, Shader RI: Human cytochromes and some newer antidepressants: Kinetics, metabolism, and drug interactions. J Clin Psychopharm 19:235–355, 1999.

low α_1 blockade may be more appropriate. Nonpharmacological management will include addressing other potential causes of orthostatic hypotension (e.g., dehydration, antihypertensive agents) and educating patients on management of orthostasis (e.g., to rise slowly from a sitting position). Pharmacological measures include use of caffeine, stimulants (methylphenidate 10–40 mg/day) or mineralocorticoids (fludrocortisone acetate, 0.05–0.2 mg/day).

Hypertension can be a side effect of venlafaxine; therefore, subjects receiving this drug should have periodic blood pressure monitoring. In unique responders to venlafaxine, hypertension related to antidepressants may be treated with medications such as doxazosin (Cardura), 1 to 2 mg/day, which also addresses other side effects, such as excessive sweating.

Sinus tachycardia may be an adverse reaction of TCAs, MAOIs, and venlafaxine; it is usually not clinically significant. TCAs or trazadone may prolong the QTc interval and exacerbate arrhythmias or conduction defects; therefore, electrocardiographic monitoring is advised during treatment with these antidepressants.

Gastrointestinal Side Effects

The SSRIs may induce nausea and dyspepsia. Dividing the dose or administering the medication with the meals may reduce the symptoms. Pharmacological measures include antacids (Maalox, Mylanta), H_2 blockers (famotidine 20–40 mg/day, ranitidine 150 mg once or twice a day), or metoclopramide (5–10 mg once daily).[11] Concomitant use of mirtazapine is useful in some subjects, presumably due to 5-HT_3 blockade as well as antihistamine effects.

Diarrhea, more common with the SSRIs, may respond to cyproheptadine (2–4 mg once daily), loperamide (2–4 mg twice daily), or *Lactobacillus acidophilus* culture.

Constipation is a side effect of anticholinergic drugs, such as TCAs. It can be managed with increased hydration, bulk laxatives (Metamucil 1–2 tsp in the morning), and stool softeners (docusate sodium, 100–200 mg/day). Bethanachol (Urecholine), a cholinergic smooth muscle stimulant, or the cholinesterase inhibitor donepezil (5–10 mg once daily) may relieve peripheral anticholinergic signs and symptoms, including constipation (10–30 mg once or twice a day).

Weight Gain

Weight gain is an adverse effect associated primarily with the use of TCAs and MAOIs, but other classes of antidepressants, including SSRIs, have been reported to induce weight gain. Management should include nutritional advice and increasing physical activity. Low doses of agents that have both antidepresssant and anorectic effects (SSRIs, stimulants, buproprion) can be added to a non-MAOI antidepressant to limit or manage weight gain. Pilot studies have reported benefit in limiting weight gain when adding H_2 blockers (famotidine 20–40 mg/day, ranitidine 150 mg once or twice daily).[10] Topiramate (50–200 mg/day) has also shown promise in reducing weight gains due to psychotropic medications, although some individuals develop cognitive side effects, which limit its use.

Adverse Effects Involving the Central Nervous System

The differential diagnosis of insomnia should include, besides an adverse reaction to the antidepressant, a residual symptom of depression, a manic episode in a bipolar disorder, or substance abuse. The management of insomnia should begin with sleep hygiene measures (e.g., avoiding daytime napping). Frequently, dosing the antidepressant earlier in the day can decrease insomnia. Pharmacological interventions include the use of trazodone (50–100 mg at bedtime), mirtazapine (15 mg at bedtime), TCAs (25–50 mg at bedtime of drugs such as amitriptyline, doxepin), benzodiazepines, zolpidem (10 mg at bedtime), zaleplon, or sedating antihistamines. Only trazodone and zolpidem have shown efficacy in placebo-controlled studies in managing antidepressant-induced insomnia.

Fatigue and sedation can be also either side effects of some antidepressants (more frequent with MAOI, TCAs, nefazodone, mirtazapine) or residual symptoms of depression. The management includes bedtime dosing of the antidepressant, adding an activating antidepressant to an SSRI (bupropion SR 100 mg once or twice daily), a psychostimulant (methylphenidate 10–20 mg twice a day), or a dopaminergic agonist (amantadine 100 mg three times a day).[11] Another strategy involves switching to a more stimulating agent (e.g., bupropion, protriptyline, or venlafaxine).

A high-frequency tremor can be a side effect of TCAs, SSRIs, and MAOIs; this can be increased by caffeine and by anxiety. Pharmacological interventions include low doses of β-blockers (propranolol 10–20 mg two or three times a day, or atenolol 25–100 mg/day) or low doses of benzodiazepines.

Anticholinergic Side Effects

The anticholinergic side effects are most significant for the TCAs (imipramine, clomipramine, amitriptyline, doxepin) and include dry mouth, blurred vision, urinary hesitancy and retention, and constipation. Pilocarpine 1% solution can be used for dry mouth or blurred vision. Sugarless candy or gum can also be helpful for dry mouth. Bethanachol (Urecholine), a cholinergic smooth muscle stimulant (10–30 mg once to three times daily), or the cholinesterase inhibitor donepezil (5–10 mg/day) may relieve peripheral anticholinergic signs and symptoms.

Sexual Side Effects

Sexual dysfunction, manifested as decreased libido, erectile dysfinction, delayed orgasm, or anorgasmia are common complaints during long-term treatment with antidepressants. Clinicians should inquire about potential sexual side effects, as they are rarely reported spontaneously. Hensley and coworkers[12] reported the results of a recent large double-blind study in which sildenafil (50 or 100 mg, taken 1–2 hours before sex) was significantly superior to placebo in improving male sexual side effects due to SSRIs. An open trial suggests possible efficacy of sildenafil in women for reducing side effects due to SSRIs.[13] Other pharmacological antidotes reported in the literature include yohimbine 5.4 mg three times a day, buproprion 100 mg once or twice a day, amantadine 100 mg twice a day, cyproheptadine 4 to 16 mg once a day.[11] The concomitant use of agents blocking 5-HT$_2$ receptors (including nefazodone or mirtazapine) has also helped reduce sexual dysfunction in some patients on SSRIs.

ANTIDEPRESSANTS IN THE TREATMENT OF MAJOR DEPRESSION

Sadness is a universally experienced emotion. However, major depression is distinguished from normal sadness by one or more episodes of depressed mood, or a loss of interest or pleasure, for a minimum of 2 weeks, associated with four or more of the following symptoms: appetite disturbance, sleep disturbance, psychomotor agitation or retardation, fatigue or loss of energy, feelings of guilt or worthlessness, poor concentration, suicide attempts, or thoughts of death.[14]

Frequently, depressed patients present with a chief complaint of chronic pain, fatigue, gastrointestinal problems, anxiety, irritability, or sleep disturbance. The lack of a medical cause for these symptoms should raise the index of suspicion for clinical depression.

Depression has a heterogeneous clinical presentation, and several subtypes of depression have been described. While a complete discussion of these subtypes is beyond the scope of this chapter, we will mention the most significant subtypes of depression: psychotic, melancholic, atypical, postpartum, seasonal, catatonic, and bipolar. The presence of such variations in clinical presentation probably underlies an also significant variability in the cause of depression.

The lifetime prevalence of major depression in US community studies ranges from 10% to 25% for women and 5% to 12% for men. The point prevalence for depression for adults in US communities is 5% to 9% for women and 2% to 3% for men.[15] The lifetime rate of suicide in patients with severe major depression has been estimated as 10% to 25%.[16] The Centers for Disease Control and Prevention reported that, in 1997, depression was the eighth leading cause of death in the United States.

The acute treatment of an episode of major depression should involve treatment with antidepressant medications or electroconvulsive treatment, sometimes associated with psychotherapy. If antidepressant medications are discontinued immediately following recovery, approximately 25% of patients will relapse within 2 months.[17] Therefore, after remission from a first episode of major depression, patients should receive at least six additional months of treatment with antidepressants, at the dosage to which they responded. Any subsequent tapering of the antidepressant should be done slowly to minimize the risk of relapse and discontinuation emergent symptoms.[18] In many settings, patients with major depression continue to receive suboptimal courses of psychopharmacology.[19]

Major depression is a recurrent disorder. Fifty to 85% of subjects who recovered after a first episode of depression will experience a recurrent episode, usually within 2 or 3 years. Subjects with several previous episodes of depression, with or without high comorbid conditions, have an even higher risk of recurrence. In addition, residual symptoms of depression frequently persist and constitute risk factors for ongoing functional impairment and full relapse of depression.[20, 21]

As many as 30% to 50% of depressed patients fail to respond to an adequate antidepressant trial with a 50% or greater reduction in the severity of their symptoms.[1] When depressive symptoms fail to remit following an initial course of pharmacotherapy, clinicians routinely confront the question of which of numerous possible next-step treatments to pursue, in what combinations and following what sequence. The range of next-step strategies includes (1) *optimizing* by pursuing a more extended trial with the initial agent using higher than usual doses; (2) *augmenting* an antidepressant with an agent without established antidepressant efficacy on its own (e.g., buspirone, lithium, or thyroid hormones); (3) *combining* an antidepressant with another antidepressant (e.g., venlafaxine and mirtazapine), with another somatic therapy (e.g., electroconvulsive treatment or phototherapy), or with some form of psychotherapy; or (4) *switching* to an antidepressant within the same class (e.g., another SSRI) or outside of class (e.g., switching from an SSRI to an atypical antidepressant), to nonpharmacological somatic therapy, or to psychotherapy.[22]

ANTIDEPRESSANTS FOR CHRONIC PAIN

Antidepressants (especially TCAs) have been shown to be effective in the treatment of a variety of conditions associated with chronic pain, even in the absence of major depression. Most studies to date have documented the efficacy of TCAs in many forms of chronic pain. These include diabetic neuropathy, fibromyalgia, chronic fatigue, post-herpetic neuralgia, trigeminal neuralgia, and migraine and tension headache prophylaxis.[23–25]

When TCAs are used to treat clinical pain conditions, effective doses are frequently lower than the antidepressant doses (e.g., amitriptyline 25–75 mg/day).[23] For imipramine, antidepressant doses usually require a combined blood level (imipramine plus its active metabolite, desipramine) or greater than 400 ng/mL. When treating chronic pain, it appears unnecessary to dose every patient to these blood levels. Measurements of blood levels may still be desirable to avoid toxicity, particularly on subjects on polypharmacy. Response rates (> 50% reduction of symptoms) are 60% to 70%. In cases of nonresponse, increasing the dose can enhance treatment response.[26]

Compared to TCAs, SSRIs appear to be less efficacious in pain control, although they are reported as superior to placebo in several studies. In a double-blind, placebo-controlled study of chronic diabetic neuropathy, amitriptyline and desipramine were found to be very effective even in nondepressed patients; fluoxetine (an SSRI) appeared to have a lower efficacy for this indication.[27] Similar findings were reported in the treatment of fibromyalgia, post-herpetic neuralgia, trigeminal neuralgia, and other peripheral neuropathies. In a large meta-analysis[28] of 94 randomized placebo-controlled trials, both TCAs and SSRIs showed a substantial benefit in achieving pain control in patients with a variety of conditions (headache, fibromyalgia, gastrointestinal pain, idiopathic pain). The TCAs studied, however, had a significantly greater likelihood of efficacy than the SSRIs.

For headaches, several double-blind studies have demonstrated that migraine prophylaxis was adequately achieved with amitriptyline. TCAs were also efficacious in treating chronic tension headache and chronic arthritis pain. The effect of SSRIs on headaches is variable: some studies report improvements whereas others report worsened symptoms.

Medications with dual serotonin and norepinephrine inhibition appear to have a very good activity in the treatment of pain. Sindrup and Jensen[26] found that tricyclics with both norepinephrine and serotonin inhibition (e.g., amitriptyline) are more effective than noradrenergic TCAs (e.g., desipramine) in providing pain relief and concluded that pain control requires a combination of serotonergic and noradrenergic inhibition. This is consistent with data indicating that both serotonin and norepinephrine exert analgesic effects via descending pain pathways.[29, 30] This finding may also explain the increased efficacy of tricyclic antidepressants, as compared with selective serotonin reuptake inhibitors, in providing pain relief, as reported by some studies.[27] Anecdotal case reports suggest that serotonin-norepinephrine reuptake inhibitors also possess analgesic properties.[31, 32] More recently, Detke and colleagues[33] reported that duloxetine, a novel SNRI, may be efficacious in treating both depression and painful physical symptoms among depressed patients.

VI. REFERENCES FOR ADDITIONAL READING

1. Fava M, Davidson KG: Definition and epidemiology of treatment-resistant depression. Psychiatr Clin North Am, 19:179–200, 1996.
2. Perry PJ: Pharmacotherapy for major depression with melancholic features: Relative efficacy of tri-

cyclic versus selective serotonin reuptake inhibitor antidepressants. J Affect Disord 39(1):1–6, 1996.

3. Sindrup SH: Antidepressants as analgesics. In: Yaksh TL, et al, eds. Anesthesia: Biologic Foundations. Lippincott-Raven, Philadelphia, 1997.

4. Sindrup SH, Jensen TS: Antidepressants in the treatment of neuropathic pain. In: Hanson PT, Fields HL, Hill RG, Marchettini P, eds. Neuropathic Pain: Pathophysiology and Treatment, Progress in Pain Research and Management, Vol. 21. IASP Press, Seattle, 2001.

5. Crown WH: Economic outcomes associated with tricyclic antidepressant and selective serotonin reuptake inhibitor treatments for depression. Acta Psychiatr Scand Suppl 403:62–66, 2000.

6. Arana GW, Rosenbaum JF: Handbook of Psychiatric Drug Therapy. Lippincott Williams & Wilkins, Philadelphia, 2000.

7. Quitkin FM, Stewart JW, McGrath PJ, et al: Columbia atypical depression: A subgroup of depressives with better response to MAOI than to tricyclic antidepressants or placebo. Br J Psychiatry Suppl 21:30–40, 1993.

8. Thase ME, Trivedi MH, Rush AJ: MAOIs in the contemporary treatment of depression. Neuropsychopharmacol 12:185–219, 1995.

9. Walker SE, Shulman KI, Tailor SA, Gardner D: Tyramine content of previously restricted foods in monoamine oxidase inhibitor diets. J Clin Psychopharmacol 16:383–388, 1996.

10. Zajecka JM: Clinical issues in long-term treatment with antidepressants. J Clin Psychiatry 61(Suppl 2):20–25, 2000.

11. Smoller JW, Pollack MH, Lee DK: Management of antidepressant-induced side effects. In: Stern TA, Herman JB, eds. Psychiatry Update and Board Preparation. McGraw-Hill, New York, 2000.

12. Hensley P, Nurnberg HG, Gelenberg AJ, et al. A double-blind, placebo-controlled, multicenter study of sildenafil citrate for the treatment of sexual dysfunction associated with serotonergic reuptake inhibitor antidepressants: Double-blind results. Presented at the 41st annual meeting of the New Clinical Drug Evaluation Unit, Phoenix, Ariz, May 28–31, 2001.

13. Fava M, Rankin MA, Alpert JE, et al: An open trial of oral sildenafil in antidepressant-induced sexual dysfunction. Psychother Psychosom 67:328–331, 1998.

14. Diagnostic and Statistical Manual of Mental Disorders, 4th ed. American Psychiatric Association, 1994.

15. Regier DA, Narrow WE, Rae DS, et al: The de facto mental and addictive disorders service system. Epidemiologic Catchment Area prospective 1-year prevalence rates of disorders and services. Arch Gen Psychiatr 50:85–94, 1993.

16. Klerman GL: Clinical epidemiology of suicide. J Clin Psychiatry 48(suppl):33–38, 1987.

17. Maj M, Veltro F, Pirozzi R, et al: Pattern of recurrence of illness after recovery from an episode of major depression: A prospective study. Am J Psychiatry 149(6):795–800, 1992.

18. American Psychiatric Association: APA practice guideline for the treatment of patients with major depressive disorder. Am J Psychiatry 157(4) suppl:1–45, 2000.

19. Lin EH, Katon WJ, Simon GE, et al: Low-intensity treatment of depression in primary care: Is it problematic? Gen Hosp Psychiatry 22:78–83, 2000.

20. Judd LL, Akiskal HS, Maser JD, et al: A prospective 12-year study of subsyndromal and syndromal depressive symptoms in unipolar major depressive disorders. Arch Gen Psychiatry 55:694–700, 1998.

21. Nierenberg AA, Keefe BR, Leslie VC, et al: Residual symptoms in depressed patients who respond acutely to fluoxetine. J Clin Psychiatry 60:221–225, 1999.

22. Rosenbaum JF, Fava M, Nierenberg AA, Sachs GS: Treatment-resistant mood disorders. In: Gabbard GO, ed. Treatments of Psychiatric Disorders, 3rd ed. American Psychiatric Press, Washington, DC, 2001, pages 1307–1384.

23. Goodnick PJ, Sandoval R: Psychotropic treatment of chronic fatigue syndrome and related disorders. J Clin Psychiatry 54:12–20, 1993.

23a. Preskorn S: Clinical Pharmacology of Selective Serotonin Reuptake Inhibitors. Professional Communications, Caddo, OK, 1996.

24. Fishbain D: Evidence based data on pain relief with antidepressants. Ann Med 32:305–316, 2000.

25. McQuay HJ, Tramer M, Nye BA: A systematic review of antidepressants in neuropathic pain. Pain 68:217–227, 1996.

26. Sindrup SH, Jensen TS: Efficacy of pharmacological treatments of neuropthic pain: An update and effect related to mechanism of drug action. Pain 83:389–400, 1999.

27. Max MB, Lynch SA, Muir J, et al: Effects of desipramine, amitriptyline, and fluoxetine on pain in diabetic neuropathy. N Engl J Med 326:1250–1256, 1992.

28. O'Malley PG, Jackson JL, Santoro J, et al: Antidepressant therapy for unexplained symptoms and syndromes. J Fam Pract 48:980–990, 1999.

29. Richardson BP: Serotonin and nociception. Ann N Y Acad Sci 600:511–519, 1990.

30. Willis WD, Westlund KN: Neuroanatomy of the pain system and the pathways that modulate pain. J Clin Neurophysiology 14:2–31, 1997.

31. Ansari A: The efficacy of newer antidepressants in the treatment of chronic pain: A review of the current literature. Harv Rev Psychiatry 7(5):257–277, 2000.

32. Lynch ME: Antidepressants as analgesics: A review of randomized controlled trials. J Psychiatry Neurosci 26(1):30–36, 2001.

33. Detke MJ, Lu Y, Goldstein DJ, et al: Duloxetine, 60 mg/day, for major depressive disorder: A randomized double-blind placebo-controlled trial. J Clin Psych 63:308–315, 2002.

Chapter 20

Glutamate Receptor Antagonists

Juan Santiago-Palma, MD / Howard Smith, MD / Christine Sang, MD

Glutamate is the major excitatory neurotransmitter of the central nervous system. The interaction of glutamate with its receptors is essential for the normal function of the central nervous system, including cognition, sensation, and memory.[1] Changes in glutamate transmission have been associated with a number of central nervous system pathologic conditions, including chronic pain, opioid tolerance, dependence, and addiction. Glutamate activates two major classes of receptors: ionotropic and metabotropic. Activation of N-methyl-D-aspartate (NMDA), α-amino-3-hydroxy-5-methyl-4-isoxazole propionate (AMPA) and kainate receptors by glutatmate causes opening of an integral ion channel, and thus these agents known as ionotropic receptors. Metabotropic receptors are directly coupled to intracellular signal trasduction systems via G proteins such as protein kinase C and cyclic adenosine monophosphate.[2]

Over the past decade, researchers have paid particular attention to the NMDA receptor. A wide body of evidence suggests that the NMDA receptor system plays an important role in the transmission of nociceptive information, including the development of central sensitization and "wind-up."[3–6] Prolonged firing of C-fiber nociceptors causes release of glutamate, which acts on NMDA receptors in the spinal cord. NMDA receptors are heavily concentrated in the neurons of the dorsal horn. Activation of these receptors by the excitatory amino acid glutamate triggers influx of calcium into the cell, which initiates a number of events that alter the neuron's response to subsequent stimuli.[7, 8] These events are thought to be at least partially responsible for facilitated pain processing, the augmentation of painful responses to subsequent stimuli and the development of mechanical hyperalgesia that might follow peripheral nerve injury or tissue inflammation.[9]

The NMDA receptor antagonists act as antihyperalgesic agents. Several investigators have shown that spinal and systemic administration of NMDA receptor antagonists in patients with neuropathic pain reduces spontaneous pain and hyperalgesia in experimental,[10] acute postoperative,[11] and chronic neuropathic pain.[12, 13] Unfortunately, most of these compounds have a narrow therapeutic window, which has limited their use. NMDA receptors cause memory impairment, sedation, psychotomimetic effects, ataxia, and motor incoordination. These side effects may limit doses to those providing only modest degrees of pain relief. In fact, the ceiling analgesic effect seen with NMDA receptor antagonists in clinical studies may be due to such dose-limiting adverse effects.

Functional inhibition of NMDA receptor complex can be achieved through actions at the multiple binding sites of the receptor complex (FIGURE 1). Such sites include the primary transmitter site (competitive), strychnine-insensitive glycine site (glycine_B), phencyclidine site located inside the cationic channel (PCP) and polyamine site (NR2B selective). Recent investigations suggest that targeting NMDA receptor subunits may provide superior analgesia with the potential of a better side effect profile, especially in patients with neuropathic pain. Selective antagonists to the NR2B subunit have recently become available and are likely to open new therapeutic windows in the clinical management of pain.[14]

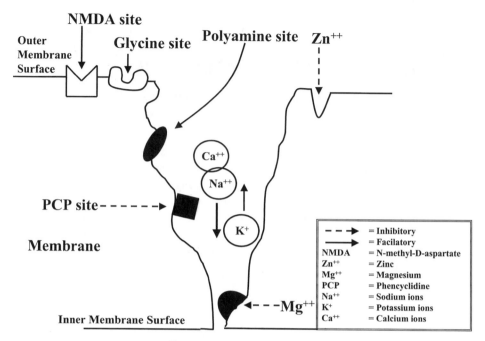

Figure 1. NMDA Receptor Complex

Metabotropic glutamate receptors (mGluRs) have also been implicated in nociceptive processing.[15–17] mGluRs modulate nociceptive processing at various levels of the nervous system and are involved in both peripheral and central sensitization associated with chronic pain.[18–21] Over the past decade, several mechanisms through which mGluRs regulate neuronal excitability and synaptic transmission have been elucidated, and a number of metabotropic glutamate receptor antagonists have been developed.

Clinically available NMDA receptor antagonists include ketamine, dextromethorphan, amantadine, memantine, magnesium sulfate, and certain opioids such as methadone. This chapter discusses the rationale for the use of the clinically available NMDA receptor antagonists in various neuropathic pain states. Clinically available non-NMDA receptor antagonists are discussed briefly.

NMDA RECEPTOR ANTAGONISTS

The currently available NMDA receptor antagonists with affinity at the phencyclidine site include ketamine and 3-(2-carboxypiperazin-4-yl)propyl-1-phosphonic acid. These drugs have been shown to modulate pain and hyperalgesia, but are limited by dose-limiting side effects. Such "uncompetitive" NMDA antagonists depend on the receptor channel to be gated in the open state. It has been suggested that the neurobehavioral toxicity of these NMDA receptor antagonists is due to their use-dependent blockade of the NMDA channel.[22]

Ketamine

Ketamine is a phencyclidine-like drug with noncompetitive NMDA receptor antagonist activity. Ketamine inhibits the NMDA receptor by binding to its phencyclidine (PCP) site. Ketamine may also function via multiple mechanisms, including enhanced peripheral monoaminergic transmission, inhibition of central and peripheral cholinergic transmission, and possibly effects on voltage-gated calcium currents. Local anesthetic qualities may be used locally at the site of injection but do not appear to be responsible for systemic effects.

Animal studies suggest that ketamine reduces nociceptive behaviors and spinal dorsal horn neuronal activity in response to tissue injury.[23–26] In humans, ketamine has been reported to relieve glossopharyngeal and neuralgia and cancer pain in subanesthetic doses.[12, 27, 28] Placebo-controlled trials in patients suffering from postherpetic neuralgia,[4, 5] acute postoperative hyperalgesia,[5, 11] phantom pain,[6] acute and chronic orofacial pain,[29] spinal cord injury,[30] chronic post-traumatic pain,[31] chronic ischemic pain,[32] and mixed neuropathic pain syndromes[4, 12] have shown that ketamine can relieve neuropathic pain and hyperalgesia. In most cases, however, appreciable symptomatic relief from ketamine develops only after the onset of unpleasant psychotomimetic side effects. Ketamine administered by the subcutaneous and intravenous route causes dose-dependent nausea, confusion, hallucinations, visual disturbances, unpleasant dreams, delirium, and other psychotomimetic adverse effects.[33] The activity of ketamine in the cortex and limbic system has been implicated in the development of such symptoms.

Oral Ketamine. A number of case reports and case series have shown the successful use of oral ketamine in experimental ischemic arm pain, post-herpetic neuralgia, neuropathic pain, and postamputation pain.[34–37] Oral ketamine may have a better side effect profile than parenteral ketamine. The administration of oral ketamine results in higher serum concentrations of norketamine, the main metabolite of ketamine. Norketamine is a noncompetitive NMDA receptor antagonist and is equipotent to its parent drug in the second phase of the formalin test. The potency of norketamine, the shorter duration of psychomotor effects of oral ketamine, and the relatively high levels of norketamine in the brain (the norketamine/ketamine AUC ratio in the brain may reach 2.9) suggest that oral ketamine may have a better therapeutic ratio for analgesia than parenteral ketamine.[38–40] Oral ketamine has been associated with hepatic damage, gastric ulcer, and memory impairment.[41]

Neuraxial Ketamine. Case reports and case series suggest that the administration of intrathecal and epidural ketamine are effective for the treatment of pain. However, ketamine has been associated with histopathological changes of the spinal cord. Stotz and colleagues[42] reported a patient with intractable cancer pain who obtained pain relief after ketamine was added to an intrathecal mixture of bupivacaine, morphine, and clonidine. Although the patients did not develop neurological deficits, focal lymphocytic vasculitis was observed close to the intratecal catheter postmortem. Karpinski and colleagues[43] reported postmortem changes of subpial spinal cord vacuolation in a terminally ill cancer patient who developed a wide-based gait after receiving a continuous infusion of intrathecal ketamine for pain control.

3-(2-carboxypiperazin-4-yl)propyl-1-phosphonic acid (CPP)

Three-((+-)-2-carboxypiperazin-4-yl)-propyl-1-phosphonic acid (CPP) is a potent and selective competitive antagonist of the NMDA receptor. CPP is not clinically available, and there is little evidence supporting its use for the management of clinical pain. Kristensen and colleagues[44] described the use of CPP in one patient with intractable neuropathic pain. In this patient, intrathecal administration of CPP abolished the spread of pain evoked by low-threshold mechanical and thermal stimuli to areas outside the territory of the injured nerve. However, continuous deep pain and allodynia in the territory of the injured nerve were unchanged. The authors suggested that CPP modulates pathological pain at the spinal level. The patient developed psychotomimetic ketamine-like side effects, which were attributed to the hydrophilicity and rostral spread of CPP.

LOW-AFFINITY CHANNEL-BLOCKING NMDA RECEPTOR ANTAGONISTS

Low-affinity NMDA receptor antagonists such as dextromethorphan, dextrorphan, remacemide, amantadine, memantine, and other adamantane analogues produce fewer neuropsychological side effects than the higher affinity antagonists. The better side effect profile of these compounds has been attributed to their low micromolar affinity for the NMDA receptor. The faster rates of block and unblock contribute in part to their more favorable toxicity profile.[45]

Dextromethorphan

Dextromethorphan and its main metabolite, dextrorphan, are low-affinity noncompetitive NMDA receptor antagonists. In addition, both compounds antagonize voltage-dependent calcium channels. The effect of dextromethorphan and dextrorphan in animal models of neuropathic pain has been variable.[46] Human studies have also yielded conflicting results.[23, 47–49] Nelson and associates[13] compared dextromethorphan to inert placebo in patients with diabetic neuropathy and post-herpetic neuralgia. Patients with diabetic neuropathy, but not patients with postherpetic neuralgia, reported better pain relief with dextromethorphan. Sang and associates[50] compared dextromethorphan with the active placebo lorazepam and obtained similar results to those of Nelson' group. However, McQuay and coworkers[5] found that dextromethorphan did not relieve pain in patients with different chronic neuropathic pain syndromes.

A potential source of variability in the analgesic studies of dextromethorphan might be the genetic polymorphism associated with the cytochrome p450-2D6 isoenzyme (CYP26).The disposition of dextromethorphan is substantially influenced by the CYP2D6 enzyme. Seven to 10% of whites and 1% of Asians have mutations in both copies of the 2D6 gene. These patients get higher drug levels than normal (poor metabolizers). Most patients have two normal copies of 2D6 gene (extensive metabolizers) and some patients may have multiple copies of the intact genes (ultra rapid metabolizers). Median elimination half life is 2.4 hours in extensive metabolizers and 19.1 hours in poor metabolizers.[51–54]

Animal and human studies have suggested that the combination of dextromethorphan with opiate analgesics may be useful for preventing opiate tolerance and dependence, while enhancing both peak and duration of opioid analgesia. Mao and colleagues,[55] in a study to evaluate the practical feasibility of the combined oral administration of morphine sulfate with dextromethorphan showed that dextromethorphan prevented the development of tolerance to the antinociceptive effects of morphine and attenuated signs of naloxone-precipitated physical dependence on morphine.

Dextromethorphan produces dose-dependent toxicity. Single doses of 30 to 60 mg produces mild side effects in less than 10% of patients. However, blockade of NMDA receptor might require doses higher than the maximum antitussive dose of 120 mg per day. In studies of patients with post-herpetic neuralgia and diabetic neuropathy, a mean dose of 400 mg was used and all patients developed adverse effects. Reported adverse effects to dextromethorphan include dizziness, fatigue, confusion, light-headedness, depression, gastrointestinal disturbances, and nystagmus.

Amantadine

Amantadine has been used as an antiviral and for the treatment of Parkinson's disease. Until recently, the mechanism of action of amantadine was speculated to be related to dopaminergic and anticholinergic activity. Recent human postmortem and in vitro studies have demonstrated that memantine may produce its pharmacological effects through noncompetitive binding to the PCP site of the NMDA receptor complex.[56–59] Investigations of the analgesic efficacy of amantidine have yielded conflicting results. Eisenberg and Pud[60] reported three patients in whom a single dose of intravenous amantadine resulted in the complete resolution of spontaneous pain, mechanical allodynia, and hyperalgesia. Pud and associates[61] also randomized 15 cancer patients with surgical neuropathic pain to receive either placebo or 200 mg of intravenous amantadine. Mean pain intensity remained significantly lower during the 48 hours following amantadine treatment as compared with the 48 hours prior to treatment, whereas no such effect was found with the placebo. However, amantadine was not analgesic in subsequent studies by Medrik-Goldberg and associates[62] and Taira[63] in patients with sciatica and different types of neuropathic pain. Amantadine produces fewer psychotomimetic side effects than ketamine and is usually well tolerated. Dose-dependent side effects include dizziness, lethargy, sleep disturbances, headache, and hallucinations as well as nausea and vomiting.

Memantine

Memantine has been used for the treatment of dementia and Parkinson's disease.[64] A number of studies have looked at memantine for the treatment of different neuropathic pain syndromes. Sang and colleagues[50] compared memantine to the active placebo lorazepam for the treatment of diabetic neuropathy and post-herpetic neuralgia and was unable to detect a treatment effect. Eisenberg and colleagues,[65] in a double-blind, randomized, placebo-controlled trial, administered memantine at a dose of 10 mg/day and 20 mg/day to patients with posptherpetic neuralgia. Reduction in spontaneous pain, mechanical and cold allodynia, mechanical hyperalgesia, and "wind-up"–like pain were found in both groups, but there were no significant differences between the placebo and the treatment group. Memantine is associated with dizziness, lethargy, sleep disturbances, headache, nausea, and vomiting.

Magnesium

A number of investigators have suggested that the administration of magnesium might be useful as an analgesic.[66] Magnesium ions prevent extracellular calcium ions from entering the cell by blocking the ion channel coupled to the NMDA receptor. Dubray and coworkers[67] showed that dietary restriction of magnesium decreased mechanical nociceptive thresholds in rats. In the same study, decreased pain threshold was reversed by the administration of MK-801, an NMDA receptor antagonist. Xiao and Bennett[68] demonstrated that spinal or subcutaneous administration of magnesium significantly reduces heat hyperalgesia and mechanical allodynia in a model of neuropathic pain. In another animal study, Takano and coworkers[66] found that intrathecal administration of magnesium sulfate caused a dose-dependent suppression of phase 2 of the formalin test. Koinig and associates,[69] in a randomized double-blind study, administered magnesium to patients undergoing arthroscopic knee surgery and found that intravenous magnesium sulfate administration reduced intraoperative and postoperative analgesic requirements. However, Felsby and associates[4] were unable to demonstrate a statistically significant reduction of pain and allodynia in patients with peripheral neuropathic pain.

Acute and chronic administration of magnesium is well tolerated. Reported adverse effects include a flushed feeling, heat sensation and pain at the injection site, and sedation.

Riluzole

Riluzole has been used for the treatment of amyotrophic lateral sclerosis. The exact mechanism of action of riluzole is unknown. It has been suggested that riluzole noncompetitively inhibits the NMDA and kainate receptors[70] as well as sodium channels.[71] Analgesic studies with riluzole have not been encouraging. Hammer and associates[72] examined the acute analgesic effect of riluzole in a human model of inflammatory pain induced by a thermal injury in 20 healthy volunteers. Riluzole had no acute analgesic effects in normal or hyperalgesic skin.

OPIOIDS WITH NMDA RECEPTOR ACTIVITY

Methadone, dextropropoxyphene, and meperidine have demonstrated low affinity for the PCP site of the NMDA receptor.[73–76] The dual action of this opioid over the NMDA and μ receptors might have important clinical implications in the treatment neuropathic pain. Because of its long half-life, excellent bioavailability, and low cost, methadone has received particular attention in recent years.

Methadone

Methadone is a racemic mixture of levorotatory (L) and dextrorotatory (D) methadone. Animal studies have shown that both D and L methadone have NMDA receptor antagonist and that both isomers bind specifically to the noncompetitive site of the NMDA receptor. However, D-methadone does not produce opioid-like locomotor activity in mice,[77] is inactive following intraventricular administration in rats,[78] and is a 50-fold less potent analgesic in humans than L-methadone. These findings suggest that D-methadone does not have opioid analgesic properties and that its analgesic activity might be mediated trough the NMDA receptor.

Besides its NMDA receptor activity, methadone differs from other opioids because of its long half-life, excellent absorption following oral and rectal administration, and lack of known active metabolites.[79] In recent years, numerous investigators have described the successful use of methadone for the treatment pain. Several reports have underscored the efficacy of methadone in the treatment of cancer pain, especially for pain refractory to high doses of other opioids.[80–85] The action of methadone over NMDA and μ receptors has important clinical implications. Because of its NMDA receptor activity, methadone may be useful for the treatment of neuropathic pain and may produce tolerance less frequently than do other opioids.

NR2B SUBUNIT ANTAGONISTS

The NMDA receptor complex encompasses many protein subunits, including NMDA R1 (NR1) and NR2 (NR2A-NR2D). Selective antagonists to the NR2B subunit have recently become available. Animal studies have demonstrated that the NR2B subunit is restricted to the forebrain and distributed in the laminae I and II of the spinal cord dorsal horn and therefore might induce anti-nociception without motor dysfunction. In a recent study, CP101,606 [(1S,2S)-1-(4-hydroxyphenyl)-2-(4-hydroxy-4-phenylpiperidino)-1-propanol], a selective NR2B subunit antagonist, was demonstrated to be antihyperalgesic in neuropathic rats without impairing rotarod performance.[14]

NON-NMDA RECEPTOR ANTAGONISTS

Kainate receptors have been associated with pain pathways, including those in primary afferents DRG neurons and, more recently, with trigeminal neurons.[86, 87] Recent studies in humans suggest that the mixed AMPA/Kainate antagonist, LY293558, can prevent capsaicin-induced hyperalgesia and allodynia with no effect on physiological nociception.[88] Similar results were reported in animal studies in which formalin-induced,[89] but not acute physiological,[90] nociceptive responses were reduced by kainate/GluR5 selective decahydroisoquinolines. In a recent randomized controlled clinical trial, Gilron and associates compared the analgesic efficacy of the AMPA/kainate antagonist, LY293558, with that of intravenous ketorolac trimethamine and placebo after oral surgery. Study drugs were administered at the onset of moderate pain; pain intensity and relief were measured for 240 minutes. LY293558 and ketorolac tromethamine were superior to placebo for pain evoked by mouth opening and in one of several measures of spontaneous pain. The potential therapeutic value of non-NMDA receptor antagonists depends on the continued development of subtype selective non-NMDA receptor antagonists. Agents that modulate AMPA and/or kainite receptors may eventually play a role as analgesics.

The anticonvulsant topiramate inhibits activity of glutamate at AMPA/kainate receptors with no effect on NMDA-evoked currents. Topiramate blocks kainate-evoked currents in patch clamp studies of hippocampal neurons, by allosterically modulating channel conductance (R.W. Johnson, PRI, 1999, data on file). In three open-label studies, 44 subjects with mixed peripheral neuropathies received topiramate doses of 250 to 300 mg/day and demonstrated reduction in VAS of 65%, 30%, and 60% in 14, 8, and 22 subjects, respectively (R.W. Johnson, PRI, 1999, data on file).

METABOTROPIC GLUTAMATE ANTAGONISTS

The metabotropic glutamate receptor antagonists (mGluRs) represent a family of G protein–coupled receptors. Eight mGluR subtypes have been cloned to date and are classified into groups I (mGluRs 1 and 5), II (mGluRs 2 and 3), and III (mGluRs 4, 6, 7, and 8) based on their sequence, signal transduction mechanisms, and pharmacological profile.[91–93] mGluRs modulate nociceptive processing at various levels of the nervous system and are involved in both peripheral and central pain sensitization. Recent investigations suggest that antagonists at group I and agonists at group II may be useful drugs to downregulate the transmission and processing of nociceptive signals.

The recent discovery of peripheral mGluRs involved in nociception may lead to peripherally acting analgesics devoid of central side effects. mGluR5 antagonists appear to be more powerful than mGluR1 antagonists in the periphery, whereas mGluR1 antagonists have significant antinociceptive effects at the spinal cord level, in the thalamus and amygdala. Noticeably, group II mGluR agonists have no effect on normal transmission in the spinal cord but reverse pain-related central sensitization.

Metabotropic glutamate receptor antagonists block secondary thermal hyperalgesia in rats with knee joint inflammation.[14] Spinal infusion of group I mGlu receptor antagonists LY393053 [(+/-)-2-amino-2-(3-cis and trans-carboxycyclobutyl-3-(9-thioxanthyl)propionic acid], LY367385 [(S)-(+)-α-amino-4-carboxy-2-methylbenzeneacetic acid], or AIDA [(R,S)-1-aminoindan-1,5-dicarboxylic acid/UPF 523] before a knee joint injection of kaolin and carrageenan, significantly reduced the development of secondary thermal hyperalgesia suggestive of sensitization of spinal neurons.[94]

CONCLUSIONS

The efficacy of NMDA receptor antagonists in animal models of neuropathic pain has been generally confirmed in human models of pain and in patients with neuropathic pain. Controlled clinical trials and multiple case reports have suggested that NMDA receptors are effective in the treatment of a variety of pain conditions. Unfortunately, most of these compounds have a narrow therapeutic window, which has limited their use. The clinically available channel-blocking NMDA receptor antagonists have consistently been associated with phencyclidine-like cognitive effects (i.e., feelings of intoxication or delirium, dissociative effects, and/or vivid dreams).

The narrow therapeutic ratio of glutamate receptor antagonists may be potentially overcome by the use of drug combinations, the development of newer low-affinity NMDA channel antagonists, and more selective systemic NMDA-receptor antagonists (which modulate binding sites within the NMDA complex, or have affinity at specific NMDA receptor subtypes). The heterogeneity of the pain state may make this approach difficult, requiring instead that the ideal analgesic interact at several selective sites with the potential for acting synergistically in terms of efficacy but not toxicity.

REFERENCES FOR ADDITONAL READING

1. Gasic GP, Hollmann: Molecular neurobiology of glutamate receptors. Annu Rev Physiol 54: 507–536, 1992.
2. Knopfel T, Kuhn R, Allgeier: Metabotropic glutamate receptors: Novel targets for drug development. J Med Chem 38:1417–1426, 1995.

3. Eide PK, Jorum E, Stubhaug A, et al: Relief of postherpetic neuralgia with the N-methyl-D aspartic acid receptor antagonist: A double-blind, cross-over comparison with morphine and placebo. Pain 58:347–354, 1994.

4. Felsby S, Nielsen J, Arendt-Nielsen L, et al: NMDA receptor blockade in chronic neuropathic pain: A comparison of ketamine and magnesium chloride. Pain 64:283–291, 1996.

5. McQuay HJ, Carroll D, Jadad AR, et al: Dextromethorphan for the treatment of neuropathic pain: A double blind randomized controlled crossover trial with integral n- or 1 design. Pain 59:127–133, 1994.

6. Nikolajsen L, Hansen CL, Nielsen J, et al: The effect of ketamine on phantom pain: A central neuropathic disorder maintained by peripheral input. Pain 67:69–77, 1996.

7. Macdermott AB, Mayer ML, Westbrook GL, et al: NMDA receptor activation increases cytoplasmic calcium concetration in cultured spinal cord neurons. Nature 321:519–522, 1986.

8. Malenka RC: The role of postsynaptic calcium in the induction of long term potentiation. Mol Neurobiol 5:289–295, 1991.

9. Sang CN: NMDA-receptor antagonists in neuropathic pain: Experimental methods to clinical trials. J Pain Symptom Manage 19:S21–S25, 2000.

10. Andersen OK, Felsby S, Nicolaisen L, et al: The effect of ketamine on stimulation of primary and secondary hyperalgesic areas induced by capsaicin: A double-blind, placebo-controlled, human experimental study. Pain 66:51–62, 1996.

11. Stubhaug A, Breivik H, Eide PK, et al: Mapping of punctuate hyperalgesia around surgical incision demonstrates that ketamine is a powerful suppressor of central sensitization to pain following surgery. Acta Anaesthesiol Scand 41:1124–1132, 1997.

12. Backonja M, Arndt G, Gombar KA, et al: Response of chronic neuropathic pain syndromes to ketamine: A preliminary study. Pain 56:51–57, 1994.

13. Nelson KA, Park KM, Robinovitz E, et al: High-dose oral dextromethorphan versus placebo in painful diabetic neuropathy and postherpetic neuralgia. Neurology 48:1212–1218, 1997.

14. Boyce S, Wyatt A, Webb JK, et al: Article title. Neuropharmacology 38:611–623, 1999.

15. Neugebauer V, Chen PS, Willis WD: Role of metabotropic glutamate receptor subtype mGluR1 in brief nociception and central sensitization of primate STT cells. J Neurophysiol 82:272–282, 1999.

16. Palecek J, Paleckova V, Dougherty PM, Willis WD: The effect of trans-ACPD, a metabotropic excitatory amino acid receptor agonist, on the responses of primate spinothalamic tract neurons. Pain 56:261–269, 1994.

17. Young MR, Blackburn-Munro G, Dickinson T, et al: Antisense ablation of type I metabotropic glutamate receptor mGluR1 inhibits spinal nociceptive transmission. J Neurosci 18:10180–10188, 1998.

18. Fundytus ME: Glutamate receptors and nociception: Implications for the drug treatment of pain. CNS Drugs 15:29–58, 2001.

19. Karim F, Bhave G, Gereau RW: Metabotropic glutamate receptors on peripheral sensory neuron terminals as targets for the development of novel analgesics. Mol Psychiatry 6:615–617, 2001.

20. Neugebauer V: Metabotropic glutamate receptors: Novel targets for pain relief. Expert Rev Neurother 1:207–224, 2001.

21. Neugebauer V: Peripheral metabotropic glutamate receptors: Fight the pain where it hurts. Trends Neurosci 24:550–552, 2001.

22. Rogawski MA: Therapeutic potential of excitatory amino acid antagonists: Channel blockers and 2,3-benzodiazepines. Trends Pharmacol Sci 14:325–331, 1993.

23. Mao J, Price DD, Hayes RL, et al: Intrathecal treatment with dextrorphan or ketamine potently reduces pain-related behaviors in a rat model of peripheral mononeuropathy. Brain Res 605:164–168, 1993.

24. Qian J, Brown SD, Carlton SM: Systemic ketamine attenuates nociceptive behaviours in a rat model of peripheral neuropathy. Brain Res 715:51–62, 1996.

25. Burton Aw, Lee DH, Saab C, Chung JM: Preemptive intrathecal ketamine injection produces a long lasting decrease in neuropathic pain behaviors in a rat model. Reg Anesthesia Pain Med 24: 208–213, 1999.

26. Hartrick CT, Wise JJ, Patterson JS: Preemptive intrathecal ketamine delays mechanical hyperalgesia in the neuropathic rat. Anesth Ana 86:557–560, 1998.

27. Eide K, Stubhaug A: Relief of glossopharyngeal neuralgia by ketamine-induced N-methyl-D-aspartate receptor blockade. Neurosurg 41:505–508, 1997.

28. Fine PG: Low-dose ketamine in the management of opioid nonresponsive terminal cancer pain J Pain Symptom Manage 17:296–300, 1999.

29. Mathisen LC, Skjelbred P, Skoglund LA, Oye I: Effect of ketamine, an NMDA receptor inhibitor, in acute and chronic orofacial pain. Pain 61:215–220, 1995.

30. Eide PK, Jorum E, Stubhaug A, Stenehjem AE: Central dysesthesia pain after traumatic spinal cord injury is dependent on N-mehtyl-D-aspartate receptor activation. Neurosurgery 37:1087, 1995.

31. Max MB, Byas-Smith MG, Gracely RH, Bennett GJ: Intravenous infusion of the NMDA antagonist, ketamine in chronic posttraumatic pain with allodynia: A double-blind comparison to alfentanyl and placebo. Clin Neuropharmacol 18:360–368, 1995.

32. Persson J, Hasselstrom J, Wiklund B, et al: The analgesic effect of racemic ketamine in patients with chronic ischemic pain due to lower extremity arteriosclerosis obliterans. Acta Anaesthesiol Scand 42:750–758, 1998.

33. Jansen KL: Ketamine: Can chronic use impair memory? Int J Addict 25:133–139, 1990.

34. Hoffman V, Coppenjans H, Vercauteren M, Adriansen H: Succeful treatment of post-herpetic neuralgia with oral ketamine. Clin J Pain 10:240–242, 1994.

35. Broadley KE, Kurowska A, Tookman A: Ketamine injection used orally. Palliat Med 10:247–250, 1996.

36. Fisher K, Hagen NA: Analgesic effects of oral ketamine in chronic neuropathic pain of spinal origin: A case report. J Pain Symptom Manage 18:61–66, 1999.

37. Haines DR, Gaines SP: Nof 1 randomised contolled trials of oral ketamine in patients with chronic pain. Pain 83:283–287, 1999.

38. Shimonaya M, Shimonaya N, Gorman AL, et al: Oral ketamine is antinociceptive in the rat formalin test: The role of the metabolite norketamine Pain 81:85–93, 1999.

39. Grant IS, Nimmo WS, Clements JA: Pharmacokinetics and analgesic effects of IM and oral ketamine. Br J Anaesth 53:805–810, 1981.

40. Leung LY, Baille TA: Comparative pharmacology in the rat of ketamine and its two principal metabolites, norketamine and (Z)-6-hydroxynorketamine. J Med Chem 29:2396–2399, 1986.

41. Klepstead P, Borchgrevink PC: Four years treatment with ketamine and a trial of dextromethorphan in a patient with severe post-herpetic neuralgia. Acta Anesthesiol Scand 41:422–426, 1997.

42. Stotz M, Oehen HP, Gerber H: Histological findings after long term infusion of intrathecal ketamine for chronic pain: A case report. J Pain Symtom Manage 18:223–228, 1999.

43. Karpinsky N, Dunn J, Hansen L, Masliah E: Subpial vacuolar myelopathy after intrathecal ketamine:report of a case. Pain 73:103–105, 1997.

44. Kristensen JD, Svensson B, Gordh T: The NMDA-receptor antagonist CPP abolishes neurogenic 'wind-up pain' after intrathecal administration in humans. Pain 51:249–253, 1992.

45. Rogawski MA: Therapeutic potential of excitatory amino acid antagonists: Channel blockers and 2,3-benzodiazepines. Trends Pharmacol Sci 14:325–331, 1993.

46. Chaplan SR, Malmberg AB, Yaksh TL: Efficacy of spinal NMDA receptor antagonism in formalin hyperalgesia and nerve injury evoked allodynia in the rat. J Pharmacol Exp Ther 280:829–838, 1997.

47. Mao J, Price DD, Mayer DJ: Mechanisms of hyperalgesia and morphine tolerance: A current view of the their possible interactions. Pain 62:259–274, 1995.

48. Tal M, Bennett GJ: Neuropathic pain sensations are differentially sensitive to dextrorphan. Neuroreport 5:1438–1440, 1994.

49. Tal M, Bennett GJ: Dextrorphan relieves neuropathic heat-evoked hyperalgesia in the rat. Neurosci Lett 151:107–110, 1993.

50. Sang CN, Booker S, Gilron I, et al: Dextromethorpahn and memantine in painful diabetic neuropathy and postherpetic neuralgia: Efficacy and dose response trials. Anesthesiology 96:1053–1061, 2002.

51. Capon DA, Bochner F, Kerry N, et al: The influence of CYP2D6 polymorphism and quinidine on the disposition and antitussive effect of dextromethorphan in humans. Clin Pharmacol Ther 60:295–307, 1996.

52. Zhang Y, Britto MR, Valderhaug KL, Wedlund: Mediated inhibition of cytochrome P4502D6. Clin Pharmacol Ther 51:647–655, 1992.

53. Preskorn SH: Clinically relevant pharmacology of selective serotonin reuptake inhibitors: An overview with emphasis on pharmacokinetics and effects on oxidative drug metabolism. Clin Pharmacokinet 32 (Suppl 1):1–21, 1997.

54. Virani A, Mailis A, Shapiro LE, Shear NH: Drug interactions in human neuropathic pain pharmacotherapy. Pain 73:3–13, 1997.

55. Mao J, Price DD, Caruso FS, Mayer DJ: Oral administration of dextromethorphan prevents the development of morphine tolerance and dependence in rats. Pain 67:361–368, 1996.

56. Kornhuber J, Bormann J, Hubers M, et al: Effects of the 1-amino-adamantanes at the MK-801-binding site of the NMDA-receptor-gated ion channel: A human postmortem brain study. Eur J Pharmacol 25:297–300, 1991.

57. Kornhuber J, Schoppmeyer K, Riederer P: Affinity of 1-aminoadamantanes for the sigma binding site in post-mortem human frontal cortex. Neurosci Lett 163:129–131, 1993.

58. Lupp A, Lucking CH, Koch R, et al: Inhibitory effects of the antiparkinsonian drugs memantine and amantadine on N-methyl-D-aspartate-evoked acetylcholine release in the rabbit caudate nucleus in vitro. J Pharmacol Exp Ther 263:717–724, 1992.

59. Stoof JC, Booij J, Drukarch B: Amantadine as N-methyl-D-aspartic acid receptor antagonist: New possibilities for therapeutic applications? Clin Neurol Neurosurg 94:S4–6, 1992.

60. Eisenberg E, Pud D: Can patients with chronic neuropathic pain be cured by acute administration of the NMDA receptor antagonist amantadine? Pain 74:337–339, 1998.

61. Pud D, Eisenberg E, Spitzer A, et al: The NMDA receptor antagonist amantadine reduces surgical neuropathic pain in cancer patients: A double blind, randomized, placebo controlled trial. Pain 75:349–354, 1998.

62. Medrik-Goldberg T, Lifschitz D, Pud D, et al: Intravenous lidocaine, amantadine, and placebo in the treatment of sciatica: A double-blind, randomized, controlled study. Reg Anesth Pain Med 24:534–540, 1999.

63. Taira T: Comments on Eisenberg and Pud. Pain 78:221–222, 1998.

64. Fleischhacker WW, Buchgeher A, Schubert H: Memantine in the treatment of senile dementia of the Alzheimer type. Prog Neuropsychopharmacol Biol Psychiatry 10:87–93, 1986.

65. Eisenberg E, Kleiser A, Dortort A, et al: The NMDA (N-methyl-D-aspartate) receptor antagonist memantine in the treatment of postherpetic neuralgia: A double-blind, placebo-controlled study. Eur J Pain 2:321–327, 1998.

66. Takano Y, Sato E, Kaneko T, Sato I: Antihyperalgesic effects of intrathecally administered magnesium sulfate in rats. Pain 84:175–179, 2000.

67. Dubray C, Alloui A, Bardin L, et al: Magnesium deficiency induces an hyperalgesia reversed by the NMDA receptor antagonist MK801. Neuroreport 8:1383–1386, 1997.

68. Xiao WH, Bennett GJ: Magnesium suppresses neuropathic pain responses in rats via a spinal site of action. Brain Res 666:168–172, 1994.

69. Koinig H, Wallner T, Marhofer P, et al: Magnesium sulfate reduces intra- and postoperative analgesic requirements. Anesth Analg 87:206–210, 1998.

70. Debono MW, Le Guern J, Canton T, et al: Inhibition by riluzole of electrophysiological responses

mediated by rat kainate and NMDA receptors expressed in Xenopus oocytes Eur J Pharmacol 235:283–289, 1993.

71. Benoit F, Escande D: Riluzole specifically blocks inactivated Na channels in myelinated nerve. Fibre Fluger Arch 419:603–609, 1991.

72. Hammer NA, Lilleso J, Pedersen JL, et al: Effect of riluzole on acute pain and hyperalgesia in humans. Br J Anaesth 82:718–722, 1999.

73. Ebert B, Andersen S, Krogegard-Larsen P: Ketobemidone, methadone and pethidine and noncompetitive N-methyl-D-aspartate (NMDA) antagonists in the rat cortex and spinal cord. Neurosci Lett 187:165–168, 1995.

74. Ebert B, Thorkeildsen C, Andersen S, et al: Opioid analgesics as noncompetitive N-methyl-D-asparate (NMDA) antagonists. Biochem Pharmeol 36:S58–S59, 1998.

75. Ebert B, Andersen S, Hjeds J, Dickenson AH: Dextropropoxyphene acts as a noncompetitive N-methyl-D-aspartate antagonist. J Pain Symptom Manage 15:269–274, 1998.

76. Gorman AL, Elliott KJ, Innutti CE: The D and L isomers of methadone bind to the noncompetitive site on the N-methyl-D-aspartate (NMDA) receptor in rat forebrain and spinal cord. Neurosci Lett 223:5–8, 1997.

77. Smits SE, Myers AB: Some comparative effects of racemic methadone and its optical isomers in rodents. Res Commun Chem Pathol Pharmacol 7:651–662, 1974.

78. Ingoglia NA, Dole VP: Localization of D- and L-methadone after intraventricular injection into rat brains. J Pharmacol Exp Ther 175:84–87, 1970.

79. Faisinger R, Schoeller T, Bruera E: Methadone in the management of cancer pain: A review. Pain 52:137–147, 1993.

80. Crews JC, Sweeney NJ, Denson DD: Clinical efficacy of methadone in patients refractory to other mu opioid receptor analgesics for the management of terminal cancer pain. Cancer 72:2266–2272, 1993.

81. Galer BS, Coyle N, Pasternak GW, Portenoy RK: Individual variability in the response to different opioids: Report of five cases. Pain 25:297–312, 1986.

82. Manfredi PL, Borsook D, Chandler SW, Payne R: Intravenous methadone for cancer pain unrelieved by morphine and hydromorphone: Clinical observations. Pain 70:99–101, 1997.

83. Morley JS, Watt JW, Wells JC, et al: Methadone in pain uncontrolled by morphine. Lancet 342:1243–1271, 1993.

84. Mercadante S, Casuccio A, Calderone L: Rapid switching from morphine to methadone in cancer patients with poor response to morphine. J Clin Oncol 17:3307–3312, 1999.

85. Sawe J: High dose morphine and methadone in cancer patients: Clinical pharmacokinetic consideration of oral treatment [review]. Clin Pharmacokinet 11:87–106, 1986.

86. Agrawal SG, Evans RH: The primary afferent depolarizing action of kainate in the rat. Br J Pharmacol 87:345–355, 1986.

87. Huettner JE: Glutamate receptor channels in rat DRG neurons: Activation by kainate and quisqualate and blockade of desensitization by Con A. Neuron 3:255–266, 1990.

88. Sang CN, Hostetter MP, Gracely RH, et al: AMPA/kainate antagonist LY293558 reduces capsaicin-evoked hyperalgesia but not pain in normal skin in humans. Anesthesiolog 89:1060–1067, 1998.

89. Simmons RM, Li DL, Hoo KH, et al: Kainate GluR5 receptor subtype mediates the nociceptive response to formalin in the rat. Neuropharmacology 37:25–36, 1998.

90. Procter MJ, Houghton AK, Faber ES, et al: Actions of kainate and AMPA selective glutamate receptor ligands on nociceptive processing in the spinal cord. Neuropharmacology 37:1287–1297, 1998.

91. Anwyl R: Metabotropic glutamate receptors: Electrophysiological properties and role in plasticity. Brain Res Rev 29:83–120, 1999.

92. Gasparini F, Kuhn R, Pin JP: Allosteric modulators of group I metabotropic glutamate receptors: Novel subtype-selective ligands and therapeutic perspectives. Curr Opin Pharmacol 2:43–49, 2002.

93. Schoepp DD, Jane DE, Monn JA: Pharmacological agents acting at subtypes of metabotropic glutamate receptors. Neuropharmacology 38:1431–1476, 1999.

94. Zhang L, Lu Y, Chen Y, et al: Group I metabotropic glutamate receptor antagonists block secondary thermal hyperalgesia in rats with knee joint inflammation. J Pharmacol Exp Therapeut 300: 149–156, 2002.

Chapter 21

Cholecystokinin as an Endogenous Mediator of Opioid-Induced Paradoxical Pain and Antinociceptive Tolerance

Todd W. Vanderah, PhD/Michael H. Ossipov, PhD/Josephine Lai, PhD/Frank Porreca, PhD

ANATOMICAL DISTRIBUTION OF CHOLECYSTOKININ AND CHOLECYSTOKININ RECEPTORS

Cholecystokinin (CCK) was first described as a hormone that was secreted from the gastrointestinal tract into the circulation and that exerted contraction of the gallbladder.[1] CCK was isolated from porcine intestine as CCK_{33}.[2] The sulfated octapeptide of CCK is heterogeneously distributed throughout the brain and spinal cord.[3–6] Notably, the distributions of CCK and CCK receptors in the central nervous system show significant overlap with the distributions of endogenous opioid peptides[7] and of opioid receptors.[8] Importantly, immunoreactivity for CCK is seen in periaqueductal gray, raphe nuclei, and the medullary reticular formation,[5,9] which are structures known to modulate nociception. CCK and enkephalins have been found to be co-localized in axonal projections from periaqueductal gray neurons and coinciding with the terminations of spinothalamic tract neurons.[10] Furthermore, nerve terminals of CCK and enkephalin-containing neurons overlap in the periaqueductal gray and rostral ventromedial medulla (RVM), strongly suggesting that these neurotransmitters are likely to exert mutually modulatory effects.[11] CCK-containing projections from the RVM to the spinal cord have been visualized.[12] Under normal conditions, CCK is not found in the dorsal root ganglia or terminals of primary afferents of nonprimates but is detected in the superficial laminae of the spinal cord.[9,13,14] It is likely that spinal CCK arises from supraspinal descending projections and spinal interneurons.[5]

Two CCK receptor subtype populations have been identified, with the CCKA subtype being predominant in visceral organs of the digestive system and CCKB being predominant in the central nervous system.[5,15–17] CCKB receptors are found throughout the entire central nervous system of rodents but only in the brain of primates.[8,18,19] In contrast, the CCKA receptor is found in the spinal cord of primates.[8,18,19]

CHOLECYSTOKININ PROMOTES NOCICEPTION

Early reports had suggested that CCK may be antinociceptive; however, such results have been inconsistent and accompanied by other behavioral signs, such as ptosis and sedation, and may therefore be inconclusive.[15] In contrast, CCK microinjected into the RVM excites dorsal horn unit activity, an action consistent with a pronociceptive role.[20–22] In keeping with this suggestion, the microinjection of CCK into the RVM of normal rats produced behavioral signs of pain, including an increased sensitivity to normally nonnoxious mechanical stimuli and to noxious thermal hyperalgesia.[23] Additionally, the RVM administration of L365,260, a CCKB receptor antagonist, produced a reversible block of pain elicited by experimental (spinal nerve ligation) nerve injury.[23] Furthermore, spinal CCK antagonists blocked hyperalgesia produced by neurotensin administered into the RVM, again demonstrating a role for CCK in promoting hyperalgesia.[24] Except where L365,260 produced a biphasic antinociceptive effect in squirrel monkeys,[25] CCK antagonists alone have not produced an antinociceptive effect, again indicating a lack of continuous CCK-mediated tonic facilitation in the normal condition.[26]

CHOLECYSTOKININ ACTS AS AN ENDOGENOUS "ANTI-ANALGESIC" PEPTIDE

Numerous studies demonstrate CCK-mediated modulation of opioid antinociception. Spinal or systemic CCK blocked endogenously opioid-mediated footshock-induced antinociception.[27] Exogenous CCK also blocked morphine-induced antinociception.[27] CCK antagonists elicited an enhancement of morphine-induced antinociception while producing no antinociceptive activity when given alone.[13,27–33] It was also shown that a systemic CCKB antagonist, inactive alone, significantly enhanced the antinociceptive effect of systemic or spinally administered morphine in rats and mice.[34,35] Knock-down of the CCKB receptor with supraspinal administration of antisense oligodeoxynucleotides also enhanced morphine antinociception.[36] Finally, antinociception mediated by endogenous opioids by blockade of "enkephalinases" was also enhanced by CCK antagonists.[36–39]

The mechanisms by which CCK acts as an "antiopioid" are currently unkown. It was suggested that CCK counteracts the opioid-induced inhibition of depolarization-induced Ca^{++} influx into primary afferent neurons by eliciting a mobilization of Ca^{++} from intracellular stores, thus maintaining nociceptive neurotransmitter release.[30] Most recently, it was found that CCK infused into the RVM blocked the antinociceptive effect of systemic morphine.[40] Although the circuitry is not fully understood, it appeared to do so by blocking the morphine-induced increase in firing of RVM "OFF"-cells.[31] These data present a model that suggests a balance between endogenous opioid and CCK activity such that they modulate each other's activity.[13,26] Opioids promote CCK release which in turn modulates the antinociceptive activity of the opioid, acting as an endogenous regulatory system.[13,26] However, the ability of opioids to elicit CCK release in the RVM is unknown.

MORPHINE ELICITS CHOLECYSTOKININ RELEASE

Whereas CCK has been shown to modulate opioid antinociceptive activity, morphine in turn has been demonstrated to promote CCK release, apparently keeping a harmonious balance between endogenous pronociceptive and antinociceptive systems.[13,38,41,42] Microdialysis techniques performed in vivo demonstrated that systemic and spinal morphine increased cerebrospinal fluid levels of CCK.[43] Systemic morphine resulted in an 89% increase in CCK levels in spinal cord perfusate.[42] Microdialysis studies also revealed a naloxone-reversible marked increase in extracellular CCK in the frontal cortex of conscious rats after systemic morphine.[44] Importantly, this effect was clearly demonstrated to be mediated through the interaction of morphine with δ opioid receptors.[44] Similar observations were made in the spinal dorsal horn using microdialysis techniques.[45]

ANTI-OPIOID ACTIONS OF CHOLECYSTOKININ MAY ACCOUNT FOR MORPHINE ANTINOCICEPTIVE TOLERANCE

Many theories have been advanced to explain the phenomenon of opioid tolerance, most of which have focused on changes occurring at the cellular level to gain an appreciation of the mechanisms that drive this phenomenon.[46–50] While these changes are clearly relevant and important to observations made using intact "physiological" systems, our current level of understanding does not allow us to directly relate cellular mechanisms with opioid-induced changes at the systems level. Mechanistic interpretation of preclinical studies of opioid antinociceptive tolerance is particularly difficult, as many substances have been shown to reverse established opioid (usually morphine) tolerance and some substances have been shown to prevent the development of opioid antinociceptive tolerance. These include, among others, CGRP antagonists,[51,52] nitric oxide synthase inhibitors,[53] calcium channel blockers,[54] cyclooxygenase inhibitors,[53] protein kinase C inhibitors,[55] competitive and noncompetitive N-methyl-D-aspartate (NMDA) antagonists (see later), α-amino-3-hydroxy-5-methyl-4-isoxazole propionate antagonists,[56] superoxide dismutase mimics (Salvemini and Porreca, unpublished observations), dynorphin antiserum,[57] and CCK antagonists.[58,59] Perhaps the most studied of these substances are the excitatory amino acid antagonists, especially the NMDA antagonists, which have led to proposed mechanisms focusing on the likely co-localization of NMDA and opioid receptors and common intracellular pathways, such as translocation of PKCγ.[55] However, given the large number of modulatory systems shown to alter opioid tolerance, it is unclear whether common cellular localization and mechanisms can account for the actions of all these substances.

One of the most intriguing hypotheses relating to morphine antinociceptive tolerance has been the suggestion of an up-regulation of endogenous antiopioids, although not specifically related to CCK.[60] In keeping with this concept, the development of antinociceptive tolerance to morphine is indeed associated with an up-regulation of CCK.[41,61] Prolonged exposure to morphine has resulted in an accelerated increase in CCK expression, which in turn further attenuated the antinociceptive effect of morphine, thus resulting in apparent antinociceptive tolerance.[42] For example, after 1, 3, and 6 days of exposure to morphine, whole brain levels of proCCK mRNA increased by 52%, 62%, and 97%, respectively.[41] It was also shown that a single subcutaneous injection of morphine produced two- to three-fold increases in CCK mRNA content in the hypothalamus and spinal cord.[61] The development of antinociceptive tolerance to morphine was accompanied by elevated CCK content in the amygdala.[62] Increased release of CCK has also been seen in cases of sustained morphine administration. Microdialysis performed in the spinal cord of morphine-tolerant rats indicated increases in K^+-evoked release of CCK *in vivo*.[63] Finally, sustained morphine administration correlated with persistent release of CCK in the frontal cortex.[64]

If elevated CCK levels and increased release of CCK underlie aspects of opioid antinociceptive tolerance, then it should be expected that CCK antagonists would block antinociceptive tolerance. Numerous studies have demonstrated that the co-administration of CCK antagonists with morphine prevents the development of antinociceptive tolerance.[28,59,65] Furthermore, behavioral signs of already established antinociceptive tolerance to morphine have been reversed by CCK antiserum or CCKB antagonists at doses that did not potentiate morphine in naive rats.[41,66–68]

An interesting and potentially important aspect of the possibility that CCK may limit opioid antinociceptive tolerance arises from the observation that morphine-induced release of CCK may be mediated by opioid δ receptors, at least in the frontal cortex[44] and in the spinal cord.[45] The possibility that δ opioid receptors may be critical for morphine-induced release of CCK may explain why opioid δ antagonists have been reported to prevent the development of antinociceptive tolerance to morphine.[64,69,70]

CONCLUSION

In summary, CCK is positioned as a prime candidate with regard to the enhancement of nociception, because (1) it acts as an endogenous pronociceptive antiopioid; (2) it is upregulated with morphine tolerance; (3) its distribution overlaps significantly with that of endogenous opioid systems, particularly with regard to nociceptive processing pathways; and (4) CCK in the RVM likely mediates facilitation and signs of abnormal pain. Currently, opioids, in particular morphine, fentanyl, and related μ-opioid receptor analgesics, remain the primary drugs of choice for the treatment of moderate to severe pain. In spite of their well-accepted clinical efficacy, the use of opioid analgesics for the treatment of many chronic or prolonged pain states is hampered by the development of tolerance to their antinociceptive effect.[71–73]

A common aspect of the action of many of these endogenous systems is their ability to promote experimental pain. From this perspective, pain might be viewed as a physiological antagonist of antinociception (or analgesia, clinically) and thus, increased pain may manifest as opioid tolerance.[57,74,75] Although this interpretation that opioid-induced abnormal pain underlies antinociceptive tolerance will require further study, there is considerable experimental and clinical evidence that opioids produce abnormal pain. Opioid-induced pain may occur at the same time as antinociception/analgesia, thus being masked under normal circumstances. Critically, opioid-induced pain seems to be mediated by different mechanisms from those necessary to produce pain relief (i.e., opioid-induced pain is readily blocked by NMDA antagonists while antinociceptive actions are not[76,77]), and this effect occurs over a time-course different from that associated with antinociception.[76,77] Therefore, one might hypothesize that opioid-induced release of CCK in the RVM activates descending pain facilitation mechanisms; yet, the precise mechanisms of descending pain facilitation are not understood and likely involve the recruitment of many different systems in the spinal dorsal horn. This may allow the antagonists/inhibitors described to block pain at the spinal level and elicit a block of the reduced opioid antinociceptive potency (i.e., the behavioral manifestation of antinociceptive tolerance), but may ultimately be related to the actions of CCK at supraspinal sites to promote pain.

REFERENCES FOR ADDITIONAL READING

1. Ivy, A.C. and Oldberg, E., A hormone mechanism of gallbladder contraction and evacuation, Am J Physiol, 86 (1928) 599–613.
2. Mutt, V. and Jorpes, J.E., Hormonal polypeptides of the upper intestine, Biochem J, 125 (1971) 57P-58P.
3. Rehfeld J.F., Immunochemical studies on cholecystokinin. I. Development of sequence-specific radioimmunoassays for porcine triacontatriapeptide cholecystokinin. J. Biol. Chem., 253,(1978) 4016–4021.
4. Larsson, L. and Rehfeld, J. F., A peptide resembling COOH-terminal tetrapeptide amide of gastrin from a new gastrointestinal endocrine cell type, Nature, 277 (1979) 575–8.

5. Baber, N.S., Dourish, C.T. and Hill, D.R., The role of CCK caerulein, and CCK antagonists in nociception, Pain, 39 (1989) 307–28.

6. Savasta, M., Palacios, J.M. and Mengod, G., Regional localization of the mRNA coding for the neuropeptide cholecystokinin in the rat brain studied by in situ hybridization, Neurosci Lett, 93 (1988) 132–8.

7. Larsson, L. I. and Stengaard-Pendersen, K., Immunocytochemical and ultrastructural differentiation between Met-enkephalin-, Leu-enkephalin-, and Met/Leu-enkephalin-immunoreactive neurons of feline gut, J Neurosci., 2 (1982) 861–78.

8. Ghilardi, J.R., Allen, C.J., Vigna, S.R., McVey, D.C. and Mantyh, P.W., Trigeminal and dorsal root ganglion neurons express CCK receptor binding sites in the rat, rabbit, and monkey: possible site of opiate-CCK analgesic interactions, J Neurosci, 12 (1992) 4854–66.

9. Hokfelt, T., Herrera-Marschitz, M., Seroogy, K., Ju, G., Staines, W.A., Holets, V., Schalling, M., Ungerstedt, U., Post, C., Rehfeld, J.F. and et al., Immunohistochemical studies on cholecystokinin (CCK)-immunoreactive neurons in the rat using sequence specific antisera and with special reference to the caudate nucleus and primary sensory neurons, J Chem Neuroanat, 1 (1988) 11–51.

10. Gall, C., Lauterborn, J., Burks, D. and Seroogy, K., Co-localization of enkephalin and cholecystokinin in discrete areas of rat brain, Brain Res, 403 (1987) 403–8.

11. Skinner, K., Basbaum, A.I. and Fields, H.L., Cholecystokinin and enkephalin in brain stem pain modulating circuits, Neuroreport, 8 (1997) 2995–8.

12. Mantyh, P.W. and Hunt, S.P., Evidence for cholecystokinin-like immunoreactive neurons in the rat medulla oblongata which project to the spinal cord, Brain Res, 291 (1984) 49–54.

13. Stanfa, L., Dickenson, A., Xu, X.J. and Wiesenfeld-Hallin, Z., Cholecystokinin and morphine analgesia: variations on a theme, Trends Pharmacol Sci, 15 (1994) 65–6.

14. Verge, V.M., Wiesenfeld-Hallin, Z. and Hokfelt, T., Cholecystokinin in mammalian primary sensory neurons and spinal cord: in situ hybridization studies in rat and monkey, Eur J Neurosci, 5 (1993) 240–50.

15. Innis, R.B. and Snyder, S.H., Distinct cholecystokinin receptors in brain and pancreas, Proc Natl Acad Sci U S A, 77 (1980) 6917–21.

16. Moran, T.H., Robinson, P.H., Goldrich, M.S. and McHugh, P.R., Two brain cholecystokinin receptors: implications for behavioral actions, Brain Res, 362 (1986) 175–9.

17. Wank, S.A., Pisegna, J.R. and de Weerth, A., Cholecystokinin receptor family. Molecular cloning, structure, and functional expression in rat, guinea pig, and human, Ann N Y Acad Sci, 713 (1994) 49–66.

18. Hill, D.R., Shaw, T.M. and Woodruff, G.N., Binding sites for 125I-cholecystokinin in primate spinal cord are of the CCK-A subclass, Neurosci Lett, 89 (1988) 133–9.

19. Mercer, L.D., Beart, P.M., Horne, M.K., Finkelstein, D.I., Carrive, P. and Paxinos, G., On the distribution of cholecystokinin B receptors in monkey brain, Brain Res, 738 (1996) 313–8.

20. Hong, E.K. and Takemori, A.E., Indirect involvement of delta opioid receptors in cholecystokinin octapeptide-induced analgesia in mice, J Pharmacol Exp Ther, 251 (1989) 594–8.

21. Jeftinija, S., Miletic, V. and Randic, M., Cholecystokinin octapeptide excites dorsal horn neurons both in vivo and in vitro, Brain Res, 213 (1981) 231–6.

22. Pittaway, K.M., Rodriguez, R.E., Hughes, J. and Hill, R.G., CCK 8 analgesia and hyperalgesia after intrathecal administration in the rat: comparison with CCK-related peptides, Neuropeptides, 10 (1987) 87–108.

23. Kovelowski, C.J., Ossipov, M.H., Sun, H., Lai, J., Malan, T.P. and Porreca, F., Supraspinal cholecystokinin may drive tonic descending facilitation mechanisms to maintain neuropathic pain in the rat, Pain, 87 (2000) 265–73.

24. Urban, M.O., Smith, D.J. and Gebhart, G.F., Involvement of spinal cholecystokininB receptors in mediating neurotensin hyperalgesia from the medullary nucleus raphe magnus in the rat, J Pharmacol Exp Ther, 278 (1996) 90–6.

25. O'Neill, M.F., Dourish, C.T., Tye, S.J. and Iversen, S.D., Blockade of CCK-B receptors by L-365,260 induces analgesia in the squirrel monkey, Brain Res, 534 (1990) 287–90.

26. Wiesenfeld-Hallin, Z. and Xu, X.J., The role of cholecystokinin in nociception, neuropathic pain and opiate tolerance, Regul Pept, 65 (1996) 23–8.

27. Faris, P.L., Komisaruk, B.R., Watkins, L.R. and Mayer, D.J., Evidence for the neuropeptide cholecystokinin as an antagonist of opiate analgesia, Science, 219 (1983) 310–2.

28. Dourish, C.T., O'Neill, M.F., Coughlan, J., Kitchener, S.J., Hawley, D. and Iversen, S.D., The selective CCK-B receptor antagonist L-365,260 enhances morphine analgesia and prevents morphine tolerance in the rat, Eur J Pharmacol, 176 (1990) 35–44.

29. Hughes, J., Hunter, J.C. and Woodruff, G.N., Neurochemical actions of CCK underlying the therapeutic potential of CCK-B antagonists, Neuropeptides, 19 Suppl (1991) 85–9.

30. Stanfa, L.C., Sullivan, A.F. and Dickenson, A.H., Alterations in neuronal excitability and the potency of spinal mu, delta and kappa opioids after carrageenan-induced inflammation, Pain, 50 (1992) 345–54.

31. Suh, H.H. and Tseng, L.F., Differential effects of sulfated cholecystokinin octapeptide and proglumide injected intrathecally on antinociception induced by beta- endorphin and morphine administered intracerebroventricularly in mice, Eur J Pharmacol, 179 (1990) 329–38.

32. Watkins, L.R., Kinscheck, I.B., Kaufman, E.F., Miller, J., Frenk, H. and Mayer, D.J., Cholecystokinin antagonists selectively potentiate analgesia induced by endogenous opiates, Brain Res, 327 (1985a) 181–90.

33. Watkins, L.R., Kinscheck, I.B. and Mayer, D.J., Potentiation of morphine analgesia by the cholecystokinin antagonist proglumide, Brain Res, 327 (1985b) 169–80.

34. Ossipov, M.H., Kovelowski, C.J., Vanderah, T. and Porreca, F., Naltrindole, an opioid delta antagonist, blocks the enhancement of morphine-antinociception induced by a CCKB antagonist in the rat, Neurosci Lett, 181 (1994) 9–12.

35. Vanderah, T.W., Bernstein, R.N., Yamamura, H.I., Hruby, V.J. and Porreca, F., Enhancement of morphine antinociception by a CCKB antagonist in mice is mediated via opioid delta receptors, J Pharmacol Exp Ther, 278 (1996) 212–9.

36. Vanderah, T.W., Lai, J., Yamamura, H.I. and Porreca, F., Antisense oligodeoxynucleotide to the CCKB receptor produces naltrindole- and [Leu5]enkephalin antiserum-sensitive enhancement of morphine antinociception, Neuroreport, 5 (1994) 2601–5.

37. Maldonado, R., Derrien, M., Noble, F. and Roques, B.P., Association of the peptidase inhibitor RB 101 and a CCK-B antagonist strongly enhances antinociceptive responses, Neuroreport, 4 (1993) 947–50.

38. Noble, F., Derrien, M. and Roques, B.P., Modulation of opioid antinociception by CCK at the supraspinal level: evidence of regulatory mechanisms between CCK and enkephalin systems in the control of pain, Br J Pharmacol, 109 (1993) 1064–70.

39. Valverde, O., Maldonado, R., Fournie-Zaluski, M.C. and Roques, B.P., Cholecystokinin B antagonists strongly potentiate antinociception mediated by endogenous enkephalins, J Pharmacol Exp Ther, 270 (1994) 77–88.

40. Heinricher, M.M., McGaraughty, S. and Tortorici, V., Circuitry Underlying Antiopioid Actions of Cholecystokinin Within the Rostral Ventromedial Medulla, J Neurophysiol, 85 (2001) 280–286.

41. Zhou, Y., Sun, Y.H., Zhang, Z.W. and Han, J.S., Accelerated expression of cholecystokinin gene in the brain of rats rendered tolerant to morphine, Neuroreport, 3 (1992) 1121–3.

42. Zhou, Y., Sun, Y.H., Zhang, Z.W. and Han, J.S., Increased release of immunoreactive cholecystokinin octapeptide by morphine and potentiation of mu-opioid analgesia by CCKB receptor antagonist L-365,260 in rat spinal cord, Eur J Pharmacol, 234 (1993) 147–54.

43. de Araujo Lucas, G., Alster, P., Brodin, E. and Wiesenfeld-Hallin, Z., Differential release of cholecystokinin by morphine in rat spinal cord, Neurosci Lett, 245 (1998) 13–6.

44. Becker, C., Hamon, M., Cesselin, F. and Benoliel, J.J., Delta(2)-opioid receptor mediation of morphine-induced CCK release in the frontal cortex of the freely moving rat, Synapse, 34 (1999) 47–54.

45. Gustafsson H., Afrah, A.W., and Stiller C.O., Morphine-induced in vivo release of spinal cholecysto-kinin is mediated by δ-opioid receptors-effect of peripheral axotomy, J Neurochem., 77, (2001) 1–10.

46. Bohn, L.M., Gainetdinov, R.R., Lin, F.T., Lefkowitz, R.J. and Caron, M.G., Mu-opioid receptor de-sensitization by beta-arrestin-2 determines morphine tolerance but not dependence, Nature, 408 (2000) 720–3.

47. He, L., Fong, J., von Zastrow, M. and Whistler, J.L. Regulation of opioid receptor trafficking and morphine tolerance by receptor oligomerization, Cell, 108 (2002) 271 – 82.

48. Childers, S.R., Opioid receptor-coupled second messenger systems, Life Sci, 48 (1991) 1991–2003.

49. Collin, E. and Cesselin, F., Neurobiological mechanisms of opioid tolerance and dependence, Clin Neuropharmacol, 14 (1991) 465–88.

50. Sabbe, M.B. and Yaksh, T.L., Pharmacology of spinal opioids, J Pain Symptom Manage, 5 (1990) 191–203.

51. Menard, D.P., van Rossum, D., Kar, S., St Pierre, S., Sutak, M., Jhamandas, K. and Quirion, R., A calcitonin gene-related peptide receptor antagonist prevents the development of tolerance to spinal morphine analgesia, J Neurosci, 16 (1996) 2342–51.

52. Powell, K.J., Ma, W., Sutak, M., Doods, H., Quirion, R. and Jhamandas, K., Blockade and reversal of spinal morphine tolerance by peptide and non- peptide calcitonin gene-related peptide receptor antagonists, Br J Pharmacol, 131 (2000) 875–84.

53. Powell, K.J., Hosokawa, A., Bell, A., Sutak, M., Milne, B., Quirion, R. and Jhamandas, K., Compar-ative effects of cyclo-oxygenase and nitric oxide synthase inhibition on the development and re-versal of spinal opioid tolerance, Br J Pharmacol, 127 (1999) 631–44.

54. Aley, K.O. and Levine, J.D., Different mechanisms mediate development and expression of toler-ance and dependence for peripheral mu-opioid antinociception in rat, Journal of Neuroscience, 17 (1997) 8018–23.

55. Mao, J., Price, D.D., Phillips, L.L., Lu, J. and Mayer, D.J., Increases in protein kinase C gamma im-munoreactivity in the spinal cord of rats associated with tolerance to the analgesic effects of mor-phine, Brain Research, 677 (1995) 257–67.

56. Kest, B., McLemore, G., Kao, B. and Inturrisi, C.E., The competitive alpha-amino-3-hydroxy-5-methylisoxazole-4-propionate receptor antagonist LY293558 attenuates and reverses analgesic tolerance to morphine but not to delta or kappa opioids, Journal of Pharmacology & Experimen-tal Therapeutics, 283 (1997) 1249–55.

57. Vanderah, T.W., Gardell, L.R., Burgess, S.E., Ibrahim, M., Dogrul, A., Zhong, C.M., Zhang, E.T., Malan, T.P., Jr., Ossipov, M.H., Lai, J. and Porreca, F., Dynorphin promotes abnormal pain and spinal opioid antinociceptive tolerance, J Neurosci, 20 (2000) 7074–9.

58. Dourish, C.T., Hawley, D. and Iversen, S.D., Enhancement of morphine analgesia and prevention of morphine tolerance in the rat by the cholecystokinin antagonist L-364,718, Eur J Pharmacol, 147 (1988) 469–72.

59. Xu, X.J., Wiesenfeld-Hallin, Z., Hughes, J., Horwell, D.C. and Hokfelt, T., CI988, a selective antag-onist of cholecystokininB receptors, prevents morphine tolerance in the rat, Br J Pharmacol, 105 (1992) 591–6.

60. Rothman, R.B., Brady, L.S., Xu, H. and Long, J.B., Chronic intracerebroventricular infusion of the antiopioid peptide, Phe- Leu-Phe-Gln-Pro-Gln-Arg-Phe-NH2 (NPFF), downregulates mu opioid binding sites in rat brain, Peptides, 14 (1993) 1271–7.

61. Ding, X.Z. and Bayer, B.M., Increases of CCK mRNA and peptide in different brain areas follow-ing acute and chronic administration of morphine, Brain Res, 625 (1993) 139–44.

62. Pu, S., Zhuang, H., Lu, Z., Wu, X. and Han, J., Cholecystokinin gene expression in rat amygdaloid neurons: normal distribution and effect of morphine tolerance, Brain Res Mol Brain Res, 21 (1994) 183–9.

63. Lucas, G.A., Hoffmann, O., Alster, P. and Wiesenfeld-Hallin, Z., Extracellular cholecystokinin lev-els in the rat spinal cord following chronic morphine exposure: an in vivo microdialysis study, Brain Res, 821 (1999) 79–86.

64. Becker, C., Pohl, M., Thiebot, M.H., Collin, E., Hamon, M., Cesselin, F. and Benoliel, J.J., Delta-opioid receptor-mediated increase in cortical extracellular levels of cholecystokinin-like material by subchronic morphine in rats, Neuropharmacology, 39 (2000) 161–71.

65. Kellstein, D.E. and Mayer, D.J., Spinal co-administration of cholecystokinin antagonists with morphine prevents the development of opioid tolerance, Pain, 47 (1991) 221–9.

66. Ding, X.Z., Fan, S.G., Zhou, J.P. and Han, J.S., Reversal of tolerance to morphine but no potentiation of morphine- induced analgesia by antiserum against cholecystokinin octapeptide, Neuropharmacology, 25 (1986) 1155–60.

67. Hoffmann, O. and Wiesenfeld-Hallin, Z., The CCK-B receptor antagonist Cl 988 reverses tolerance to morphine in rats, Neuroreport, 5 (1994) 2565–8.

68. Singh, L., Field, M.J., Hunter, J.C., Oles, R.J. and Woodruff, G.N., Modulation of the in vivo actions of morphine by the mixed CCKA/B receptor antagonist PD 142898, Eur J Pharmacol, 307 (1996) 283–9.

69. Schiller, P.W., Fundytus, M.E., Merovitz, L., Weltrowska, G., Nguyen, T.M., Lemieux, C., Chung, N.N. and Coderre, T.J., The opioid mu agonist/delta antagonist DIPP-NH(2)[Psi] produces a potent analgesic effect, no physical dependence, and less tolerance than morphine in rats, J Med Chem, 42 (1999) 3520–6.

70. Wells, J.L., Bartlett, J.L., Ananthan, S. and Bilsky, E.J., In vivo pharmacological characterization of SoRI 9409, a nonpeptidic opioid mu-agonist/delta-antagonist that produces limited antinociceptive tolerance and attenuates morphine physical dependence, J Pharmacol Exp Ther, 297 (2001) 597–605.

71. Foley, K.M., Opioids, Neurol Clin, 11 (1993) 503–22.

72. Foley, K.M., Misconceptions and controversies regarding the use of opioids in cancer pain, Anticancer Drugs, 6 Suppl 3 (1995) 4–13.

73. Way, E.L., Loh, H.H. and Shen, F.H., Simultaneous quantitative assessment of morphine tolerance and physical dependence, J Pharmacol Exp Ther, 167 (1969) 1–8.

74. Vanderah, T.W., Ossipov, M.H., Lai, J., Malan, T.P. and Porreca, F., Mechanisms of opioid-induced pain and antinociceptive tolerance: descending facilitation and spinal dynorphin, Pain, 92 (2001a) 5–9.

75. Vanderah, T.W., Suenaga, N.M., Ossipov, M.H., Malan, T.P., Jr., Lai, J. and Porreca, F., Tonic Descending Facilitation from the Rostral Ventromedial Medulla Mediates Opioid-Induced Abnormal Pain and Antinociceptive Tolerance, J Neurosci, 21 (2001b) 279–286.

76. Celerier, E., Laulin, J., Larcher, A., Le Moal, M. and Simonnet, G., Evidence for opiate-activated NMDA processes masking opiate analgesia in rats, Brain Res, 847 (1999) 18–25.

77. Laulin, J.P., Celerier, E., Larcher, A., Le Moal, M. and Simonnet, G., Opiate tolerance to daily heroin administration: an apparent phenomenon associated with enhanced pain sensitivity, Neuroscience, 89 (1999) 631–6.

Chapter 22

Cholecystokinin Receptor Antagonists

Gary J. McCleane, MD

With an increased selection of pharmacologic agents now available for pain management, the ability to provide good-quality pain relief with minimal side effects has improved. Analgesia, or analgesia in the absence of excessive side effects, is still not achieved in some patients, however. Consequently, clinicans must be aware of as many therapeutic modalities as possible so that the ultimate goal of pain relief is achieved more consistently. Currently, clinicians interested in pain management fall into two broad categories: (1) those who advocate the use of strong opioids in long-term pain management and (2) those who do not because of fears of partial efficacy (particularly with neuropathic pain) and tolerance to the analgesic effect of strong opioids. Any stratagem for enhancing the analgesic effect and preventing tolerance to these opioids should reduce the understandable anxiety of this latter group and improve patient satisfaction.

In 1928, Ivy and Oldberg[12] described the existence of a hormone with an action on the gallbladder. They named it *cholecystokinin* (CCK), and it is now known to be a peptide present in the gastrointestinal tract (CCK A) and central nervous system (CCK B).[11, 15, 25] Much evidence exists for an important role for CCK in pain modulation and tolerance to opioid analgesics, yet the use of CCK-active agents is infrequent, with no licensed preparations currently available. Although the basic scientific understanding of the exact role of CCK and CCK antagonists is described in many excellent reviews,[26, 31, 32] the human clinical perspective has not been adequately addressed.

This chapter examines a selection of the available evidence of the role of CCK in pain management and discusses how this knowledge can be extrapolated into clinical practice. The pathway from the knowledge of the presence of CCK in the central nervous system to the ultimate clinical application of CCK antagonists as proanalgesic agents is a logical, stepwise progression. A selection of the evidence for this pathway is considered.

CHOLECYSTOKININ

CCK is a naturally occurring peptide in the central nervous system and alimentary tract. Many factors can influence the concentration in which it is found *in vivo*. Xu et al[34] showed in a rodent model that CCK-like immunoreactivity is approximately equal in control and spinally injured rats who do not show allodynia (approximately 2 to 3 ppm of CCK). In spinally injured rats who do have allodynia, the concentration of CCK-like immunoreactivity is substantially elevated (>10 ppm of CCK).

Given this apparent association between an elevation of CCK levels and one of the cardinal symptoms of neuropathic pain, the issue of the relevance of these elevated levels arises. Schafer et al[27] examined the effect of CCK injection on fentanyl-induced analgesia in rats with induced paw inflammation and showed that there were distinctly reduced paw pressure thresholds in these animals when CCK was injected compared with control animals, with the implication that CCK had an antiopioid effect. These investigators further examined the effect of CCK A and CCK B injection and showed that CCK B had a greater antiopioid effect than CCK A, although this finding has not been confirmed in human subjects.

Similarly, Faris et al[7] examined the effect of CCK injection on front paw shock–induced opiate antinociception in rats and showed that CCK injection significantly reduced this induced antinociception. These pieces of evidence suggest that if CCK is elevated by administration of the peptide, analgesia is reduced, and elevated endogenous levels are associated with increased pain.

Are CCK levels elevated when pain is experienced, and do clinical interventions have an effect on CCK levels? The answer to both questions seems to be yes. Xu et al[35] examined rats that had a unilateral section of the sciatic nerve and found that there was a dramatic increase in the number of dorsal root ganglia neurons synthesizing CCK after sciatic nerve division compared with controls. Although administration of morphine or the CCK receptor antagonist CI 988 alone had little effect on autotomy (a sign of neuropathic pain or dysesthesia in animal models), when they were given together there was a significant reduction in autotomy behavior.

Not only neural injury leads to elevated CCK/CCK mRNA levels. It seems that long-term opioid administration has a similar effect. Tang et al[28] showed that if morphine is added to artificial spinal fluid perfusing the subarachnoid space, there is an increase in CCK content of the spinal fluid. In a similar vein, Ding and Bayer[3] examined the content of CCK mRNA and CCK immunoreactivity in rats before and after acute and long-term morphine administration. They found that the mRNA and immunoreactivity were not altered by single-dose administration of morphine but were increased significantly after long-term administration of morphine.

CHOLECYSTOKININ ANTAGONISTS: ANTINOCICEPTION

If CCK has an antiopioid effect, this would be substantiated if antagonism of elevated CCK levels produced an improvement in the quality of pain relief. Dourish et al[5] examined the effect of intrathecal injection of saline, morphine, L365 260 (a CCK B antagonist), and combinations of each on the rat tail flick test. They showed that saline had little effect, whereas morphine alone had a greater effect on the percentage maximum pressure effect in this pain model. The addition of L365 260 to morphine produced a further marked increase in the percentage maximum pressure effect, implying that this CCK antagonist had an augmented antinociceptive effect with morphine.

Wiesenfeld-Hallin et al[33] used the rat hot plate test model and examined the effect of morphine, PD134 308 (a CCK B antagonist), and both together on the percentage increase in flick latency and had similar results: Morphine alone caused some increase in flick latency, which was substantially increased by the addition of PD134 308 to the morphine. Similarly, Lavigne et al[17] showed in a rat model that the CCK A antagonist devazepide and the CCK B antagonist L365 260 enhanced the antinociceptive effect of morphine when measured using a thermal sensorimotor tail flick test, whereas Watkins et al[29] showed that the nonspecific CCK A and CCK B antagonist proglumide enhanced the antinociceptive effect of morphine again in a rat tail flick test model.

Coudore-Civiale et al[2] studied the effect of morphine and CI 988 (a CCK B antagonist) on mechanical hyperalgesia and allodynia in normal, mononeuropathic, and diabetic rats. They found that CI 988 had no antinociceptive effects in normal rats but had antinociceptive effects in the mononeuropathic and diabetic animals. The combination of CI 988 and morphine had a superadditive effect in the diabetic rats. Similarly, Nichols et al[22] again studying rats with induced mechanical allodynia showed that morphine and L365 260 (a CCK B antagonist) had no antiallodynic activity when given alone, but when administered together, a significant antiallodynic effect was observed.

In contrast to these positive findings, Kellstein and Mayer[13] found that although acute intrathecal administration of CCK antagonists (proglumide and lorglumide) enhanced the analgesic effect of intrathecal morphine, when they were administered on a long-term basis there was a loss of this facilitation of opioid antinociception as judged by rat tail flick assays. As can be seen, most of the animal evidence is suggestive of a potential beneficial application to the human clinical situation. If CCK antagonists do have a proanalgesic effect, however, may they also potentiate opioid-related side effects, in particular respiratory depression? If this were so, their use could be limited. Dourish et al[6] examined the effect of a CCK A antagonist (devokade) on respiratory rates in squirrel monkeys. They found that injection of vehicle (control) had no effect, whereas the decrease in respiratory rate was approximately equal in monkeys given morphine and morphine/devokade. This reassuring finding is borne out in clinical practice, in which no adverse effect on respiratory function is seen when CCK antagonist/opioid combinations are used. In a study of nine human subjects who had been receiving long-term treatment with sustained-release morphine, the addition of L365 260 on two occasions had no effect on respiratory or cardiovascular variables.[19]

HUMAN EVIDENCE

The human literature on CCK antagonists is surprisingly sparse when compared with that available for animal models. Lavigne et al[16] examined subjects undergoing third molar extraction and found that 4 mg of morphine had little analgesic effect, whereas 8 mg produced more marked analgesia. Addition of proglumide (a nonspecific CCK A and CCK B antagonist) to a 4-mg dose of morphine produced similar analgesia to an 8-mg dose of morphine administered alone and prolonged its duration of action in a useful fashion.

Price et al[24] used an experimental human thermal pain model. Morphine, 0.04 mg/kg, failed to produce analgesia, as did proglumide, 100 μg, when administered separately. When these agents were given together, there was definite pain relief.

McCleane[20] studied 40 adults with chronic benign pain of mixed origin. All were taking sustained-release morphine (mean dose, 50 mg daily) for a median duration of 7.4 months (range, 0.3 to 72 months). All subjects were deriving less than optimal analgesia. Subjects were challenged in a double-blind crossover fashion with placebo and proglumide. Median pain scores were altered insignificantly by addition of placebo, but fell by 2 units on a 0 to 10 visual analog scale with addition of proglumide. Side effects were minimal, and the subjects' prestudy duration of pain and morphine consumption had no relationship to the analgesia apparent when proglumide was added.

In a randomized, double-blind crossover study of 40 subjects taking a stable dose of sustained-release morphine for chronic neuropathic pain, subjects received placebo; L365 260, 40 mg; and L 365 260, 120 mg, daily for 2 weeks (with a 2-week washout period between treatments) in varying orders. Pain, activity, and sleep quality and concomitant analgesic consumption were recorded for 2 weeks before the study (baseline) and throughout the study period.[19] There were no differences in any of the measured variables throughout the study period. It does seem that although the rodent and murine evidence suggests CCK B antagonists should be of most relevance, there are species variations, and the CCK A antagonists are of more relevance in primate/human pain models. Dourish et al,[6] as mentioned previously, showed a useful antinociceptive effect of addition of a CCK A antagonist to morphine in a primate (squirrel monkey) model, contrary to what the rodent models would have predicted.

Currently, there are no CCK antagonists licensed for their proanalgesic effects. Off-label use of CCK antagonists is with experimental compounds apart from proglumide (MILLID, Rottapharma, Italy), a nonspecific CCK A and CCK B antagonist that is available and has been shown to have a positive effect on the symptoms of gastric ulceration.[8]

CHOLECYSTOKININ ANTAGONISTS: PREVENTION OF TOLERANCE TO OPIOIDS

In addition to evidence for an antinociceptive effect of CCK antagonists, there is evidence that this class of drug can prevent tolerance to the analgesic effect of opioids. Kissin et al[14] studied acute tolerance to alfentanil infusion in rats. The rats had an alfentanil infusion for 4 hours, followed by boluses of alfentanil alone, alfentanil and L365 260, and alfentanil with proglumide at times 60, 120, and 240 minutes after alfentanil infusion was begun. The antinociceptive responses after these administrations were assessed using a tail pressure design. The cumulative reduction in analgesic effect increased in the rats that received alfentanil alone from around 55% at T = 60 minutes to 95% at T = 240 minutes. In contrast, the rats that received L365 260 boluses with alfentanil had a cumulative reduction in analgesic response of around 18% at T = 60 minutes, 31% at T = 120 minutes, and 72% at T = 240 minutes. Corresponding reductions in the rats that received alfentanil and proglumide were 20%, 28%, and about 50%, showing a significant attenuation of the acute tolerance to alfentanil infusion.

Dourish et al[5] examined rats pretreated with morphine for 6 days. Rat tail flick tests were examined. Neither saline (control) nor morphine injections had a noticeable effect on tail flick latencies. There were significant increases in latencies, however, when morphine injection was accompanied by the CCK B antagonist L365 260. Similarly, Dourish et al[4] showed in a rat model that the CCK A antagonist L364 718 enhanced the antinociceptive efficacy of morphine, as shown in a rat tail flick test. After 6 days of treatment with morphine and L364 718, tolerance to the antinociceptive effect of morphine had not occurred.

Panerai et al[23] examined the effect of the nonspecific CCK A and CCK B antagonist proglumide on tolerance to the antinociceptive effect of chronically administered morphine using rat tail flick and hot plate tests. They showed that proglumide prevented tolerance to morphine, but they were unable to show any reduction in physical dependence, as judged by acute withdrawal reactions, when proglumide and morphine were coadministered.

Idanpaan-Heikkila et al[10] studied rats treated with morphine for 12 days after surgical infliction of a unilateral peripheral mononeuropathy. Nociception was assessed using a vocalization threshold to paw pressure technique. At day 12, rats were treated with varying combinations, including L365 260 and morphine, for a further 4 days. By day 16, all animals receiving morphine alone or morphine and placebo were tolerant to the antinociceptive effect of acutely administered morphine. In rats that had been treated with L365 260 and morphine, tolerance was completely prevented. In this well-established model of neuropathic pain, coadministration of a CCK B antagonist completely prevented tolerance.

Tang et al[28] showed that in rats administration of morphine subcutaneously causes tolerance after seven to eight injections. This tolerance to morphine is partially blocked if proglumide also is administered.

Zarrindast et al[37] approached the topic of tolerance in a slightly different fashion. They used a mouse hot plate test. The mice received morphine for 3 to 5 days. All became tolerant to it. Mice that were given the CCK agonist caerulein (a peptide closely related to CCK) had a potentiation of the antinociceptive effect of subsequently administered morphine. L365 260 and MK 329, both CCK antagonists, decreased tolerance to morphine. These workers suggested that the results show an important role for the CCK receptor in antinociceptive tolerance to morphine, but the fact that the agonist and antagonists reduced tolerance confuses the matter. They also found that CCK agonists and antagonists had no effect on the occurrence of morphine dependence. They confirmed their findings in another report in which caerulein, MK 329 (a CCK A antagonist), and L365 260 (a CCK B antagonist) when administered to mice who had received morphine on a chronic basis all diminished tolerance to acutely administered morphine, suggesting that both CCK subtypes, A and B, are implicated in tolerance to morphine.[36] Conversely, Lu et al,[18] using a rat model, found that caerulein increased the naloxone-induced withdrawal reaction, whereas pretreatment with the CCK antagonists L365 260 and MK 329 attenuated this withdrawal reaction. Mitchell et al[21] examined the relationship of tolerance to morphine and certain environmental cues. When morphine administration was paired with particular environmental cues, these cues could act as conditioned stimuli that elicit a conditioned response opposing the agonist effect of morphine—this is known as *associative tolerance*. When morphine was administered in the absence of these cues, nonassociative tolerance developed. These investigators found that when L365 260 was injected into the amygdala, associative, but not nonassociative, tolerance was blocked. These results suggest that antinociceptive tolerance to short-acting and long-acting opioids can be reduced if a CCK antagonist is coadministered.

CHOLECYSTOKININ ANTAGONISTS: REVERSAL OF ESTABLISHED TOLERANCE TO OPIOIDS

If coadministration of an opioid and CCK antagonist can prevent tolerance to the antinociceptive effect of the opioid, is it possible that the use of a CCK antagonist could reverse established tolerance to that opioid? Several workers addressed this issue in animal models. Hoffmann and Wiesenfeld-Hallin[9] studied the results of hot plate tests in rats that had become tolerant to morphine's antinociceptive effect because of repeated administration. The rats were challenged with further morphine, with saline (control) or morphine and CI 988 (a CCK B antagonist). The rats that received morphine/saline continued to exhibit tolerance. The rats that received the CCK antagonist had significant antinociception when morphine was given.

Watkins et al[30] similarly studied the effect of CCK antagonists using a rat model. They found that the nonspecific CCK A and CCK B antagonist proglumide potentiated morphine-induced antinociception and seemed to reverse established tolerance. There currently are no published human studies that examine the effect of CCK antagonists on analgesic tolerance.

CHOLECYSTOKININ ANTAGONISTS: EFFECT ON TRICYCLIC-INDUCED ANALGESIA

Coudore-Civiale et al[1] published an intriguing insight into the effect of CCK antagonists on tricyclic-induced antinociception. They used a diabetic rat model and measured the paw pressure vocalization threshold. Administration of CI 988 (a CCK B antagonist) alone caused a small increase in vocalization threshold when compared with saline (control). The threshold was slightly greater when clomipramine was given. When clomipramine and CI 988 were coadministered, there was a marked increase in vocalization threshold, suggesting that this CCK antagonist can augment the antinociceptive effect of this tricyclic antidepressant. No human controlled trial evidence exists to verify this effect in the clinical setting, but the scope for investigation of this therapeutic possibility exists.

CONCLUSION

The evidence presented in this chapter suggests that CCK levels are elevated when neural injury occurs and with long term opioid administration. CCK has an antiopioid effect, and elevated levels are associated with reduced antinociceptive efficacy of opioids. If these elevated levels are antagonized, antinociceptive efficacy of the opioid is increased. Administration of CCK antagonists in the animal model may prevent the onset of, or reduce the extent of, antinociceptive tolerance to opioids. CCK antagonists also may reverse established tolerance.

Further human study is desirable to substantiate the proanalgesic effect of CCK antagonists and to determine if the prevention of tolerance and the reversal of established tolerance shown in animal models is reproduced in the human clinical situation. This work is particularly needed because it seems that CCK antagonists have few side effects and yet may be used to maximize the analgesic potential and minimize the dose of opioids that have more pronounced side-effect profiles.

REFERENCES

1. Coudore-Civiale MA, Courteix C, Boucher M, et al: Potentiation of morphine and clomipramine analgesia by cholecystokinin B antagonist CI 988 in diabetic rats. Neurosci Lett 286:37–40, 2000.
2. Coudore-Civiale M-A, Courteix C, Fialip J, et al: Spinal effect of the cholecystokinin B receptor antagonist CI 988 on hyperalgesia, allodynia and morphine induced analgesia in diabetic and mono neuropathic rats. Pain 88:15–22, 2000.
3. Ding XZ, Bayer BM: Increases of CCK mRNA and peptide in different brain areas following acute and chronic administration of morphine. Brain Res 625:139–144, 1993.
4. Dourish CT, Hawley D, Iverson SD: Enhancement of morphine analgesia and prevention of morphine tolerance in the rat by the cholecystokinin antagonist L364 718. Eur J Pharmacol 147:469–472, 1988.
5. Dourish CT, O'Neill MF, Coughlan J, et al: The selective CCK B receptor antagonist L365 260 enhances morphine analgesia and prevents morphine tolerance in rats. Eur J Pharmacol 176:35–44, 1990.
6. Dourish CT, O'Neill MF, Schaffer LW, et al: The cholecystokinin receptor antagonist Devazepide enhances morphine induced analgesia but not morphine induced respiratory depression in the squirrel monkey. J Pharmacol Exp Ther 255:1158–1165, 1990.
7. Faris PL, Komisaruk BR, Watkins LR, Mayer DJ: Evidence for the neuropeptide cholecystokinin as an antagonist of opiate analgesia. Science 219:310–312, 1983.
8. Galeone M, Moise G, Ferrante F, et al: Double-blind clinical comparison between a gastrin recep-

tor antagonist, proglumide, and a histamine H$_2$ blocker, cimetidine. Curr Med Res Opin 5:376–382, 1978.

9. Hoffmann O, Wiesenfeld-Hallin Z: The CCK B receptor antagonist CI 988 reverses tolerance to morphine in rats. Neuroreport 5:2565–2568, 1994.

10. Idanpaan-Heikkila JJ, Guilbaud G, Kayser V: Prevention of tolerance to the antinociceptive effects of systemic morphine by a selective cholecystokinin B receptor antagonist in a rat model of peripheral neuropathy. J Pharmacol Exp Ther 282:1366–1372, 1997.

11. Innis RB, Snyder SH: Distinct cholecystokinin receptors in brain and pancreas. Proc Natl Acad Sci U S A 77:6917–6921, 1980.

12. Ivy AC, Oldberg E: A hormone mechanism for gallbladder contraction and evacuation. Am J Physiol 86:599–613, 1928.

13. Kellstein DE, Mayer DJ: Chronic administration of cholecystokinin antagonists reverses the enhancement of spinal morphine analgesia induced by acute pre-treatment. Brain Res 516:263–270, 1990.

14. Kissin I, Bright CA, Bradley EL: Acute tolerance to continuously infused alfentanil: The role of cholecystokinin and N-methyl-D-aspartate-nitric oxide systems. Anesth Analg 91:110–116, 2000.

15. Larsson LI, Rehfeld JF: Localization and molecular heterogeneity of cholecystokinin in the central and peripheral nervous system. Brain Res 165:201–218, 1979.

16. Lavigne GJ, Hargreaves KM, Schmidt EA, Dionne RA: Proglumide potentiates morphine analgesia for acute postsurgical pain. Clin Pharmacol Ther 45:666–673, 1989.

17. Lavigne GJ, Millington WR, Mueller GP: The CCK A and CCK B receptor antagonists, Devazepide and L365 260, enhance morphine antinociception only in non-acclimated rats exposed to a novel environment. Neuropeptides 21:119–29, 1992.

18. Lu L, Huang M, Liu Z, Ma L: Cholecystokinin B receptor antagonists attenuate morphine dependence and withdrawal in rats. Neuroreport 11:829–832, 2000.

19. McCleane GJ: A phase 1 study of the CCK antagonist L365 260 in human subjects taking sustained release morphine for intractable pain. (in press).

20. McCleane GJ: The cholecystokinin antagonist proglumide enhances the analgesic efficacy of morphine in humans with chronic benign pain. Anesth Analg 87:1117–1120, 1998.

21. Mitchell JM, Basbaum AI, Fields HL: A locus and mechanism of action for associative morphine tolerance. Nat Neurosci 3:47–53, 2000.

22. Nichols ML, Bian D, Ossipov MH, et al: Regulation of morphine anti allodynic efficacy by cholecystokinin in a model of neuropathic pain in rats. J Pharmacol Exp Ther 275:1339–1345, 1995.

23. Panerai AE, Rovati LC, Cocco E, et al: Dissociation of tolerance and dependence to morphine: A possible role for cholecystokinin. Brain Res 410:52–60, 1987.

24. Price DD, von der Gruen A, Miller J, et al: Potentiation of systemic morphine analgesia in humans by proglumide, a cholecystokinin antagonist. Anesth Analg 64:801–806, 1985.

25. Rehfeld JF: Immunochemical studies on cholecystokinin. J Biol Chem 253:4022–4030, 1978.

26. Roques BP, Noble F: Association of enkephalin catabolism inhibitors and CCK B antagonists: A potential use in the management of pain and opioid addiction. Neurochem Res 21:1397–1410, 1996.

27. Schafer M, Zhou L, Stein C: Cholecystokinin inhibits peripheral opioid analgesia in inflamed tissue. Neuroscience 82:603–611, 1998.

28. Tang J, Chou J, Iadarola M, et al: Proglumide prevents and curtails acute tolerance to morphine in rats. Neuropharmacology 23:715–718, 1984.

29. Watkins LR, Kinscheck LB, Mayer DJ: Potentiation of morphine analgesia by the cholecystokinin antagonist proglumide. Brain Res 327:169–180, 1985.

30. Watkins LR, Kinscheck IB, Mayer DJ: Potentiation of opiate analgesia and apparent reversal of morphine tolerance by proglumide. Science 224:395–396, 1984.

31. Wettstein JG, Bueno L, Junien JL: CCK antagonists: Pharmacology and therapeutic interest. Pharmacol Ther 62:267–282, 1994.

32. Wiesenfeld-Hallin Z, Xu X-J: The role of cholecystokinin in nociception, neuropathic pain and opiate tolerance. Regul Pept 65:23–28, 1996.

33. Wiesenfeld-Hallin Z, Xu X-J, Hughes J, et al: PD134308, a selective antagonist of cholecystokinin type B receptor, enhances the analgesic effect of morphine and synergistically interacts with intrathecal galanin to depress spinal nociceptive reflexes. Proc Natl Acad Sci U S A 87:7105–7109, 1990.

34. Xu X-J, Alster P, Wu W-P, et al: Increased level of cholecystokinin in cerebrospinal fluid is associated with chronic pain-like behaviour in spinally injured rats. Peptides 22:1305–1308, 2001.

35. Xu X-J, Puke MJ, Verge VM, et al: Up regulation of cholecystokinin in primary sensory neurones is associated with morphine insensitivity in experimental neuropathic pain in the rat. Neurosci Lett 152:129–32, 1993.

36. Zarrindast M-R, Nikfar S, Rezayat M: Cholecystokinin receptor mechanism(s) and morphine tolerance in mice. Pharmacol Toxicol 84:46–50, 1999.

37. Zarrindast M-R, Zabihi A, Rezayat M, et al: Effects of Caerulein and CCK antagonists on tolerance induced to morphine antinociception in mice. Pharmacol Biochem Behav 58:173–178, 1997.

Chapter 23

Miscellaneous Analgesic Agents

Howard S. Smith, MD

TRAMADOL

Tramadol hydrochloride (Ultram) is a centrally acting analgesic that has essentially become a "new class of analgesic." It was first introduced in Germany in 1977. Tramadol HCl, ±*cis*-2-[(dimethylamino) methyl]-1-(3-methoxyphenyl) cyclohexanol hydrochloride, is a racemic mixture with a molecular weight of 299.8, a chemical formula of $C_{16} H_{25} NO_2 HCl$, and a pKa of 9.41 at 23°C. It is a white, crystalline powder that is readily soluble in water and ethanol, with solubility exceeding 200 mg/mL over the pH range of 1 to 8.

PHARMACOKINETICS

Absorption. Tramadol is almost completely absorbed in a rapid fashion (roughly 85%) from the gastrointestinal tract.[1] Tramadol has a strong tissue affinity and a large volume of distribution (based on an average of a 70 kg person). In healthy volunteers, peak plasma tramadol concentrations are attained about 2 hours after ingestion of a 100 mg oral dose.[2] Steady-state plasma concentrations tend to be reached after 2 days of dosing. Administration of tramadol with food does not significantly affect its rate or extent of absorption.[3]

Bioavailability. The bioavailability of oral tramadol is about 75% (showing first-pass metabolism). Bioavailability rises above 90% with multiple dosing, which could be secondary to saturation of first-pass hepatic biotransformation mechanisms.[2] Administration of tramadol with food does not significantly affect its bioavailability.[3]

Distribution. Tramadol is uniformaly distributed diffusely throughout the body (Vol = 2.7 L/Kg for average 70 Kg person). Plasma protein binding of tramadol is low (20.2%) and saturation of binding sites does not occur in the clinically dosing range, suggesting that it does not significantly affect medications that are highly bound to plasma proteins (e.g., warfarin).

Metabolism. After oral administration, tramadol is metabolized primarily by N and O-dethylation (phase I reactions) and conjugation of O-demethylated compounds (phase II reactions).[4] Eleven metabolites have been identified, five from phase I and six from phase II reactions.[4] The formation of many metabolites of tramadol (including M1) is dependent on metabolism via CYP2D6 of the cytochrome p450 family. Of the 11 known metabolites, only M1 exhibits antinociceptive activity in animals.[5]

Excretion. Tramadol and its metabolites are eliminated primarily via renal excretion (90%), with the remainder excreted in the feces.[4] Less than 1% of tramadol and its metabolites is eliminated via biliary excretion. The mean elimination half-life of tramadol is

6.3 hours after a single, oral 100 mg dose and increases to roughly 7 hours after multiple oral doses. The elimination of the M1 metabolite after a single oral dose of tramadol is 7.4 hours.[4]

Mechanism of Action

Tramadol is thought to provide analgesia via at least two mechanisms: Some analgesia may be derived from the relatively weak interaction of tramadol with the μ-opioid receptor. The second and major mechanism, which is thought to account for at least 70% of tramadol's analgesic activity, is via inhibiting the reuptake of norepinephrine and serotonin.[6] Norepinephrine and serotonin reuptake inhibition is roughly two orders of magnitude less than that of the tricyclic antidepressant imipramine.[6] However, these proposed mechanisms still do not seem to fully explain all of tramadol's analgesic actions. In studies with attempts to reverse tramadol-induced analgesia with naloxone, an estimated 30% of the analgesia produced by tramadol was believed to be contributed by effects from its interaction at the μ-opioid receptor.[7] Although some practitioners have considered tramadol to be an opioid or an "atypical opioid," I do not share this belief. There does not appear to be a clear clinical concensus of what defines an opioid medication (for clinical purposes). Therefore, I will attempt to provide a working definition.

Binding to the μ-Opioid Receptor. Clearly, merely binding to the μ, κ, or δ receptors is not enough. To be considered an opioid medication, an agent should bind to and interact with at least one opioid receptor and produce significant analgesia. I propose that, to be considered an opioid medication, an agent must meet these two criteria: (1) At least 50% more of the agent's significant analgesic action should be due to its binding and interaction with an opioid receptor. (This can be estimated by giving naloxone). Note: naloxone will antagonize all three opioid receptors; however, the doses to do this are not equal, μ receptors being the most susceptible to naloxone antagonism. (2) The opioid receptor binding inhibition constant (Ki; in μM) should be less than 1, as it is for traditional opioids such as codeine (0.2), D-propoxyphene (0.034), and morphine (0.00034) (TABLE 1).

TABLE 1

Opioid Receptor Binding Inhibition Constant of Various Analgesic Agents

Compound	$K_1(\mu M)$				
	μ	δ	κ	Norepinephrine	5 Serotonin
($\pm$)Tramadol (Ultram)	2.1	57.6	42.7	0.78	0.99
(+)Tramadol	1.3	62.4	54.0	2.51	0.53
(−)Tramadol	24.8	213	53.5	0.43	2.35
($\pm$)M1	0.0121	0.911	0.242	1.52	5.18
Codeine	0.2	5.1	6.0	IA	IA
Morphine	0.00034	0.092	0.57	IA	IA
D-Propoxyphene	0.034	0.38	1.22	IA	IA
Imipramine	3.7	12.7	1.8	0.0066	0.021

Modified with permission from Raffe RB, Friederichs E, Reimann E, et al: Complementary and synergistic antinociceptive interaction between the enantiomers of tramadol. J Pharmacol Exp Ther 1993;267:331–340.

Tramadol does not meet either of these criteria. In fact, comparing tramadol to imipramine, a tricyclic antidepressant (TCA), tramadol actually looks more like a TCA than an opioid. The Ki of tramadol at the μ-opioid receptor is 2.1 μM versus 3.7 for imipramine (both greater than 1). Looking at the Ki of noreipinephrine and serotonin receptors, both tramadol and imipramine have values less than 1, whereas the opioids codeine, propoxyphene, and morphine are inactive at both these receptors, even at 10 μM. Of course critics may draw attention to the M1 metabolite which does "look like an opioid" by Ki values; however, clinically, M1 may not provide significant analgesia. Inhibition of tramadol metabolism to M1 in humans had no effect on the extent of tramadol-induced analgesia.[8] The contribution of M1 to the analgesic effect of tramadol in humans appears minimal following a single oral dose.[9] After multiple oral doses, the analgesic contribution of M1 is unknown. Enggaard et al presented evidence at the 10th World Congress on Pain suggesting that the opioid-like effect of (+)-M1 appeared to contribute to the acute analgesic effects of tramadol analgesia seems also to be provided by the monoaminergic effect of tramadol itself.[104]

Also, in mice and rats, there appears to be a preferential brain versus plasma distribution of tramadol over M1,[10] which, if present in humans, would go along with the parent compound (tramadol), affecting the descending pain pathways as a significant analgesic mechanism. The binding of tramadol to the μ-opioid receptor is at least 6000-fold less than that of morphine, 60-fold less than that of dextropropoxyphene, and 10-fold less than that of codeine.[9]

Reuptake of Norepinephrine and Serotonin. In laboratory animals, mono-O-desmethyl tramadol (M1; the major active metabolite of tramadol) binds up to 200-fold more potently at the μ-opioid receptor than the parent compound.[11] Also, in laboratory animals, the antinociception produced by M1 is three times more potent than that of the parent compound.[5]

Racemic tramadol is more potent that the theoretical additive effects of the individual enantiomers, thus demonstrating synergistic antinociceptive effects.[12] Enantiomers of tramadol interact less than synergistically regarding adverse effects (e.g., constipation).[12] The weak opioid-like properties of tramadol are largely confined to the (+)enantiomer of tramadol. The (+)enantiomer of tramadol is almost five-fold more potent at inhibiting serotonin reuptake as compared to norepinephrine reuptake; conversely, the (−)enantiomer of tramadol is roughly five- to 10-fold more potent at inhibiting norepinephrine reuptake than serotonin reuptake.[12]

Sagata and colleagues[13] provided evidence that much of tramadol's antinociceptive effects in clinically relevant concentrations is due to inhibition of norepinephrine transporter (NET) function by blocking desipramine-binding sites. NETs located in the presynaptic membranes of noradrenergic nerve terminals regulate neurotransmission by taking up no release into the synaptic cleft.[14] Thus, NET suppression facilitates noradrenergic neurotransmission of the descending inhibitory system of the brain and spinal cord.[15] Bohn and colleagues[16] reported that the tricyclic antidepressant enhanced morphine-induced analgesia in wild-type mice but not in NET knockout mice, suggesting that the antinociceptive effect of desipramine is chiefly due to NET blockade. Additionally, it is conceivable that some of the mechanism of tramadol-induced analgesia is due to effects on acetycholine receptors. Brain muscarinic and nicotinic acetylcholine receptors may play a role in antinociception.[17,18] Tramadol has been shown to suppress the function of nicotinic receptors in cells[19] and M1 muscarinic receptors expressed in *Xenopus laevis* oocytes.[20]

Note: M1 is muscarinic receptor subtype 1 and not a specific receptor for the M1 metabolite of tramadol.

Tramadol is clinically available in the United States only in the oral form. In Europe, the

TABLE 2

Tramadol Dosing Adjustments

Condition	Maximal Daily Dose
Concommittment therapy with Carbamazepine in healthy patients ≤ 75 years old	800 mg
Healthy patient ≤ 75	400 mg
Age > 75	300 mg
Renal insufficiency (creatinine clearance <30 mL/min)	200 mg (q12hr dosing interval)
Hepatic insufficiency	100 mg (q12hr dosing interval)

parenteral form is available, and it has been studied in children using drops.[21] Dosing adjustments are required in patients with advanced age, hepatic disease, or renal disease (TABLE 2).

Apaydin and associates[22] demonstrated the antinociceptive effect of tramadol in a model of neuropathic pain in rats.

Tramadol has been studied in conjunction with local anesthetics for nerve blocks (it blocks nerve conduction with local anesthetic type action),[23] intravenous regional anesthesia,[24] and intravenous (boluses,[25] continuous drip,[25] patient-controlled analgesia[26]) and epidural analgesia.[27] Also, in an animal study, intrathecal tramadol performed exceptionally well as an intrathecal analgesic.[28] The use of patient-controlled analgesia with tramadol plus injectable aspirin (lysine acetyl salicylate) may offer advantages in certain patients and situations.[26]

Adverse Effects

The most common adverse effects with tramadol are nausea and vomiting, constipation, headache, dizziness and lightheadedness, and drowsiness.[29] Adverse effects seem to be dose-related and transient. Tramadol may be much better tolerated with the use of an extremely slow and gradually increasing titration schedule.[30] Unlikely side effects (using appropriate doses) include respiratory depression and a very low risk of seizures.[31,32] Although tramadol may lower the seizure threshold and seizures have occurred in patients on tramadol alone and without apparent other risk factors for seizures, it is extremely unlikely to lead to seizures by itself. Tramadol may enhance the seizure risk in patients taking monoamine oxidase inhibitors, neuroleptics, or other drugs that lower the seizure threshold, in patients with epilepsy, or in patients otherwise at increased risk for seizure. When used concurrently with tricyclic antidepressants (agents that may lower the seizure threshold), there is also an increased risk of seizure, however, this seems to be commonly done in clinical practice without a significant problem. Adding a selective serotonin reuptake inhibitor to a tricyclic antidepressant and tramadol may also lead to an increased risk of seizures. Patients taking this combination of drugs should be followed carefully, although the risk even in this situation is not high. The antidepressant that may pose the most increased risk of seizure in patients already on tramadol is bupropion (Wellbutrin), which is also used as an adjunct for smoking cessation.

The development of tolerance to analgesia may be lower with tramadol than with opioids. The "abuse potential" of tramadol has continued to be a controversial topic. In vivo microdialysis measures demonstrating release of dopamine within the nucleus accumbens shell (which may contribute to the "rewarding" properties of tramadol), together with the results of conditioned place preference studies, both performed in rats, are consistent with an abuse potential to tramadol.[33] There is no question that tramadol can lead to physical dependence (withdrawal symptoms may occur if it is discontinued abruptly) as well as psychological dependence or addiction, even in the absence of a history of substance abuse.[24] This information is clearly written in the approved product label, which was revised in August 2001 to state that dependence and abuse, including drug-seeking behavior and taking illicit actions to obtain tramadol, are not limited to patients with a prior history of opioid dependence. The current product label also states that tramadol is not recommended for patients with a history of drug abuse or dependence, as these patients are at high risk for abuse or dependence with tramadol.

Brinker and coworkers,[35] who work at the Food and Drug Administration's MedWatch database of adverse event reports, state that the Food and Drug Administration has received 912 domestic adverse-event reports from March 1995 through June 2001, classified under the coding terms "drug dependence" (426), "drug withdrawal" (407), or "drug abuse" (241) in association with tramadol (the sum exceeds 912, since a report may have included more than one adverse event coding term). However, most of these reports include a history of drug or substance abuse, and clinicians may not have appreciated the phenomenon of pseudotolerance in some other cases.

The World Health Organization Expert Committee on Drug Dependence (32nd report) recommend a critical review for tramadol and four other agents at a future meeting.[36] Cicero and coworkers[37] reported the results of a post-marketing surveillance program to monitor tramadol abuse in the United States. Rates of tramadol abuse or dependence were roughly 2 per 100,000 patients exposed the first year after launch and, since early 1996, have been less than 0.75 per 100,000 patients. Ninety-seven percent of cases of tramadol abuse and dependence involved patients with histories of alcohol and drug abuse. Sustained exclusive use of tramadol to produce intoxication was rare.

Overall, considering the enormous widespread use of tramadol and relative ease of access, it seems that the "true" incidence of psychological dependence on or addiction to tramadol by the Diagnostic and Statistical Manual of Mental Disorders (DSM-IV) criteria in patients without histories of alcohol or drug abuse, although unknown, is low. Therefore, clinicians should be aware that abuse is a possibility with tramadol use (even in a patient without a history of substance abuse), but they certainly should not be concerned in the least about writing appropriate prescriptions for appropriate patients as long as they continue to monitor their patients using sound medical doctrines and judgement.

Drug Interactions

The use of tramadol in patients receiving monoamine oxidase inhibitors should be avoided. Concurrent therapy of cimetidine with tramadol caused a statistically significant decrease in total body clearance (14% versus 22%) of tramadol as well as significant increases in the area under the serum concentration versus time curve (AUC) (15% to 27%) and terminal elimination half-life (up to 19%). However, since these changes are not considered clinically significant, no dosage adjustment is recommended. Concurrent therapy of carbamazepine and tramadol seems to result in significant reductions in maximum concentration (C_{max}) (49%), AUC (74%) and terminal elimination half-life (46%) of tramadol. The decreased plasma concentration of tramadol is thought to be the result of increased metabolism secondary to enzyme induction. Coagulation parameters, although usually reasonably stable, should probably be monitored when tramadol is administered to patients on oral anticoagulants.

Clinical Aspects

Although tramadol seems to be a broad-spectrum analgesic and has been used for treating diabetic neuropathy, fibromyalgia, and so on, it seems particularly useful in treating musculoskeletal pain.[38] Additionally, tramadol may be useful in the perioperative period at wound closure to prevent postanesthetic shivering,[39] which, aside from being quite uncomfortable, can increase oxygen consumption 300% to 400%, an unwanted occurrence in patients with diminished cardiopulmonary reserves. Tramadol in doses of 0.75 mg/kg and 1.0 mg/kg IV does not affect intracranial pressure or cerebral perfusion pressure in adult postcraniotomy patients and seems to be a safe and effective analgesic at a dose of 1.0 mg/kg for postcraniotomy pain control.[40]

Other differences in tramadol versus traditional opioids may include relatively less effect on biliary system pressure or the sphincter of Oddi, less respiratory depressant activity, less itching, less tolerance, and a stimulatory effect on natural killer cells, perhaps mediated through serotonergic mechanisms.[41]

The analgesic efficacy of tramadol may be impaired by concurrent administration of ondansetron.[42,43] Raffa[44] has outlined the potential rationale for the use of combination analgesics, which includes multiple sites of action targeting multiple pain pathways, complementary pharmacokinetic activity, and synergistic analgesic effects leading to reduced adverse event profile with comparable efficacy.

Tramadol and acetaminophen (as well as probably traditional nonsteroidal antiinflammatory drugs [NSAIDs] show synergy in animals studies.[45] A tramadol/acetaminophen combination product (Ultracet) is currently available in the United States.[46–48]

With few exceptions, N-oxides of most centrally acting analgesics (e.g., opioids) have little or no analgesic activity. One exception, tramadol N-oxide, appears to produce dose-related antinociception, probably by acting as a prodrug for tramadol.[49] A longer duration of action, fewer side effects, and less toxicity, possibly because of a blunted plasma spike, are two potential advantages of tramadol N-oxide over tramadol.

A long-acting formulation of tramadol may be available in the future.[50]

MEXILETINE

Mexiletine (Mexitil) is an "oral" antiarrhythmic analog of lidocaine that has been structurally modified to reduce first-pass hepatic metabolism and enable chronic oral therapy to achieve efficacy. It has electrophyiological properties similar to those of lidocaine, and, as with lidocaine, the side effects of mexilitine are predominantly gastrointestinal and central nervous system (CNS) effects. The bioavailability after oral administration is relatively high (> 80%), and the elimination half-life is roughly 9 to 15 hours. The dose for a healthy adult can be started at 150 mg PO tid, and the drug should be taken with meals. Tremor and nausea are the major dose-related adverse affects and are usually minimized by taking the medication with food. The use of mexilitine in patients with significant preexisting tremor should be avoided if possible. A baseline electrocardiogram (ECG) should be obtained, although at low doses mexiletine generally does not have significant electrophysiologic effects.

Mexiletine undergoes hepatic metabolism, which is inducible by phenytoin and various other drugs. Galer and colleagues[51] suggested that a positive response to intravenous lidocaine (e.g., diminished pain) indicates patients who might benefit from analgesic effects of mexilitine. Backonja[52] has highlighted five randomized placebo-controlled trials of mexilitine in the literature, four involving painful diabetic neuropathy,[53–56] and one involving central pain from spinal cord injury.[57] Oskarsson and associates,[55] in a relatively large study, showed no effect of mexilitine for painful diabetic neuropathy. The primary outcome assessed global pain with a visual analog scale, using a parallel design. However, there was relief of burning and stabbing pain, heat sensation, and formication.[55,52] Two studies with a smaller number of patients[56,57] as well as other studies are essentially negative (NNY=10).[52]

In spite of these findings, anectodotal cases, and criticisms of the design of the mentioned studies (e.g., using predetermined dose and pushing the dose high enough to side effects of efficacy), clinicians continue to use mexilitine for selected clinical circumstances.

NEUROLEPTICS

Phenothiazine neuroleptics, and possibly some other neuroleptic agents, may be analgesic (e.g., chlorpromazine, fluphenazine, perphenazine, trifluoperazine, methotrimeprazine [L-mepromazine]). The analgesic effects of parenteral methotrimeprazine are better established than those of oral neuroleptics, for which there is a dearth of well-controlled evidence.[58]

MUSCLE RELAXANTS

"Muscle relaxants" are clinically considered to encompass a wide variety of heterogeneous agents, which are used with the intent to diminish heightened muscular tone and are often employed in pharmacological approaches to the treatment of chronic musculoskeletal pain.[59] Most "muscle relaxants" (not to be confused with nondepolarizing or depolarizing muscle relaxants, which produce neuromuscular blockade with resultant paralysis, including respiratory muscles) do not possess specific direct muscle relaxation properties but rather are thought to work through general CNS depressant activities (TABLE 3). Most are for short-term

TABLE 3

Standard Drugs Used for Musculosketal Conditions

Drug	Dose	Frequency Reported Side Effects
Baclofen	PO: Initial dose 5 mg tid. May increase every 3 days up to 40–80 mg/daily	Drowsiness, psychiatric disturbances, urinary frequency, retention, constipation, vomiting, hypersensitivity reactions
Carisoprodol	PO: 350 mg tid-qid	Drowsiness, dizziness, ataxia, tremor, gastrointestinal upset
Cyclobenzaprine	PO: 10 mg tid	Drowsiness, dry mouth, dizziness
Diazepam (benzodiazepine)	PO: 2–10 mg bid-tid	Drowsiness, sedation, dizziness
Metaxolone	PO: 400–800 mg tid-qid	Drowsiness, dizziness, nausea
Methocarbamol	PO: 750–1500 mg qid for 2–3 days IV/IM: 1 g, may repeat every 8 hours for maximum of 3 days	Drowsiness, dizziness, gastrointestinal upset
Orphenadrine citrate	PO: 100 mg bid IV/IM: 60 mg q12 hrs	Anticholinergic affects, restlessness, agitation
Tizanidine	PO: Initial dose 2 mg qhs; may titrate slowly up to 8 mg tid	Dry mouth, dizziness, fatigue, possible hypotension

Modified with permission from Smith HS, Barton AE: Pharmaceutical update: Tizanidine in the management of spasticity and musculoskeletal complaints in the palliative care population. Am J Hospic Palliat Care 2000;17:50–58.

use and, although used clinically for the treatment of chronic musculoskeletal pain, have no specific antinociceptive qualities. Exceptions to this are baclofen and tizanidine, agents that can be used on a chronic basis and seem to possess specific antinociceptive qualities. It remains to be seen whether orphenadrine may also be among these agents.

Muscle cramps, spasms, and stiffness are distinct from spasticity and can have numerous causes including abnormalities of lower motor neurons and spinal inhibitor mechanisms, abnormalities of the sarcolemma of muscle fibers or of the intrinsic muscle fiber conducting system (e.g., volleys of impulses across neuromuscular junctions), and abnormalities of muscle relaxation (e.g., inability to relax, partial relaxation, delayed or slowed relaxation). Abnormalities of any structural or functional component of the neuromuscular junction and sarcomere may contribute to muscular symptoms.[60]

Glycine and γ-aminobutyric acid (GABA) are the neurotransmitters for the two major spinal inhibitory systems and seem to function tonically as one in the modulation of low threshold mechanical input.[61] Removal of either of these systems may lead to an allodynic state; however, the simultaneous removal of both system appears to induce a synergistic allodynia.[61]

Baclofen

Baclofen (Lioresal) is the p-chlorophenyl derivative of GABA. Baclofen is a GABA-B agonist that has been used for muscle spasms and spasticity, neuropathic pain, and so on. Baclofen may enhance the effectiveness of antiepileptic drugs in certain neuropathic pain states. Side effects include sedation, weakness, and confusion. Abrupt cessation may cause a withdrawal syndrome, such as hallucinations, anxiety, tachycardia, or seizures.

Baclofen may not be very well tolerated in elderly patients, but it certainly can be given a trial. The initial dose in an elderly patient should probably be 5 mg orally twice a day. Peak serum concerntrations occur within 3 to 8 hours after oral ingestion. The half-life of baclofen is about 4 hours. It is excreted by the kidney and should not be used in patients with renal failure. The usual initial adult dose is 10 mg orally, three times a day, and generally 80 mg/day is considered a maximum dose for routine clinical use. However, some clinicians will go much higher for cases of refractory spasticity.[60]

Baclofen has both presynaptic and post-synaptic actions. At the presynaptic site, baclofen decreases calcium conduction with resultant decreased excitatory amino acid release. At the post-synaptic site, baclofen increases potassium conductance, leading to neuronal hyperpolarization. Additionally, baclofen may inhibit the release of substance P. Use of baclofen appears to lead to marked facilitation of segmental inhibition.

Steardo and coworkers,[62] in an open-label study of 16 patients, concluded that baclofen was effective for trigeminal neuralgia. Fromm and coworkers[63] reported a pilot study of 10 patients with paroxysms of trigeminal neuralgia who were followed for 1 year. Seven patients were pain free to almost pain free with a dose of 60 to 80 mg per day. Fromm and coworkers compared baclofen and carbamazepine in 10 patients with a double-blind protocol and with 50 patients in an open-label study design. They found that carbamazepine was more effective than baclofen alone.[63] Additionally, when baclofen was combined with phenytoin, it was more effective than by itself. The combination of baclofen and carbamazepine yielded the greatest efficacy. This finding suggested synergism between baclofen and carbamazepine.

Baclofen is a racemic mixture, with L-baclofen being the active form.[64] Terrence and colleagues[65] found that L-baclofen may antagonize the actions of L-baclofen; therefore, "pure" L-baclofen may be more advantageous than the racemate. Fromm and Terrence[66] compared

L-baclofen to racemic baclofen in 15 patients in a double-blind cross-over study. L-Baclofen was more effective in nine patients, six of whom remained pain free 4 to 17 months; (mean, 10 months) later. L-Baclofen was also better tolerated. They concluded that L-baclofen was significantly better than racemic baclofen in the treatment of trigeminal neuralgia.

Future studies could be undertaken to study whether the combination of oxcarbazepine and L-baclofen yields potential therapeutic benefits in certain patients with intractable trigeminal neuralgia.

The precise mechanisms by which baclofen produces skeletal muscle relaxation are unknown but may involve its activity at both pre- and post-synaptic GABA-B receptors, which diminishes neurotransmitter release from presynaptic terminals.

Mann-Metzer and Yarom[67] concluded that both the pre- and post-synaptic effects of baclofen are mediated by GABA-B receptors that decrease calcium currents. This contrasts with old tenets that presynaptic receptor effects involved calcium currents and post-synaptic receptor effects involved potassium currents. Baclofen has convincingly demonstrated antinociceptive properties in animal neuropathic pain models.[68]

Baclofen can be used orally or via an implantable intrathecal pump. Baclofen is renally excreted as the parent drug; therefore, dosage reductions may be necessary in patients with impaired renal function.

In addition to its effects on spasticity and as a "muscle relaxant," in which it has been used orally for chronic low back pain and muscular spasms and intrathecally for conditions that may exhibit refractory spasticity (e.g., multiple sclerosis),[69] baclofen has been used for various chronic pain states, including orally for trigeminal neuralgia,[70] atypical facial pain and cluster headaches,[71] and intrathecally for complex regional pain syndrome type I.[72] Additionally, other potential uses seem to be growing: the presence of GABA and its receptor, GABA-B, suggests that this system may be relevant in the production or management of endodontic pain.[73]

An underappreciated potential use of baclofen is as a therapeutic agent for the management of gastroesophageal reflux disease (GERD).[74] It could be employed as an adjunct for patients with poorly controlled GERD, as single-agent therapy, or for patients with spasticity and musculoskeletal conditions and significant GERD.

Benzodiazepines

The benzodiazepines are commonly used in the treatment of spasticity associated with spinal cord injury. These agents work by binding to specific benzodiazepine receptors located on the terminals of primary afferent fibers. This binding increases the flux of chloride across the terminal membrane, resulting in an increase in membrane potential. Typically, longer acting benzodiazepines, such as diazepam and clonazepam, are used to control spastic symptoms.[75-77] The benzodiazepines may be effective as alternative or adjunctive agents but cause significant sedation and are associated with problematic withdrawal syndrome. Unlike various other benzodiazepines, clonazepam may possess analgesic qualities in certain chronic pain conditions not associated with muscle spasm/spasticity. In most clinical situations, clonazepam and baclofen should not be used together, as they are both GABA-B agonists.

Botulinum Toxin

Efforts to directly "relax" tight or spastic muscle has led to attempts to dampen the synaptic release of acetylcholine, thereby inducing a state of "relaxation" or "flaccid paralysis."

Botulinum toxins, by affecting the exocytosis of acetylcholine-containing vesicles, seem to be able to accomplish this. The processes involved in vesicle exocytosis have begun to be elucidated.

As the vesicle fuses to the membrane, it forms helical "coils." The proposed process is a zippering process,[78] in which the coil from VAMP (associated with the vesicle) lies parallel to the other coils and membrane immediately adjacent to the synaptosome-associated protein (SNAP)-25 coils, which also lie parallel to and immediately adjacent to the syntaxin coil, which lies parallel to and immediately adjacent to the membrane. This docking "helical sandwich" (as I refer to it) then eventually contributes (as the SNARE [soluble N-ethylmaleimide-sensitive-factor attachment protein receptor] complex) to veiscle fusion and exocytosis.

The role of botulinum toxin (BTX) can be appreciated by understanding the events associated with the release of acetylcholine into the synapse. The BTX heavy chain binds to the presynaptic terminal and is internalized along with the light chain. The BTX light chain acts as a zinc endopeptidase and is the active part interfering with acetylcholine release.

There are at least seven antigenically distinct BTX neurotoxins. BTX-A acts predominantly at the SNAP, where BTX-B appears to act primarily at the VAMP/synaptobrevin site. BTX-C is thought to act primarily at syntaxin and the SNAP.

The two clinically available botulinum toxins in the United States are botulinum toxin type A (Botox) and botulinum toxin type B (Myobloc) (Elan San Diego, CA, US) [In Europe it is marketed as Neurobloc]. A different formulation of botulinum toxin A known as Dysport is used in Europe as well as a version used in China (Lanzhou Biological Products Institute) but are currently not available in the United States. Effects seem to last for roughly 3 to 6 months after injection, at which point a repeat injection generally reproduces the effects. Botulinum toxins are beginning to be used for more and more chronic pain states (in addition to painful conditions, e.g. cervical dystonia), including chronic headaches, low back pain, abdominal pain secondary to sphincter of Oddi dysfunction and so on. The mechanism of botulinum toxin-induced analgesia remains elusive.

Botulinum Toxin–Induced Analgesia

Although it is generally accepted that botulinum toxins may lead to diminished pain in patients with painful muscle spasm or cervical dystonia by diminishing muscle tone, it is also felt that botulinum toxin may itself possess analgesic properties. The mechanisms of botulinum toxin-induced analgesia are unknown.

The most evident mechanisms of botulinum toxin–induced analgesia are via reduction of muscle spasm by cholinergic chemodenervation at motor end plates and by inhiition of gamma motor endings in muscle spindles.[79]

It is conceivable that subcutaneous injection of botulinum toxins may contribute to antinociception by inhibition of local neurotransmitter release from primary sensory neurons in the area of the injection.[80]

Future uses of botulinum toxins for analgesia may lead to redesigned toxins for intrathecal use. Conjugating erythrina cristagallu lectin (ELC), a protein with high affinity for the carbohydrate moieties, on nociceptive fibers (C and A deltas) to a fragment of botulinum toxin A lacking the binding domain (LHn/A) resulted in a novel analgesic that displayed long-lasting analgesic properties when administered intrathecally.[80] Since this new conjugate retained its endopeptidase activity, a significant possible mechanism of action for analgesia could be inhibition of neurotransmitter release by inhibition of exocytosis via interference with the SNARE complex (cleaving SNAP-25).

Murakami and coworkers[81] have proposed various antiepileptic drugs (e.g., carbamazepine, valproate, zonisamide) that may affect the SNARE complex and therefore various exocytosis processes.[81]

Carisoprodol

Carisoprodol may be useful for the short-term treatment of acute musculoskeletal disorders, especially in combination with acetaminophen, aspirin, or NSAIDs. Carisoprodol (Soma) is primarily metabolized in the liver to several metabolites, including meprobamate. This metabolic conversion, although relatively small, has been postulated to be the reason that carisorpodol may have abuse potential.[82–85] The formation of meprobamate from carisoprodol is by N-dealkylation via CYP2C19.[86] Poor metabolizers of mephenytoin have a diminished ability to metabolize carisoprodol and therefore may be at increased risk of developing concentration-dependent side effects (e.g., drowsiness, hypotension, CNS depression) at "usual" adult doses.[86]

Davis and Alexander,[87] in a retrospective study of 24 deaths with the presence of carisoprodol detected at autopsy, concluded that carisoprodol may cause significant respiratory depression and that the simultaneous use of propoxyphene and carisoprodol may be especially dangerous. (It would have been interesting to know if any of these 24 people were poor metabolizers of mephenytoin).

Although the precise mechanisms of action of carisoprodol (as well as meprobamate) are uncertain, one theory is that they act as indirect agonists at the GABA-A receptor, yielding CNS chloride ion channel conduction effects similar to benzodiazepines. Therefore, flumazenil may be a potentially useful antidote to carisoprodol toxicity.[88]

Cyclobenzaprine

Cyclobenzaprine (Flexeril) is structurally similar to TCAs and, as such, demonstrates significant anticholinergic side effects. It differs from amitriptyline by only one double bond.[89] Additionally, if musculoskeletal doses are exceeded, cyclobenzaprine exhibits a side-effect profile similar to that of the TCAs, including lethargy and agitation, although it usually does not appear to produce significant dysrhythmias beyond sinus tachycardia. It is generally used for musculoskeletal conditions, including fibromyalgia[90] and low back pain.[91] Cyclobenzaprine is best used in short-term treatment but may be used intermittently for chronic pain.[58]

Elderly patients seem to tolerate cyclobenzaprine less well and may develop hallucinations[92] as well as significant anticholinergic side effects, such as sedation. The use of significant lower dosing schedules in elderly patients may be prudent.[93]

Metaxolone

Metaxolone (Skelaxin) is an oxazolidone derivative that is useful for the acute management of peripheral musculoskeletal complaints but is not very effective in the treatment of spasticity related to neurological disorders.[94] Although the benefit of this agent in the treatment acute musculoskeletal syndromes may be related to its sedative effects, it seems to be well tolerated and offers a reasonable therapeutic option for a wide variety of musculoske-tal complaints.

Methocarbamol

Methocarbamol (Robaxin) is a carbamate derivative of guaifenisin. This agent is available both orally and parenterally and is indicated for the short-term management of muscu-loskeletal conditions. Schneider[95] reported on the use of intraoperative and postoperative methocarbamol providing significant analgesia for 62 patients undergoing manipulation of the pectoralis major muscle associated with breast implant surgery.

Orphenadrine

Orphenadrine citrate, a monomethylated derivative of diphenhydramine, has been used by clinicians as a "muscle relaxant" and seems to possess analgesic qualities as well.[96–98] Al-though peripheral H_1 and H_2 receptor antagonists do not appear to be analgesic, centrally acting antihistamines may be.[99] The analgesic mechanisms of orphenadrine may be multi-factorial, and modulation of the raphe-spinal serotonergic systems may contribute.[100]

Orphenadrine (Norflex) may exhibit characteristics of a noncompetitive N-methyl-D-asparate type of glutamate antagonist.[98] In addition to its use alone, orphenadrine has been used with acetaminophen, aspirin, and NSAIDs. During a post-marketing surveillance study, 641 patients with painful musculoskeletal conditions were treated with a parenteral combination infusion of diclofenac (75 mg) and orphenadrine (30 mg) for 7 days (neither the parenteral formulation of diclofenac nor the combination is available in the United States).[101] The global evaluation at the end of treatment on a scale of 1 (very good) to 4 (insufficient) was 1.6, the tolerability score was 1.3, and the acceptability score was 1.5, with 3.1% of patients noting adverse effects (pre-dominantly gastrointestinal).[101] Adverse effects associated with this agent are mainly related to its anticholinergic action (dry mouth, blurred vision, urinary retention, and constipation). This agent is available orally as well as parenterally. (see Table 3 for doses)

Tizanidine

Tizanidine (Zanaflex) is an imidazoline derivative that is structurally related to clonidine. Ti-zanidine's action is primarily derived from agonism at the α_2-adrenoreceptor. This activity results in direct inhibition of excitatory release of amino acids and a concomitant inhibition of facilitory coeruleospinal pathways.[102] Reduction in spasticity produced by tizanidine is believed to be mediated presynaptically in the spinal cord.[103] Ultimately, reduction of sym-pathetic outflow reduces facilitation of spinal motor neurons and produces a myotonolytic effect.[60]

After oral administration, the bioavailability of tizanidine is estimated to be 21%, secondary to extensive first-pass metabolism by the liver.[60] Peak plasma concentrations following an 8 mg dose are generally achieved 1.5 hours after administration.[60] The elimination half-life is reported to range between 1.2 and 3 hours.[60] Tizanidine exhibits linear pharmacokinetics over a dose range of 10 to 20 mg. This agent does not exhibit extensive protein-binding properties. Approximately 30% of the total serum concentration of this agent is bound to plasma proteins and blood cells.[60] Metabolism of tizanidine occurs primarily in the liver through oxidative processes, and metabolites of the parent compound have no known pharmacological activity. Excretion of tizanidine and its metabolites occurs primarily via the kidneys (53–66%).[60]

REFERENCES FOR ADDITIONAL READING

1. Lintz W, Barth H, Osterloh G, et al: Bioavailability of enteral tramadol formulations. First communication: capsules. Arzneimitt Forsch Drug Res 1986;36:1278–1283.

2. Liao S, Hill JF, Nayak RK: Pharmacokinetics of tramadol following single and multiple oral doses in man [abstract]. Pharm Res 1992;9(suppl 10):S–308.

3. Liao S, Hills J, Stubbs RJ, et al: The effect of food on the bioavailability of tramadol [abstract]. Pharm Res 1992;9(suppl 10):S–308.

4. Lintz W, Erlacin S, Frankus E, et al: Biotransformation of tramadol in man and animal: Arzneimitt Forsch Drug Res 1981;31:1932–1943.

5. Hennies H-H, Friderichs E, Schneider J: Receptor binding, analgesic and antitussive potency of tramadol and other selective opioids. Arzneimitt Forsch Drug Res 1988;38:877–880.

6. Raffa RB, Friderichs E, Reimann E, et al: Opioid and nonopioid components independently contribute to the mechanism of action of tramadol, an "atypical" opioid analgesic. J Pharmacol Exp Ther 1992;260:275–285.

7. Collart L, Luthy C, Dayer P: Partial inhibition of tramadol antinociceptive effect by naloxone in man [abstract]. Br J Clin Pharmacol. 1993;35:73P.

8. Collart L, Luthy C, Dayer P: Multimodal analgesic effect of tramadol [abstract]. Clin Pharmacol Ther 1993;53:223.

9. Collart L, Luthy C, Dayer P: Tramadol concentration-effect relationship [abstract]. Clin Pharmacol Ther 1994;55:208.

10. Tao Q, Stone DJ, Borenstein MR, et al: Differential tramadol and O-desmethyl metabolite levels in brain vs. plasma of mice and rats administered tramadol hydrochloride orally. J Clin Pharm Ther 2002; 27:99–106.

11. Codd EE, Raffa RB, Shank RP, Vaught JL: Opioid and nonopioid activity of the analgesic tramadol and its major metabolite mono-O-desmethyltramado. Abstract presented at FASEB/International Narcotics Research Conference, June 30–July 5, 1991; Copper Mountain, CO.

12. Raffa RB, Friederichs E, Reimann E, et al: Complementary and synergistic antinociceptive interaction between the enantiomers of tramadol. J Pharmacol Exp Ther 1993;267:331–340.

13. Sagata K, Minami K, Yanagihara N, et al: Tramadol inhibits norepinephrine transporter function at desipramine-binding sites in cultured bovine adrenal medullary cells. Anesth Analg 2002;94:901–906.

14. Barker EL, Blakely RD: Norepinephrine and serotonin transporters. In: Bloom FE, Kupfer DJ, eds. Psychopharmacology, 4th ed. New York, Raven Press, 1995:321–333.

15. Monks R, Merskey H: Psychotropic drugs. In: Wall PD, Melzack R, eds. Textbook of Pain, 4th ed. Edinburgh, Churchill Livingstone, 1999:1155–1186.

16. Bohn LM, Xu F, Gainetdinov RR, et al: Potentiated opioid analgesia in norepinephrine transporter knock-out mice. J Neurosci 2000;20:9040–9045.

17. Naguib M, Yaksh TL: Characterization of muscarinic receptor subtypes that mediate antinociception in the rat spinal cord. Anesth Anal 1997;85:847–853.

18. Picciotto MR, Caldarone BJ, King SL, et al: Nicotinic receptors in the brain: Links between molecular biology and behavior. Neuropsychopharmacology 2000;22:451–465.

19. Shiraishi M, Minami K, Yanagihara N, et al: Inhibitory effects of tramadol on nicotinic acetylcholine receptors in cultured bovine adrenal chromaffin cells [abstract]. Anesthesiology 2001;95:A706.

20. Shiraishi M, Minami K, Uezono Y, et al: Inhibition by tramadol of muscarinic receptor-induced responses in cultured adrenal medullary cells and in Xenopus laevis oocytes expressing cloned M1 receptors. J Pharmacol Exp Ther 2001;299:255–260.

21. Payne KA, Roleofse JA: Tramadol drops in children: Analgesic efficacy, lack of respirator effects, and normal recovery times. Anesth Prog 1999;46:91–96.

22. Apaydin S, Uyar M, Karabay N, et al: The antinociceptive effect of tramadol on a model of neuropathic pain in rats. Life-Sci 2000; 66:167–137.

23. Mert T, Gunes Y, Guven M, et al: Comparison of nerve conduction blocks by an opioid and a local anesthetic. Eur J Pharmacol 2002;439:77–81.

24. Acalovschi I, Cristea T, Margarit S, et al: Tramadol added to lidocaine for intravenous regional anesthesia. Anesth Analg 2001; 92:209–214.

25. Rud U, Fischer MV, Mewes R, et al: Postoperative analgesia with tramadol: Continuous infusion versus repetitive bolus administration. Anaesthesist 1994; 43:316–321.

26. Pany E-E, Huang S, Tung C-C, et al: Patient-controlled analgesia with tramadol versus tramadol plus lysine acetyl salicylate. Anesthe Analg 2000;91:1226–1229.

27. Vercauteren M, Vereecken K, La Malfa M, et al: Cost-effectiveness of analgesia after caesarean section: A comparison of intrathecal morphine and epidural PCA. Acta Anaesthesiol Scand 2002;46: 85–89.

28. Dhasmana KM, Banerjee AK, Rating W, et al: Analgesic effect of tramadol in the rat. Zhongguo Yao Li Xue Bao 1989;10:289–293.

29. Edwards JE, McQuay HJ, Moore RA: Combination analgesic efficacy: Individual patient data meta-analysis of single-dose oral tramadol plus acetaminophen in acute postoperative pain. J Pain Symptom Manage 2002;23:121–130.

30. Petrone PD, Kamin M, Olson W: Slowing the titration rate of tramadol HCl reduces the incidence of discontinuation due to nausea and/or vomiting: A double-blind randomized trial: J Clin Pharmacol Ther 1999;24:115–123.

31. Gassa C, Derby L, Vasilakis-Scaramozza C, et al: Incidence of first-time seizures in users of tramadol. Pharmacotherapy 2000;20:629–634.

32. Gardiner JS, Blough D, Drinkard CR, et al: Tramadol and seizures: Surveillance study in a managed care population. Pharmacotherapy 2000;20:1423–1431.

33. Sprague JE, Leifheit M, Selken J, et al: In vivo microdialysis and conditioned place preference studies in rats are consistent with abuse potential of tramadol. Synapse 2002;43:118–121.

34. Yates WR, Nguyen MH, Warnock JK: Tramadol dependence with no history of substance abuse [letter]. Am J Psychiatry 2001:158:964.

35. Brinker A, Bonnel RA, Beitz J: Abuse, dependence, or withdrawl associated with tramadol. Am J Psychiatry 2002;159:881.

36. WHO Expert Committee on Drug Dependence: Thirty-second report. World Health Organ Tech Rep Ser 2001;903:i–v, 1–26.

37. Cicero TJ, Adams EH, Geller A, et al: A post marketing surveillance program to monitor Ultram (tramadol hydrochloride) abuse in the United States. Drug Alcohol Depend 1999;57:7–22.

38. Reig E: Tramadol in musculoskeletal pain: a survey. Clin Rheumatol 2002;21(Suppl 1):S9–12.

39. Mathews A, Al Mulla A, Varghese PK, et al: Postanesthetic shivering: A new look at tramadol. Anaesthesia. 2002;57:394–398.

40. Ferber J, Juniewicz H, Glogowska E, et al: Tramadol for postoperative analgesia in intracranial surgery: Its effect on ICP and CPP. Neurol Neurochir Pol. 2000;34:70–79.

41. Sacerdote P, Bianchi M, Gaspani L, et al: The effects of tramadol and morphine on immune responses and pain after surgery in cancer patients. Anesth Analg 2000;90:1411–1414.

42. De Witte JL, Schoenmaekers B, Sessler DI, et al: The analgesic efficacy of tramadol is impaired by concurrent administration of ondansetron. Anesth Analg 2001:92:1319–1321.

43. Arciono R, della Rocca M, Romano S, et al: Ondansetron inhibits the analgesic effect of tramadol: A possible 5-HT3 spinal receptor involvement in acute pain in humans. Anesth Analg 2002;94: 1553–1557.

44. Raffa RN: Pharmacology of oral combination analgesics: Rational therapy for pain. J Clin Pharmacol Ther 2001;26:257–264.

45. Tallarida RJ, Radda RB: Testing for synergism over a range of fixed ration drug combinations: Replacing the isobologram. Life Sci 1996;58:PL23–28.

46. Medve RM, Wang J, Karim: Tramadol and acetaminophen tablets for dental pain. Anest Prog 2001; 48:79–81.

47. Silverfield JC, Kamin M, Wu SC, et al: Tramadol/acetaminophen combination tablets for the treatment of osteoarthritis flare pain: Multicenter, outpatient, randomized, double-blind, placebo-controlled, parallel-group, add-on study. Clin Ther 2002;24:282–297.

48. Mullican WS, Lacy JR: Tramadol/acetaminophen combination tablets and codeine/acetaminophen combination capsules for the management of chronic pain: A comparative trial: Clin Ther 2001; 23:1429–1445.

49. Raffa RB, Haslego ML, Maryanoff CA, et al: Unexpected antinociceptive effect of the N-oxide (RWJ 38705) of tramadol hydrochloride. J Pharmacol Exp Ther 1996;278:1098–1104.

50. Petzke F, Radbruch L, Sabatowski R, et al: Slow-release tramadol for treatment of chronic malignant pain: An open multicenter trial. Support Care Cancer 2001;9:48–54.

51. Galer BS, Harle J, Rowbotham MC: Response to intravenous lidocaine infusion—a new subsequent response to oral mexiletine: A prosoective study. J Pain Symptom Manage 1996:12:161–167.

52. Bacjonja M: Anticonvulsants and antiarrhythmics in the treatment of neuropathic pain syndromes. In: Hansson PT, Fields HL, Hill RG, Marchettini P, eds. Neuropathic Pain: Pathophysiology and Treatment, Progress in Pain Research and Management, vol. 21. Seattle, IASP Press, 2001.

53. Dejgard A, Petersen P, Kastrup J: Mexiletine for treatment of chronic painful diabetic neuropathy. Lancet 1988;1:9–11.

54. Stracke H, Meyer UE, Schumacher HE, Federlin K: Mexiletine in the treatment of diabetic neuropathy. Diabetes Care 1993;15:1550–1555.

55. Oskarsson P, Ljunggren JG, Lins PE: Efficacy and safety of mexiletine in the treatment of painful diabetic neuropathy. The Meciletine Study Group. Diabetic Care 1997;20:1594–1597.

56. Wright JM, Oki JC, Graves L: Mexiletine in the symptomatic treatment of diabetic peripheral neuropathy. Ann Pharmacother 1997;31:29–34.

57. Chiou-Tan FY, Tuel SM, Johnson JC, et al: Effect of mexiletine on spinal cord injury dysesthetic pain. Am J Phys Med Rehabil 1996:75:84–87

58. Merskey H: Pharmacological approaches other than opioids in chronic non-cancer pain management. Acta Anaesthesiol Scand 1997;41:187–190.

59. Moulin DE: Systemic drug treatment for chronic musculoskeletal pain. Clin J Pain 2001;17 (4 Suppl):S86–93.

60. Smith HS, Barton AE: Pharmaceutical update: Tizanidine in the management of spasticity and musculoskeletal complaints in the palliative care population. Am J Hosp Palliat Care 2000;17:50–58.

61. Loomis CW, Khandwala H, Osmond G, et al: Coadministration of ontrathecal strychnine and bicuculline effects synergistic allodynia in the rat: An isobolographic analysis. J Pharmacol Exp Ther 2001;296:756–761.

62. Steardo L, Leo A, Marano E: Efficacy of baclofen in trigeminal neuralgia and some other painful conditions. Eur Neurol 1984;23:51–55.

63. Fromm GH, Terrence CF, Chattha AS, et al: Baclofen in trigeminal neuralgia: Its effect on the spinal trigeminal nucleus—a pilot study. Arch Neurol 1980;37:768–771.

64. Olpe HR, Demieville H, Baltzer V: The biologic activity of D- and L- baclofen (lioresal). Eur J Pharmacol 1978;52:133–136.

65. Terrence CF, Sax M, Fromm GH, et al: Effect of baclofen enantiomorphs on the spinal trigeminal nucleus and steric similarities of carbamazepine. Pharmacology 1983;37:88–94.

66. Fromm GH, Terrence DF: Comparison of L-baclofen and racemic baclofen in trigeminal neuralgia. Neurology 1987;37:1725–1728.

67. Mann-Metzer P, Yarom Y: Pre- and post synaptic inhibition mediated by GABA(B) receptors in cerebellar inhibitory interneurons. J Neurophysiol 2002;87:183–190.

68. Patel S, Maeem S, Kesingland A, et al: The effects of GABA(B) agonists and gabapentin on me-

chanical hyperalgesia in models of neuropathic and inflammatory pain in the rat. Pain. 2001;90: 217–226.

69. Shapiro RT: Management of spasticity, pain, and paroxysmal phenomena in multiple sclerosis. Curr Neurol Neruosci Rep 2001;1:299–302.

70. Turp JC, Gobetti JP: Trigeminal neuralgia: An updtate. Compend Contin Educ Dent 2002;21: 279–282.

71. Hering-Hanit R, Gadoth N: The use of baclofen in cluster headache. Curr Pain Headache Rep 2001; 5:79–82.

72. Zuniga RE, Perera S, Abram SE: Intrathecal baclofen: A useful agent in the treatment of well-established complex regional pain syndrome. Reg Anesth Pain Med 2002;27:90–93.

73. Wurm C, Richardson JD, Bowles W, et al: Evaluation of functional GABA(B) receptors in dental pupl. J Endod 2001;27:620–623.

74. Lidums I, Lehmann A, Checklin H, et al: Control of transient lower esophageal sphincter relaxations and reflux by the GABA(B) agonist baclofen in normal subjects. Gastroenterology 2000, 118:7–13.

75. Broderick CP, Radnitz CL, Bauman WA: Diazepam usage in veterans with spinal cord injury. J Spinal Cord Med 1997;20:406–409.

76. Cendrowski W, Sobczyk W: Clonazepam, baclofen, and placebo in the treatment of spasticity. Eur Neurol 1997;16:257–262.

77. Roussan M, Terrance C, Fromm G: Baclofen versus diazepam for the treatment of spasticity and long-term follow-up of baclofen therapy. Pharmatherapeutical 1987;4:278–284.

78. Finley MF, Patel SM, Madison DV, et al: The core membrane fusion complex governs the probability of synaptic vesicle fusion but not transmitter release kinetics. J Neurosci 2002;22:1266–1272.

79. Parpura V, Haydan PG: Physiological astrocytic calcium level stimulate glutamate release to modulate adjacent neurons. Proc Natl Acad Sci U S A 2000;97:8629–8634.

80. Cui M, Chaddock JA, Rubino J, et al: Targeted destridiul and endopeptidase: Antinociceptive activity in preclinical models of pain. Arch Pharmacol 2002;365(suppl) 2:R16.

81. Murakami T, Okada M, Kawata Y, et al: Determination of effects of antiepileptic drugs on SNAREs mediated hippocampal monoamine release using in vivo microdialysis. Br J Pharmacol 2001;134: 507–520.

82. Reeves RR, Pinkofsky HB, Carter OS: Carisoprodol: A drug of continuing abuse. J Am Osteopathic Assn. 1997;97:723–724.

83. Dougherty RJ: Carisoprodol should be a controlled substance. Arch Fam Med 1995;4:582.

84. Rust GS, Hatch R, Gums JG: Carisoprodol as a drug of abuse. Arch Fam Med 1993;2:429–432.

85. Chop WM Jr: Should carisoprodol be a controlled substance? Arch Fam Med. 1993;2:911.

86. Dalen P, Alvan G, Wakelkamp M, et al: Formation of meprobamate from carisoprodol is catalyzed by CYP2C19. Pharmacogenetic 1996;6:387–394.

87. Davis GG, Alexander CB: A review of carisoprodil deaths in Jefferson County, Alabama. South Med J 1998;91:726–730.

88. Roberge RJ, Lin E, Krenzelok EP: Flumazenil reversal of carisoprodol (Soma) intoxication. J Emerg Med 2000;18:61–64.

89. Lofland JH, Szarlej D, Buttaro R, et al: Cyclobenzaprine hydrochloride is a commonly prescribed centrally acting muscle relaxant, which is structurally similar to tricyclic antidepressants (TCAs) and differs from amitriptyline by only one double bond. Clin J Pain 2001;17:103–104.

90. Reynolds WJ, Moldofsky H, Saskin P, et al: The effects of cyclobenzaprine on sleep physiology and symptoms in patients with fibromyalgia. J Rheumatol 1991;18:452–454.

91. Browing R, Jackson JL, O'Malley PG: Cyclobenzaprine and back pain: A meta-analysis. Arch Intern Med 2001;161:1613–1620.

92. Douglass MA, Levine DP: Hallucinations in an elderly patient taking recommended doses of cyclobenzaprine. Arch Intern Med 2000;160:1373.

93. Spiller HA, Winter ML, Mann KV, et al: Five-year multicenter retrospective review of cyclobenzaprine toxicity. J Emerg Med 1995;13:781–785.

94. McEvoy GK, ed: AHFS Drug information. Bethesda, MD. American Society of Health-Systems, Pharmacists, 1999.

95. Schneider MS: Pain reduction in breast augmentation using methocarbamol. Aesthetic Plast Surg 1997;21:23–24.

96. Hunskaar S, Donnell D: Clinical and pharmacological review of the efficacy of orphenadrine and its combination with paracetamol in painful conditions. J Intern Med Res 1991;19:71–87.

97. Hunskaar S, Berge OG, Hole K: Orphenadrine citrate increases and prolongs the antinociceptive effects of paracentamol in mice. Acta Pharmacol Toxicol 1986;59:53–59.

98. Hunskaar S, Berge OG, Hole K: Antinociceptive effects of orphendrine citrate in mice. Eur J Pharmacol 1985;111:221–226.

99. Berthold CW, Dionne RA: Clinical evaluation of H1-receptor and H2-receptor antagonists for acute postoperative pain. J Clin Pharmacol 1993;33:944–948.

100. Hunskaar S, Rosland JH, Hole K: Mechanisms of orphenadrine-induced antinociception in mice: Role for serotonergic pathways. Eur J Pharmacol 1989;160:83–91.

101. Aglas F, Fruhwald FM, Chlud K: Results of efficacy study with diclofenac/orphenadrine infusions in patients with musculoskeletal disease and functional disorders. Acta Med Austria 1998; 25:86–90.

102. Coward DM: Tizanidine: Neuropharmacology and mechanism of action. Neurology 1994; 44(suppl 9):S6–S11.

103. Milanov I, Georgiev D: Mechanisms of tizanidine action on spasticity. Acta Neurol Scand 1994; 89:274–279.

Chapter 24

Novel Routes of Analgesic Administration

James C. Crews, MD

HISTORY OF ANALGESIC ADMINISTRATION

Historically, analgesic medications were administered most commonly by topical application or oral routes. A variety of herbs and plant extracts were used medicinally for their analgesic properties, including opium, mandragora, hebane, and hemp. The ancient Sumerians described the use of opium as an analgesic more than 5,000 years ago. The description of the use of analgesic tablets dates back to the first century A.D. in a reference by Celsus, in his *De Medicina*. Topical and oral routes of administration were used throughout the Middle Ages and the Renaissance with little alternative developments until the latter part of the eighteenth century, when Joseph Priestly discovered nitrous oxide, and Sir Humphrey Davy observed the analgesic properties of inhalation of the gas.[7]

In the nineteenth century, morphine and codeine were isolated from crude opium, and salicylic acid was produced from willow bark leading to the subsequent introduction of aspirin. Morton's public demonstration of the anesthetic properties of ether in 1846 led to the development of inhalation anesthesia. The development of the hollow needle by Rynd and the syringe by Wood permitted the injection of analgesics. Development of these devices together with the isolation and pharmacologic exploration of cocaine initiated the development of local anesthetics and regional anesthetic and analgesic techniques.[7]

In the twentieth century, many synthetic chemical analgesic compounds were developed, including acetaminophen, nonsteroidal antiinflammatory drugs, aminoamide local anesthetics, and a variety of synthesized opioid analgesics. During the first three quarters of the twentieth century, routine analgesic delivery was limited largely to the oral and intramuscular routes.

The discovery, development, and description of a variety of novel analgesic delivery systems and routes of administration occurred in the last 25 to 30 years of the twentieth century. The first generation of the microprocessor-based patient-controlled infusion device for patient-controlled analgesia (PCA) was developed in the late 1960s and early 1970s. The patient-controlled opioid analgesic delivery system has become a standard of care for systemic opioid analgesic administration.[5] The discovery of analgesia produced by the spinal administration of morphine in rats by Yaksh and Rudy[16] in 1976 led to spinal opioid analgesia for humans. Spinal analgesic delivery for hospitalized patients with acute pain and for inpatient and outpatient management of severe chronic and cancer-related pain syndromes is a relatively routine modality throughout the world.[36] This chapter discusses other more recent developments in novel analgesic delivery systems, novel routes of administration, and some novel analgesic compounds that are in current clinical practice or in clinical development.

NOVEL ANALGESIC DELIVERY SYSTEMS

Transdermal Fentanyl Delivery System

The transdermal fentanyl delivery system (Duragesic, Janssen Pharmaceuticals) was developed as a noninvasive continuous opioid delivery alternative to intravenous or subcutaneous opioid infusion. Advantages of this noninvasive transdermal delivery system included no requirement for intravenous or subcutaneous access and no costly and bulky infusion pump. Fentanyl was determined to be a good candidate for transdermal application because of its physiochemical properties of low molecular weight, adequate lipid solubility, and high analgesic potency.[18]

The system is composed of a series of thin, flexible films: a backing layer, a drug reservoir, a rate-limiting membrane, and an adhesive (Fig. 1). The drug is dissolved in ethanol (to increase drug-skin flux) and gelled with hydroxyethyl cellulose. Drug delivery is proportional to the surface area of the system in contact with the skin. Elevation of body temperature to 40°C can increase absorption by one third.[18] The system was designed to provide continuous transcutaneous delivery of fentanyl for 72 hours. Residual fentanyl remaining within the system after 72 hours of continuous application may range from 28% to 84% of the original fentanyl content.[31]

Serum concentrations of fentanyl have been reported to plateau approximately 14 hours after placement of the system.[40] Other studies reported a delay in peak plasma levels until 17 to 48 hours after application.[27] The terminal half-life value for plasma levels after removal of the device is approximately 17 hours,[40] with a range of 13 to 25 hours.[27] The device is supplied in four different doses approximately equal to an intravenous fentanyl delivery of 25, 50, 75, or 100 μg/h, although wide interpatient variability in absorption of drug and plasma concentrations has been reported. Potential disadvantages of this passive transdermal delivery system include no mechanism for intermittent rescue dose administration, the delay in onset of analgesia after initial application of the device, and the cutaneous depot of drug that continues to be absorbed after removal of the device.

This system is especially attractive as an alternative opioid delivery system in patients unable to tolerate oral administration of opioids. As mentioned, however, this device does not

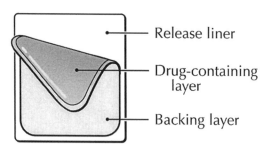

Figure 24–1. Schematic drawing of the D-TRANS system (ALZA Corporation) as used in the Duragesic Transdermal Fentanyl Delivery System. An adhesive layer is placed on the underside of the system to adhere to the patient's skin. (Courtesy of ALZA Corporation: D-TRANS technology: How does it work? HTTP://www.alza.com/wt/how.zoo?page_name=transdermal_how; Available at accessed Nov 13, 2001.)

address the requirement for administration of intermittent rescue doses of opioid for incident pain. Patients still may require intermittent administration of subcutaneous, intravenous, intramuscular, oral, or rectal doses of drug for rescue analgesia while using this system. This device also has been used as an alternative to oral opioid administration with the potential benefits of less frequent dosing intervals (every 72 hours compared with every 8 to 12 hours). Some patients report better analgesia with transdermal fentanyl compared with oral opioid administration, with improved quality of life and a slightly lower incidence of constipation.[1, 2, 34, 35] Other drug-related adverse events are similar to other routes of opioid administration. Some patients report local skin irritation at the application site either from the adhesive or from other components of the device. The passive transdermal fentanyl delivery system should be used in patients with long-term continuous opioid dosing requirements.

Electrophoretic Transdermal Fentanyl Delivery System

Electrotransport or iontophoresis as a means of enhancing the transport of charged molecules across the skin has been studied extensively. An electrotransport transdermal system for fentanyl (E Trans, ALZA Corporation) has been developed that combines the noninvasive advantage of passive transdermal drug delivery with the ability to allow patient-controlled intermittent demand dosing of drug. In this system, drug delivery is enhanced by application of a small electrical current. A patient-controlled (on-demand) button activates the electrical current–enhanced transdermal transport of drug, allowing intermittent drug delivery in response to patient demand. The design of the device makes it capable of a variety of dosing patterns, including continuous, patterned, or on-demand drug delivery.[3]

The electrotransport transdermal fentanyl delivery system currently in clinical development is a small, lightweight, self-contained system approximately the width and length of the passive transdermal fentanyl device with a depth (height) of about 5 mm. The plastic device adheres to the skin with a pressure-sensitive adhesive layer. The device housing has a light emitting diode, which indicates the device status and dose count, and a patient-activated on-demand button. The internal components consist of a drug-containing anode hydrogel (ionized fentanyl), an inert cathode hydrogel, a battery, and the electronic circuitry (Fig. 2). The delivered dose is preset and based on the intensity and duration of the applied electrical current. Preclinical trials have reported no or barely perceptible skin erythema 24 hours after removal of the system.[19]

There is essentially no significant passive drug delivery of the electrotransport system. On activation of the device, time to detection of appreciable blood levels and analgesic effect ranges from 10 to 30 minutes. This device may have applications for acute pain states, such as postoperative analgesia in adults and children, and may be suitable for outpatient use. This device also may have applications for incident pain for patients with chronic or cancer-related pain and perhaps as a coanalgesic delivery system with the passive transdermal fentanyl system.

Oral Transmucosal Fentanyl Citrate Delivery System

The oral transmucosal (buccal and sublingual) route of administration has been studied as a potential site of opioid drug delivery because of the relatively rapid absorption possible through the oral mucosa and the fact that orally absorbed drugs are not subject to first-pass

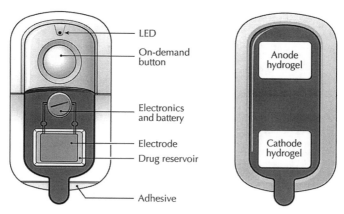

Figure 24–2. Schematic cutaway drawing of top of the E-TRANS system (ALZA Corporation) as used in the electrophoretic transport Fentanyl delivery system. (Courtesy of ALZA Corporation: E-TRANS technology: How does it work? Available at HTTP://www.alza.com/wt/how.zoo?page_name=tech_electro_how; accessed Aug 22, 2001.)

hepatic metabolism as are enterically absorbed drugs.[38] Buccal and sublingual administration of morphine and buprenorphine was studied compared with oral systemic administration with variable results (see later).[13, 15, 37, 41] The small molecular size and the lipophilic characteristic of fentanyl facilitate buccal and sublingual absorption.[38]

Oral transmucosal fentanyl citrate (OTFC, Anesta Corporation; brand name, ACTIQ, Abbott Laboratories) is a fentanyl delivery system that incorporates the drug in a sucrose matrix on a plastic handle.[30] The patient places the sucrose/drug matrix into the mouth, and as the matrix dissolves, the drug is released for rapid absorption across the oral mucosa. The remaining portion of the drug is swallowed, then absorbed in the stomach and intestine. The total systemic bioavailability (oral mucosal and gastrointestinal) of fentanyl from the OTFC delivery system is approximately 50%.[39] The system is available in 200-, 400-, 600-, 800-, 1,200-, and 1,600-μg units.[14] The unit typically is dissolved in the mouth over 10 to 15 minutes. Time to meaningful pain relief has been reported as between 2 and 14 minutes. Peak plasma concentrations of fentanyl occur at approximately 20 minutes after dosing.[30]

The OTFC delivery system is especially attractive as a treatment option for patients with breakthrough pain from cancer. This delivery system offers a solution to the treatment of breakthrough pain in patients using a transdermal fentanyl delivery system for continuous opioid analgesic requirements.[10, 12, 14] The OTFC delivery system was shown to be superior to immediate-release oral morphine for treatment of breakthrough cancer pain with respect to time to onset, total pain relief, and patient satisfaction.[12] The OTFC delivery system may be used in patients who are unable to tolerate the traditional oral route of administration. This delivery system also has been used for patients with acute pain states, such as postoperative pain and procedure-related pain.[4, 30]

Sublingual and Buccal Opioid Administration

Buccal and sublingual delivery routes have been used for opioids in patients unable to tolerate oral-enteral routes of administration. Various opioids have been used for the buccal and sublingual routes, including morphine, hydromorphone, methadone, levorphanol, fentanyl, oxycodone, diacetyl morphine, and buprenorphine.[42] Potential advantages of the oral mucosal route of administration compared with the oral enteral route include easy access, the potential for more rapid onset, and the possible avoidance of hepatic first-pass elimination. Problems encountered with the administration of tablet or solution preparations of opioids via the buccal or sublingual route included a lack of palatability of the drug preparation and poor or highly variable absorption.[37, 42]

In a study of oral absorption of various opioid analgesics, buprenorphine (55%), fentanyl (51%), and methadone (34%) were absorbed to a significantly greater extent than morphine (18%). Levorphanol, hydromorphone, oxycodone, heroin, and naloxone were absorbed more poorly compared with morphine. In general, this study showed that more lipophilic drugs were absorbed better through the oral mucosa than were more hydrophilic drugs. Increasing the oral pH to 8.5 increased the oral mucosal absorption of methadone to 75%. Methadone and fentanyl were absorbed in a contact time–dependent fashion, whereas buprenorphine was not.[42]

Morphine has been used through the buccal or sublingual route in patients with cancer-related pain unable to tolerate oral-enteral routes of administration. Some patients show adequate absorption for this route to be an alternative to oral-enteral administration. Bioavailability of the oral mucosal route can approach that of the oral-enteral route in some individuals and theoretically could result in more rapid onset of analgesia.[37] An aerosolized morphine preparation for sublingual administration also was studied but was found to have no particular advantages compared with oral morphine administration, with a mean bioavailability of 20%.[41] Buprenorphine was studied with some success as a candidate for oral mucosal drug delivery because of its relatively high absorption.[15]

Nebulized Drug Delivery Systems

The inhalation of nebulized morphine has been explored as an alternative noninvasive delivery route, which offers the potential for rapid onset of analgesic activity. Nebulized morphine has been described as a treatment for dyspnea associated with end-stage cardiopulmonary disease or cancer. As noted with other transmucosal delivery systems, absorption of nebulized morphine is limited, and interpatient bioavailability is highly variable. Mean bioavailability of nebulized morphine in a study in healthy subjects was reported as 5%.[32] Another study of nebulized morphine in anesthetized and intubated patients reported a relative bioavailability ranging from 9% to 35%, with a mean of 17% compared with an intramuscular dose of morphine.[11] Acute respiratory depression was reported in a patient after a relatively small dose of nebulized morphine suggesting that patients be monitored closely while receiving morphine by this route of administration.[25] A study in a small group of postoperative patients reported favorable analgesia scores and side-effect profiles for nebulized morphine, doses every 4 hours compared with intravenous PCA.[13a]

Additional studies with nebulized opioid delivery systems seem to be warranted to improve the interindividual variability and relatively low absorption shown in preliminary studies using nebulized morphine. The use of more lipophilic opioids or changes in nebulization technique may produce more consistent and favorable results.

Subcutaneous Implant Delivery Systems

Osmotic Infusion Pumps Implantable osmotic infusion pumps are currently in clinical development for long-term, continuous, subcutaneous drug delivery. The first approved use of the

DUROS Implant System is for the administration of leuprolide for treatment of prostate cancer.[43] The DUROS implant consists of a titanium alloy cylinder, 4 mm in diameter by 45 mm in length (Fig. 3). Inside the titanium case is an end cap with a rate-controlling diffusion moderator and a tiny delivery orifice, a drug reservoir, a piston device, an osmotic engine, and a semipermeable polyurethane diffusion membrane. The membrane allows a water permeation rate into the osmotic engine (hyperosmotic sodium chloride medium) that results in the required piston movement and drug delivery rate.[43]

Osmotic infusion pump technology is based on the principle of osmosis. A semipermeable membrane is placed over the osmotic engine compartment of the pump. Water is drawn through the membrane into the engine compartment in response to the osmotic gradient between the osmotic engine and the surrounding subcutaneous tissue. The osmotic engine, composed of a hyperosmotic sodium chloride solution, expands as it imbibes water and exerts pressure on the piston, resulting in movement of the piston. This piston movement forces the drug formulation through the orifice in the diffusion moderator at a rate corresponding to the rate of water permeation into the osmotic engine.[43]

Osmotic delivery systems are placed into the subcutaneous tissue of the inner upper arm through a small trocar implanter under local anesthesia. Osmotic delivery systems have been shown to exhibit precise, zero-order kinetics for continuous drug delivery in humans for a 1-year delivery lifetime. The system is designed with a specific continuous delivery rate. Dose adjustments are made on the basis of the device delivery rate and the number of devices implanted. At the end of the osmotic delivery system's lifetime, the device is removed and replaced with a new device.

Implanted subcutaneous osmotic infusion pumps for continuous delivery of sufentanil (DUROS sufentanil, Durect Corporation) are currently in clinical development. This device is being developed for the continuous subcutaneous delivery of sufentanil for 3 months. A second device, DUROS hydromorphone (Durect Corporation), is in development for the continuous spinal delivery of hydromorphone (DURECT Corporation Product Pipeline; DUROS Sufentanil; DUROS Hydromorphone http://www.durect.com/wt/sec.php?page_name=pipeline).

Ethylene Vinyl Acetage Polymer Implants. Nonbiodegradable polymer implants have been studied for continuous drug delivery for a variety drugs, including prednisolone, insulin, dopamine, contraceptives, antibiotics, and cancer chemotherapy drugs. Polymer implants also have been studied as a long-term opioid analgesic delivery system with hydromorphone. EVA copolymer disks containing hydromorphone and coated in polymethyl methacrylate were shown capable of producing sustained hydromorphone drug delivery for 4 weeks.[29]

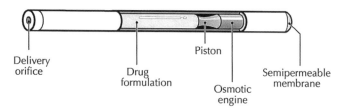

Figure 24–3. Schematic cutaway drawing of the DUROS osmotic infusion pump implant (ALZA Corporation). The cylinder is approximately 45 mm in length and 4 mm in diameter. (Courtesy of ALZA Corporation: DUROS technology: How does it work? Available at HTTP://www.alza.com/wt/print.zoo?page_name=nonerodible_how; accessed Aug 22, 2001.)

Significant advantages of these implantable subcutaneous drug delivery systems include their ability to provide continuous dosing without external pumps, catheters, or support services and a minimal risk of drug diversion. Disadvantages include the requirement of the minor placement procedure and the requirement for some other administration system for dosing of medication for breakthrough pain.

Liposomal Encapsulation Systems

Inability to maintain sustained therapeutic drug concentration at or near the target tissue is one limitation of traditional analgesic delivery systems. Local anesthetics require a minimum effective concentration at or near the target neural tissue to maintain prolonged analgesic effects. Opioids require a minimum effective concentration at the level of the spinal dorsal horn or in the spinal cerebrospinal fluid to maintain spinal analgesic activity. The encapsulation of drugs in aqueous solution inside multivesicular lipid microspheres is one method to provide sustained, localized drug delivery at or near a target tissue.

Drugs encapsulated in lipid microspheres or liposomes, when administered regionally, remain at the site of injection and are released slowly from the lipid vesicles into the surrounding tissue. The liposomes function as vehicles to deliver drugs in high concentrations to specific tissue targets, while avoiding systemic drug toxicity because only a portion of the total drug is bioavailable at a given time. The residence time and the release rate of the drug are determined by the composition and size of the lipid microsphere formulation. Liposomal drug delivery systems have been developed for the antineoplastics doxorubicin and daunorubicin and for the antifungal amphotericin B. Liposomal encapsulation analgesic delivery systems are currently in development for morphine[20] and bupivacaine.[17]

One liposomal encapsulated delivery system is the DepoFoam (SkyePharma PLC) technology. DepoFoam consists of microscopic spherical particles composed of numerous nonconcentric internal aqueous chambers containing the encapsulated drug (Fig. 4). Each chamber is separated from adjacent chambers by a single bilayer lipid membrane made of synthetic analogs of naturally occurring lipids (dioleolyl phosphatidylcholine, dipalmitoyl phosphatidylglycerol, cholesterol, and a triglyceride such as triolein). The DepoFoam particles containing the drug in the encapsulated aqueous phase, when suspended in physiologic saline and stored at 4° to 8°C, retain their structure, and little drug is released. On injection, reorganization and deterioration of the membranes allows slow, incremental release of the drug.[20] Other liposomal drug delivery formulations have been described.[17]

Several animal studies showed the potential utility of liposomal drug encapsulation systems for producing prolonged analgesic effects for morphine[23, 44, 45] and bupivacaine.[9, 17] Two preliminary reports describing the epidural administration of liposomal encapsulated bupivacaine in humans have been published.[8, 24]

The safety of repeated epidural injections with the DepoFoam delivery system was studied in dogs, and no significant pathologic effects were found.[45] In a study of the efficacy of epidurally delivered morphine using the DepoFoam system, time to onset of analgesia was 0.4 ± 0.2 hours for 5 mg of plain morphine compared with 1.3 ± 0.3 hours for 30 mg of liposomally encapsulated morphine. Duration of action was 27 ± 2 hours for plain morphine compared with 62 ± 0.3 hours for the 30-mg liposomal encapsulated morphine preparation.[44]

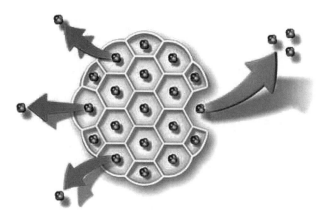

Figure 24–4. Illustration of the DepoFoam system of liposomal drug encapsulation. Spherical particles of non-concentric aqueous chambers contain the drug in an aqueous phase. Bilayer lipid membranes separate the chambers. Drug is released from the chambers after injection to produce sustained localized drug delivery. Sustained release *in vivo* or postinjection occurs through reorganization of lipid membranes resulting in pore formation and erosion. (From SkyePharma. Injectables: DepoFoam Technology. Available at HTTP://www.skyepharma.com/injectable.html; accessed Aug 22, 2001.)

Bupivacaine 0.25% encapsulated in multilamellar liposomes administered to a patient with cancer-related pain was reported to produce analgesia of 11 hours' duration compared with 4 hours' duration for plain bupivacaine 0.25%.[24] Onset, duration, and quality of analgesia were assessed in a preliminary study of postoperative patients receiving an epidural dose of 0.5% bupivacaine with epinephrine 1:200,000 compared with patients receiving a liposomal 0.5% bupivacaine formulation.[8] Onset times were reported as similar, but duration of pain relief was reported as 3.2 ± 0.4 hours with bupivacaine compared with 6.25 ± 1.13 hours with liposomal bupivacaine. No motor block was recorded in any of the patients in the liposomal bupivacaine group.

The development of liposomal drug delivery systems for local anesthetics and opioids as techniques to produce longer duration of analgesic activity with a single injection seems to hold great promise for clinical use. Questions regarding prolonged motor blockade and tissue toxicity with local anesthetic liposomal formulations and prolonged opioid-related side effects (especially respiratory depression) with liposomal opioid formulations need to be addressed in the development of this technology for widespread clinical use. The ability to extend the duration of action for a local anesthetic block from several hours to a few days without the requirement of catheter or infusion pump systems would be an attractive option in the management of postoperative pain. The use of longer duration formulations of either local anesthetics or opioids may have significant utility in patients with chronic and cancer-related pain.

Sustained-Release Oral Delivery Systems

Efforts to prolong the analgesic effect (prolongation of the blood concentration-time profile) for a relatively short-acting, enterally absorbed drug such as morphine, oxycodone, or hydromorphone would require alteration of the distribution, metabolism, or excretion characteristics of the drug. A more practical choice would be to design a formulation to modify the absorption rate of the drug within the gastrointestinal tract. Different formulation approaches have been used to control the rate of morphine dissolution from the controlled-release or sustained-release oral delivery systems.

One formulation involves the adsorption of the drug onto a hydrophilic polymer (e.g., hydroxy-alkyl cellulose), which is embedded in some form of a wax or hydrophobic matrix (higher molecular weight aliphatic alcohols), granulated, and compressed into tablets. After oral administration, fluid within the gastrointestinal tract dissolves the tablet surface and hydrates the hydrophilic polymer to produce a gel, the formulation of which is controlled by the aliphatic alcohols. The rate of drug release from this formulation depends on the rate of diffusion of the dissolved drug through the gel layer at the surface of the tablet. The depth of the gel layer increases over time as fluid gains access to the deeper regions of the tablet. The release rate is controlled by variations in the hydrophilic polymer, the type of hydrophobic matrix, or the ratio of the two. Different dosage strengths require different formulations. The tablet must be taken whole and not be chewed or crushed to retain the sustained-release characteristics of the formulation. Variations of this formulation approach are used for delivery systems for morphine and oxycodone: MS Contin and OxyContin (Purdue Pharma) and OraMorph SR (Roxane Laboratories).[16, 28]

An alternative approach involves creation of a pellet or granule that is composed of an inert core onto which is sequentially sprayed a defined small dose of drug, then application of a polymer coat of a defined porosity and thickness. These pellets or granules are placed within a gelatin capsule for a single dose unit. After oral administration, the gelatin capsule is dissolved releasing the pellets or granules. Fluid in the gastrointestinal tract diffuses through the outer polymer coat to dissolve the drug. The nature of the inert core and the composition and thickness of the polymer coat control the rate of dissolution. Because all the pellets or granules are identical, the number or amount of pellets or granules determines the dosage. After dissolution of the outer gelatin capsule, the small granules behave similar to a liquid rather than a single large particle or tablet, which on occasion may be retained in the stomach for some time. The nature of the small granules when removed from the gelatin capsule also allows for taking the dose as sprinkles on a soft food (e.g., apple sauce) or through a feeding tube without disruption of the sustained-release properties of the formulation. This formulation approach is used for morphine (Kadian; F. H. Faulding & Co, Ltd.).[16]

Several studies have reported pharmacokinetic and pharmacodynamic comparisons of the various sustained-release preparations. The ideal characteristics of a sustained-release opioid preparation would include equal bioavailability of drug compared with the immediate-release formulation, with relatively linear release characteristics, avoiding peak-and-trough effects associated with dosing. Comparisons made between equal dose strengths of MS Contin and OraMorph SR showed a greater peak morphine concentration (greater C_{max}) and slightly greater total bioavailability (AUC [area under the concentration-time curve]) for MS Contin compared with OraMorph SR (167.4 and 152.3 ng-h/mL). The release characteristics of OraMorph SR seem to be more linear than that of MS Contin, however.[21] Both preparations show release characteristics supporting an 8- to 12-hour dosing interval. In studies of MS Contin comparing an 8-hour versus 12-hour dosing interval, it was found that fewer than 10% of patients are likely to require a dosing interval less than 12 hours.[22, 26, 33]) In my clinical experience, side effects in some patients related to peak blood levels of drug that occur 1 to 2 hours after dosing and the incidence of breakthrough pain 10 to 12 hours after dosing with the Contin delivery system can be reduced by dividing the 24-hour drug dose requirement into three 8-hourly doses compared with two 12-hourly doses.

Studies comparing MS Contin and Kadian indicated similar efficacy and side-effect profiles for the same doses of the two formulations with MS Contin administered on a 12-hour dosing interval and Kadian administered either on a 12-hour or a 24-hour dosing interval.[6] In a study of the pharmacokinetic differences between 12-hourly doses of MS Contin and 24-hourly doses of Kadian, significantly less fluctuation in plasma morphine concentration was shown for Kadian despite a dosing interval double that of MS Contin.

Other sustained-release opioid formulations have been described, including a controlled-release morphine suspension and rectally administered formulations.[16] Sustained-release preparations for oxycodone (OxyContin; Purdue Pharma) also are available, and a sustained-release codeine preparation (Codeine Contin; Purdue Pharma) is available in Canada. Sustained-release preparations of other opioids, including hydromorphone and hydrocodone, are currently in clinical development.

NOVEL ANALGESIC DRUGS

Clinical development of novel analgesic delivery systems has been paralleled by the clinical development of many structurally or mechanistically novel analgesic drugs. In the area of local anesthetic agents, the single-isomer local anesthetics S-ropivacaine (Naropin; Astra/Zeneca) and S- or levo-bupivacaine (Chirocaine; Purdue Pharma) have been developed on the basis that the S-isomer local anesthetics are safer with respect to cardiovascular and central nervous system toxicity in the case of unintentional overdose or intravascular injection than the R-isomer or the racemic mixture. In the area of nonsteroidal antiinflammatory drugs, after the discovery of a second isoform of the cyclo-oxygenase (COX) enzyme, the COX-2 selective inhibitors were developed. The drugs have been shown to have equal analgesic efficacy with a much better safety profile with respect to gastrointestinal ulceration and erosion and a lack of platelet effects compared with the nonselective COX inhibitors.

In terms of mechanistically novel analgesic agents, the α_2-agonist clonidine, after receiving approval for use as an analgesic in cancer-related pain, is being used as a spinal analgesic and local anesthetic adjuvant in selected cases. Neostigmine has been studied as spinal analgesic acting through a mechanism involving spinal muscarinic receptors. Adenosine, through agonist activity at spinal A1 receptors, may diminish glutamate release from spinal systems. Ziconotide, an N-type calcium channel blocker, has been studied as a spinal analgesic in acute, chronic, and cancer-related pain. The γ-aminobutyric acid analog gabapentin has seen an expanding role as an analgesic agent in neuropathic pain states.

CONCLUSIONS

Of the more traditional opioid delivery systems, the oral route of administration has the advantage of relatively noninvasive administration but the disadvantages of slow onset of activity, requirement for adequate enteral absorption, and the effects of first-pass hepatic metabolism. The intravenous route of administration is associated with rapid onset of action and ease of titration of drug dose to effect but is more invasive and dependent on catheters, pumps, and skilled nursing care for continuous delivery. The ideal analgesic delivery system would have the ability to produce rapid onset of analgesia on patient demand through a painless, noninvasive means. It also would be able to provide stable but titratable continuous administration of analgesics when needed for longer term administration. The novel analgesic delivery systems discussed in this chapter attempt, in a variety of ways, to bridge the gap between the advantages and disadvantages of the traditional oral and intravenous routes of administration toward the goal of meeting the challenges of the ideal analgesic delivery system.

REFERENCES

1. Ahmedzai S, Brooks D: Transdermal fentanyl versus sustained-release oral morphine in cancer pain: Preference, efficacy, and quality of life. The TTS-Fentanyl Comparative Trial Group. J Pain Symptom Manage 13:254–261, 1997.

2. Allan L, Hays H, Jensen NH, et al: Randomised crossover trial of transdermal fentanyl and sustained release oral morphine for treating chronic non-cancer pain. BMJ 322:1154–1158, 2001.

3. ALZA Corporation: E-TRANS technology: how does it work? Available at http://www.alza.com/ wt/print.zoo?page_name+nonerodible_how; accessed Oct 22, 2001.

4. Ashburn MA, Lind GH, Gillie MH, et al: Oral transmucosal fentanyl citrate (OTFC) for the treatment of postoperative pain. Anesth Analg 76:377–381, 1993.

5. Ashburn MA, Ready LB: Postoperative pain. In: Loeser JD (ed): Bonica's Management of Pain. Philadelphia: Lippincott Williams & Wilkins, 2001, pp 765–823.

6. Bloomfield SS, Cissell GB, Mitchell J, et al: Analgesic efficacy and potency of two oral controlled-release morphine preparations. Clin Pharmacol Ther 53:469–478, 1993.

7. Bonica JJ, Loeser JD: History of pain concepts and therapies. In: Loeser J (ed): Bonica's Management of Pain. Philadelphia: Lippincott Williams & Wilkins, 2001, pp 3–25.

8. Boogaerts JG, Lafont ND, Declercq AG, et al: Epidural administration of liposome-associated bupivacaine for the management of postsurgical pain: A first study. J Clin Anesth 6:315–320, 1994.

9. Boogaerts JG, Lafont ND, Luo H, Legros FJ: Plasma concentrations of bupivacaine after brachial plexus administration of liposome-associated and plain solutions to rabbits. Can J Anaesth 40: 1201–1204, 1993.

10. Christie JM, Simmonds M, Patt R, et al: Dose-titration, multicenter study of oral transmucosal fentanyl citrate for the treatment of breakthrough pain in cancer patients using transdermal fentanyl for persistent pain. J Clin Oncol 16:3238–3245, 1998.

11. Chrubasik J, Wust H, Friedrich G, Geller E: Absorption and bioavailability of nebulized morphine. Br J Anaesth 61:228–230, 1988.

12. Coluzzi PH, Schwartzberg L, Conroy JD, et al: Breakthrough cancer pain: A randomized trial comparing oral transmucosal fentanyl citrate (OTFC) and morphine sulfate immediate release (MSIR). Pain 91:123–130, 2001.

13. Davis T, Miser AW, Loprinzi CL, et al: Comparative morphine pharmacokinetics following sublingual, intramuscular, and oral administration in patients with cancer. Hosp J 9:85–90, 1993.

13a. Fagraeus L, Fulda G, Lange A, Giberson F: Nebulized morphine in acute thoracic pain (abstr). Anesthesiology 93:A851, 2000.

14. Farrar JT, Cleary J, Rauck R, et al: Oral transmucosal fentanyl citrate: Randomized, double-blinded, placebo-controlled trial for treatment of breakthrough pain in cancer patients. J Natl Cancer Inst 90:611–616, 1998.

15. Gaitini L, Moskovitz B, Katz E, et al: Sublingual buprenorphine compared to morphine delivered by a patient-controlled analgesia system as postoperative analgesia after prostatectomy. Urol Int 57:227–229, 1996.

16. Gourlay GK: Sustained relief of chronic pain. Pharmacokinetics of sustained release morphine. Clin Pharmacokinet 35:173–190, 1998.

17. Grant GJ, Barenholz Y, Piskoun B, et al: DRV liposomal bupivacaine: preparation, characterization, and in vivo evaluation in mice. Pharm Res 18:336–343, 2001.

18. Grond S, Radbruch L, Lehmann KA: Clinical pharmacokinetics of transdermal opioids: Focus on transdermal fentanyl. Clin Pharmacokinet 38:59–89, 2000.

19. Gupta SK, Sathyan G, Phipps B, et al: Reproducible fentanyl doses delivered intermittently at different time intervals from an electrotransport system. J Pharm Sci 88:835–841, 1999.

20. Howell SB: Clinical applications of a novel sustained-release injectable drug delivery system: De-poFoam technology. Cancer J 7:219–227, 2001.

21. Hunt TL, Kaiko RF: Comparison of the pharmacokinetic profiles of two oral controlled-release morphine formulations in healthy young adults. Clin Ther 13:482–488, 1991.

22. Kaiko RF, Grandy RP, Oshlack B, et al: The United States experience with oral controlled-release morphine (MS Contin tablets): Parts I and II. Review of nine dose titration studies and clinical pharmacology of 15-mg, 30-mg, 60-mg, and 100-mg tablet strengths in normal subjects. Cancer 63:2348–2354, 1989.

23. Kim T, Murdande S, Gruber A, Kim S: Sustained-release morphine for epidural analgesia in rats. Anesthesiology 85:331–338, 1996.

24. Lafont ND, Legros FJ, Boogaerts JG: Use of liposome-associated bupivacaine in a cancer pain syndrome. Anaesthesia 51:578–579, 1996.

25. Lang E, Jedeikin R: Acute respiratory depression as a complication of nebulised morphine. Can J Anaesth 45:60–62, 1998.

26. Lazarus H, Fitzmartin RD, Goldenheim PD: A multi-investigator clinical evaluation of oral controlled-release morphine (MS Contin tablets) administered to cancer patients. Hospice J 6:1–15, 1990.

27. Lehmann KA, Zech D: Transdermal fentanyl: Clinical pharmacology. J Pain Symptom Manage 7:S8–16, 1992.

28. Leslie S: The Contin delivery system: Dosing considerations. Allergy Clin Immunol 78:768–773, 1986.

29. Lesser GJ, Grossman SA, Leong KW, et al: In vitro and in vivo studies of subcutaneous hydromorphone implants designed for the treatment of cancer pain. Pain 65:265–272, 1996.

30. Lind GH, Marcus MA, Mears SL, et al: Oral transmucosal fentanyl citrate for analgesia and sedation in the emergency department. Ann Emerg Med 20:1117–1120, 1991.

31. Marquardt KA, Tharratt RS, Musallam NA: Fentanyl remaining in a transdermal system following three days of continuous use. Ann Pharmacother 29:969–971, 1995.

32. Masood AR, Thomas SH: Systemic absorption of nebulized morphine compared with oral morphine in healthy subjects. Br J Clin Pharmacol 41:250–252, 1996.

33. Mignault GG, Latreille J, Viguie F, et al: Control of cancer-related pain with MS Contin: A comparison between 12-hourly and 8-hourly administration. J Pain Symptom Manage 10:416–422, 1995.

34. Nugent M, Davis C, Brooks D, Ahmedzai SH: Long-term observations of patients receiving transdermal fentanyl after a randomized trial. J Pain Symptom Manage 21:385–391, 2001.

35. Payne R, Mathias SD, Pasta DJ, et al: Quality of life and cancer pain: Satisfaction and side effects with transdermal fentanyl versus oral morphine. J Clin Oncol 16:1588–1593, 1998.

36. Ready LB: Regional analgesia with intraspinal opioids. In: Loeser JD (ed): Bonica's Management of Pain. Philadelphia: Lippincott Williams & Wilkins, 2001, pp 1954–1966.

37. Robison JM, Wilkie DJ, Campbell B: Sublingual and oral morphine administration: Review and new findings. Nurs Clin North Am 30:725–743, 1995.

38. Stanley TH, Hague B, Mock DL, et al: Oral transmucosal fentanyl citrate (lollipop) premedication in human volunteers. Anesth Analg 69:21–27, 1989.

39. Streisand JB, Varvel JR, Stanski DR, et al: Absorption and bioavailability of oral transmucosal fentanyl citrate. Anesthesiology 75:223–229, 1991.

40. Varvel JR, Shafer SL, Hwang SS, et al: Absorption characteristics of transdermally administered fentanyl. Anesthesiology 70:928–934, 1989.

41. Watson NW, Taylor KM, Joel SP, et al: A pharmacokinetic study of sublingual aerosolized morphine in healthy volunteers. J Pharm Pharmacol 48:1256–1259, 1996.

42. Weinberg DS, Inturrisi CE, Reidenberg B, et al: Sublingual absorption of selected opioid analgesics. Clin Pharmacol Ther 44:335–342, 1988.

43. Wright JC, Tao LS, Stevenson CL, et al: An in vivo/in vitro comparison with a leuprolide osmotic implant for the treatment of prostate cancer. J Control Release 75:1–10, 2001.

44. Yaksh TL, Provencher JC, Rathbun ML, Kohn FR: Pharmacokinetics and efficacy of epidurally delivered sustained-release encapsulated morphine in dogs. Anesthesiology 90:1402–1412, 1999.

45. Yaksh TL, Provencher JC, Rathbun ML, et al: Safety assessment of encapsulated morphine delivered epidurally in a sustained-release multivesicular liposome preparation in dogs. Drug Deliv 7:27–36, 2000.

46. Yaksh TL, Rudy TA: Analgesia mediated by a direct spinal action of narcotics. Science 192:1357–1358, 1976.

Chapter 25

Synergistic Epidural Analgesia*

Leonard S. Bushnell, MD

TWO PRINCIPLES

If you learn and *do* two things from this time forward, you will be in the top 98th percentile of physicians who treat patients with pain. It does no good simply to know these two things; you must apply them daily with each patient you treat. The first principle is *always use analgesic drugs in synergistic combinations of two or more*. The basis for this principle is pharmacologic. The second principle is *never allow analgesic gaps*. The basis for this principle is physiologic.

To obtain useful synergistic interactions, choose drugs from different classes that overlap for the desired effect—analgesia—and that do not overlap for underdesired side effects. Using two or more synergistic drug classes together (e.g., μ agonist opioids, such as morphine, and cyclooxygenase (COX) inhibitors, such as nonsteroidal anti-inflammatory drugs [NSAIDS] provides better analgesia, allows reduction in dose and reduction in side effects, and increases safety. This is straightforward pharmacology.[30]

Do not allow analgesic gaps. If the battery on an epidural pump goes dead, the bag runs dry, or the catheter dislodges, unless such a mishap is corrected promptly, breakthrough pain will occur. Bombardment of the spinal cord dorsal horn by C fiber stimulation produces wind-up, central sensitization, and hyperalgesia.[28] A similar series of events occurs if PRN (*as needed*) orders are written for intravenous or oral analgesics for patients who have ongoing clinical pain.

PAIN STATES

Although in their writings, clinicians recognize a seemingly endless variety of pain syndromes, basic scientists recognize three pain states. The first is *normal pain*, required for reflex withdrawal from noxious, potentially harmful, stimuli (i.e., "too hot," "too sharp"). Withdrawal from such noxious stimuli is necessary to prevent injury in everyday life. Normal pain should be preserved at least partially during the provision of prolonged analgesia.

Hyperalgesia occurs from a kind of two-dimensional amplification in noxious pain signals. Noxious signals arriving at the spinal cord are amplified and increased in duration. The patient reports, "it's sore."

---

*Throughout this chapter, results and conclusions determined by studies or intrathecal administration of drugs in *rats* are applied *unqualified* to clinical observation of drug therapy by the epidural, intravenous, and oral routes in *humans*. The verbs *is* and *are* are used instead of *may be*. The reasons for presenting material in this way are threefold: simplicity; clarity; and, in nearly 10 years' experience with pain treatment in postoperative patients, it is the author's experience that human responses to drugs at the spinal level are *as if* rat data for one route apply in humans by other routes, at least qualitatively. This parallelism is used most in discussion of synergy and relative strength of synergy. Rigorous proof in humans is not likely to be forthcoming for years.

The third pain state is *allodynia*. This pain occurs when normally nonnoxious stimuli are transformed and interpreted as noxious. The patient reports, "it's tender."

Hyperalgesia typically is described as occurring after injury, including surgery. Allodynia typically is described in association with neuropathic pain states. It is difficult to perform surgery, however, without cutting nerves, usually smaller fibers, and allodynia is normally present after surgery.

TWO DEFINITIONS

The following definitions help to clarify clinical thinking about drug classes that provide analgesia. *Analgesics* are drugs that *block transmitter release*. The two drug classes currently available that block transmitter release from the primary afferent in the dorsal horn of the spinal cord are μ agonist opioids (e.g., morphine, fentanyl) and α_2-agonists (clonidine, dexmedetomidine, and tizanidine). Future drug classes, not yet available, that are analgesics because they block transmitter release are δ agonists and N-calcium channel blockers. *Antihyperalgesics* are drugs that block the *effects* of transmitter release. They block the consequences of transmitter release in second-order neurons: projection neurons from the spinal cord to the higher central nervous system or interneurons in the spinal cord. Drugs in this category include COX inhibitors (NSAIDs), nitric oxide synthetase (NOS) inhibitors, and N-methyl-D-aspartate (NMDA) receptor blockers.

YAKSH RAT

In 1976, Yaksh and Rudy described an intrathecal drug delivery system in a rat preparation. An intrathecal catheter is introduced just below the occiput of the rat and advanced caudad through the intrathecal space, under fluoroscopic control, until the catheter tip lies opposite the lumbosacral swelling of the spinal cord. The catheter is fixed at the occiput, originally by epoxy glue, to prevent subsequent catheter movement. Noxious stimuli are presented to the rat's hindlimb, to the rat's tail, or by infusing noxious substances (e.g., AMPA, NMDA, substance P) through the catheter. Analgesics or antihyperalgesics are infused, either singly or in combination, through the catheter to the lumbosacral region of the spinal cord to ascertain analgesic effects. This rat drug delivery system is the basis for the determination of virtually all knowledge obtained of the spinal action of analgesic effects of drugs in the 1980s and 1990s (Fig. 1).

ANALGESIC SYNERGY

Drug *classes* should be chosen that overlap for analgesia but not for side effects.[18,30] Drug classes that largely fit these requirements are μ agonist opioids, COX inhibitors, α_2-agonists, NOS inhibitors, NMDA receptor blockers, and local anesthetics (when delivered by thoracic epidural catheters) (Fig. 2).

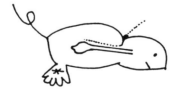

Figure 1. The Yaksh rat.

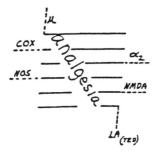

Figure 2. Overlap for analgesia, not for side effects (dotted lines).

Bupivacaine, Not Any μ Agonist Opioid, Is the Spread-Limiting Drug

In the early 1990s, there was much discussion of the pros and cons of using, for epidural analgesia, a relatively hydrophilic μ agonist opioid (e.g., morphine) versus a relatively lipophilic μ agonist (e.g., fentanyl).[4] Much of the discussion concerned spread of the drug along the neuraxis: morphine spreads more, and fentanyl spreads less (i.e., is relatively segmental in its effects). Examination of the literature from the mid-1990s shows that when lumbar epidural catheter placement is used,[18] adequate analgesia may be obtained with either morphine or fentanyl, but the addition of bupivacaine does not improve the analgesia or lower the μ agonist dose requirement. This is not the case for thoracic catheter placement at the appropriate spinal cord segments corresponding to the spinal level of incoming noxious stimuli.[4] Analgesia is improved substantially by the addition of local anesthetic, particularly analgesia with movement, and the dose of μ agonist opioid is decreased substantially.

The aforementioned principles are presented by Penning and Yaksh.[24] When the catheter tip is placed adjacent to the appropriate spinal cord segments, the following results are obtained. Morphine and bupivacaine are synergistic. The strength of analgesic synergy of the combination of the two drugs is approximately 10 times that of either drug used alone. Synergy is for the μ agonist opioid effect, not for the local anesthetic effect. The location of the synergistic effect is in the dorsal horn of the spinal cord. Analgesic synergy is obtained at local anesthetic concentrations too low to block sodium channels. The mechanism of action of the local anesthetic at these low concentrations is debated, but currently unknown.

Clinical Illustration of Analgesic Synergy

On numerous occasions on our acute pain service, patients have been encountered who were receiving morphine via patient-controlled analgesia as the sole postoperative analgesic. Commonly the analgesia is marginal, and the patient is sedated and nauseated. The surgeon may object strongly to the use of COX inhibitors (NSAIDs). On these occasions, we have added oral clonidine, an α_2-agonist, in the lowest dose tablet available, 0.1 mg. Several hours later, analgesia is improved, the patient is more mobile, the nausea is gone, and the patient is alert. Morphine and clonidine both cause sedation; why is the patient more alert?

The patient's use of morphine via the patient-controlled analgesia machine has dropped substantially. Morphine and clonidine are synergistic for their analgesic action, yielding better analgesia and allowing reduction of the μ agonist opioid dose.

Prediction of Synergy

Synergy will occur if drugs from two classes are used, both of which act presynaptically[30] (Fig. 3). That is, both act as analgesics to block transmitter release from the primary afferent in the dorsal horn of the spinal cord. Examples are μ agonists, α_2-agonists, δ agonists, and N-channel blockers. Every paired combination of these four drug classes that has been tested is synergistic.

Synergy may or may not occur when drugs from two classes are used together, one of which acts presynaptically and one postsynaptically. μ agonists plus COX inhibitors are strongly synergistic. A μ agonist plus adenosine is merely additive. If two drug classes both of which act postsynaptically are used, synergy will not occur—at least in all pairs tested. An example is COX inhibitors plus adenosine.

Relative Strength of Synergy

Relative strength of synergy has been established for several pairs of drug classes using the Yaksh rat intrathecal delivery system.[10,18,30] Relative analgesic strengths compared with the use of either drug alone are shown in Figure 4.

In 1981, Yeung and Rudy showed physiologic (as opposed to pharmacologic) synergy between spinal and supraspinal μ agonist receptor sites. Spinal lumbar and supraspinal catheters were placed. Morphine was administered by the spinal lumbar catheter only. This produced profound analgesia. A tiny amount of naloxone, too small to have any systemic effect, administered by the spinal lumbar catheter reversed the analgesia. A similarly tiny amount of naloxone administered by the supraspinal catheter also abolished the analgesia produced by spinal lumbar morphine. The strength of physiologic synergy between spinal and supraspinal μ agonist receptor sites (both activated by morphine) was approximately 30-fold. Similar effects have been shown for fentanyl. It is questionable whether the selective spinal action of relatively hydrophilic μ agonists touted in the 1990s is of consequence.

DRUG CLASSES

Many physicians expend huge mental energy sorting out minor differences in drugs within a given class (e.g., μ agonist opioids, COX inhibitors). Textbooks often lump analgesic and antihyperalgesic drugs into two classes, opioids and adjuvants. This classification reflects archaic thinking about pharmacology, which drug companies in their marketing encourage. In consulting on inpatients with chronic pain problems, we have encountered patients with seven μ agonist opioid commercial prescriptions ordered but no prescription written for an analgesic or antihyperalgesic drug from any other drug class.

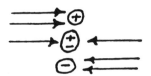

Figure 3. Two presynaptic drugs yield synergy. Two post synaptic drugs yield additive effect—one pre-, one post-: effect not predictable.

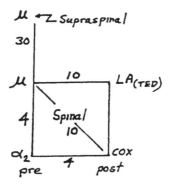

Mu + COX   ten-fold
Mu + *local anesthetic   ten-fold
Mu + alpha-2   four-fold
Alpha-2 + COX   four-fold

* Local anesthetic delivered via *thoracic* catheter, i.e., opposite the relevant spinal cord segments.

Figure 4. Relative strength of synergy for pairs of drug classes.

A more sensible approach, in light of contemporary pharmacology, is to learn well two or three drugs in *each* of the available classes—*particularly dose versus anticipated side effects*. Currently available, useful drug classes for analgesia include μ agonist opioids, α_2-agonists, COX inhibitors, perhaps an NOS inhibitor, NMDA receptor antagonists, and local anesthetics (when delivered via a thoracic epidural catheter). The gabapentanoids also look promising.

DRUG DOSES

Drug dose, particularly in the case of μ agonist opioids, can spell the difference between inadequate analgesia and adverse side effects, including death. For μ agonists, the line between adequate analgesic and hazardous side effects can be thin.

By contrast, physicians are frequently passionate about choice of drugs within a given class. This is particularly true for the μ agonist opioids. Decades ago, arguments raged about the relative merits of morphine versus meperidine versus hydromorphone delivered orally or parenterally. In the 1990s, arguments commonly centered on the merits of morphine versus hydromorphone versus meperidine versus fentanyl delivered via epidural catheter.

For the past decade, we have used fentanyl for our epidural solutions for one reason: *dosing safety*. Fentanyl [16,27] is overwhelmingly the most commonly used μ agonist opioid in the operating room by anesthesiologists. The intravenous and epidural doses are identical. Tell any first year resident with only 2 months' experience that you are going to relieve severe pain in a 50-year-old patient with 10 μg of fentanyl delivered either intravenously or via epidural catheter, and he or she will view you as a fool. Tell the same resident that you are about to administer 100 μg of fentanyl to a 100-year-old patient via either route, and the resident will know that you are proposing an absurdly dangerous dose. But ask an expert anesthesiologist with 10 to 20 years' experience to cite for you equally absurd doses of those two ends of the spectrum for morphine, for hydromorphone, and for meperidine, and you probably will be greeted with a blank stare.

Familiarity with dosing is crucial to patient safety. In 10 years' experience on our acute pain service, we have not encountered a single huge dosing error for fentanyl in epidural prescriptions written by first-year residents or others. With the other μ agonists just mentioned, we have seen frequent errors by seasoned anethesiologists ranging up to four-fold overdosing.

Doses can be kept low by using synergy. We keep the dosing levels of fentanyl/bupivacaine epidural solutions low by the addition of oral or parenteral COX inhibitors, α_2-agonists, and NMDA receptor blockers.

FORMALIN TEST

Before discussing the formalin test, let's consider an appropriate human analogy. Have you ever touched a hot stove and hurt yourself but not harmed yourself? Of course the answer is yes. Your fingertips hurt for a few minutes, then the pain subsides. After that, your fingertips begin to hurt, burn, ache, throb, and are exquisitely sensitive to touch. This goes on for an hour or more, then it subsides. Your fingertips now feel funny, then that too goes away. All the while, when you look at your fingers, there is no visible burn injury (Fig. 5).

The formalin test has similarities. A tiny amount of formalin is injected into the rat's hind paw pad (see asterisk in Fig. 1). Each time the rat places its foot down it hurts, and the rat flinches (i.e., lifts its paw). It is easy to count the flinches and to time flinches per minute. Consistently, each rat exhibits two flinching phases. In phase 1, flinching rapidly accelerates and subsides virtually completely at about 10 minutes. In phase 2, after 10 minutes, flinching again accelerates, and the rate of flinching usually overshoots that of phase 1 and continues for more than an hour. Phase 1 results from transmitter release, is analogous to normal pain, and can be blocked by an drug class that blocks transmitter release (e.g., μ agonist opioids and α_2-agonists given in a sufficient dose). Phase 2 arises from the result of transmitter release in the second-order neuron, be it a projection neuron such as one in the spinothalamic tract or a spinal interneuron. Phase 2 can be blocked completely with a sufficient dose of NMDA antagonist.

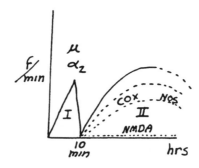

Figure 5. The formalin test.

The discussion of the effect of drugs on the formalin test pertains to drugs delivered intrathecally in the Yaksh rat preparation. A major discovery in 1992, by Malmberg and Yaksh,[17] was that COX inhibitors, long known to work in the periphery, also work in the central nervous system. COX inhibitors, in tiny doses too small to have any peripheral effect, exhibit a dose-dependent *partial* inhibition of phase 2 of the formalin test (by analogy, of wind-up, of central sensitization, of hyperalgesia—all of which are overlapping concepts and phenomena). NOS inhibitors exhibit a similar dose-dependent partial blockade of phase 2 and the aforementioned related phenomena.[19]

NEUROTRANSMISSION OF PAIN SIGNALS IN THE CENTRAL NERVOUS SYSTEM

Figure 6 represents current concepts of pain signal transmission in the dorsal horn. Imagine an old-fashioned, two-pronged electrical plug as representing the terminal of a primary afferent (e.g., C fiber) in the dorsal horn of the spinal cord. Now imagine a modern, three-holed electrical socket as representing the first neuron, across the synapse, in the central nervous system, whether this neuron be a projection neuron in the spinothalamic tract or an interneuron within the spinal cord. The *two prongs* of the plug represent the two principal pain transmitter classes: (1) excitatory amino acids, principally glutamate; and (2) neuropeptides (neurokinins), the principal representative substance P (there is a large family of neuropeptides of as yet incompletely determined relevance). The *three socket holes* represent receptors: (1) The NMDA receptor; (2) non-NMDA receptors (this family of receptors has difficult names: AMPA [amino methyl propionic acid], quisqualate, and kainate; all of them operate sodium potassium channels, are superfast [i.e., in milliseconds], and are activated for normal protective pain that triggers withdrawal reflexes); and (3) neurokinin receptors (these receptors are activated by substance P and are G protein linked).

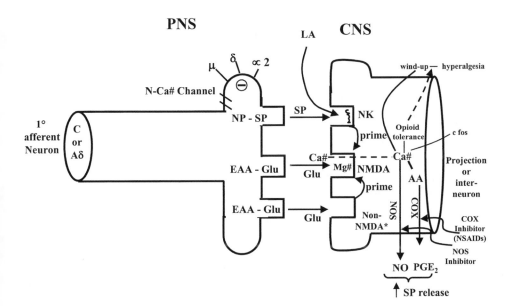

Figure 6. Pain neurotransmission in the dorsal horn.

How does this system work? Action potentials arriving along C fibers operate presynaptic N-calcium channels, which leads to the release of glutamate and substance P. Glutamate activates non-NMDA channels as described previously. Substance P activates neurokinin receptors, but glutamate cannot itself activate the NMDA receptor.

NMDA Receptor

Most receptors are either voltage gated (i.e., operated by action potentials or sufficient accumulation of end plate potentials) or ligand gated (i.e., operated by transmitter chemicals). The NMDA receptor is voltage gated and ligand gated, and the gating sequence must be in that order. Two keys are required to open the lock. First, a so-called priming voltage must be developed at non-NMDA receptors or neurokinin receptors to remove a voltage-dependent block exerted by the presence of magnesium. When this priming occurs, glutamate can activate the NMDA receptor and open its calcium channel.

Calcium entry initiates several events of great clinical importance in the central nervous system:

1. The wind-up–central sensitization–hyperalgesia sequence. Pain signals entering the central nervous system from the periphery are now increased greatly in amplitude and in duration.
2. c-fos gene activation. c-fos is a so-called intermediate early gene. It produces a protein product called FOS. FOS can be stained in experimental animals. The stain shows up as brown spots in the nuclei of certain neurons in the dorsal horn of the spinal cord. FOS is a marker of neuronal activity. After a given peripheral pain stimulus, the FOS reaction begins in about 5 minutes and peaks at 2 hours. The FOS reaction and the wind-up hyperalgesia phenomenon are believed to occur in the same neurons in the spinal cord. They occur in patients during surgery unless the spinal cord is protected. Volatile general anesthetics do not protect the spinal cord. Thoracic epidurals with synergistic drug combinations can protect the spinal cord.
3. Calcium entry also leads to activation of COX, yielding prostaglandins, most importantly prostaglandin E_2.
4. NOS also is activated by calcium entry, yielding nitric oxide.

Prostaglandins and nitric oxide accelerate the release of substance P from the primary afferent, yielding a positive feedback mechanism that further amplifies pain signals.

The pharmacologic tools necessary to prevent this hyperalgesic sequence are available: use of thoracic epidural analgesia with synergistic drugs and the epidural infusion supplemented with intravenous or oral drugs that also are synergistic. As always with synergistic analgesia, this approach provides better analgesia, decreased dose requirement, decreased side effects, and increased safety.

PHARMACOLOGY

Presynaptic Acting Drugs

μ *Agonist Opioids.* Morphine and the other μ agonist opioids block transmitter release from the primary afferent in the spinal cord. μ agonists also have a postsynaptic effect: hyperpolarization of the postsynaptic membrane. Clinically, this effect is trivial compared with the presynaptic effect. Spinal opioids used alone have limitations in blocking responses such as wind-up.[6]

α_2-agonists. Clonidine is currently the only α_2-agonist approved by the Food and Drug Administration for neuraxial (spinal) use. It is useful via the oral and intravenous (available in Europe) routes and the epidural route. Presynaptic and postsynaptic actions are parallel with those of the μ agonists.

Future Presynaptic Drug Classes

δ Agonists. Presynaptic and postsynaptic actions of δ agonists are similar to μ agonists. Results in animals indicate, however, that this drug class will be of immense importance not because of the nature of the drugs or the nature of the receptors, but rather because of the *location* of the receptors. δ receptors are located primarily in the *spinal cord*. There are comparatively few δ receptors in the brain and the gut. Animal studies indicate that δ agonists will be potent analgesics with minimal respiratory depression, addiction potential, and gastrointestinal side effects such as constipation.

N-Calcium Channel Blockers. N-calcium channel blockers currently are not approved by the Food and Drug Administration. Representatives so far are all omega conopeptides. These neuropeptides are derived from cone shells found in the Pacific and Indian Oceans. N-channel blockers are extremely potent, presynaptic-acting analgesics that block transmitter release. They have the advantage of exhibiting *no tolerance* in animal experiments in which morphine exhibits extreme tolerance. They have the disadvantage that analgesic doses may produce *motor block*. They seem unlikely to be useful as sole analgesic agents. The opening of voltage gated N-calcium channels by C and A delta fiber action potentials is thought to be the normal mechanism triggering pain transmitter release. More familiar calcium channel blockers, such as nifedipine, block so-called L-calcium channels and have little analgesic effect.

Postsynaptic Acting Drugs

Cyclooxygenase Inhibitors. COX inhibitors block prostaglandin release and block the positive feedback mechanism—the accelerated release of substance P—caused by prostaglandins. Ketorolac is the available parenteral COX inhibitor. For oral use, we prefer ibuprofen for three reasons. First, ibuprofen is in a first-place tie with ketorolac and ketoprofen for central nervous system *analgesic efficacy*.[23] Ketorolac has major gastrointestinal side effects. Second, in a meta-analysis of many COX inhibitors, ibuprofen had the fewest gastrointestinal side effects. Third, ibuprofen is inexpensive. COX inhibitors are strongly synergistic with μ agonists.

Nitric Oxide Synthetase Inhibitors. There is no available drug that is surely in the category of NOS inhibitors. There is some evidence, however, that acetaminophen exerts its action by inhibition of nitric oxide production.[3] A long-standing practice by primary care physicians of using aspirin and acetaminophen together for a sprained ankle may be rational because the two drug classes are likely to be additive.

N-Methyl-D-Aspartate Receptor Blockers. Dextromethorphan is the most readily available NMDA blocker. It is available in the form of Robitussin DM or generic analog preparations. Dextromethorphan is not a clean drug because it has other actions. The clinically useful dose range seems to be 30 to 60 mg every 4 to 6 hours. We have seen sedation with the 60-mg dose in elderly patients. Some hospital pharmacies make up 30-mg dextromethorphan gel caps.

Ketamine in low dose, 10 mg, followed by an infusion of 10 mg/h (i.e., 1.5 mg/kg), can be a useful NMDA blocker for postoperative pain. So far, it has been used more commonly in Europe.

Magnesium is an NMDA blocker. It exerts a voltage-dependent block at the NMDA calcium channel. It can be useful via infusion. The dose is half that used for preeclampsia.

A finding of immense potential clinical importance is that opioid tolerance—a hyperalgesic state—can be prevented and reversed by NMDA receptor blockade.[2,20,21] We have seen a fourfold reduction in μ agonist requirements after a 36-hour infusion of magnesium, ketamine, and oral dextromethorphan. This reduction occurred in a patient who had extraordinary neuropathic pain, opioid tolerance, and associated hyperalgesia, who before the administration of NMDA receptor antagonists required 700 μg of fentanyl per hour.

Local Anesthetics. In 1992, Penning and Yaksh[24] showed that intrathecal morphine and bupivacaine are synergistic, the strength of synergistic interaction is 10 times that of either drug used alone, the synergy is for the opioid, not the local anesthetic effect; and the location of the synergy is in the spinal cord. The bupivacaine concentration in this study was too low to block sodium channels. The mechanism by which local anesthetics at such low doses interact synergistically in the dorsal horn of the spinal cord with μ agonists is not known. Bupivacaine has been shown, in vitro to block the attachment of substance P to its receptor, the neurokinin receptor.[13] For this reason, local anesthestics are placed arbitrarily in this position on the spinal cord pain transmission diagram.

SUMMARY

1. The spinal cord is in the thorax; true, except for a few sacrococcygeal segments.
2. The spinal cord is the target for opioids and low-dose local anesthetics.
3. μ agonists and local anesthetics act synergistically if thoracic epidural catheters are used. Local anesthetics (e.g., bupivacaine) are the spread-limiting drugs. Several studies indicate that with lumbar catheter placements, the addition of bupivacaine does not improve analgesia.
4. The eleventh commandment of regional anesthesia, based on almost a century of subarachnoid anesthesia, previously was, "Don't go above L2 because that's where the spinal cord is." In a decade from now, standard practice for epidural analgesia may well be "don't go below L2 because that's where the spinal cord is."
5. The paraspinous approach, rather than the midline approach, for thoracic epidurals will result in fewer failed epidurals and fewer instances of inadequate analgesia. This occurs for anatomic and geometric reasons beyond the scope of this chapter.
6. COX inhibitors, α_2-agonists, and NMDA receptor blockers administered intravenously or orally can improve analgesia, decrease the required epidural dose (especially opioid requirements), decrease side effects, and increase safety.

7. Future analgesics and antihyperalgesics include COX II inhibitors (COX I inhibitors cause gastrointestinal disturbances, platelet dysfunction, and renal dysfunction), pure α_2-agonists, δ agonists, pure NMDA receptor blockers, blockers at the glycine site of the NMDA (such drugs do not cause PCP-like side effects, a potential problem with most NMDA receptor blockers such as ketamine), NOS inhibitors, N-calcium channel blockers, AMPA/kainate (non-NMDA) receptor antagonists, and NK-I receptor antagonists.

REFERENCES AND ANNOTATED BIBLIOGRAPHY

1. Austin KL, Stapleton JU, Mather LI: Relationship between block meperidine concentrations and analgesic response. Anesthesiology 53:460–466, 1980. Probably the most careful opioid dose-response titrations ever done in postoperative patients: fourfold variation in analgesic requirements; very steep dose-response slope between severe pain and comfort (MEAC); above MEAC, only increased side effects.
2. Basbaum A: Insights into the development of opioid tolerance. Pain 61:349–352, 1995. Editorial perspective on the Mao, Price, and Mayer papers on morphine tolerance and related hyperalgesia.
3. Bjorkman R, Hallman KM, Hedner J, et al: Acetaminophen blocks spinal hyperalgesia induced by NMDA and substance P. Pain 57:259–264, 1994. The block of hyperalgesia is partial, it is reversed by flooding the system with arginine. Acetaminophen seems to act clinically by block of nitric oxide production.
4. Breivik H, Niemi G, Haugtomt H, Hogstrom H: Optimal epidural analgesia: Importance of drug combinations and correct segmental site of injection. In: Post-operative Pain Management. Clinical Anesthesiology, Vol 9. London, 1995.
   Bupivacaine, not any of the μ agonist opioids, is the spread-limiting drug. This fact, in combination with the information in Penning and Yaksh's 1992 article, constitutes a primary pharmacologic rationale for thoracic epidural catheter placement.
5. Carpenter RL: Does outcome change with pain management? Annual Refresher Course Lectures, American Society of Anesthesiologists, 1995.
   Effect of thoracic epidural analgesia on organ systems and outcome.
6. Chapman V, Haley JE, Dickenson AH: Electrophysiologic analysis of preemptive effects of spinal opioids on N-methyl-D-aspartate receptor-mediated events. Anesthesiology 81:1429–1435, 1994.
   NMDA receptor–mediated neuronal responses, such as wind-up and the established second phase of the formalin response, are poorly responsive to opioids.
7. deLeon-Casasola OA, Lema MJ: Epidural bupivacaine/sufentanyl therapy for postoperative pain control in patients tolerant to opioid and unresponsive to epidural bupivacaine/morphine. Anesthesiology 80:303–309, 1994. A μ agonist with low fractional occupance (high efficacy) (e.g., sufentanyl) can provide adequate analgesia in patients tolerant to a low-efficacy μ agonist (e.g., morphine).
8. deLeon-Casasola OA, Parker B, Lema MJ, et al: Postoperative epidural bupivacaine-morphine therapy, experience with 4,227 surgical cancer patients. Anesthesiology 81:368–375, 1994.
   A Roswell Park series with methods and results.
9. Dirig DM, Yaksh TL: Differential right shifts in the dose-response cursve for intrathecal morphine and sufentanil as a function of stimulus intensity. Pain 62:321–328, 1995.
   Clarity concerning μ agonist efficacy and fractional receptor occupancy. Morphine, in contrast to sufentanil, becomes a partial agonist at high stimulus intensity.
10. Eisenach JC: Aspirin, the miracle drug: Spinally, too? Anesthesiology 79:211–213, 1993.
    An easy introduction to isobolograms to test for analgesic synergy; contained in a worthy editorial.
11. Kehlet H: Postoperative pain relief. Reg Anesth 19:369–377, 1994.
    An easy overview of contemporary acute pain management emphasizing the uses of excellent analgesia and partial sympathectomy.

12. Kehlet H, Dahl BD: The value of "multimodal" or "balanced analgesia" in postoperative pain treatment. Anesth Analg 1977:1048–1056, 1993.

Review article comparing the last decade's world experience with epidural local anesthetics, versus opiods, versus the combination of both. One summary: combination, A minus; opioids, C plus; local anesthetics alone, D. Worth reading to form your own opinion. (If a low-dose local anesthetic alone were more efficacious one might have seen the development of acute pain services in the 1960s.)

13. Li YM, Wingrove DE, Phon Too H, et al: Local anesthetic inhibit substance P binding and evoked increases in Intracellular Ca $^{2+}$ Anesthesiology 82:166–173, 1995.

A mechanism of action of low-dose local anesthetics in the spinal cord.

14. Liu SS, Carpenter R, Mackey D, et al: Effects of perioperative analgesic technique on rate of receovery after colon surgery. Anesthesiology 83:757–765, 1995.

15. Liu S, Carpenter RL, Mulroy MF, et al: Intravenous versus epidural administration of hydromophone. Anesthesiology 82:682–688, 1995.

T10–L1 catheters. No difference in analgesia, gastrointestinal function, length of stay. More itching in epidural group. Twice total dose in intravenous group. Both groups got ketorolac. Blinded.

16. Lubenow TR, Tank EN, Hopkins EM, et al: Comparison of patient-assisted epidural analgesia with continuous-infusion epidural analgesia for postoperative patients. Reg Anesth 19:206–211, 1994.

Patient-controlled epidural analgesia is dose-sparing and improves analgesia for fentanyl-bupivacaine epidurals.

17. Malmberg AB, Yaksh TL: Hyperalgesia medicated by spinal glutamate or substance P receptor blocked by spinal cyclooxygenase inhibition. Science 257:1276–1279, 1992.

The original proof of the direct spinal action of NSAIDs.

18. Malmberg AB, Yaksh TL: Pharmacology of the spinal action of ketorolac, morphine, ST-91, U50488H and L-PIA on the formalin test and an isobolographic analysis of the NSAID interaction. Anesthesiology 79:270–281, 1993.

Demonstration of the synergistic and nonsynergistic actions of various drug combinations. The great strength of synergy between cyclooxygenase inhibitors and μ agonists. This issue of anesthesiology has a clear companion editorial by Eisenach on isobolograms, the most commonly used test for drug synergy.

19. Malmberg AB, Yaksh TL: Spinal nitric oxide synthesis inhibition blocks NMDA-induced thermal hyperalgesia and produces antinociception in the formalin test in rats. Pain 54:291–300, 1993.

Blocking nitric oxide synthetase partially blocks windup.

20. Mao J, Price DD, Mayer DJ: Experimental mononeuropathy reduces the antinociceptive effects of morphine: Implications for common intracellular mechanisms involved in morphine tolerance and neuropathic pain. Pain 61:353–364, 1995.

Neuropathic pain produces opioid tolerance *before* exposure to opioids. Mechanisms of neuropathic pain and opioid tolerance show great overlap.

21. Mao J, Price DD, Mayer DJ: Mechanism of hyperalgesia and morphine tolerance: A current view of their possible interactions. Pain 62:259–274, 1995.

Morphine tolerance, hyperalgesia, and neuropathic pain have overlapping mechanisms. Opioid tolerance *produces* hyperalgesia.

22. Marlowe S, Engstrom R, White PF: Epidural patient-controlled analgesia (PCA): An alternative to continuous epidural infusions. Pain 37:97–101, 1989. The original presentation of patient-controlled epidural analgesia hydromophone (no local anesthetic).

(lumbar) versus continuous infusion resulted in 50% dose sparing.

23. McCormack K: Non-steroidal anti-inflammatory drugs and spinal nociceptive processing. Pain 59:9–43, 1994.

An exhaustive review.

24. Penning JP, Yaksh TL: Interaction of intrathecal morphine with bupivacaine and lidocaine in the rat. Anesthesiology 77:1186–1200, 1994. Demonstration of opioid local anesthetic effect and that the side of synergy is in the dorsal horn of the spinal cord.

25. Ready LB, Oden R, Chadwick HS, et al: Development of an anesthesiology-based postoperative pain management service. Anesthesiology 68:100–106, 1988.
    A classic article on APS organization; emphasis on epidural bolus morphine technique.

26. Saeki S, Yaksh L: Suppression of nociceptive responses by spinal mu opioid agonists: Effects of stimulus intensity and agonist efficacy. Anesth Analg 77:265–274, 1993.
    Pharmacodynamics of sufentanil, a drug with high efficacy, blocks strong stimuli. Morphine, with low efficacy, does not (i.e., with strong stimuli—such as might be encountered in the operating room—morphine becomes a partial agonist). Efficacy is an expression of the occupancy-effect relationship, the fraction of receptors occupied to produce full effect (e.g., analgesia). Efficacy and potency are not the same thing: Buprenorphine, more potent than morphine, is a partial μ agonist at all doses.

27. Scott DA, Beilby DSN, McClymont C: Postoperative analgesia using epidural infusions of fentanyl with bupivacaine: A prospective analysis of 1,014 patients. Anesthesiology 83:727–737, 1995.
    An Australian series with methods and results similar to BIH.

28. Woolf CJ, Chong MS: Preemptive analgesia—treating postoperative pain by preventing the establishment of central sensitization. Anesth Analg 77:362–379, 1993.
    Review article. Perhaps of more value for presentation of the physiology of central sensitization (p. 364–366) than for lending clarity to preemptive analgesia. Without *continuous* analgesia, central sensitization develops.

29. Yaksh TL: Neuropathic pain mechanisms. ASRA Comprehensive Review of Pain Management, 1995.
    Why α_2-agonists, NMDA antagonists, NMDA glycine binding site antagonists, and systemic local anesthetics may become the mainstays of neuropathic pain mechanisms.

30. Yaksh TL, Malmberg AB: Interaction of spinal modulatory receptor systems. In: Fields HL, Liebeskind JC (eds): Progress in Pain Research and Management, Vol 1. Seattle, IASP Press, 1994.
    Excellent review of spinal drug synergy.

Chapter 26

Spinal Analgesics

Wolfgang C. Ummenhofer, MD

One of the primary aims of anesthesia is to provide the patient analgesia, permitting the performance of surgical procedures without discomfort and decreasing postoperative pain to a tolerable level. After the introduction of modern general anesthetic techniques with potent volatile and intravenous anesthetic drugs and neuromuscular blocking agents, academic focus and anesthetic training programs concentrated mainly on the efferent side of the nociceptive reflex arc. In the 1990s, a great deal of medical literature and political effort were devoted to the management of pain, to reassess the postulate expounded by Crile in 1915:[17] Functional restoration after injury will be accelerated if defense reflexes (appropriate in nature but inappropriate in the therapeutic context) can be held in abeyance by blockade of neural nociceptive input from the injured area.[92] Regional anesthetic techniques have gained general acceptance within anesthetic practice, but postoperative or therapeutic opioid administration is controversial.

Opioids are perhaps the oldest and most studied drugs. The use of opium for its euphoric effects can be traced back more than 4,000 years, and its respiratory depressant effects first were noted approximately 600 years ago.[24] Systemic opioids have a limited therapeutic index. Pain relief and side effects, the worst of them being respiratory depression, cannot be separated completely by choice of dose or opioid, and one aim of spinal drug administration is to deliver drugs to specific sites in the spinal cord at lower concentrations that are not generally attainable after systemic delivery of the drug. A goal of epidural and subarachnoid administration of opioids is to separate analgesic from respiratory effects by delivering the drug directly to the spinal cord, where there are receptors for analgesia but none for respiratory depression.

Although spinal application of morphine is reported to date back to 1901,[74] it was not until the discovery of the opiate receptors that the technique aroused widespread interest. In 1971, highly specific opioid receptors were described[45]; in 1973, opioid receptors were localized in mammalian brain,[91] and in 1976, they were found to exist in primate spinal cord.[70] Also in 1976, Yaksh and Rudy[113] first showed the effectiveness of intrathecal opioids in abolishing experimental pain in an animal model. When Kitahata and Collins[69] reviewed the spinal action of opioid analgesics in 1981, there was only one controlled study of intrathecal opioid analgesic activity in humans,[109] one study of epidural opioid effects,[38] and about a dozen case reports[37] including the preliminary communication by Behar and colleagues,[4] which acted as a catalyst to promote further studies. Such rapid and widespread use in diverse clinical applications followed that more than 100 case reports were published in 1981.[37] Never in the history of medicine has a concept progressed so rapidly from laboratory experimentation in animals to widespread clinical application in humans.[81]

The early rush to empirical clinical application of subarachnoid and epidural injections of morphine brought early fatalities from unexpected late-onset respiratory depression.[27,43] An increasing number of investigations tried to identify safer opioids than morphine and safer ways of using them, to justify spinal application of opioids outside the constraints imposed by conventional wisdom. Opioids such as meperidine,[85] fentanyl,[47] alfentanil,[31, 32] sufentanil,[46, 52, 71] and, in rats, remifentanil[19] have been investigated for spinal administration, but respiratory depression was not restricted to the use of morphine.[34, 83]

Regarding desired action and possible side effects, pharmacodynamic and pharmacokinetic parameters could be used to identify an *ideal* epidural and intrathecal opioid[29]; contrary to an increasing number of clinical investigations, however, there are only a few comprehensive kinetic data available comparing different opioids in well-controlled in vivo models. Anatomic structures within the different neuraxial compartments largely influence distribution processes and determine the bioavailability of a drug delivered to reach a specific target within the spinal cord.

This chapter presents what is known about anatomic and physiologic prerequisites that govern drug distribution across the blood-brain barrier (BBB) and across the barrier of the spinal meninges and within the cerebrospinal fluid (CSF). The chapter delineates the current knowledge of the fate of drugs administered into the epidural and intrathecal spaces and describes which physical and chemical properties direct redistribution processes from these spaces into the spinal cord.

BARRIER FUNCTION WITHIN CENTRAL NEURAXIAL ANATOMY

Before addressing the physicochemical properties of opioids and their implications more thoroughly, some pharmacokinetic aspects of their penetration across the BBB, distribution within the CSF, and redistribution to the central nervous system (CNS) and to the systemic circulation are considered. Investigation of opioid action on the brain, discovery of cerebral opiate receptors, and studies on BBB mechanisms have preceded the corresponding features on the spinal cord.

Blood-Brain Barrier and Brain Opioid Delivery

Because of its unique functions within the body, the brain is separated from the chemical environment of the other organs by the BBB. Only brain areas with a defined neuroendocrine function, such as the hypothalamus or the circumventricular organs, lack a tight BBB. The anatomy of brain capillaries is the main reason for the permeability characteristics not encountered with other organs.[62] Brain capillaries lack fenestrations, and so-called tight junctions that have high electrical resistance connect the endothelial cells. Even small electrolytes do not readily pass between them. Brain capillary endothelial cells are surrounded by extensions of astrocytes called *foot processes*, which seem to be responsible for inducing and maintaining BBB properties within the adjacent endothelial cells.[1]

Although the anatomic barrier presented by the BBB has been known for nearly 100 years, the physiologic barrier presented by brain endothelial cells is a more recent discovery. Several investigators identified multiple enzyme systems (e.g., cytochrome P-450, UDP-glucuronosyltransferase) capable of metabolizing opioids and other xenobiotics.[43, 78] It is unknown whether drug metabolism occurs to an appreciable extent in brain endothelial cells.

Another physiologic component of the BBB are the membrane-bound transporters that can transport various drugs. One of the most interesting of these transporters, with respect to opioid pharmacology, is P-glycoprotein (*MDR1* gene product). P-glycoprotein is a nonspecific transporter for a variety of dissimilar xenobiotics,[41] including morphine-6-glucuronide.[59] Morphine-6-glucuronide is a morphine metabolite that is much more potent than morphine as an analgesic (47 to 360 times) when administered intracerebroventricularly but not when administered intravenously.[42] Active exclusion of morphine-6-glucuronide by P-glycoprotein, and not simply its hydrophilic character, may be responsible for morphine-6-glucuronide's low BBB permeability[111] and consequently its low intravenous potency. More direct evidence that P-glycoprotein may be responsible for excluding opioids from the CNS comes from the work of Schinkel et al.[95] These investigators administered loperamide, a peripherally acting, antidiarrheal opiate that does not cross the BBB, to wild-type and knock-out mice (the latter lack the gene coding for P-glycoprotein). Oral loperamide induced typical opiate-like behavior in the knock-out mice but no such behavior in the wild-type mice. It seems that loperamide normally is prevented from crossing the BBB by active P-glycoprotein–mediated exclusion.

The physicochemical properties, if any, that make opioids potential targets for either metabolism by brain endothelial cells or active exclusion by P-glycoprotein remain to be determined. Both of these mechanisms need to be considered, however, as potentially important determinants of opioid bioavailability and analgesic efficacy.

In 1971, Herz and Teschemacher[54] reviewed activities and sites of antinociceptive action of morphine-like analgesics and kinetics of distribution after intravenous, intracerebral, or intraventricular application. Drug effects on the CNS included a series of problems not encountered with other organs. The BBB impedes or prevents the penetration of drugs with low lipid solubility into the brain, and the distribution of substances between octanol and water can define values for their relative hydrophilicity or lipophilicity.

After intravenous administration, the brain concentration of morphine and dihydromorphone increases to a maximum of only about 5% of their corresponding plasma concentrations, whereas the concentration of fentanyl was found to be about 10 times greater in the brain than in the plasma.[54] For lipophilic substances, the BBB is no obstacle, and such drugs can reach their receptors easily from the capillaries. Because most of the neurons are located within a distance of not more than 50 μ from a capillary, there is no significant distance to be overcome. Because of the high blood supply to the brain, substantial amounts of lipophilic substances pass into brain tissue during their first passage through the brain's vasculature. The substances are retained to a great extent in the brain, resulting in concentrations far above plasma levels. At the same time, the plasma concentration drops quickly, and the substance leaves the brain again.

With intraventricular application, lipophilic compounds leave the ventricular system rapidly. Within a few minutes after injection, a large amount of substance leaves the CSF compartment through the choroid plexus; the remainder of the drug permeates initially into the brain and to its receptors, then passes rapidly into the blood circulation. Because of its large number of capillaries, the brain can act like a sieve through which these substances readily fall; this explains why the doses required to bring about a given antinociceptive effect by either mode of application do not differ much. In contrast, when hydrophilic compounds are injected into the ventricular system, they are retained in the CSF to a much greater degree. The speed of permeation into periventricular tissue is slower than it is with lipophilic substances, as shown by delayed onset of drug action. This slower penetration most likely is related to diffusion of these substances mainly through the intercellular clefts, whereas lipophilic drugs also can take a transcellular route. Hydrophilic compounds remain in the ventricular system for a long time, ensuring the maintenance of a high concentration gradient and further permeation of the substance into the tissue. Out of an applied quantity of fentanyl, not more than 10% was found 15 minutes after administration, but 40% to 60% of applied morphine was found at this time, and more than 10% of morphine was present in the CSF even after 1 hour. Fentanyl appeared in the blood quickly, whereas morphine entered the systemic circulation much more slowly. There is an inverse relationship between the rate of appearance in blood and the duration of the drug in the ventricular system. Within 5 minutes after intraventricular application, 40% to 50% of fentanyl but only 3% to 6% of morphine was found in the blood.

These different kinetics are not due to a structural impediment of diffusion. A CSF-brain barrier comparable to the BBB does not exist. The ependyma seems to be relatively easily penetrated by lipophilic and hydrophilic compounds. Using autoradiographic techniques, the amount of radiolabeled substance found in brain tissue at various time points after intraventricular application was determined. Although for morphine the quantity did not change much with time, for fentanyl there was a rapid decline during the first hour after injection. The two substances had different distribution patterns. Morphine preferentially diffused into gray matter, whereas fentanyl exhibited a pronounced preference for fiber structures. It was suggested that these differences reflected the different lipid solubilities of the compounds. Morphine continued its penetration into the brain, whereas the activity of fentanyl decreased quickly and, 120 minutes after injection, was scarcely detectable in a small zone at the periventricular wall. The delayed onset of morphine antinociceptive action corresponded to its slow permeation into the deeper layers ($> 800 \mu m$) of the ventricular wall. At 15 minutes after injection, the time of first evaluation of the diffusion depth, the penetration front of fentanyl already was beyond the maximum point and in the process of withdrawal. This observation corresponds well with antinociceptive animal data, which show the maximum analgesic effect of fentanyl occurs before this time.[54]

After intracerebral microinjection, the passage of the compounds into the blood circulation is similar to that obtained by intraventricular injection. The lipophilicity of the substance determines the speed of passage into the circulation.

For intraventricular administration, the different distribution kinetics of hydrophilic and lipophilic opioids can be described by the relative importance of two factors: (1) fast diffusion into brain tissue and fast migration into the blood with lipophilic substances and (2) slow diffusion into the brain tissue and slow migration into the blood with hydrophilic substances. The hydrophilic or lipophilic character of intraventricularly applied compounds largely determines the differences in their duration of action.

Herz and Teschemacher[54] determined the dose producing the maximum effect by each route of administration for many opioids and found that the intravenous-to-intraventricular dose ratios were as follows: morphine, 892; hydromorphone, 531; meperidine, 8.5; and fentanyl, 5.8. They found a high correlation between the lipid solubility of each drug and the intravenous-to-intraventricular dose ratios, and they postulated that hydrophilic drugs, such as morphine and hydromorphone, remain in the CSF for long periods, maintaining a concentration gradient from the ventricles to the brain. Lipid-soluble drugs diffuse rapidly from the CSF to the brain, but they diffuse with equal rapidity from the brain to the blood vessels. There is rapid equilibration from the CSF to the intravascular compartment, minimizing the differences between intraventricular and intravenous effects.

This discussion of brain opioid pharmacokinetics is best considered in the context of the parallelism to the spinal cord with the comparable compartments of the epidural space, CSF, and spinal cord white and gray matter. Similar explanations are likely to hold true for the transfer of drugs from the spinal subarachnoid space to the spinal cord.

Anatomy of the Spinal Meninges and Their Role in Spinal Drug Delivery

Comparable to the brain and the BBB, the spinal cord is separated from the surrounding blood compartment by a protecting layer of meninges. The outermost and thickest of the three meninges is the dura mater, which, until more recently, was held to be the principal meningeal permeability barrier. Consequently, although data were not consistent, most studies investigating meningeal drug permeation used isolated dura preparation and found molecular weight and shape of drugs to be determinants of opioid penetration.[80, 94] Bernards and Hill[8] showed, however, that the dura mater is actually the most permeable of the three spinal meninges. Composed of collagen and elastin fibers, the dura mater is largely acellular except for a layer of cells that form the border toward the arachnoid mater. These so-called dural border cells and their large extracellular spaces form a virtual *subdural space* that does not exist *in situ*.[106] The dural border cells strongly adhere to the outer cell layer of the arachnoid mater, but because of rare intercellular connections and the absence of collagen reinforcement, this region is particularly friable. It is estimated that 10% of intended spinal injections[63] and 1% of intended epidural injections[73] are made into this posttraumatic intradural space. Arterial, venous, and lymphatic vessels copiously supply the dura mater and may provide nutrients and metabolic exchange to the avascular arachnoid mater.[106] Epidurally administered drugs may be cleared partly into the systemic circulation by this vascular bed before reaching the spinal cord.

In contrast to the dura mater, the arachnoid membrane has little substance and neither can be seen on imaging nor can be perceived as the needle penetrates it. It has a filmy, elastic consistency and recedes from an advancing needle. Dissection of a fresh specimen shows that the arachnoid readily separates from the inner surface of the dura or even delaminates and splits between its different layers.[55] The arachnoid mater consists of overlapping layers of flattened cells with closely adherent cell membranes connected together by frequent tight junctions, desmosomes and gap junctions.[106] These tight junctions are believed to be the basis for the arachnoid, and not the dura mater, being the principal meningeal permeability barrier, accounting for more than 90% of the resistance to drug diffusion from the epidural space to the CSF.[8] Where the spinal nerve roots traverse the dura and arachnoid membranes, arachnoid herniations through the dura mater into the epidural space form arachnoid granulations. Comparable with cranial arachnoid granulations, spinal arachnoid granulations may serve as a site for material in the CSF to exit the subarachnoid space. It is reasonable to speculate that these arachnoid granulations also may serve as a preferred route for epidural drugs to reach the spinal cord, but experimental data suggest this is not the case.[9]

Between the arachnoid and the pia mater is the subarachnoid space containing CSF. This compartment is connected with the cranial CSF and contains the unmyelinated spinal nerve roots. The pia mater consists of a cellular layer bordering the subarachnoid space and a connective tissue layer interspersed with collagen on the surface of the spinal cord. It covers the blood vessels lying on the surface of the spinal cord, but in contrast to the arachnoid mater, the pia is fenestrated so that the spinal cord is in direct communication with the subarachnoid space. CSF may be looked on as an extension of the spinal extracellular fluid.[14] On histologic grounds alone, the pia mater seems to be unimportant as a barrier to drug movement, which is confirmed by experimental observations.[8]

Barrier and Metabolic Functions of the Spinal Meninges

As noted earlier, drugs can diffuse across the spinal meninges.[7, 8, 80, 94, 103] Contrary to in vitro studies on human tissue obtained from the autopsy,[80, 94] Bernards and Hill[8] showed in an in vitro diffusion cell model with live spinal meninges from monkeys and dogs that the arachnoid mater is the principal meningeal barrier to drug diffusion. Permeability coefficients through intact monkey spinal meninges are 6.2×10^{-4} cm/min for morphine and 2.3×10^{-3} cm/min for alfentanil (Table 1); active transport or facilitated diffusion mechanisms did not seem to play any role in the transmeningeal diffusion of these drugs.

The absence of drug transport through the arachnoid villi from the epidural space to the CSF[9, 21] reflects material traversing the villi by micropinocytosis. This process was shown to be unidirectional from the CSF to the epidural space or venous system.[2, 114] From a teleo-

TABLE 1

Physicochemical Characteristics and Pharmacokinetics of Commonly Used Opioid Agonists

Parameter	Morphine	Meperidine	Fentanyl	Sufentanil	Alfentanil	Remifentanil
pKa	7.9	8.5	8.4	8.0	6.5	7.26
% nonionized (pH 7.4)	23	7	8.5	20	89	58
λow	1	39	955	1,737	129	NA
Protein binding (%)	35	70	84	93	92	66–93
Clearance (ml·min^{-1})	1,050	1,020	1,530	900	238	4,000
Vd$_{ss}$*	224	305	335	123	27	30
Rapid distribution half-life ($T_{1/2}$D, min)	—	—	1.2–1.9	1.4	1.0–3.5	0.4–0.5
Slow redistribution half-life ($T_{1/2}\alpha$, min)	1.5–4.4	4–16	9.2–19	17.7	9.5–17	2.0–3.7
Elimination half-life ($T_{1/2}\beta$, h)	1.7–3.3	3–5	3.1–6.6	2.2–4.6	1.4–1.5	0.17–0.33
Meningeal permeability coefficient (cm/min $\times 10^{-3}$)	0.6	NA	0.9	0.75	2.3	NA
MEAC (ng·ml^{-1})	10–15	200	0.6	0.03	15	NA

λow, octanol:water partition coefficient; Vd$_{ss}$, steady-state volume of distribution; MEAC, minimum effective analgesic concentration, defined in most studies as the plasma opioid concentration with just-perceptible analgesia. (MEAC represents a range of plasma levels, not a specific value. MEAC plasma levels may vary up to fivefold between different patients and with time and activity in a specific patient.) NA, not available.
Data from Bernards CM, Hill HF: Physical and chemical properties of drug molecules governing their diffusion through the spinal meninges. Anesthesiology 77:750–756, 1992.
Adapted from Coda BA: Opioids. In: Barash PG (ed): Clinical Anesthesia, 3rd ed. Philadelphia: Lippincott-Raven, 1996, pp 329–358.

logic point of view, it is reasonable not to select evolutionarily for a complex BBB and, at the same time, to develop transport systems for foreign material from the epidural space to the CNS, circumventing this barrier.

Besides mere diffusion through the spinal meninges or preferential transport through the spinal nerve root cuff, diffusion through the walls of spinal radicular arteries and subsequent delivery to the spinal cord via radicular blood flow was proposed as a third possible mechanism of drug movement from the epidural space.[37] This hypothetical vascular route subsequently was identified as active in drug removal but not drug transport to the spinal cord.[12]

The only mechanism by which drugs move from the epidural space to the spinal cord seems to be by diffusion, mainly governed by arachnoid mater permeability. Understanding this principal factor that determines drug permeation across the meninges offers the potential of influencing the redistribution of spinally administered drugs and altering their spinal bioavailability.

For epidural catheterization that is either long-term or temporary, bacterial colonization and an increasing incidence of catheter-related infections have been described.[58, 90] Meningeal permeability for hydrophilic and lipophilic drugs was shown *in vitro* to be increased by *Staphylococcus aureus* bacteria and bacterial toxins.[105]

The barrier function of the spinal meninges has been considered to be solely anatomic. More recent evidence suggests, however, that the meninges may serve as metabolic barriers limiting the spinal bioavailability of different pharmacologically active compounds. The cranial[43, 79, 108, 116] and the spinal meninges[51, 65, 66, 104] were shown to have enzyme systems capable of metabolizing endogenous neurotransmitters and exogenous drug molecules. The role of these enzyme systems in the meninges is unclear. Similar to the BBB, which serves as a structural and a metabolic shield protecting the CNS from the rest of the body, the spinal meninges also may remove stray neurotransmitters from the CSF or prevent permeation of undesirable chemicals present in the blood or epidural space. These findings may have clinical relevance. Epinephrine, an endogenous neurotransmitter and an adjuvant commonly added to local anesthetics and opioids administered into the epidural and intrathecal spaces, was shown to be 75% metabolized through local catechol-O-methyltransferase while diffusing across the spinal meninges.[66] Research on the pharmacology of nociception showed the involvement of cholinergic transmission at the spinal level and the safe use of intrathecal neostigmine for spinal pain modulation.[57] The cholinesterase activity of the spinal meninges, as shown for monkeys and pigs,[104] also may contribute to the endogenous spinal cord/CSF acetylcholine metabolism and the incidence of untoward effects after therapeutic intrathecal neostigmine administration.

Future clinical directions point to the inhibition of enzymes responsible for metabolizing desirable drugs or neurotransmitters, increasing drug bioavailability in the spinal cord. Enzymes responsible for metabolizing undesirable neurotransmitters, such as substance P in chronic pain stages, could be induced so as to decrease the amount of neurotransmitter available within the spinal cord. The meninges could metabolize inactive prodrugs, designed to be cleared rapidly from the blood to the CSF, to yield pharmacologically active compounds within the CSF.

A discussion of the barrier function of the spinal meninges often tends to be unidirectional, focusing only on the limited bioavailability of epidurally administered drugs. The meninges may play a crucial role in redistributing intrathecally administered drugs to the epidural space, reducing their availability for their intended target in the CSF or spinal cord. An ideal drug for epidural administration would diffuse rapidly across the spinal meninges, whereas an ideal drug for intrathecal administration would have low meningeal permeability.

PHYSIOLOGY OF THE CEREBROSPINAL FLUID AND INTRATHECAL DRUG DISTRIBUTION

As mentioned previously, the CSF may be looked on as an extension of the spinal extracellular fluid.[14] Similarly, reflecting its role as medium between neuronal tissue and circulation, the CSF has been regarded as an ultrafiltrate of blood plasma having similar composition except for a considerably lower protein content. The main functions of the CSF are to cushion the CNS against trauma and to clear waste products of neuronal metabolism from the CNS; this includes removal of endogenous transmitters, drugs and their metabolites, and all other substances entering the brain and spinal cord by blood or epidural space.

Produced within the choroid plexus of the brain's lateral ventricles, the CSF reaches the spinal cord through the central ventricular system connected to the subarachnoid spaces of the brain and spinal cord. Approximately 400 to 500 mL of fluid is produced each day, at a rate of about 0.35 mL/min. CSF is exchanged two to three times a day, reflecting the total amount of 140 to 150 mL in normal adults.[110] Of approximately 75 mL that is intracranial, 23 mL is located within the ventricles. The remaining 75 mL of CSF lies within the spinal subarachnoid space and represents the potential volume of CSF within which spinally administered drugs can be distributed. The volume of spinal CSF within which anesthetic solutions are distributed under most clinical conditions is, however, substantially less than 75 mL. A considerable portion of this 75 mL must be in the area of the subarachnoid space occupied by the cauda equina distal (i.e., caudad) to L2.[48] In vivo measurement of lumbosacral CSF volume showed a nearly threefold variability of CSF volume in healthy adults.[56] Using magnetic resonance imaging, Carpenter et al[23] measured lumbosacral CSF volumes from 42.7 to 81.1 mL.[23] Obese individuals have substantially less CSF, which is caused partly by compression of the neural foramina.[71] CSF is absorbed into the venous circulation through herniations of the arachnoid that protrude into the lumina of veins through gaps in the dura. These herniations, the arachnoid villi, are particularly numerous in the superior sagittal sinus but also are present in other intracranial veins. Arachnoid villi are found adjacent to spinal nerve roots as they emerge through the dura. The quantitative significance of spinal arachnoid villi in the absorption of CSF is unknown but has been considered to be minor compared with the role played by intracranial arachnoid villi.[49]

The driving force of CSF movement is the pressure head within the producing lateral ventricles, with posture being an important factor of distribution. Patients in the lateral position have a CSF pressure of 60 to 100 mm Hg in the lumbar region, which increases to 200 to 250 mm Hg when patients change to a sitting position. High CSF pressures accelerate the passive clearance across the arachnoid villi toward the venous system; when CSF pressure exceeds venous pressure by 2 to 4 mm Hg, the arachnoid villi serve as one-way valves releasing CSF into the dural sinuses. When venous pressure exceeds CSF pressure, the leaf-like valves close, preventing blood from entering the CSF compartment. The main direction of flow of the 500 mL of CSF produced per day is intracranial; only a small portion of CSF (perhaps <10%[49]) flows downward through the spinal subarachnoid space. On its way from the brain to the sacral cul-de-sac, CSF flows caudally along the dorsal aspect of the spinal cord and returns rostrally along the ventral surface of the cord to reach the basilar cisterns. In humans, this round trip is estimated to take approximately 2 to 2.5 hours. In addition to the flow of CSF, a pulsatile to-and-fro motion is imparted to the CSF by the normal pulsatile motion of the brain, which occurs with each heartbeat. Observations from magnetic resonance imaging confirmed that the CSF is not a still lake of fluid but vigorously oscillates with arterial pulsations.[71] These two mechanisms of CSF movement and effects of posture and positioning are principally responsible for the rostral spread of drugs that are dissolved in CSF. Changes in transabdominal and transthoracic pressures and turbulence produced in the CSF by injections of solutions with volumes exceeding 10% of the spinal CSF volume also are important factors. The cranial movement of colored dyes and radio-labeled tracers introduced into the spinal subarachnoid space depends on these factors.[89]

The conventional wisdom is that hydrophobic drugs are less likely to undergo significant rostral spread within the CSF compared with more hydrophilic drugs. The movement of the CSF has an effect on both classes of drugs, however, as soon as they dissolve within the CSF. Gourlay et al[46] found detectable concentrations of the relatively hydrophobic fentanyl in cervical CSF within 3 minutes after lumbar epidural administration in humans. There is evidence that hydrophobic drugs have a much faster clearance from the CSF than more hydrophilic ones.[102] Consequently, owing to their more rapid removal, a relatively smaller fraction of the administered dose of hydrophobic compounds reaches cephalad sites; lipid solubility itself does not alter the rate at which drugs spread rostrally.

Initial intrathecal drug distribution may depend on the route of application. Epidural administration requires diffusion across the meninges, whereas direct subarachnoid deliverance results in a primarily high intrathecal concentration. Injection speed, composition of the drug solution (i.e., specific gravity and volume of the bolus), site of injection, pH of the CSF, intraabdominal pressure, patient age, and position of the patient determine the degree of mixing or drug expansion within the CSF.[48, 49]

For spinally administered anesthetic solutions, the force or rate of injection had no clinically significant effect on the spread in CSF.[18, 76, 84] The resistance of the application systems (i.e., long catheters or thin spinal needles) reduces significantly the amount of kinetic energy exerted by forceful injection. A low internal cross-sectional area of the delivering needle or catheter results in little mixing of the injected solution with CSF during intrathecal administration.[92] The viewpoint that *true* low injection speed should be in the order of 1 mL/8 min[15] seems to be of little clinical relevance.

A second crucial factor affecting the initial distribution of intrathecal drugs is the *baricity* of the injectant.[5, 89] The density of a solution is the weight in grams of 1 mL of solution (i.e., g/mL). The specific gravity of a solution is a ratio: the density of the solution divided by the density of water. Baricity is defined as the ratio of the density of the injected solution compared with the density of CSF, which averages 1.0003 g/mL at 37°C.[49] Solutions with a baricity greater than 1.000, typically prepared by adding dextrose 5% to 8%, are called *hyperbaric*, whereas solutions with a baricity less than 1.000, prepared by mixing drugs in water, are *hypobaric*. Solutions that are the same density as CSF are termed *isobaric*; truly isobaric solutions are difficult to prepare because one rarely knows an individual's exact CSF density at a given temperature. For isobaric solutions, the position of the patient has no effect on drug distribution, whereas hyperbaric solutions move down the spinal column in response to gravity, and hypobaric solutions rise within the CSF. As a function of time, baricity of a solution affects drug distribution only until the solution is diluted sufficiently by CSF so that it becomes isobaric. Closely related to baricity of the injected solution, the patient's position is the most important factor determining the initial distribution of intrathecally administered drugs. Composition of epidurally administered drug solutions, contrary to the situation with intrathecal delivery, has little if any effect on drug movement within the CSF because drugs pass the arachnoid mater as individual molecules and not as a solution.

For local anesthetic solutions, Greene[49] identified 25 factors that could affect distribution in the CSF, and he divided them into two groups. Factors that had no clinically demonstrable significant effects included patient's weight, patient's gender, direction in which the bevel of a standard lumbar puncture needle faces, turbulence created by alterations in rate of injection or by barbotage, diffusion of local anesthetic in CSF, composition of CSF, CSF circulation, CSF pressure, concentration of local anesthetic in the solution injected, and addition of vaso-constrictors to the local anesthetic solution. Factors that demonstrably affected distribution of local anesthetic solutions in CSF, although of widely varying clinical significance, included patient's age; patient's height, anatomic configuration of the spinal column; site of injection; direction of the needle during injection, volume of CSF; density of CSF; density and baricity of the anesthetic solution injected, position of the patient (with hypobaric or hyper-baric solutions), dosage of local anesthetic; and volume of anesthetic solution injected. Car-penter et al[23] showed that variability in lumbosacral CSF volume is the most important factor identified to date that contributes to the variability in the spread of spinal sensory anesthesia, corresponding to the clinical observation that repeated spinal anesthesia in the same person produces relatively consistent spread and duration of spinal anesthesia. In contrast to the corre-lations between CSF volume and measures of sensory anesthesia, CSF volume did not correlate with the duration of motor blockade. These findings probably would not be helpful for guid-ing clinical practice, however, because CSF volume is not measured before anesthesia, is highly variable, and is not predicted easily by patient characteristics.[23]

For epidural opioid administration, the volume of injectant seems to be most important for lipophilic opioids but has been shown to be unimportant for morphine.[82, 85, 98] Move-ment and position of the patient have been discussed as possible reasons for cephalad mi-gration of opioid-containing CSF with consecutive respiratory depression,[34] and prophylaxis has been suggested if the patient is kept in the head-up position. This position may not al-ways be possible, however, because it is uncomfortable for the patient and may contribute to cardiovascular instability.[68]

PHYSICOCHEMICAL PROPERTIES OF DRUG MOLECULES GOVERNING THEIR DIFFUSION THROUGH THE SPINAL MENINGES

Drugs administered into the epidural space for selective spinal analgesia must diffuse through the spinal meninges to gain access to their sites of action in the spinal cord. Knowledge of the physical and chemical properties of drug molecules (see Table 1) that govern their diffusion through the meninges is important for understanding the pharmacokinetics of epidural anal-gesia.[10, 31]

Hydrophilicity and Hydrophobicity

Penetration of a solute through any tissue is a complex process in which the solute first must partition into the tissue, then diffuse through the tissue, and finally partition out of the tis-sue's opposite surface. This process of partitioning and diffusion is described by the solute's permeability coefficient (P), expressed mathematically by the equation $P = K \times D/L$, where K = the solute's tissue:water partition coefficient; D = the diffusivity of the solute within the tissue; and L = the thickness of the tissue.[10] The solute's tissue:water partition coefficient is a measure of the solute's relative solubility in tissue and water and largely depends on the rel-ative hydrophobicity of the solute. The solute's relative hydrophobicity often is measured by its octanol:water distribution coefficient, and the solute's diffusivity largely depends on phys-ical properties such as size, shape, or mass.[100] Which of these physical parameters correlates best with diffusivity depends on the nature of the tissue and the diffusion path taken by the solute (e.g., water-filled pores, intercellular channels, transcellular diffusion). The relative ease with which a drug molecule penetrates through the spinal meninges depends on one or more of that drug's physical and chemical properties—molecular weight, molecular radius, molecular volume, molecular surface area, or hydrophobicity.

Moore et al[80] reported that molecular weight is the principal determinant of drug flux across the dura mater. If so, morphine and meperidine, with molecular weights of 285 and 247, should penetrate the dura with equal speed, which is not the case.[98] An in vivo study in dogs showed that the large-molecular weight inulin passed the dura as rapidly as morphine,[40] and it has been suggested that the observed in vivo difference in pharmacokinetics of drugs is due primarily to the difference in lipophilicity.[98] Bernards and Hill[8] showed that the arachnoid mater, and not the dura mater, is the principal permeability barrier to drugs diffusing through the spinal meninges, and the results of Moore et al[80] may not apply to the meninges as a whole.

Lipid solubility was suggested as an important chemical property determining a drug's permeability through the meninges.[16, 36, 37] In an in vitro model using monkey spinal meninges, Bernards and Hill[10] found a biphasic relationship between the octanol:buffer distribution coefficient and the drug's measured permeability coefficients but no relationship between a drug's permeability coefficient and any measure of drug mass, molecular shape, or molecular size. Drugs of intermediate hydrophobicity seem to move more readily between the lipid and the aqueous phases of the tissue, and their partition coefficients are correspondingly greater. This finding is consistent with data describing an optimal distribution coefficient for BBB penetration,[52] and a similar biphasic relationship was shown for other living tissues, such as cornea[67, 96] or skin.[115]

In addition to opioids, a biphasic relationship has been shown for penetration-enhancing drugs, such as acylcarnitines (see later), to promote hydrophilic drug permeation across the spinal meninges.[11] Acylcarnitines must surpass a crucial chain length (10 carbon units) but should not exceed 16 carbon units, and the ability of the acylcarnitines to increase the transmeningeal flux of morphine in vitro is reduced on either side of this range.[103]

Enhancement of Meningeal Permeability

The barrier function of the spinal meninges can be altered to increase the permeability of hydrophilic and hydrophobic drugs, improving a drug's bioavailability. As described earlier, hydrophobic drugs have relatively low meningeal permeability, presumably because they are sequestered in the lipophilic environment of the arachnoid mater cell membranes. Lowering the energy requirements to their entering the aqueous cellular phase theoretically could increase their penetration of the hydrophilic interior of the arachnoid cell. Hydrophilic drugs, conversely, can penetrate the interior of the arachnoid cell easily, but they have difficulties entering the lipid bilayer of the cell membrane on either side of the arachnoid.

Cyclodextrins, cyclic oligosaccharides, have been used for years to solubilize hydrophobic compounds otherwise insoluble in aqueous solutions.[101] They possess a ring structure with a hydrophobic interior, whereas the exterior is hydrophilic because of numerous hydroxyl groups. Hydrophobic molecules are effectively shielded by cyclodextrin from surrounding water molecules, and because no bonds are formed between shield and hydrophobic compound, movement in and out of the cyclodextrin is fast. For spinal drug delivery, cyclodextrin has been shown to improve transport of lipophilic compounds,[61, 112] and Bernards showed in vitro that combining sufentanil with cyclodextrin more than doubled sufentanil's meningeal permeability.[7]

Hydrophilic compounds such as morphine cannot enter the lipid bilayer of the arachnoid cell membrane easily, which presumably limits their meningeal permeability. In vitro studies showed that addition of acylcarnitines to a hydrophilic drug solution increased its ability to traverse the hydrophobic exterior of the arachnoid membrane.[11, 103] Acylcarnitines are naturally occurring amphipathic molecules found in all mammalian cells. Within cellular metabolism, they are essential compounds to shuttle fatty acids across the inner mitochondrial membrane for subsequent oxidation.

The use of permeability-increasing adjuncts such as cyclodextrins or acylcarnitines offers a theoretical chance to improve transport processes across the spinal meninges of epidurally administered drugs. In the future, *drug design* taking into account physicochemical properties may increase the bioavailability of spinally administered drugs to their target cells by combining a specific compound with a suitable adjunct as a shuttle.

NEURAXIAL OPIOID PHARMACOKINETICS

Despite widespread use, little is known about the comparative pharmacokinetics of spinally administered opioids. Pharmacokinetic characteristics of the *ideal* opioid for neuraxial use include rapid distribution from epidural administration across the spinal meninges or from the CSF to the cord after intrathecal administration. Ideally, this distribution should be combined with slow clearance back from the cord to plasma (i.e., high integral exposure of the spinal cord to the opioid) and moderate rostral CSF distribution. At least in an animal model on intrathecal drug administration, neither lipophilic nor hydrophilic opioids had the physicochemical properties to achieve this purpose.[102] It may not be possible to design a drug with an *ideal* constellation of pharmacokinetic properties. We may have to rethink spinal drug administration to localize drug delivery to the spinal target.

Basic Considerations

Opioid/receptor activity is governed mainly by pharmacodynamic rules, but the amount of an initially administered opioid dose available at its site of action depends largely on pharmacokinetic variables. Pharmacokinetics determine the relationship between drug dose and its concentration at the effector sites. Because spinal opiate receptors bind δ and κ opioid agonists with high affinity, one theoretically could administer a smaller dose of a selective agonist (e.g., D-ala^2-D-leu^5 enkephalin, a stable analog of leucine-enkephalin with hydrophilic properties comparable to morphine) instead of a *nonselective* agonist (e.g., morphine) to produce comparable effects. Theoretically, administration of a smaller (but more potent) intrathecal dose would decrease CSF and plasma concentrations and minimize effects at supraspinal analgesic sites activated as a result of vascular or CSF redistribution of the opioid. δ or κ receptor selectivity alone is not sufficient, however, to produce selective spinal effects because a hydrophilic δ agonist (e.g., D-ala^2-D-leu^5 enkephalin) was associated with supraspinal redistribution and side effects similar to morphine.[89] This illustrates the importance of CSF distribution in the production of toxic and therapeutic effects, even with a relatively selective opioid agonist, and underlines, at least for clinical conditions, the superiority of pharmacokinetics when compared with pharmacodynamic conditions.

Changes in drug concentration over time in the various compartments such as blood, epidural space, CSF, and at the effector site within the brain or spinal cord are determined by physicochemical properties of the drug and by a multitude of biologic functions involved in the processes of absorption, redistribution, biotransformation, and elimination. Two-compartment or three-compartment models are used to characterize opioid distribution after different routes of application: intravenous, epidural, intrathecal, and, although rare, intracerebroventricular.[3] Figure 1 shows a simplified pharmacokinetic model for spinally administered opioids superimposed on a conventional three-compartment open mammillary model.

For intravenous administration of opioids, the initial effects are mainly cerebral and are determined by blood flow per unit weight that is about twice that for the spinal cord.[75] After the distribution phases, there is a more equal concentration of opioid at both sites, and spinal analgesia can participate fully in the overall analgesic effect.

Epidural administration aims at selective spinal analgesia, but opioids can move in at least three possible directions: There may be a *local* distribution to epidural fat, relatively direct

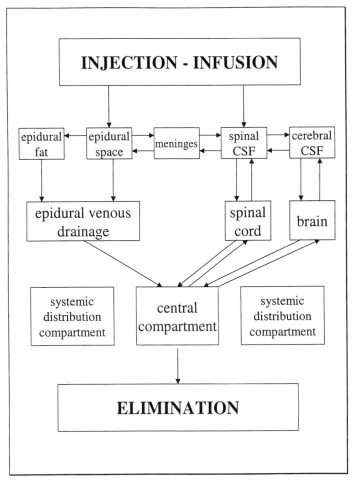

Figure 1. Pharmacokinetic model for spinal drug administration (Adapted from Chrubasik J, Chrubasik S, Martin E: The ideal epidural opioid—fact or fantasy? Eur J Anaesthesiol 10:79–100, 1993.)

access to the central compartment via the epidural venous drainage, or less direct access across the spinal meninges to the CSF and CNS. The desired effect compartment (spinal cord) is reached through the spinal CSF, but the brain (the *side-effect compartment* of greatest concern) still can be accessed through both the central compartment and the CSF. No more than 5% of any opioid is ever likely to reach the CSF,[87, 98] but this amount is located in a small volume of distribution. For morphine, the volume of distribution is about 1 mL·kg^{-1} [88] so that the CSF concentrations of morphine are between 40 and 200 times those of plasma during the distributive phases after an epidural injection.[50, 64] With more lipophilic opioids, the ratio of CSF to plasma concentrations is much less (e.g., only 14:1 for sufentanil).[86] This is because of faster distribution within and from the CSF.[39]

The intent of subarachnoid administration is to achieve selective spinal analgesia by placing a small dose of opioid in a small volume of distribution to access the spinal effector compartment without reaching the brain via the central compartment. High concentrations of opioid still may be carried to the brain, however, by the unpredictable movements of the CSF. Redistribution across the spinal meninges, especially for lipophilic drugs, also can occur.

In contrast to opioids administered into the plasma, epidural or intrathecal opioids must diffuse relatively long distances to reach their site of action in the spinal cord dorsal horn. In so doing, they are subject to the same laws of thermodynamics that govern the movement of molecules in any other chemical environment. Specifically, they diffuse in random directions from their site of administration, and they partition into the chemical microenvironments in which they are thermodynamically most stable. The epidural space, intrathecal space, and spinal cord contain many different microenvironments, including epidural fat, collagen, arachnoid cell membranes, intracellular organelles, CSF, axons, myelin, neuronal cell bodies, extracellular fluid, and glycocalix. Which of these microenvironments a given molecule preferentially partitions into depends on that molecule's particular physicochemical properties, and the pattern of partitioning plays a crucial role in determining its bioavailability in the spinal cord.

Epidural Pharmacokinetics

To understand how physicochemical properties govern the rate and extent to which epidurally administered opioids redistribute to the spinal cord, it is necessary to understand how opioids get to the spinal cord from the epidural space.[6] Several mechanisms have been proposed: (1) diffusion through the spinal meninges, (2) preferential diffusion through the spinal nerve root cuff,[35] and (3) diffusion through the walls of spinal radicular arteries with subsequent carriage to the spinal cord via radicular blood flow.[37] Experimental animal studies showed, however, that epidurally administered drugs do not preferentially diffuse through the spinal nerve root cuff,[9] and they are not carried to the spinal cord by radicular blood flow.[12] To date, the only mechanism shown to be responsible for drug movement between the epidural space and the spinal cord is diffusion through the spinal meninges[8, 10] with subsequent diffusion through the CSF and the spinal cord white matter to reach the spinal cord dorsal horn. Epidurally administered drugs that reach the CSF also can diffuse back across the meninges into the epidural space, but unless and until the drug's concentration in the epidural space falls below that in the CSF, net drug transfer will be directed from the epidural space into the CSF. Diffusion depends mainly on an opioid's physicochemical properties (e.g., its degree of hydrophobicity) (see earlier).

Meningeal permeability is not the only determinant of an opioid's spinal cord bioavailability after epidural administration. Drugs can partition into various environments in the epidural space and be unavailable for transfer across the spinal meninges. In particular, epidural fat may serve as a sequestration site for lipid-soluble drugs, such as fentanyl or sufentanil.[102] Consequently, much less sufentanil is bioavailable to cross the spinal meninges than is the more hydrophilic drug morphine. It also has been suggested that epidurally administered drugs can be cleared from the epidural space by direct uptake through the wall of epidural veins; despite claims to the contrary, this mechanism for drug clearance has never been shown clearly.[37]

In comparing the parameters of 50 μg of sufentanil administered epidurally, intramuscularly, or intrathecally in dogs, the rank order of maximum plasma concentration was intrathecal > epidural > intramuscular, and for the time to reach maximum plasma concentration was intrathecal = intramuscular > epidural (i.e., epidural resulted in the fastest absorption). After 90 minutes, the plasma concentration was epidural = intrathecal > intramuscular. For alfentanil, the redistribution into the plasma after delivery by the three different routes was essentially indistinguishable.[93] In humans, an identical kinetic profile also was found.[25] Morphine absorbs more slowly into the plasma after intrathecal injection compared with epidural or intramuscular injection. The order of maximum concentration was epidural > intramuscular = intrathecal.[93] In humans, vascular absorption also was shown to be faster after epidural administration and was similar for intrathecal and intramuscular injection.[26]

For epidural opioid administration, the volume of injectant is a variable that is easily manipulated and can influence the efficacy of the drug. This seems to be most important for lipophilic opioids; when epidural fentanyl, 50 μg, was given in different concentrations after cesarean section, analgesic efficacy was reduced for diluent volumes less than 5 mL,[13] and an animal model showed that analgesia from epidural sufentanil improved as a function of diluent volume.[107] In contrast to more lipophilic opioids, injectant volume does not seem to be an important factor affecting analgesia from epidural morphine.[82, 98] Epidural injection of morphine in a volume of 1 mL gave analgesia equivalent to injection in a volume of 10 mL.[28] For meperidine, an opioid with intermediate lipophilicity (see Table 29–1), the onset and quality of analgesia after cesarean section were better when an epidural dose of 25 mg was diluted to a volume of 5 mL or 10 mL compared with 2 mL.[85] Because injection of epidural opioids in large volumes increases the potential risk of respiratory depression from cephalad spread of the drug,[30] a dilution of epidural meperidine to 5 mL was recommended.[85]

Intrathecal Pharmacokinetics

Opioids injected directly into the CSF are cleared by two competing mechanisms: diffusion into the spinal cord and diffusion into the epidural space. It is important to understand what fraction of an intrathecally administered opioid dose is cleared into the epidural space because this amount of drug is essentially unavailable in the spinal cord. The necessary investigations have not been done in humans because it is not possible to measure drug concentrations in spinal cord or epidural space. As shown in a pig model connected with a 16-compartment pharmacokinetic model,[102] the four opioids (morphine, fentanyl, alfentanil, and sufentanil) studied showed markedly different pharmacokinetic behavior, which correlates well with their pharmacodynamic features (dose potency, onset, and duration) observed clinically. The spinal cord showed a high exposure to morphine relative to alfentanil, fentanyl, and sufentanil after intrathecal administration. This high exposure to morphine is attributed to its limited volume of distribution in the spinal cord and slow clearance into the systemic circulation. The relatively low spinal cord exposure to the three other opioids occurs for different reasons. Alfentanil is cleared rapidly from the spinal cord into the systemic circulation. Fentanyl is routed largely into the epidural space, followed by sequestration in epidural fat. Given its high lipophilicity, sufentanil has limited free drug availability within the spinal cord, despite its long residence time and sequestration in spinal cord tissue.

In their large-animal model of spinal delivery of sufentanil, alfentanil, and morphine for long-term administration, Sabbe et al[93] found no changes in the calculated pharmacokinetic parameters between day 1 and day 28 of the treatment.[93] Their findings suggest that there is no change in the absorption of the drug over time from the intrathecal space into the plasma. In this dog model, all drugs were absorbed rapidly into the plasma with alfentanil > sufentanil = morphine. These findings coincide with the relative duration of action observed with these respective agents after intrathecal delivery and the propensity for producing an early onset of supraspinal effects. Similar plasma kinetics after intrathecal administration of morphine and sufentanil were reported in human studies.[26, 53, 60, 89, 99] After intrathecal administration of sufentanil in humans, fast absorption into the plasma was found. Ionescu et al[60] reported the time to reach the maximum plasma concentration was 6 ± 3 minutes. Hansdottir et al[53] reported 39 ± 10 minutes as the time to reach the maximum plasma concentration, but sufentanil was cleared rapidly from the CSF. After intrathecal administration of morphine in humans, low morphine plasma concentrations and a typically slow onset of peak concentration in blood were reported.[22, 99]

The spinal cord is arranged anatomically into an outer mantle of white matter surrounding the core of gray matter. Because opioid receptors are buried in lamina I, II, and V of gray matter, lipid-soluble substances could be sequestered in the hydrophobic domain of the myelin surrounding axons in the white matter and would be unavailable to move extensively through the aqueous extracellular space. In rabbit brains, Herz and Teschemacher[54] reported that fentanyl preferentially accumulated in white matter after intraventricular CSF administration, whereas morphine preferentially accumulated in gray matter (see earlier).

These pharmacokinetic studies suggest that extremes of lipid solubility limit the bioavailability of opioids at their target receptors in the spinal cord dorsal horn because they are sequestered either in epidural fat or in the hydrophobic environment of spinal cord white matter. Consistent with these data, McQuay et al[77] showed that the analgesic potency of intrathecally administered opioids in rats is inversely proportional to a drug's lipid solubility. This finding clearly contradicts earlier theoretical calculations for distribution of opioids between CSF and the spinal cord; Bullingham et al[20] had concluded that the percentage of the initial dose of intrathecally administered opioid taken up into the spinal cord is related to lipid solubility and postulated a theoretical percentage of about 4% for morphine and greater than 95% for lipophilic compounds such as fentanyl; they neglected possible redistribution and sequestration processes. It may be underappreciated that a large fraction of intrathecally administered drug is lost into the epidural space and epidural fat and is unavailable to target sites in the spinal cord.[102] The rank order for the transfer rate constants from the CSF to the epidural space is the same as the meningeal permeability coefficients determined in previous in vitro studies by Bernards and Hill[10]—alfentanil > fentanyl > morphine

> sufentanil. Drugs of intermediate hydrophobicity (alfentanil's octanol:buffer distribution coefficient = 129) are more permeable across the spinal meninges than are drugs of greater (fentanyl's octanol:buffer distribution coefficient = 955, and sufentanil's octanol:buffer distribution coefficient = 1,737) or lesser hydrophobicity (morphine's octanol:buffer distribution coefficient = 1).

CONCLUSION

The systemic circulation is a complex network of blood vessels flowing through many tissues and organs. Some of these organs take up drugs and eliminate them from the body, whereas other organs act as large reservoirs that can absorb or release drugs depending on the concentration gradients.

The spinal intrathecal space seems to be an *easy* environment with a bag of fluid surrounded by the meninges and neural tissue dangling within it, the target site—the spinal parenchyma—only several millimeters distant from the administered drug and easily accessed by simple diffusion process. The *simple* intrathecal space does not resolve easily into mammillary models. The slow flow of drug in the spinal space, combined with the rapid uptake by intrathecal tissues and redistribution to the epidural space, produces large drug gradients. Redistribution of drugs after epidural or intrathecal administration is a complex process because molecules partition within and among the many microenvironments they encounter. As pointed out by Shafer and Eisenach,[97] the spinal space is by no means pharmacokinetically homogeneous in the way the arterial blood is homogeneous, and the future key to understanding of intrathecal pharmacokinetics may be similar to the three most important things in real estate: location, location, location.

REFERENCES

1. Abbott NJ, Revest PA, Romero IA: Astrocyte-endothelial interaction: Physiology and pathology. Neuropathol Appl Neurobiol 18:424–433, 1992.
2. Alksne JF, Lovings ET: The role of the arachnoid villus in the removal of red blood cells from the subarachnoid space: An electron microscope study in the dog. J Neurosurg 36:192–200, 1972.
3. Ballantyne JC, Carr DB, Berkey CS, et al: Comparative efficacy of epidural, subarachnoid, and intracerebroventricular opioids in patients with pain due to cancer. Reg Anesth 21:542–556, 1996.
4. Behar M, Magora F, Olshwang D, Davidson JT: Epidural morphine in treatment of pain. Lancet 1:527–529, 1979.
5. Bernards C: Epidural and spinal anesthesia. In: Barash PG, Cullen BF, Stoelting RK (eds): Clinical Anesthesia, 3rd ed. Philadelphia: Lippincott-Raven, 1996, pp 645–668.
6. Bernards C: Clinical implications of physicochemical properties of opioids. In: Stein C (ed): Opioids in Pain Control. Cambridge: University Press, 1999, pp 166–187.
7. Bernards CM: Effect of (hydroxypropyl)-beta-cyclodextrin on flux of morphine, fentanyl, sufentanil, and alfentanil through the spinal meninges of monkey. J Pharm Sci 83:620–622, 1994.
8. Bernards CM, Hill HF: Morphine and alfentanil permeability through the spinal dura, arachnoid, and pia mater of dogs and monkeys. Anesthesiology 73:1214–1219, 1990.
9. Bernards CM, Hill HF: The spinal nerve root sleeve is not a preferred route for redistribution of drugs from the epidural space to the spinal cord. Anesthesiology 75:827–832, 1991.
10. Bernards CM, Hill HF: Physical and chemical properties of drug molecules governing their diffusion through the spinal meninges. Anesthesiology 77:750–756, 1992.
11. Bernards CM, Kern C: Palmitoyl carnitine increases the transmeningeal flux of hydrophilic but not hydrophobic compounds in vitro. Anesthesiology 84:392–396, 1996.

12. Bernards CM, Sorkin LS: Radicular artery blood flow does not redistribute fentanyl from the epidural space to the spinal cord. Anesthesiology 80:872–878, 1994.

13. Birnbach DJ, Johnson MD, Arcario T, et al: Effect of diluent volume on analgesia produced by epidural fentanyl. Anesth Analg 68:808–810, 1989.

14. Bonati M, Kanto J, Tognoni G: Clinical pharmacokinetics of cerebrospinal fluid. Clin Pharmacokinet 7:312–335, 1982.

15. Bourke DL, Sprung J, Harrison C, Thomas P: The dribble speed for spinal anesthesia. Reg Anesth 18:326–327, 1993.

16. Bromage PR: Epidural anaesthetics and narcotics. In: Wall PD (ed): Textbook of Pain, 2nd ed. Edinburgh: Churchill Livingstone, 1989, pp 744–753.

17. Bromage PR: 50 Years on the wrong side of the reflex arc. Reg Anesth 21:1–4, 1996.

18. Bucx MJ, Kroon JW, Stienstra R: Effect of speed of injection on the maximum sensory level for spinal anesthesia using plain bupivacaine 0.5% at room temperature. Reg Anesth 18:103–105, 1993.

19. Buerkle H, Yaksh TL: Continuous intrathecal administration of shortlasting mu opioids remifentanil and alfentanil in the rat. Anesthesiology 84:926–935, 1996.

20. Bullingham RES, McQuay HJ, Moore RA: Extradural and intrathecal narcotics. In: Recent Advances in Anaesthesia and Analgesia. Edinburgh: Churchill Livingstone, 1982, pp 141–156.

21. Byrod G, Olmarker K, Konno S, et al: A rapid transport route between the epidural space and the intraneural capillaries of the nerve roots. Spine 20:138–143, 1995.

22. Camu F, Debucquoy F: Alfentanil infusion for postoperative pain: A comparison of epidural and intravenous routes. Anesthesiology 75:171–178, 1991.

23. Carpenter RL, Hogan QH, Liu SS, et al: Lumbosacral cerebrospinal fluid volume is the primary determinant of sensory block extent and duration during spinal anesthesia. Anesthesiology 89:24–29, 1998.

24. Chaney MA: Side effects of intrathecal and epidural opioids. Can J Anaesth 42:891–903, 1995.

25. Chauvin M, Salbaing J, Perrin D, et al: Clinical assessment and plasma pharmacokinetics associated with intramuscular or extradural alfentanil. Br J Anaesth 57:886–891, 1985.

26. Chauvin M, Samii K, Schermann JM, et al: Plasma concentration of morphine after i.m., extradural and intrathecal administration. Br J Anaesth 53:911–913, 1981.

27. Christensen V: Respiratory depression after extradural morphine. Br J Anaesth 52:841, 1980.

28. Chrubasik J: Low-dose epidural morphine by infusion pump. Lancet 1:738–739, 1984.

29. Chrubasik J, Chrubasik S, Martin E: The ideal epidural opioid—fact or fantasy? Eur J Anaesthesiol 10:79–100, 1993.

30. Chrubasik S, Chrubasik J: Selection of the optimum opioid for extradural administration in the treatment of postoperative pain. Br J Anaesth 74:121–122, 1995.

31. Coda BA: Opioids. In: Barash PG, Cullen BF, Stoelting RK (eds): Clinical Anesthesia, 3rd ed. Philadelphia: Lippincott-Raven, 1996, pp 329–358.

32. Coda BA, Brown MC, Schaffer R, et al: Pharmacology of epidural fentanyl, alfentanil, and sufentanil in volunteers. Anesthesiology 81:1149–1161, 1994.

33. Coda BA, Brown MC, Schaffer RL, et al: A pharmacokinetic approach to resolving spinal and systemic contributions to epidural alfentanil analgesia and side-effects. Pain 62:329–337, 1995.

34. Cornish PB: Respiratory arrest after spinal anesthesia with lidocaine and fentanyl. Anesth Analg 84:1387–1388, 1997.

35. Cousins MJ, Bromage PR: Epidural neural blockade. In: Cousins MJ, Bridenbaugh PO (eds): Neural Blockade in Clinical Anesthesia and Management of Pain, 2nd ed. Philadelphia: JB Lippincott, 1987, pp 253–360.

36. Cousins MJ, Cherry DA, Gourlay GK: Acute and chronic pain: Use of spinal opiates. In: Cousins MJ, Bridenbaugh PO (eds): Neural Blockade in Clinical Anesthesia and Management of Pain, 2nd ed. Philadelphia: JB Lippincott, 1988, pp 955–1029.

37. Cousins MJ, Mather LE: Intrathecal and epidural administration of opioids. Anesthesiology 61: 276–310, 1984.
38. Cousins MJ, Mather LE, Glynn CJ, et al: Selective spinal analgesia. Lancet 1:1141–1142, 1979.
39. De Sousa H, Stiller R: Cisternal CSF and arterial plasma levels of fentanyl, alfentanil, and sufentanil after lumbar epidural injection (abstr). Anesthesiology 71:A839, 1989.
40. Durant PA, Yaksh TL: Distribution in cerebrospinal fluid, blood, and lymph of epidurally injected morphine and inulin in dogs. Anesth Analg 65:583–592, 1986.
41. Ford JM, Hait WN: Pharmacology of drugs that alter multidrug resistance in cancer. Pharmacol Rev 42:155–199, 1990.
42. Frances B, Gout R, Monsarrat B, et al: Further evidence that morphine-6 beta-glucuronide is a more potent opioid agonist than morphine. J Pharmacol Exp Ther 262:25–31, 1992.
43. Ghersi-Egea JF, Leininger-Muller B, Suleman G, et al: Localization of drug-metabolizing enzyme activities to blood-brain interfaces and circumventricular organs. J Neurochem 62:1089–1096, 1994.
44. Glynn CJ, Mather LE, Cousins MJ, et al: Spinal narcotics and respiratory depression. Lancet 2:356–357, 1979.
45. Goldstein A, Lowney LI, Pal BK: Stereospecific and nonspecific interactions of the morphine congener levorphanol in subcellular fractions of mouse brain. Proc Natl Acad Sci U S A 68:1742–1747, 1971.
46. Gourlay GK, Murphy TM, Plummer JL, et al: Pharmacokinetics of fentanyl in lumbar and cervical CSF following lumbar epidural and intravenous administration. Pain 38:253–259, 1989.
47. Grass JA, Sakima NT, Schmidt R, et al: A randomized, double-blind, dose-response comparison of epidural fentanyl versus sufentanil analgesia after cesarean section. Anesth Analg 85:365–371, 1997.
48. Greene NM: Uptake and elimination of local anesthetics during spinal anesthesia. Anesth Analg 62:1013–1024, 1983.
49. Greene NM: Distribution of local anesthetic solutions within the subarachnoid space. Anesth Analg 64:715–730, 1985.
50. Gustafsson LL, Grell AM, Garle M, et al: Kinetics of morphine in cerebrospinal fluid after epidural administration. Acta Anaesthesiol Scand 28:535–539, 1984.
51. Haninec P, Grim M: Localization of dipeptidylpeptidase IV and alkaline phosphatase in developing spinal cord meninges and peripheral nerve coverings of the rat. Int J Dev Neurosci 8:175–185, 1990.
52. Hansch C, Bjorkroth JP, Leo A: Hydrophobicity and central nervous system agents: On the principle of minimal hydrophobicity in drug design. J Pharm Sci 76:663–687, 1987.
53. Hansdottir V, Hedner T, Woestenborghs R, Nordberg G: The CSF and plasma pharmacokinetics of sufentanil after intrathecal administration. Anesthesiology 74:264–269, 1991.
54. Herz A, Teschemacher H-J: Activities and sites of antinociceptive action of morphine-like analgesics and kinetics of distribution following intravenous, intracerebral, and intraventricular application. In: Harper NJ, Simmonds AB (eds): Advances in Drug Research. London: Academic Press, 1971, pp 79–119.
55. Hogan Q: Anatomy of spinal anesthesia: some old and new findings. Reg Anesth Pain Med 23: 340–347, 1998.
56. Hogan QH, Prost R, Kulier A, et al: Magnetic resonance imaging of cerebrospinal fluid volume and the influence of body habitus and abdominal pressure. Anesthesiology 84:1341–1349, 1996.
57. Hood DD, Eisenach JC, Tuttle R: Phase I safety assessment of intrathecal neostigmine methylsulfate in humans. Anesthesiology 82:331–343, 1995.
58. Hunt JR, Rigor BM, Collins JR: The potential for contamination of continuous epidural catheters. Anesth Analg 56:222–225, 1977.
59. Huwyler J, Drewe J, Klusemann C, Fricker G: Evidence for P-glycoprotein-modulated penetration

of morphine-6-glucuronide into brain capillary endothelium. Br J Pharmacol 118:1879–1885, 1996.

60. Ionescu TI, Taverne RH, Houweling PL, et al: Pharmacokinetic study of extradural and intrathecal sufentanil anaesthesia for major surgery. Br J Anaesth 66:458–464, 1991.

61. Jang J, Yaksh TL, Hill HF: Use of 2-hydroxypropyl-beta-cyclodextrin as an intrathecal drug vehicle with opioids. J Pharmacol Exp Ther 261:592–600, 1992.

62. Janzer RC: The blood-brain barrier: Cellular basis. J Inherit Metab Dis 16:639–647, 1993.

63. Jones M, Newton T: Inadvertent extra-arachnoid injections in myelography. Radiology 80:818–822, 1963.

64. Jorgensen BC, Andersen HB, Engquist A: CSF and plasma morphine after epidural and intrathecal application. Anesthesiology 55:714–715, 1981.

65. Kern C, Bernards CM: Ascorbic acid inhibits spinal meningeal catechol-o-methyl transferase in vitro, markedly increasing epinephrine bioavailability. Anesthesiology 86:405–409, 1997.

66. Kern C, Mautz DS, Bernards CM: Epinephrine is metabolized by the spinal meninges of monkeys and pigs. Anesthesiology 83:1078–1081, 1995.

67. Kishida K, Otori T: A quantitative study on the relationship between transcorneal permeability of drugs and their hydrophobicity. Jpn J Ophthalmol 24:251–259, 1980.

68. Kitahata LM: Spinal analgesia with morphine and clonidine. Anesth Analg 68:191–193, 1989.

69. Kitahata LM, Collins JG: Spinal action of narcotic analgesics. Anesthesiology 54:153–163, 1981.

70. Lamotte C, Pert CB, Snyder SH: Opiate receptor binding in primate spinal cord: Distribution and changes after dorsal root section. Brain Res 112:407–412, 1976.

71. Liu SS, McDonald SB: Current issues in spinal anesthesia. Anesthesiology 94:888–906, 2001.

72. Lu JK, Schafer PG, Gardner TL, et al: The dose-response pharmacology of intrathecal sufentanil in female volunteers. Anesth Analg 85:372–379, 1997.

73. Lubenow T, Keh-Wong E, Kristof K, et al: Inadvertent subdural injection: A complication of an epidural block. Anesth Analg 67:175–179, 1988.

74. Matsuki A: Nothing new under the sun—a Japanese pioneer in the clinical use of intrathecal morphine. Anesthesiology 58:289–290, 1983.

75. Matsumiya N, Dohi S: Effects of intravenous or subarachnoid morphine on cerebral and spinal cord hemodynamics and antagonism with naloxone in dogs. Anesthesiology 59:175–181, 1983.

76. McClure JH, Brown DT, Wildsmith JA: Effect of injected volume and speed of injection on the spread of spinal anaesthesia with isobaric amethocaine. Br J Anaesth 54:917–920, 1982.

77. McQuay HJ, Sullivan AF, Smallman K, Dickenson AH: Intrathecal opioids, potency and lipophilicity. Pain 36:111–115, 1989.

78. Minn A, Ghersi-Egea JF, Perrin R, et al: Drug metabolizing enzymes in the brain and cerebral microvessels. Brain Res Rev 16:65–82, 1991.

79. Mitro A, Lojda Z: Histochemistry of proteases in ependyma, choroid plexus and leptomeninges. Histochemistry 88:645–646, 1988.

80. Moore RA, Bullingham RE, McQuay HJ, et al: Dural permeability to narcotics: In vitro determination and application to extradural administration. Br J Anaesth 54:1117–1128, 1982.

81. Morgan M: Quidquid agas, prudenter agas, et respice finem (editorial). Anaesthesia 37:527–529, 1982.

82. Morgan M: The rational use of intrathecal and extradural opioids. Br J Anaesth 63:165–188, 1989.

83. Negre I, Gueneron JP, Ecoffey C, et al: Ventilatory response to carbon dioxide after intramuscular and epidural fentanyl. Anesth Analg 66:707–710, 1987.

84. Neigh JL, Kane PB, Smith TC: Effects of speed and direction of injection on the level and duration of spinal anesthesia. Anesth Analg 49:912–918, 1970.

85. Ngan Kee WD, Lam KK, Chen PP, Gin T: Epidural meperidine after cesarean section: The effect of diluent volume. Anesth Analg 85:380–384, 1997.

86. Nordberg G, Hedner T, Mellstrand T: Sufentanil pharmacokinetics in plasma and CSF following epidural administration. Clin Pharmacol Ther 43:53, 1988.

87. Nordberg G, Hedner T, Mellstrand T, Dahlstrom B: Pharmacokinetic aspects of epidural morphine analgesia. Anesthesiology 58:545–551, 1983.
88. Nordberg G, Hedner T, Mellstrand T, Dahlstrom B: Pharmacokinetic aspects of intrathecal morphine analgesia. Anesthesiology 60:448–454, 1984.
89. Payne R: CSF distribution of opioids in animals and man. Acta Anaesthesiol Scand Suppl 85:38–46, 1987.
90. Pegues DA, Carr DB, Hopkins CC: Infectious complications associated with temporary epidural catheters. Clin Infect Dis 19:970–972, 1994.
91. Pert CB, Snyder SH: Opiate receptor: Demonstration in nervous tissue. Science 179:1011–1014, 1973.
92. Ross BK, Coda B, Heath CH: Local anesthetic distribution in a spinal model: A possible mechanism of neurologic injury after continuous spinal anesthesia. Reg Anesth 17:69–77, 1992.
93. Sabbe MB, Grafe MR, Mjanger E, et al: Spinal delivery of sufentanil, alfentanil, and morphine in dogs: Physiologic and toxicologic investigations. Anesthesiology 81:899–920, 1994.
94. Sato J, Sato H, Yamamoto T, et al: [The mechanism of dural permeability to narcotics and local anesthetics]. Masui 35:917–923, 1986.
95. Schinkel AH, Wagenaar E, Mol CA, van Deemter L: P-glycoprotein in the blood-brain barrier of mice influences the brain penetration and pharmacological activity of many drugs. J Clin Invest 97:2517–2524, 1996.
96. Schoenwald RD, Ward RL: Relationship between steroid permeability across excised rabbit cornea and octanol-water partition coefficients. J Pharm Sci 67:786–788, 1978.
97. Shafer SL, Eisenach JC: Location, location, location. Anesthesiology 92:641–643, 2000.
98. Sjostrom S, Hartvig P, Persson MP, Tamsen A: Pharmacokinetics of epidural morphine and meperidine in humans. Anesthesiology 67:877–888, 1987.
99. Sjostrom S, Tamsen A, Persson MP, Hartvig P: Pharmacokinetics of intrathecal morphine and meperidine in humans. Anesthesiology 67:889–895, 1987.
100. Stein WD: Transport and Diffusion Across Cell Membranes. New York: Academic Press, 1986.
101. Szejtli J: Cyclodextrin Technology. Boston: Kluwer Academic Publishers, 1988.
102. Ummenhofer WC, Arends RH, Shen DD, Bernards CM: Comparative spinal distribution and clearance kinetics of intrathecally administered morphine, fentanyl, alfentanil, and sufentanil. Anesthesiology 92:739–753, 2000.
103. Ummenhofer WC, Bernards CM: Acylcarnitine chain length influences carnitine-enhanced drug flux through the spinal meninges in vitro. Anesthesiology 86:642–648, 1997.
104. Ummenhofer WC, Brown SM, Bernards CM: Acetylcholinesterase and butyrylcholinesterase are expressed in the spinal meninges of monkeys and pigs. Anesthesiology 88:1259–1265, 1998.
105. Ummenhofer WC, Stapleton AE, Bernards CM: Effect of Staphylococcus aureus bacteria and bacterial toxins on meningeal permeability in vitro. Reg Anesth Pain Med 24:24–29, 1999.
106. Vandenabeele F, Creemers J Lambrichts I: Ultrastructure of the human spinal arachnoid mater and dura mater. J Anat 189:417–430, 1996.
107. Vercauteren M, Meert T, D'Hooghe R, et al: Spinal sufentanil in rats: Part III. Effect of diluent volume on epidural sufentanil. Acta Anaesthesiol Scand 36:305–308, 1992.
108. Volk B, Hettmannsperger U, Papp T, et al: Mapping of phenytoin-inducible cytochrome P450 immunoreactivity in the mouse central nervous system. Neuroscience 42:215–235, 1991.
109. Wang JK, Nauss LA, Thomas JE: Pain relief by intrathecally applied morphine in man. Anesthesiology 50:149–151, 1979.
110. Wood JH: Physiology, pharmacology and dynamics of cerebrospinal fluid. In: Wood JH (ed): Neurobiology of Cerebrospinal Fluid. New York, 1980, pp 1–16.
111. Wu D, Kang YS, Bickel U, Pardridge WM: Blood-brain barrier permeability to morphine-6-glucuronide is markedly reduced compared with morphine. Drug Metab Dispos 25:768–771, 1997.
112. Yaksh TL, Jang JD, Nishiuchi Y, et al: The utility of 2-hydroxypropyl-beta-cyclodextrin as a vehicle for the intracerebral and intrathecal administration of drugs. Life Sci 48:623–633, 1991.

113. Yaksh TL, Rudy TA: Analgesia mediated by a direct spinal action of narcotics. Science 192:1357–1358, 1976.

114. Yamashima T: Functional ultrastructure of cerebrospinal fluid drainage channels in human arachnoid villi. Neurosurgery 22:633–641, 1988.

115. Yano T, Nakagawa A, Tsuji M, Noda K: Skin permeability of various non-steroidal anti-inflammatory drugs in man. Life Sci 39:1043–1050, 1986.

116. Zajac JM, Charnay Y, Soleilhic JM, et al: Enkephalin-degrading enzymes and angiotensin-converting enzyme in human and rat meninges. FEBS Lett 216:118–122, 1987.

Chapter 27

Clinical Applications of Spinal Analgesia

Steven P. Cohen, MD/Salahadin Abdi, MD, PhD

HISTORY

The first neuraxial injections of local anesthetic were described by Leonard Corning in 1885, first in a dog, and then in a man afflicted with "seminal incontinence."[1] Following this landmark paper, 14 years elapsed before Augustus Bier, a surgeon, used the technique of spinal cocainization to provide anesthesia for surgical patients.[2] In the year 1901, the French physician Sicard applied local anesthetic via the caudal route to treat a patient with low back pain.[3] Another major breakthrough came in 1942 when Manalan first used a catheter to provide continuous access to the epidural space during labor analgesia.[4] The epidural injection of steroids to treat sciatica was first reported in the year 1953 by Lievre.[5] In 1979, several years after the first identification of opioid receptors in the central nervous system and the endogenous opioid enkephalin, Wang and colleagues[6] reported treating cancer pain with the intrathecal injection of morphine. Currently, a number of agents are administered neuroaxially to treat both acute and chronic pain.

LOCAL ANESTHETICS

The most widely used spinal analgesics are local anesthetics, which are used both for surgical anesthesia and for pain relief. The mechanism of action by which local anesthetics provide analgesia is via the blockade of sodium channels, the sentinel event in the depolarization of neurons. As such, local anesthetics are capable of blocking the transmission of all nerve fibers, not just the A delta and C fibers responsible for pain. One local anesthetic that may selectively target sensory neurons, however, is ropivicaine. In addition to their own inherent analgesic effects, there is also evidence to suggest that neuraxial local anesthetics may act synergistically with opioids. By virtue of the large volumes required for epidural analgesia and the ability of sodium channel blockers to suppress ectopic discharges from damaged neurons, the systemic absorption of certain local anesthetics administered epidurally may be of added benefit in the treatment of neuropathic pain states.[7]

The major limitations to the use of local anesthetics for treatment of chronic pain are as follows:

- Sensory blockade
- Motor blockade
- Local anesthetic toxicity during epidural infusion
- Cardiovascular depression

Other side effects of neuraxial local anesthetics include urinary retention and diarrhea.

OPIOIDS

Opioid analgesics exert their actions through inhibition of target cell activity. Mediating these effects are three endogenous opioid receptors: μ, δ, and κ. Although peripherally located opioid receptors have been identified, the predominant analgesic sites are believed to reside in the central nervous system. In the brain, these receptor sites include the brainstem, thalamus, forebrain, and mesencephalon. In the substantia gelatinosa, they include post-synaptic receptors located on cells originating in the dorsal horn of the spinal cord as well as presynaptic receptors found on the spinal terminals of primary afferent fibers. Some of the proposed mechanisms of cell inhibition include the following:

- Membrane hyperpolarization via activation of potassium channels
- Suppression of voltage-gated calcium channels resulting in the diminished terminal release of neurotransmitters
- Receptor-mediated inhibition of adenylate cyclase

The effects of opioids are determined not only by their affinity for endogenous receptors but also by their ability to reach those receptors. The onset of analgesia is similar for intrathecal and epidural narcotics, suggesting that the penetration of neural tissue (and not dura) is the rate-limiting step. Whereas intrathecal opioids exert their analgesic properties by presynaptically inhibiting the release of substance P and calcitonin gene–related peptide, which are neuropeptides believed to be responsible for transmitting nociceptive signals across synapses, and by hyperpolarizing post-synaptic neurons, epidurally administered narcotics may work by an additional mechanism. Since the systemic absorption of an epidural bolus of some narcotics is similar to that which follows an intramuscular injection, it is likely that the plasma levels of these drugs produced during an epidural infusion contribute to their analgesic effects.[8] The importance of this effect varies according to the drug's lipophilicity.

Lipid solubility determines in part several other important characteristics of intraspinal opioids, including the spread of analgesia and side effects. Highly water-soluble opioids such as morphine exhibit a greater degree of rostral spread when injected into the subarachnoid or epidural space than lipid-soluble compounds so that in pain conditions requiring higher spinal levels or more extensive coverage, the degree of analgesia they confer may be better. Conversely, since many side effects of spinal opioids, such as pruritus and nausea and vomiting, and life-threatening complications, such as delayed respiratory depression, are the result of interaction with opioid receptors in the brain, the more water-soluble compounds are associated with a higher incidence of adverse effects. Table 1 lists the recommended conversion ratios between different opioids.

The earliest studies on intraspinal opioids were conducted on patients suffering from cancer pain, but more recent studies have found intrathecal and epidural narcotics to be effective in nonmalignant pain as well.[9,10] These conditions include not only nociceptive pain but also neuropathic pain, a heterogeneous group of disorders originally believed to be resistant to narcotics. However, certain aspects of neuropathic pain such as tactile allodynia may be less responsive to the effects of spinal opiates. This may stem from the absence of opiate receptors on the spinal terminals of low-threshold mechanoreceptors thought to mediate the allodynic state. In fact, many neuropathic conditions may require nonopioid adjuvants such as local anesthetics or α_2 agonists to be added to spinal opioids for successful pain relief.

When opioids are administered directly into the cerebrospinal fluid, only a fraction of the systemic dose is required because there are no anatomic barriers to be crossed, and vascular

TABLE 1.

Conversion Ratios between Opioid Agents

Equianalgesic Doses of Opioids, mg

Drug	Oral	Parenteral	Epidural	Intrathecal	Water Solubility
Morphine	300	100	10	1	High
Hydromorphone	60	20	2	0.2	Intermediate
Meperidine	3000	1000	100	10	Low
Fentanyl	—	1	0.1	0.01	Low
Sufentanil	—	0.1	0.01	0.001	Low

reuptake is slow. In addition, when administered intrathecally, the ratio of two of morphine's main metabolites, morphine-3-glucoronide and morphine-6-glucuronide, to the parent compound is less than when morphine is given orally.[11] Although not all side effects of intrathecal opioids are dose-related, in many instances this drastic reduction in dosage translates into reduced side effects. In fact, one of the primary indications for a trial with intrathecal or epidural narcotics is a good analgesic response to opioids coupled with intractable side effects. Among the adverse opioid effects reduced by switching from oral formulations to spinal administration are sedation and constipation. Those that are increased include pruritus, urinary retention, and edema.

The mechanisms contributing to the various adverse effects of opioids are incompletely understood but probably are multifactorial. These include those that are mediated via interaction with specific opioid receptors, and those that are not. Undesirable effects not mediated by opioid receptors, such as central nervous system excitation and hyperalgesia, cannot be reversed with naloxone. The incidence of the various opioid-induced side effects depends on a number of different factors, including the opioid infused, the route of administration and dosage, the patient's age, the extent of the disease, concurrent drug use to include oral narcotics, concomitant medical problems, and prior exposure to opioids. The most frequent side effects of intrathecal morphine are listed in Table 2.[12] With the possible exceptions of sweating, peripheral edema and constipation, most of these adverse effects tend to diminish with time.

Rare side effects of intrathecal narcotics include nystagmus, thermoregulatory dysfunction, arrhythmias, hair loss, neurotoxicity, reactivation of herpes simplex infections, and anaphylaxis.

α_2-ADRENERGIC AGONISTS

The intraspinal administration of α_2-agonists to provide analgesia has been used since 1985. Although several different subtypes of α_2 receptors have been identified that may play a role in antinociception, recent studies have suggested that it is the α_{2_A} receptor that is primarily responsible for analgesia.[13] The mechanism of action of spinally administered α_2-agonists is similar to that of opioids.[14] Presynaptically, they bind to α_2-adrenergic receptors on small primary afferent neurons, thus decreasing the release of neurotransmitters involved in relaying pain signals. On post-synaptic neurons, α_2-agonists hyperpolarize the cell by increasing potassium conductance through Gi-coupled K^+ channels. They have also been

TABLE 2

Incidence of Side Effects with Long-Term Intrathecal Morphine

Side Effect	Incidence, %
Constipation	50
Urinary retention	42.7
Nausea	36.6
Impotence	26.8
Vomiting	24.4
Nightmares	23.2
Pruritus	14.6
Sweating	8.5
Edema	6.1
Disturbance of libido	4.9
Fatigue	3.7
Dry mouth	3.7
Hypothyroidism	2.4
Dizziness	2.4
Amenorrhea	2.4
Convulsions	1.2
Loss of appetite	1.2
Provocation of asthma	1.2

From Winkelmuller M, Winkelmuller W: Long-term effects of continuous intratracal opioid treatment in chronic pain of nonmalignment etiology. J Neurosurg 1996; 85:459–467.

shown to activate spinal cholinergic neurons, which may contribute to their analgesic effects. In addition to their antinociceptive properties, α_2-agonists produce dose-dependent sedation, presumably by inhibitory mechanisms involving the locus coeruleus in the brainstem.

The most studied α_2-agonist is the antihypertensive medication clonidine. Although it is currently approved by the Food and Drug Administration for epidural use only in cancer pain, clinical reports have shown it to be effective both intrathecally and epidurally for nonmalignant pain as well. Several studies show that clonidine may prolong and enhance the effects of spinal and epidural anesthesia with local anesthetics and that adding it to opioids for labor analgesia may extend the duration of pain relief.[15–17] Unlike spinal opioids, clonidine may be effective against tactile allodynia. It has also been reported to be effective in treating spasticity and central pain following spinal cord injury.[18] In the largest study to date done by Eisenach and colleagues[19] in 85 patients with severe cancer pain, the authors found that while pain relief was better in the clonidine-epidural group than in the placebo group, there was no difference in rescue epidural morphine requirements. Although neuraxial clonidine has been found to be effective in treating all types of pain, it may be most effective in patients with neuropathic or sympathetically maintained pain.[20]

The most common side effects of neuraxial clonidine are sedation, hypotension, and bradycardia.[19] These are more frequent following the larger doses needed to provide epidural analgesia than with intrathecal administration and may in part be due to systemic absorption of the drug. In low doses by either route, these effects are usually well tolerated. In many cases, the opioid-sparing properties of α_2-adrenergic agonists far outweigh the side effects.

Whereas clonidine is the most studied α_2-adrenergic agonist and the only one that is approved by the Food and Drug Administration for epidural use, there are several other α_2-agonists with similar properties. These include dexmedetomidine, detomidine, and tizanidine. Although preclinical studies indicate that some of these may be effective for spinal and epidural analgesia in humans, more research needs to be carried out before they become readily available in clinical practice.

N-METHYL-D-ASPARTATE RECEPTOR ANTAGONISTS

The most studied N-methyl-D-aspartate (NMDA) receptor antagonist for neuraxial use is ketamine, a noncompetitive NMDA antagonist that has been administered both epidurally and intrathecally in humans for acute and chronic pain relief. Following tissue injury, the activation of spinal NMDA receptors can induce a state of facilitated processing from repetitive small afferent fiber stimulation, leading to an increased response to high- and low-threshold stimulation and enhanced receptor field size. This process, known as wind-up, is responsible for such phenomena such as allodynia and hyperalgesia. When delivered spinally, NMDA receptor antagonists have little effect on acute activation but may block wind-up induced by small afferent input.

In a randomized, double-blind study by Choe and associates,[21] when combined with epidural morphine for upper abdominal surgery, ketamine was found to prolong the duration of analgesia and decrease the number of patients requiring supplemental injections. In combination with intrathecal morphine alone or with other agents in patients suffering from cancer pain, the addition of intraspinal ketamine has been shown to enhance the analgesic effects of opioids and the other drugs while reducing the development of tolerance.[22] In other several studies examining the effects of adding ketamine spinally or epidurally to the local anesthetic bupivacaine for surgical anesthesia, however, researchers have not been able to demonstrate any additional benefit.[23,24] Although intrathecal ketamine was reported as providing adequate short-term anesthesia by Bion in 1984,[25] a more recent study by Hawksworth and Serpell[26] found that the high frequency of psychomimetic disturbances, its short duration of action, and the high incidence of incomplete anesthesia precluded its use as a sole anesthetic agent. In a case report by Kristensen and coworkers[27], the spinal administration of CPP (3-(2-carboxypoperazin-4-yl) propyl-1-phosphonic acid), a competitive NMDA antagonist, was noted to suppress wind-up but not spontaneous pain or allodynia in a patient with a peripheral nerve injury. Four hours after the last injection of CPP, psychomimetic ketamine-like side effects developed that were attributed to the rostral spread of medication.

In the doses used to provide epidural or spinal analgesia, the frequent side effects encountered with ketamine may limit its usefulness.[26] These side effects are similar to those occurring with parenteral administration and include nystagmus, nausea and vomiting, and psychomimetic disturbances such as hallucinations. In addition, cardiovascular changes may be encountered, with the directional change in blood pressure depending on the patient, dosage used, and spinal level obtained.

There are questions that remain unanswered regarding the neurotoxicity of intraspinal ketamine, both with and without preservatives. Karpinski and coworkers[28] reported a case of a terminal cancer patient who received a 3-week intrathecal infusion of ketamine and was found to have subpial vacuolar myelopathy on autopsy. At present, ketamine is not approved by the Food and Drug Administration for neuraxial use in the United States.

CALCIUM CHANNEL BLOCKERS

Voltage-sensitive calcium channel conduction is essential for the transmission of pain. In clinical studies, both N- and L-type calcium channel antagonists have been shown to contain analgesic properties. N-type calcium channels are found in high concentrations in the substantia gelatinosa and dorsal root ganglion cells, where they play a role in the release of transmitters such as substance P involved in nociceptive pathways.

In one double-blind, randomized study examining the effects of a continuous intrathecal infusion of the N-type calcium channel blocker ziconotide started prior to surgical incision and continued for 48 to 72 hours postoperatively in patients who had received spinal anesthesia, patients in the treatment groups had lower pain scores and decreased postoperative patient-controlled analgesia morphine requirements than those who had received a placebo infusion.[29] In four out of six patients receiving the high dose of ziconotide (7 μg/hour as opposed to 0.7 μg/hour), adverse effects such as blurred vision, nystagmus, dizziness, and sedation necessitated discontinuing the infusion. These adverse effects, which disappeared after discontinuing the infusion, were likely due to delayed clearance of ziconotide from neural tissues. There was no difference in postoperative pain scores between patients who had received the high-dose ziconotide infusion and those receiving the low dose. Even during prolonged delivery, there is no development of tolerance with intrathecal ziconotide use.[30]

In another double-blind study, adding the L-type calcium channel blocker verapamil to epidural bupivacaine both before and after surgical incision was found to reduce postoperative analgesic requirements in patients undergoing abdominal surgery.[31] In this paper, the authors reported no increased incidence of sedation or mood disturbances in the treatment group. However, animal studies have failed to show independent antinociceptive effects for the intrathecal administration of various L-type calcium channel blockers, although in combination with morphine, their interactions appear to be synergistic.[32]

ADENOSINE

Adenosine A1 receptors are found in high concentrations in the substantia gelatinosa, primarily on nonprimary afferent terminals. In both animal and human experiments, neuraxial adenosine has been found to have antinociceptive activity. This effect appears to be mediated by A1 receptors. Proposed mechanisms include a reduction in glutamate release from spinal afferents, and a decrease in substance P concentrations in the cerebrospinal fluid. The analgesic effects of both systemic and intrathecal adenosine may be abolished by adenosine receptor antagonists such as methylxanthines.

In a phase I clinical safety study published in 1998 by Rane and coworkers in healthy human volunteers,[33] the intrathecal injection of adenosine reduced areas of secondary allodynia after skin inflammation and decreased forearm ischemic tourniquet pain. Ice water–induced cold pain was unchanged by adenosine. No adverse side effects were noted, although one patient who received a 2000 μg injection (ranges of adenosine tested were from 500 μg to 2000 μg) experienced transient low back pain. In a case report on a patient with neuropathic leg pain and tactile-allodynia, an A1 adenosine agonist administered intrathecally provided long-term relief of the patient's stimulus-dependent pain.[34] Pain relief has also been reported following intrathecal administration in a patient suffering from secondary erythromelalgia.[35] In a later randomized, double-blind study by Rane and coworkers[36] evaluating the effects of intrathecal adenosine on anesthetic and postoperative analgesic requirements in women undergoing hysterectomies, however, no difference was found between the adenosine and placebo groups. In a recent assessment done with a different formulation of adenosine that is marketed in the United States (the one utilized by Ranes was formulated in Sweden), Eisenach and colleagues[37] found that intrathecal adenosine reduced the hyperalgesia and allodynia associated with intradermal capsaicin injection but had no effect on acute noxious chemical or thermal stimulation. These findings are actually consistent with those of Rane's group,[33,36] and indicate that adenosine may be more effective for chronic neuropathic pain due to central sensitization than it is for acute nociceptive pain. The only side effects noted in this study were headache and back pain.[38]

CHOLINERGIC AGONISTS

In animal models, the spinal administration of cholinergic agonists and acetylcholinesterase inhibitors results in antinociception. When administered neuraxially, nicotinic agonists can initially produce paradoxical nociceptive behavior, followed by a subsequent increase in nociceptive thresholds. The spinal delivery of cholinesterase inhibitors has been similarly demonstrated to increase pain thresholds. The analgesic effects of neuraxial cholinergic drugs may in part be mediated by muscarinic M1 and M3 receptors, found in dorsal root ganglia and superficial laminae of the dorsal horn. Furthermore, studies have shown that the stimulation of muscarinic receptors in the spinal cord can enhance the release of γ-amino butyric acid (GABA) and nitric oxide. In animal models, tolerance to the analgesic effects of cholinergic agents develops rapidly.

In a phase I safety assessment done in healthy human volunteers by Hood and associates,[39] the administration of intrathecal neostigmine reduced visual analog pain scores to painful cold stimulation. In a study examining the drug's postoperative analgesic effects in women undergoing abdominal hysterectomies both with and without narcotics, the administration of intrathecal neostigmine reduced postoperative pain scores and opioid requirements comparable to the fentanyl group, with the greatest effect seen in patients receiving both fentanyl and the high dose (25 μg) of neostigmine.[40] These results support those of another study demonstrating synergistic effects between intrathecal neostigmine and opioids.[41] Some studies have suggested that intrathecal neostigmine is more effective for somatic than visceral pain.[42] In a clinical trial performed in healthy volunteers, combining spinal neostigmine with epidural clonidine provided additive but not synergistic analgesic effects, with the authors attributing part of neostigmine's antinociceptive properties to α_2-adrenergic enhancement.[43] In this study, adding neostigmine diminished clonidine-induced reductions in blood pressure and norepinephrine levels. In an experiment comparing different combinations of neuraxial analgesics for labor analgesia in healthy parturients, patients receiving bupivacaine, fentanyl, clonidine, and neostigmine had significantly longer analgesia than those receiving bupivacaine and fentanyl, or bupivicaine, fentanyl, and clonidine.[44]

The most common side effects of intrathecal neostigmine are nausea, vomiting, and, at doses exceeding 150 μg, sedation and leg weakness. At low doses, neostigmine is not associated with significant hemodynamic effects. At higher doses (750 μg), however, increases in blood pressure, heart rate, respiratory rate and anxiety may occur.[39] When combined with other spinal analgesics, the drug-sparing effects of neostigmine may actually decrease side effects. Since the mid 1990s, the only form of neostigmine available in the United States contains the preservative methyl-propylparaben.

γ-AMINOBUTYRIC ACID AGONISTS

In clinical studies, both GABA-A and GABA-B agonists have been shown to contain analgesic effects when injected neuraxially. The GABA-A receptor is part of a chloride channel ionophore complex modulated by barbiturates, benzodiazepines, alcohol, propofol, and etomidate. Stimulation of this receptor increases chloride conductance and may prevent afferent neuronal discharges by shunting electrical currents that would otherwise depolarize the membrane. This alteration in neuronal function changes the spinal cord processing of nociceptive input in such a way that animals receiving intrathecal midazolam exhibit a dermatomal level of decreased pinprick sensation. Since the antinociceptive effect of intrathecal midazolam can be reversed in rats by the administration of naloxone, an additional mechanism of action may involve a spinal cord-opioid pathway that does not involve μ-receptors.

The GABA-B receptor is a G-protein–linked complex whose activation results in augmentation of potassium channel currents. This results in the hyperpolarization of the neuronal cell membrane, leading to a decrease in opening of voltage-sensitive calcium channels, and a reduction in transmitter release. Although GABA-B receptors are found throughout the spinal cord, they are present in the highest concentrations in the substantia gelatinosa, being located both pre- and post-synaptically. The GABA-B agonist most studied in humans is the muscle relaxant baclofen.

Clinical studies are not consistent in demonstrating antinociceptive effects of neuraxially administered GABA-A and B agonists. The addition of both intrathecal and epidural midazolam to local anesthetics with and without opioids was found in several studies to enhance postoperative analgesia and reduce the need for narcotics.[45–47] In a double-blind study evaluating the effects of adding intrathecal midazolam to bupivacaine in patients undergoing hemorrhoidectomy, the addition of midazolam was found to expedite the onset of spinal analgesia in a dose-dependent manner.[48] Other studies have found intrathecal midazolam to be effective in treating chronic mechanical low back pain, musculoskeletal pain, and neurogenic pain.[49,50] However, the administration of subarachnoid midazolam was not shown to be effective in treating pain associated with peripheral vascular disease and malignancy.[50] The potential side effects of spinal midazolam include dose-dependent sedation and amnesia.

A plethora of literature attests to the safety of intrathecal baclofen in humans, with most of the research done on patients with spinal spasticity. There are numerous studies showing the effectiveness of intrathecal baclofen to treat central pain states, including those following stroke, spinal cord injury, cerebral palsy, and multiple sclerosis.[51–53] Interestingly, intrathecal baclofen has also been found to be an effective treatment for noncentral neuropathic pain conditions, including complex regional pain syndrome and phantom limb pain.[54, 55] Since the most common use of baclofen is as a muscle relaxant, it is not surprising that several authors report intrathecal baclofen to be beneficial for spasm-related pain.[56, 57] However, not all studies assessing the effects of intrathecal baclofen for pain have been uniformly positive. In one study involving 16 spinal cord injury patients and a 12-month follow-up period, intrathecal baclofen was found to reduce musculoskeletal but not neurogenic pain.[58] In view of the results of this study and the temporal disparity regarding its analgesic effects on central pain and muscle spasm, it is likely that different pain-relieving mechanisms exist for these two conditions. Potential side effects of neuraxial baclofen include weakness and sedation.

SOMATOSTATIN

There is extensive literature on the use of spinal somatostatin for pain relief. To date, at least six somatostatin receptors have been identified that are dispersed throughout the periacqueductal gray, ventral horn, primary afferent neurons, and substantia gelatinosa. The antinociceptive effects of somatostatin result from presynaptic inhibition. Stimulation of somatostatin receptors results in hyperpolarization of the cell via a G-protein–coupled inwardly rectifying potassium current. This serves to block coupled calcium channels, reduce transmitter release, and decrease the synthesis of cyclic AMP.

Epidural somatostatin has been demonstrated in several studies to provide postoperative pain relief for patients undergoing abdominal and other surgical procedures.[59–61] There are also reports of intrathecal and epidural somatostatin providing pain relief for patients with cancer.[62,63] In a study performed by Mollenholt and associates[63] examining the efficacy of continuous intrathecal and epidural infusions of somatostatin in patients with intractable cancer pain unresponsive to opioids, the authors described demyelination of spinal nerve roots and dorsal columns in two of their eight patients at autopsy, although none demonstrated any clinical signs of neurological deficits. As the patients were receiving other treatments for cancer, including chemotherapy and radiation treatment, these pathological changes could not definitively be attributed to somatostatin. Furthermore, all patients in this investigation required a rapid escalation of dose over a relatively short period, perhaps indicating the development of tolerance. In another report, octreotide, a synthetic analog of somatostatin with a longer half-life, was noted to provide long-term relief in two patients with intractable nonmalignant pain from pseudohypertrophic muscular dystrophy and multiple sclerosis.[64] However, not all studies examining spinal somatostatin for pain relief have found the drug to be of benefit.[65] Aside from the aforementioned possibility of neurotoxicity, the neuraxial use of somatostatin is associated with minimal side effects.

NEUROLEPTICS

When administered parenterally, neuroleptic drugs have been demonstrated to have analgesic as well as sedative and antiemetic effects in humans. Similarly, in several clinical studies, including two randomized controlled trials, the butyrophenone droperidol has been shown to potentiate epidural analgesia with opioids.[66–68] In one of these trials, the addition of epidural droperidol significantly reduced the duration of analgesia obtained with epidural sufentanil.[66]

The mechanism by which neuraxial droperidol exerts its antinociceptive effects has not been fully delineated but may involve descending dopaminergic tracts in the spinal medulla. Additional benefits of combining epidural droperidol with narcotics may include a reduction in adverse side effects, including nausea, vomiting, urinary retention, and hypotension. Side effects of epidural droperidol include sedation, respiratory depression, and parkinsonian effects. One report noted a case of akathisia after long-term use of epidural droperidol.[69]

ASPIRIN

As with oral administration, the mechanism of action for spinally administered aspirin is inhibition of prostaglandin synthesis, most likely at the spinal level. In humans, there have been several studies examining the analgesic effects of intrathecal aspirin in patients with chronic, refractory pain.[70, 71] In a large study conducted in 60 cancer patients with intractable pain, a single dose of isobaric lysine acetylsalicylate (doses ranged from 120 to 720 mg) resulted in excellent relief in 78% of cases, with the duration of analgesia lasting from 3 weeks to 1 month on average.[70] Side effects of intrathecal aspirin tend to be short-lived, consisting of generalized fatigue and occasional hallucinations at night. However, owing to the lack of toxicological studies, its use for long-term continuous infusion in humans should be limited to cancer patients with short life expectancies who present with refractory pain unresponsive to conventional therapy.

CONCLUSION

The use of spinal analgesics to modulate pain is a rapidly expanding field, with broad implications in the management of acute and chronic pain. While there are numerous compounds currently available that have been shown to contain antinociceptive properties in preclinical studies, only those that have been examined in humans are discussed in this chapter. Other substances that have shown promise for future study in humans include nitric oxide inhibitors, dynorphins, calcitonin, neurotensin, tricyclic antidepressants, β-blockers, and cannabinoids.

REFERENCES FOR ADDITIONAL READING

1. Corning JL: Spinal anaesthesia and local medication of the cord. N Y Med J 42:483–485, 1885.
2. Bier A: Versuche über Cocainisirung des Ruckenmarkes. Dtsch Z Chir 51:361–369, 1899.
3. Manalan SA: Caudal block anesthesia in obstetrics. J Indiana Med Assoc 35:564–565, 1942.
4. Sicard A: Les injections medicamenteuses extra-durales par voie sacrococcygienne. CR Soc Biol Paris 53:396–398, 1901.
5. Lievre J-A, Bloch-Michel H, Pean G, Uro J: L'hydrocortisone en injection locale. Rev Rhumat Mal Osteo-Articul 4:310–311, 1953.
6. Wang JK, Nauss LA, Thomas JE: Pain relief by intrathecally applied morphine in man. Anesthesiology 50:149–151, 1979.
7. Devor M, Wall PD, Catalan N: Systemic lidocaine silences ectopic neuroma and DRG discharge without blocking nerve conduction. Pain 1992;48:261–268.
8. Nordberg G: Pharmacokinetic aspects of spinal morphine analgesia. Acta Anaesthesiol Scand 28:1–38, 1984.
9. Paice JA, Winkelmuller W, Burchiel K: Clinical realities and economic considerations: Efficacy of intrathecal pain therapy. J Pain Symptom Manage 14:S14–26, 1997.
10. Yue SK, St Marie B, Henrickson K: Initial clinical experience with the SKY epidural catheter. J Pain Symptom Manage 6:107–114, 1991.
11. Faura CC, Collins SL, Moore RA, McQuay HJ: Systematic review of factors affecting the ratios of morphine and its major metabolites. Pain 74:43–53, 1998.
12. Winkelmuller M, Winkelmuller W: Long-term effects of continuous intrathecal opioid treatment in chronic pain of nonmalignant etiology. J Neurosurg 85:459–467, 1996.
13. Lakhlani PP, MacMillan LB, Guo TZ, et al: Substitution of a mutant alpha 2a-adrenergic receptor via 'hit and run' gene targeting reveals the role of this subtype in sedative, analgesic, and anesthetic-sparing responses in vivo. Proc Natl Acad Sci U S A 94:9950–9955, 1997.
14. Wallace M, Yaksh TL: Long-term spinal analgesic delivery: A review of the preclinical and clinical literature. Reg Anesth Pain Med 25:117–157, 2000.
15. Dobrydnjov I, Samarutel J: Enhancement of intrathecal lidocaine by addition of local and systemic clonidine. Acta Anaesthesiol Scand 43:556–562, 1999.
16. Milligan KR, Convery PN, Weir P, et al: The efficacy and safety of epidural infusions of levobu-

pivicaine with and without clonidine for postoperative pain relief in patients undergoing total hip replacement. Anesth Analg 91:393–397, 2000.

17. Gautier PE, De Kock M, Fanard L, et al: Intrathecal clonidine combined with sufentanil for labor analgesia. Anesthesiology 88:651–656, 1998.

18. Middleton JW, Siddall PJ, Walker S, et al: Intrathecal clonidine and baclofen in the management of spasticity and neuropathic pain following spinal cord injury: A case study. Arch Phys Med Rehabil 77:824–826, 1996.

19. Eisenach JC, DuPen S, Dubois M, et al: Epidural clonidine analgesia for intractable cancer pain: The epidural clonidine study group. Pain 61:391–399, 1995.

20. Rauck RL, Eisenach JC, Jackson K, et al: Epidural clonidine treatment for refractory reflex sympathetic dystrophy. Anesthesiology 79:1163–1169, 1993.

21. Choe H, Choi YS, Kim YH, et al: Epidural morphine plus ketamine for upper abdominal surgery: Improved analgesia from preincisional versus postincisional administration. Anesth Analg 84:560–563, 1997.

22. Muller A, Lemos D: Cancer pain: Beneficial effect of ketamine addition to spinal administration of morphine-clonidine-lidocaine mixture. Ann Fr Anesth Reanim 15:271–276, 1996.

23. Weir PS, Fee JP: Double-blind comparison of extradural block with three bupivicaine-ketamine mixtures in knee arthroplasty. Br J Anaesth 80:299–301, 1998.

24. Kathirvel S, Sadhasivam S, Saxena A, et al: Effects of intrathecal ketamine added to bupivacaine for spinal anaesthesia. Anaesthesia 55:899–904, 2000.

25. Bion JF: Intrathecal ketamine for war surgery: A preliminary study under field conditions. Anaesthesia 39:1023–1028, 1984.

26. Hawksworth C, Serpell M: Intrathecal anaesthesia with ketamine. Reg Anesth Pain Med 23:283–288, 1998.

27. Kristensen JD, Svensson B, Gordh T Jr: The NMDA-receptor antagonist CPP abolishes neurogenic 'wind-up pain' after intrathecal administration in humans. Pain 51:249–253, 1992.

28. Karpinski N, Dunn J, Hansen L, Masliah E: Subpial vacuolar myelopathy after intrathecal ketamine: Report of a case. Pain 73:103–105, 1997.

29. Atanassoff PG, Hartmannsgruber MWB, Thrasher J, et al: Ziconotide, a new N-type calcium channel blocker, administered intrathecally for acute postoperative pain. Reg Anesth Pain Med 25:274–278, 2000.

30. Jain KK: An evaluation of intrathecal ziconotide for the treatment of chronic pain. Expert Opin Investig Drugs 9:2403–2410, 2000.

31. Choe H, Kim JS, Ko SH, et al: Epidural verapamil reduces analgesic consumption after lower abdominal surgery. Anesth Analg 86:786–790, 1998.

32. Omote K, Sonoda H, Kawamata M, et al: Potentiation of antinociceptive effects of morphine by calcium-channel blockers at the level of the spinal cord. Anesthesiology 79:746–752, 1993.

33. Rane K, Segerdahl M, Goiny M, Sollevi A: Intrathecal adenosine administration. Anesthesiology 89:1108–1115, 1998.

34. Karlsten R, Gordh T Jr: An A_1-selective adenosine agonist abolishes allodynia elicited by vibration and touch after intrathecal injection. Anesth Analg 80:844–847, 1995.

35. Lindblom U, Nordfors L-O, Sollevi A, Sydow O: Adenosine for pain relief in a patient with intractable secondary erythromelalgia. Eur J Pain 1:299–302, 1997.

36. Rane K, Sollevi A, Segerdahl M: Intrathecal adenosine administration in abdominal hysterectomy lacks analgesic effect. Acta Anaesth Scand 44:868–872, 2000.

37. Eisenach JC, Hood DD, Curry R: Preliminary efficacy assessment of intrathecal injection of an American formulation of adenosine in humans. Anesthesiology 96:29–34, 2002.

38. Eisenach JC, Hood DD, Curry R: Phase I safety assessment of intrathecal injection of an American formulation of adenosine in humans. Anesthesiology 96:24–28, 2002.

39. Hood DD, Eisenach JC, Tuttle R: Phase I safety assessment of intrathecal neostigmine methylsulfate in humans. Anesthesiology 82:331–343, 1995.

40. Lauretti GR, Mattos AL, Reis MP, Pereira NL: Combined intrathecal fentanyl and neostigmine: Therapy for postoperative abdominal hysterectomy pain relief. J Clin Anesth 10:291–296, 1998.

41. Chung CJ, Kim JS, Park HS, Chin YJ: The efficacy of intrathecal neostigmine, intrathecal morphine, and their combination for post-cesarean section analgesia. Anesth Analg 87:341–346, 1998.

42. Lauretti GR, Lima ICPR: The effects of intrathecal neostigmine on somatic and visceral pain: Improvement by association with a peripheral anticholinergic. Anesth Analg 82:617–620, 1996.

43. Hood DD, Mallak KA, Eisenach JC, Tong C: Interaction between intrathecal neostigmine and epidural clonidine in human volunteers. Anesthesiology 85:315–325, 1996.

44. Owen MD, Ozsarac O, Sahin S, et al: Low-dose clonidine and neostigmine prolong the duration of intrathecal bupivicaine-fentanyl for labor analgesia. Anesthesiology 92:361–366, 2000.

45. Batra YK, Jain K, Chari P, et al: Addition of intrathecal midazolam to bupivacaine produces better post-operative analgesia without prolonging recovery. Int J Clin Pharmacol Ther 37:519–523, 1999.

46. Nishiyama T, Matsukawa T, Hanaoka K: Continuous epidural administration of midazolam and bupivacaine for postoperative analgesia. Acta Anaesthesiol Scand 43:568–572, 1999.

47. Valentine JM, Lyons G, Bellamy MC: The effect of intrathecal midazolam on post-operative pain. Eur J Anaesthesiol 13:589–593, 1996.

48. Kim MH, Lee YM: Intrathecal midazolam increases the analgesic effects of spinal blockade with bupivacaine in patients undergoing haemorrhoidectomy. Br J Anaesth 86:77–79, 2001.

49. Serrao JM, Marks RL, Morley SJ, Goodchild CS: Intrathecal midazolam for the treatment of chronic mechanical low back pain: A controlled comparison with epidural steroid in a pilot study. Pain 48:5–12, 1992.

50. Borg PA, Krijnen HJ: Long-term intrathecal administration of midazolam and clonidine. Clin J Pain 12:63–68, 1996.

51. Taira T, Kawamura H, Tanikawa T, et al: A new approach to control central deafferentation pain: spinal intrathecal baclofen. Stereotact Funct Neurosurg 65:101–105, 1995.

52. Van Schaeybroeck P, Nuttin B, Lagae L, et al: Intrathecal baclofen for intractable cerebral spasticity: a prospective, placebo-controlled, double-blind study. Neurosurgery 46:603–609, 2000.

53. Dario A, Scamoni C, Bono G, et al: Functional improvement in patients with severe spinal spasticity treated with chronic intrathecal baclofen infusion. Funct Neurol 16:311–315, 2001.

54. Zuniga RE, Perera S, Abram SE: Intrathecal baclofen: a useful agent in the treatment of well-established complex regional pain syndrome. Reg Anesth Pain Med 27:90–93, 2002.

55. Zumiga RE, Schlicht CR, Abram SE: Intrathecal baclofen is analgesic in patients with chronic pain. Anesthesiology 92:876–880, 2000.

56. Thompson E, Hicks F: Intrathecal baclofen and homeopathy for the treatment of painful muscle spasms associated with malignant spinal cord compression. Palliat Med 12:119–121, 1998.

57. Meythaler JM, Guin-Renfroe S, Brunner RC, Hadley MN: Intrathecal baclofen for spastic hypertonia from stroke. Stroke 32:2099–2109, 2001.

58. Loubser PG, Akman NM: Effects of intrathecal baclofen on chronic spinal cord injury pain. J Pain Symptom Manage 12:241–247, 1996.

59. Taura P, Planella V, Balust J, et al: Epidural somatostatin as an analgesic in upper abdominal surgery: A double-blind study. Pain 59:135–140, 1994.

60. Bagarani M, Amodei C, Beltramme P, et al: Effects of somatostatin peridurally administered in the treatment of postoperative pain. Minerva Anestesiol 55:513–516, 1989.

61. Chrubasik J, Meynadier J, Scherpereel P, Wunsch E: The effect of epidural somatostatin on postoperative pain. Anesth Analg 64:1085–1088, 1985.

62. Meynadier J, Chrubasik J, Dubar M, Wunsch E: Intrathecal somatostatin in terminally ill patients: A report of two cases. Pain 23:9–12, 1985.

63. Mollenholt P, Rawal N, Gordh T Jr, Olsson Y: Intrathecal and epidural somatostatin for patients with cancer. Anesthesiology 81:534–542, 1994.

64. Paice JA, Penn RD, Kroin JS: Intrathecal octreotide for relief of intractable nonmalignant pain: 5-year experience with two cases. Neurosurgery 38:203–207, 1996.

65. Desborough JP, Edlin SA, Burrin JM, et al: Hormonal and metabolic responses to cholecystectomy: Comparison of extradural somatostatin and diamorphine. Br J Anaesth 63:508–515, 1989.

66. Wilder-Smith CH, Wilder-Smith OH, Farschtschian M, Naji P: Epidural droperidol reduces the side effects and duration of analgesia of epidural sufentanil. Anesth Analg 79:98–104, 1994.

67. Naji P, Farschtschain M, Wilder-Smith OH, Wilder-Smith CH: Epidural droperidol and morphine for postoperative pain: Epidural droperidol and morphine for postoperative pain. Anesth Analg 70:583–588, 1990.

68. Bach V, Carl P, Ravlo O, et al: Potentiation of epidural opioids with epidural droperidol: A one year retrospective study. Anaesthesia 41:1116–1119, 1986.

69. Athanassiadis C, Karamanis A: Akathisia after long-term epidural use of droperidol: A case report. Pain 50:203–204, 1992.

70. Pellerin M, Hardy F, Abergel A, et al: Chronic refractory pain in cancer patients: Usefulness of intrathecal lysine acetylsalicylate in 60 cases. Presse Med 16:1465–1468, 1987.

71. Devoghel J-C: Small intrathecal doses of lysine-acetylsalicylate relieve intractable pain in man. J Int Med Res 11:90–91, 1983.

Chapter 28

A Peripheral Basis for Neuropathic Pain

Frank L. Rice, PhD / Michel Paré, PhD / Howard S. Smith, MD

Peripheral neuropathies occur in a wide variety of medical conditions with heterogenous etiologies and a wide range of sensory, motor and autonomic symptoms.[1,2] Those neuropathies involving cutaneous innervation cover a gamut, including numbness, hyperalgesia, allodynia, spontaneous pain, skin dryness, and excessive sweating. Pain can even occur in a territory that is devoid of "feeling" or sensation (anesthesia dolorosa). The epidemiology of painful neuropathies is uncertain. Monticelli and Beghi[3] reported a prevalence of symmetrical polyneuropathies of 1% in the general population of Italy and roughly 13% in patients older than 55 years of age who are followed by a general practitioner. The prevalence of neuropathy in patients with diabetes mellitus type II has been reported to be about 8% at the time of diagnosis and up to 50% after 25 years.[4] Guillain-Barré syndrome an inflammatory polyneuropathy, has an annual incidence rate of 1.7 per 100,000[5] with pain and/or dysethesia occurring in about 40% to 75% of Gullain-Barré syndrome patients.[6] Moulin and coworkers[7] reported that 75% of Guillain-Barré syndrome patients required opioids to provide adequate analgesia in a prospective study.

Overall, Dyck and associates[1] classified painful neuropathies according to cause in six general groupings: toxic-metabolic, post-traumatic, compressive, autoimmune, infectious, and hereditary. Estimates of neuropathies that cannot be accurately diagnosed range from about 32% to 70%.[8,9] Dyck and Lambert[10] have suggested that intensive re-evaluation with comprehensive techniques (e.g., exhaustive work-up) will improve diagnostic rates. Out of 205 patients with unclassified neuropathies originally, 42% were found to have an inherited disorder, 21% autoimmune disorders, 13% inflammatory demyelinating polyradiculoneuropathy, and 13% other causes. However, 24% remained without a diagnosis.[10] McLeod and coworkers[11] found about 13% of patients without a specific diagnosis in a series of 519 patients with chronic polyneuropathy. However, even when a precipitating factor is clear, little is known about the mechanism of most peripheral neuropathies, and their prevention and treatment are generally unpredictable and ineffective. Pain relief is typically partial and temporary at best.

At one extreme, the origin of neuropathic pain is hypothesized to originate in central nervous system neurons that have increased sensitization due to loss of primary afferent input referred to as *deafferentation*.[12,13] At the other extreme, neuropathic pain is hypothesized to originate in nociceptive primary sensory neurons that have become more irritable.[12,13] Such a condition might be referred to as *dysafferentation*. These two hypotheses are not mutually exclusive, and a combination of both mechanisms may contribute to some types of neuropathic pain. In this review, we discuss the normal organization, development, and biochemistry of cutaneous innervation as they may relate to the origin and symptoms of peripheral neuropathies, such as diabetic neuropathy[14] and post-herpetic neuralgia (PHN).[13]

In the late 1800s, the use of reduced heavy metal and supravital methylene blue techniques revealed the presence of different morphologically distinct types of endings in the skin (FIGURE 1), such as Pacini corpuscles, Ruffini corpuscles, Meissner corpuscles, Merkel cell-ending complexes, and hair-related lanceolate endings.[15–20] These were typically supplied by the larger-caliber axons seen in nerves. Although bundles of smaller caliber axons were also discovered, they were not reliably and completely stained by the techniques available at the time. Thus, their cutaneous terminations were elusive, and any observed endings had no distinctive morphology or associated terminal capsule.[21] As such, the cutaneous terminals of small-caliber axons have been collectively referred to as *free nerve endings* (FNEs).

Importantly, the cell bodies of the sensory cutaneous innervation were shown to be located in dorsal root ganglia and cranial ganglia, primarily the trigeminal ganglion of the fifth cra-

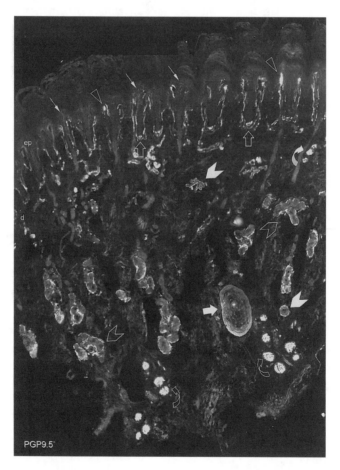

FIGURE 1. A montage of 12 digital micrographs taken with a 10 × objective of anti-protein gene product (PGP)9.5 immunofluorescence labeling of innervation in a 14 μm thick section cut perpendicular to the skin surface of the distal volar pad of the index finger. Free nerve endings are densely distributed in the epidermis (*thin arrows*). Meissner corpuscles (*open arrowheads*) are located in dermal papillae that bud off the primary epidermal ridges. Merkel cells and endings (*open broad arrows*) are located at the base of the primary epidermal ridges. Pacini corpuscles are located deeper in the dermis (*filled broad arrows*). Filled and *open chevrons* indicate innervated blood vessels and sweat glands, respectively. *Open* and *filled curved arrows* indicate deep and superficial nerves bundles; respectively, cut in cross-section: d, dermis; ep, epidermis.

nial nerve with some contribution from ganglia of the seventh, ninth, and tenth cranial nerves. As such, these "primary sensory neurons" have long axons running through the nerves, which require nutrition from the cell bodies located in the ganglia near the spinal cord and brainstem. Thus, these neurons are vulnerable to physical insults anywhere along their length, which could result in deterioration of the axons and endings distal to the site of the insult. Although the peripheral axons of primary sensory neurons have the capacity to regenerate, this process is partial and imperfect, resulting in disorganization at the site of the physical insult and often in painful neuromas as well as incomplete and disorganized cutaneous innervation resulting in losses of sensation and/or hyperalgesia and allodynia.[22,23] Although often related to disease conditions such as an acute herpes zoster attack or diabetes, symptoms of peripheral neuropathy can also occur with no known basis.

Early studies of electrical impulses applied to nerves recognized different rates of conduction and reasoned that the rate increased with the caliber of the axon as well as the presence and increased thickness of a myelin sheath. Such studies of compound action potentials recognized that some symptoms of various peripheral neuropathies could be correlated with problems associated with particular calibers of axons. Larger caliber, faster conducting axons were associated with low-threshold, highly discriminative mechanical transduction, and smaller caliber axons were implicated in more diffuse perceptions of pain, thermal sensation, and high threshold mechanical transduction.[24–28]

With the invention of the electron microscope and more powerful amplifiers for neurophysiology, a burst of research occurred in the 1950s, 1960s and early 1970s that greatly elucidated the structure and potential function of various types of cutaneous nerve endings.[29–40] Importantly, this research verified an earlier proposal by Adrian[41] that each primary sensory neuron had a preferred response to a specific modality or submodality among the spectrum of physical stimuli that contribute to our total somatosensory perception. As such, different components contributing to the spectrum of physical stimuli were being extracted and transmitted to the central nervous system by specific parallel sets of primary sensory neurons. In one case, high-frequency vibration was directly identified as the preferred response for rapidly conducting, large-caliber, thickly myelinated axons whose endings terminate in pacinian corpuscles.[42–44] Low-frequency vibration, pressure, and stretch were detected as the preferred stimuli for other thickly myelinated axons with a range of rapid conduction velocities and large-caliber collectively classified as A alpha-beta to A beta fibers. The axons for these preferred stimuli were respectively correlated with Meissner corpuscles, Merkel cell-ending complexes, and Ruffini corpuscles.[37,39,45–48] However, a critical evaluation of these correlations reveals that they are indirect and need to be re-evaluated. Indeed, recent analyses raise questions about whether Ruffini corpuscles even exist, at least in monkey and human glabrous skin.[48a,49] Meissner corpuscles were found to be multi-afferented structures that may have multiple functions, including nociception.[50,51] Moreover, Merkel endings have different terminal arborization patterns that may result in different mechanical functions such as pressure and stretch perception.[49,52]

A wide range of preferred stimuli were also detected among the relatively slowly conducting, thin-caliber, unmyelinated C fibers as well as slightly faster conducting, slightly thicker caliber, lightly myelinated A delta fibers as a range of cold to warm temperatures as well as nonnoxious skin contact across a range of low to high threshold intensities.[36,40,53,54] Importantly, both the C fiber and the A delta fiber populations included nociceptive primary sensory neurons whose preferred stimuli result in perceptions ranging from slow, diffuse, burning pain to sharp, discrete, stabbing pain. The preferred responses of such nociceptive afferents run a gamut from those that respond to extreme hot or cold temperatures, noxious chemicals, physical tissue injury, or extreme pressure as well as various combinations characterized as polymodal. In these cases, the cutaneous endings of such afferents were presumed to be among the FNEs that lack morphologically distinct characteristics. However, at the time that these various functional properties were being elucidated, as well as through the 1980s, available techniques failed to reveal the vast majority of C fiber and A delta fiber terminations.[21] Most of these fibers were thought to be located in the dermis. Little innervation was evident in the epidermis or on the vasculature.

The full extent of C fiber and A delta fiber endings was only revealed by immunochemistry following the development in the late 1980s of an antibody against a ubiquitous neuronal cytoplasmic enzyme referred to as protein-gene-product 9.5 (PGP9.5).[55-57] Anti-PGP9.5 labeling has revealed that the most extensive C-fiber and A delta fiber terminations are FNEs in the epidermis and on the cutaneous arterioles (see FIGURE 1). Additional FNEs have been found around hair follicles, in Meissner corpuscles, and among sweat glands. Beginning with antibodies against neuropeptides such as substance P, subtypes of C fibers and A delta fibers have been characterized immunochemically with an increasingly wide variety of antibodies against ligands, receptors, and ion channels that have been functionally implicated in various aspects of nociception.[51] These include opioid, vanilloid, purinergic, peptidergic, and histaminergic receptors and several types of acid-sensing ion channels. Some ion channels, such as the vanilloid-like receptor 1 (VRL1), are activated by high temperature known to elicit pain perception.[58] Purinergic receptors are activated by ATP, which is released by stressed and damaged tissue associated with pain.[59,60] Especially interesting, the vanilloid receptor 1 (VR1) is an ion channel activated by capsaicin, acidic pH, and elevated temperature, consistent with the features of polymodal nociception.[61-63]

Although more than one nociceptive chemical characteristic is known to exist on different neurons within the sensory ganglia, the full range of characteristics on any given neuron has been difficult to assess. This is because the identical neurons cannot be located in sections from the same ganglia harvested from different animals, to conduct different label combinations. Also, techniques have not yet been perfected and applied to directly correlate specific cutaneous endings with their specific cells in the ganglia in mature skin. Consequently, the full variety and functional capabilities of normal nociceptive primary sensory neurons is unknown, as well as how they may contribute to neuropathic pain.

Some indication of the potential complexity of peripheral innervation with regard to potential nociceptive mechanisms has recently been shown by taking advantage of the predictable structure of the Meissner corpuscles in monkey.[51] Although long regarded as a rapidly adapting, low-threshold mechanoreceptor innervated by A beta fibers, Meissner corpuscles have now been shown to also contain two types of C fiber innervation that have different immunochemical characteristics (FIGURE 2). One set contains calcitonin gene-related peptide (CGRP) and substance P, and the other lacks peptides but expresses the polymodal VR1 receptor. The peptidergic C fiber terminals are closely intermingled with endings of the A beta fibers, whereas the VR1 C fibers are segregated to stratified gaps between the A beta endings. Interestingly, the A beta endings also contain low levels of CGRP and substance P. Both these A beta endings and their closely related peptidergic C fiber endings also co-express a wide variety of biochemical properties, including immunolabeling for adrenergic, purinergic, and opioid receptors as well as one or more acid-sensing ion channels. In addition, the A beta endings also express the thermally activated ion channel, VRL1, as well as the substance P receptor, NK1. In contrast, the VR1 C-fibers lack substance P and CGRP but also express a

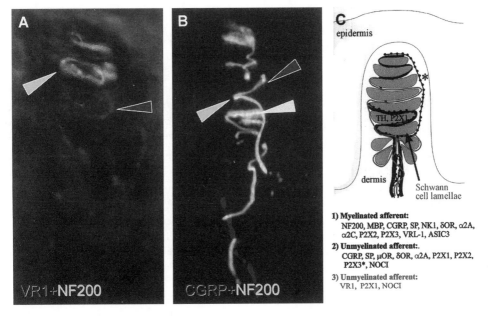

FIGURE 2. Multiple varieties of innervation to Meissner corpuscles expressing biochemical properties associated with nociceptors as seen in double-labeled conventional immunofluorescence digital images of 14 μm thick sections cut perpendicular to the skin surface in monkey digital glabrous skin. *A,* The segregated, interdigitated relationship between the VR1-positive C-fiber innervation (*right arrowhead*) and NF200-positive A beta fiber innervation (*left arrowhead*) as seen by epifluorescence microscopy. VR1-positive innervation in the Meissner corpuscle is segregated from and interdigitated with NF200-positive innervation. *B,* The close relationship between the peptidergic C-fiber (*right upper arrowhead*) and A beta fiber (*left arrowhead*) in the Meissner corpuscle double-labeled with sheep anti-CGRP and rabbit anti-NF200 as seen by confocal microscopy. Innervation having high levels of CGRP (*right upper arrowhead*) is intertwined with the NF200-positive innervation (*left arrowhead*) and is especially located along the inferior border of the NF-positive endings. In digitally merged double-labeled images, *yellow* symbols indicate the innervation definitively labeled with both primary antibodies. *C,* Schematic representation of other biochemical characteristics revealed by double label combinations (Note: Original figures are in color; adapted from Paré M, Elde R, Mazurkiewicz JE, et al: The Meissner corpuscle revised: A multiafferented mechanoreceptor with nociceptor immunochemical properties. J Neurosci 21:7236–7246, 2001.)

purinergic receptor and potential opioid receptors. Likewise, different types of C fibers are also closely affiliated with A beta fiber lanceolate endings arranged as a palisade around hair follicles in hairy skin.

Importantly, these observation indicate several previously unknown aspects of peripheral innervation that may be related to the variability and complexity of peripheral neuropathies as well as difficulty in their treatment. First, a given primary sensory afferent can have a highly complex biochemistry that can include several different nociceptive-implicated molecular mechanisms. These mechanisms may include those that presumably increase nociceptive processing—such as neuropeptides, purinergic receptors, vanilloid receptors, and acid-sensing ion channels— as well as decrease nociceptive processing, such as opioid receptors. As such, the relative sensitivity of an afferent to a potentially noxious stimulus may depend on the relative balance of its molecular components, which may increase or decrease nociception.

Second, A beta fibers that were only thought to be low-threshold mechanotransducers may also have nociceptive properties. Under abnormal conditions such A beta fibers may contribute to such pain perceptions as allodynia, which can be mediated by relatively large-caliber myelinated afferents.[64] Perhaps contributing to such allodynia, the peptidergic C fibers in Meissner corpuscles and affiliated with hair follicles may augment the sensitivity of the low-threshold A beta fibers whose endings express the NK1 receptor, especially under pathological conditions. In the spinal cord, A beta fibers have been generally shown to terminate in deeper laminae of the dorsal horn, whereas C fibers generally terminate in lamina II with collaterals to deeper laminae. In the deeper laminae, both the A beta fibers and C fiber collaterals can converge on the same second-order neurons that have been physiologically characterized as wide-dynamic range due to their presumed mechanoreceptive and nociceptive input.[53,54,65,66] It has been hypothesized that large-fiber mediated pain perception may be mediated by sprouting of A beta fiber central terminals to more superficial laminae or excess C fiber central terminals to deeper laminae.[53,54,65,66] To date, the specific sites of central termination of the C fibers and A beta fibers from the same Meissner corpuscles and same hair follicles has not been determined. Because of the close affiliation of their peripheral terminals, perhaps their central terminals normally have a close affiliation that would contribute to increased activation of wide-dynamic range neurons under pathological conditions.

Interestingly, the morphology of the Meissner corpuscles does not appear to be static under normal conditions or, especially, under pathological conditions or with aging. Instead, the proportion of C fiber and A beta fiber endings can vary among different Meissner corpuscles with a shift primarily to C fibers in aged monkeys or monkeys with naturally occurring type II diabetes.[67] Moreover, some monkeys in relatively early stages of diabetes actually have an increase in the total number of Meissner corpuscles, of which a disproportionately high number have an abnormal morphology (FIGURE 3).

Assessments of the recently discovered extensive C fiber and A delta fiber endings in the epidermis are also revealing a wide variety of mixed immunochemical properties (Paré and Rice, unpublished data).[56] Unlike in the Meissner's corpuscles, a lack of predictable anatomical landmarks precludes the identification of identical epidermal FNEs in different sections prepared with different antibody combinations. Consequently, the range of immunochemical characteristics for specific epidermal endings cannot be as thoroughly elucidated as in the Meissner corpuscles. Nonetheless, it is clear that some epidermal FNEs also can express multiple neuropeptides, receptors, and ion channels implicated in increasing and decreasing nociception. Thus, even though the epidermal FNEs may seem morphologically similar, a molecular diversity exists, consistent with the known physiological diversity among nociceptors.

The wide variety of cutaneous innervation, especially among C fiber and A delta fibers raises questions about the mechanisms that regulate the type and density of innervation during and after development and whether such mechanisms may also be involved in peripheral neuropathies. The nerve growth factor (NGF)–related family of neurotrophins and other families of trophic factors clearly play a major role in this development and maintenance.[68–70]

Since the late 1800s, it has been known that the density of cutaneous endings is higher in locations with greater tactile sensitivity, such as the face, hands, and feet. Consistent with such higher innervation density, trigeminal ganglia as well as dorsal root ganglia at cervical and lumbosacral levels were found to have especially high numbers of primary sensory neurons. Although it was initially assumed that more neurons were being produced for sites with higher innervation density, studies in the early to mid-1900s discovered that a similar

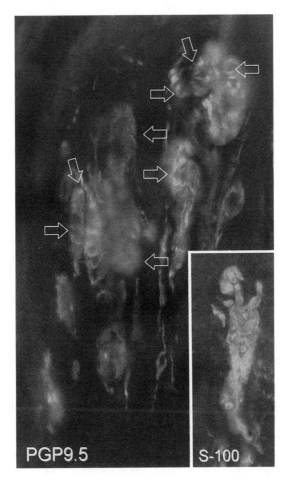

FIGURE 3. Anti-protein gene product (PGP)9.5 labeling of Meissner corpuscles (*arrows*) located in adjacent dermal papillae. Compared with age-matched normal monkeys, diabetic monkeys showed an increase in the number of Meissner corpuscles. Moreover, numerous papillae contained multiple Meissner corpuscles, which is rarely seen normally. The increased number and presence of multiple Meissner corpuscles was especially noticeable in the early-stage diabetic monkey. However, the Meissner corpuscles in the diabetic monkeys were abnormal, with fewer axons, disrupted endings, and increased Schwann cell S-100 immunoreactivity (*inset*).

excessive number of neurons was being produced in dorsal root ganglia at all spinal levels and that resulting differences at maturity were due to a process of elimination through cell death. Although neurons were being eliminated in all ganglia during development, a process called *apoptosis*, more neurons were being eliminated at thoracic levels than at lumbosacral levels. Limb elimination and transplantation in embryonic chicks revealed that the cutaneous targets were regulating the relative survival of primary afferent neurons.[71,72] Studies by Cohen and associates[73] resulted in the discovery of neuronal survival factor, NGF, and the hypothesis that primary sensory neuron survival and cutaneous innervation density was regulated by competition for NGF produced in the skin.

Subsequent studies demonstrated that not all types of sensory neurons were responsive to NGF and that other related molecules–brain-derived neurotrophic factor (BDNF), neurotrophin 3 (NT3), and neurotrophin (NT4)—were survival factors for other types of neurons.[69,70] Some types of neurons were dependent on more than one of these NGF-related neurotrophins. Within the last 10 years, the effects of the NGF-related neurotrophins have been found to be mediated by three types of tyrosine kinase receptors (trks) that may have high affinity binding for one or more of the neurotrophins and lower affinities for others.[69,70] In particular, trkA has a high affinity for NGF and lower affinity for NT3. TrkB has a comparably high affinity for BDNF and NT4, and a lower affinity for NT3. And trkC has a high affinity only for NT3. Moreover, a fourth non-kinase receptor, p75, binds all four receptors, generally at relatively lower affinity than trk receptors. Lacking a kinase domain, p75 was originally hypothesized to facilitate or interfere with neurotrophin access to the kinase receptors. However, the small intracellular domain of p75 was shown to be similar to that of transforming growth factor receptors with the capability to signal through different second messenger pathways than the kinase receptors.

The discovery of additional neurotrophins and the variety of the receptors helped explain differences in survival mechanisms for many types of cutaneous innervation. However, even taking these additional factor into account, a major problem with the neurotrophin hypothesis was that many different types of innervation are dependent on the same neurotrophins. Of particular relevance to nociceptive mechanisms, knockout studies of the neurotrophins and their receptors revealed that every type of cutaneous C fibers and A delta fibers was dependent on NGF and trkA.[74–77] However, since different types of C fibers and A delta fibers terminating in the skin develop at different times, simple competition could not explain how limited quantities of NGF would regulate the density of early developing types of NGF-dependent innervation but then allow for the development of later sets that were also dependent on NGF.

Some insight to this problem has been achieved by using the highly detailed and highly predictable microanatomy of mouse whisker pad innervation[78–80] to assay the impact of a wide variety of NGF-related knockouts and transgenic overproduction (FIGURE 4).[76,77] Importantly, these studies have demonstrated that some types of C fibers may depend only on NGF and trkA for their development; others on NGF and trkA as well as p75; others on NGF and NT3 but only trkA; and still others on NGF and NT3 but both trkA and trkC. Thus, some types of endings may initially compete for NGF but then switch to NT3, thereby potentially allowing other sets of innervation to compete for NGF. The presence of p75 in combination with trkA may enable some types of C fiber innervation to compete more efficiently for lower levels of NGF. Moreover, these studies demonstrated that BDNF and NT4 could act as survival factors for some types of A beta fiber innervation but could suppress many types of NGF-dependent C fiber innervation. Therefore, the production of BDNF or NT4 or both in the epidermis and upper dermis may act to reduce some early types of NGF-dependent innervation below the density that NGF levels would be capable of supporting. This may, in turn, make more NGF available for later sets of innervation to develop (FIGURE 5).

Still other studies revealed that some types of C fiber neurons are initially dependent on NGF, then switch their dependency to an entirely different type of trophic factor, glial-derived neurotrophic factor.[81] Glial-derived neurotrophic factor is now known to be one of several related neurotrophins, including neurturin, artemin, and persipin, that operate through an entirely different set of coreceptor molecules than the receptors for the NGF-family of neurotrophins.[82] Still other classes of trophic factors as well as isoforms among the NGF family of neurotrophins and receptors have become known as participants in establishing the normal mix of cutaneous innervation.[69,70,83]

Normal Upper Dermal and Epidermal Innervation

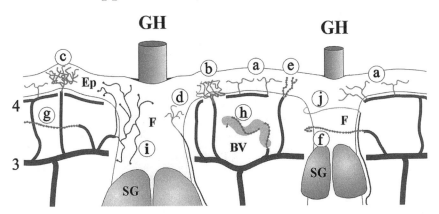

■ **Nonpeptidergic Sensory:**
   a. Penicillate endings, thin C axons
   b. Cluster endings, Aδ axons
   c. Bush endings, Aδ and C axons

■ **CGRP/SP Sensory:**
   d. Follicle neck endings, thin C axons

■ **CGRP/SP Sensory:**
   e. Epidermal endings, thick C axons
   f. Circular follicle endings, thick C axons
   g. Upper dermal endings, thick C axons
   h. Vascular endings, thick C axons

Autonomic:
■ i. Sympathetic, unmyelinated axons
▨ j. Parasympathetic?, unmyelinated axons

FIGURE 4. Schematic illustration of unmyelinated and A delta fiber innervation that arises from the dermal plexus in the intervibrissal fur of the mouse. This innervation supplies the epidermis (Ep), necks and mouths of intervibrissal hair follicles (F) and blood vessels (BV) in the upper dermis. The epidermis and the follicles (which are derived from the epidermis) are separated from the underlying dermis by a continuous basement membrane. The colors indicate the nature of the various sets of innervation. The fourth tier (4) of the dermal plexus gives rise to very thin nonpeptidergic penicillate endings (a) in the epidermis and in the mouth of the intervibrissal follicles. The third tier (3) is the source of varicose peptidergic innervation to the epidermis (e), the upper dermis (g), encircling the neck of follicles (f), and on superficial blood vessels (h); nonpeptidergic multiaxonal cluster endings (b) adjacent to the mouth of follicles and multiaxonal bush endings (c) in epidermal hillocks; and presumptive sympathetic innervation (i) to the neck of follicles. The second tier (not shown) is the source of two sets of axons that ascend along the basement membrane and sebaceous gland (SG) of follicles to terminate at their mouths and necks. One set is nonvaricose peptidergic sensory (d) and the other is presumptive parasympathetic (g). (Note: Original figure is in color; from Rice FL, Albers KM, Davis BM, et al: Differential effects of various neurotrophin and trk receptor deletions on the unmyelinated innervation of the epidermis in the whisker pad of the mouse. Dev Biol 198:57–81, 1998.)

Taken together, the developmental studies indicate that the normal variety and density of cutaneous innervation is an equilibrium achieved through competition involving a mix of promoting and suppressing effects by, and differential dependencies on, various trophic factors operating through mixed affinities among different full-length and truncated receptors (FIGURE 6). Moreover, many of these mechanisms may continue to operate at more subliminal levels to maintain the normal mix of cutaneous innervation. Consequently, some forms of peripheral neuropathy may be due to a disturbance in the normal equilibrium, which may shift the competitive balance to a new equilibrium, in which some types of innervation may be lacking and others increased. The new equilibrium may in turn account for the adverse symptoms regarded as a form of peripheral neuropathy.

Impact of Homozygous Knockouts
2-4 weeks postnatal

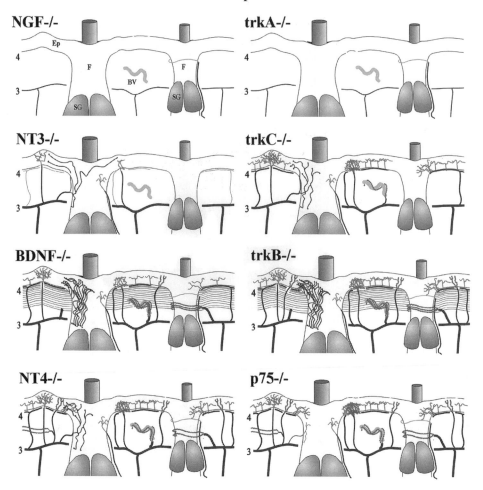

FIGURE 5. Schematic illustrations summarizing the impact of the various neurotrophin or receptor knockouts on the unmyelinated and A delta fiber innervation in the epidermis, upper dermis, and upper portion of hair follicles as seen in the mystacial pads of 2–4 week old mice. The color schemes and ending symbols are the same as in FIGURE 4. Endings symbols are removed or are reduced or increased in size, number, or density to indicate the consequences of a particular knockout. For example, penicillate endings and the fourth tier of the dermal plexus are missing in NGF and trkA knockouts. Only some remnants of the fourth tier is evident in NT-3 knockouts. The penicillate endings are increased in trkC, trkB, NT4, and p75 knockouts but seem normal in the absence of BDNF. Sympathetic innervation is missing to the necks of follicles in NGF and trkA knockouts and is reduced in the absence of p75. Sympathetic innervation is increased in BDNF and trkB knockouts but is relatively unaffected in the absence of trkC and NT4. The BDNF and trkB knockouts also have a dense aberrant stratum of sympathetic axons in the upper dermis. In the absence of NT3, the density of the sympathetic innervation is reduced but the distribution increases into the adjacent epidermis. The impacts on other sets of innervation are described in the source article (Rice et al.[77]). (Note: Original figure is in color; from Rice FL, Albers KM, Davis BM, et al: Differential effects of various neurotrophin and trk receptor deletions on the unmyelinated innervation of the epidermis in the whisker pad of the mouse. Dev Biol 198:57–81, 1998.)

Hypothesized Expression and Function
of trkA, trkB, trkC and p75

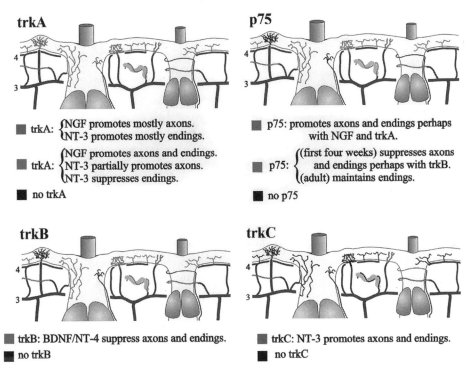

trkA

- ■ trkA: { NGF promotes mostly axons.
          NT-3 promotes mostly endings.

- ■ trkA: { NGF promotes axons and endings.
          NT-3 partially promotes axons.
          NT-3 suppresses endings.

- ■ no trkA

p75

- ■ p75: promotes axons and endings perhaps
        with NGF and trkA.

- ■ p75: { (first four weeks) suppresses axons
         and endings perhaps with trkB.
         (adult) maintains endings.

- ■ no p75

trkB

- ■ trkB: BDNF/NT-4 suppress axons and endings.
- ■ no trkB

trkC

- ■ trkC: NT-3 promotes axons and endings.
- ■ no trkC

FIGURE 6. Schematic illustrations summarizing hypothesized expressions of neurotrophin receptors and the impact of the neurotrophins on the unmyelinated and A delta fiber innervation in the epidermis, upper dermis, and upper portion of hair follicles in the mystacial pads of mice. The symbols and locations for the various sets of innervation are the same as in FIGURE 4. The color scheme has been changed to indicate which receptors are hypothesized to be expressed on each type of innervation and what the neurotrophin impact is hypothesized to be at some point during development. For example, in the *upper left panel*, sensory neurons that supply the endings labeled with green are hypothesized to express trkA through which NGF signaling primarily promotes the development of the axons and NT3 primarily promotes the development of endings. Sympathetic neurons that supply the endings labeled with *red* are hypothesized to express trkA through which NGF signaling promotes the development of the axons and endings, whereas NT3 signaling supports the development of some axons but suppresses the endings. Endings shown in *black* in each panel are hypothesized not to express the particular receptor. As shown in all four panels, the CGRP/SP sets of innervation to the epidermis, upper dermis, and necks of follicles are hypothesized to express trkA, trkB, trkC, and p75 at some time during their development. In contrast, sensory neurons that supply bush endings to the epidermis and CGRP/SP endings to the necks of follicles may only express trkA, whereas presumptive parasympathetic innervation to the necks of follicles may only express trkC. Other hypotheses are discussed in the text. (Note: Original figure is in color.)

An example of such a shift in equilibrium was seen in an evaluation of the whisker pads in mice with homozygous knockouts of NGF, NT3, trkA, or trkC.[77] In this case, every type of C fiber innervation was eliminated in NGF and trkA knockouts (see FIGURE 5). Moreover, virtually every type was also eliminated in a trkA knockout. In contrast, knockouts of trkC only had losses of some peptidergic C fibers, while some nonpeptidergic C fiber innervation in the epidermis actually increased compared to normal. These results indicated that the non-peptidergic epidermal C fiber innervation was dependent on NGF and NT3 signaling through only the trkA receptor. However, the peptidergic C-fiber innervation depended on NGF signaling through trkA but NT3 signaling through trkC. Consequently, the trkC knockout eliminated the peptidergic innervation, presumably reducing competition for NT3. In turn, more NT3 presumably was available to promote the development of the nonpeptidergic innervation. Thus, the new equilibrium of epidermal innervation lacked peptidergic C fiber endings but had excess nonpeptidergic C fiber endings.

The recent assessment of the cutaneous innervation in a patient (referred to as JW) with especially severe post-herpetic neuralgia provides an example of how a shift in biochemical characteristics and in the balance of cutaneous innervation may contribute to a variety of severe pain symptoms.[84] Several recent prior assessments of innervation in skin biopsies revealed that the occurrence of PHN following an acute herpes zoster attack was associated with a reduction in epidermal innervation as revealed by anti-PGP9.5 labeling. Such a reduction supports the hypothesis that the neuropathic pain may have its origin in the deafferentation of second-order neurons in the spinal cord. JW is a patient who had an acute herpes attack that resulted in severe intractable pain consisting of intense allodynia and extremely increased sensitivity to thermal stimuli and capsaicin. Following more than 6 years of unsuccessful treatment, this desperate patient had the entire large area of painful thoracic skin excised by a private physician despite the warning that the few prior attempts at this procedure produced widely different results.[85] In some cases, the patients obtained substantial pain relief; in other cases, pain was exacerbated. In this case, JW was fortunate to obtain substantial relief, indicating that the neuropathic pain was originating from cutaneous sensory endings. The PHN skin was generously donated for immunochemical analysis, along with a 3 mm punch biopsy from the contralateral unaffected dermatome (FIGURE 7).

The analysis with anti-PGP9.5 revealed that JW's PHN skin had reduced epidermal innervation like that reported in prior studies.[13,86] However, double-label assessments with anti-PGP9.5 and antibodies against various other antigens revealed substantial changes in the structure of the skin and the remaining endings that were consistent with JW's PHN symptoms. First, the epidermis was abnormally thin and dermal papillae were enlarged and irregularly shaped. Second, all innervation to the epidermis funneled through the dermal papillae. Epidermal endings were lacking that normally penetrate along the base of the epidermis. Third, the remaining endings were more highly branched, extended more superficially, and were longer, being oriented more parallel instead of perpendicular to the skin surface. These features indicate that, in the absence of some types of endings, the remaining endings may have sprouted so that they may be more exposed to surface stimuli and have increased surface areas. The increased surface area of the endings presumably would result in more receptors or channels per axon, which in turn would presumably lower their response thresholds to a given stimulus.

Fourth, the remaining endings in the PHN skin had increased substance P, CGRP, and VR1 immunoreactivity compared with contralateral skin innervation. Moreover, many endings co-expressed the neuropeptides with VR1, which was rarely observed in the contralateral biopsy. Fifth, antibodies for 200 kD neurofilament protein (NF200) normally label A beta fibers and their endings, as well as A delta fibers. Anti-NF200 rarely labels the endings of A delta fibers or any C fibers and their endings. As such, in the biopsy contralateral to the PHN skin, NF200 was detected almost exclusively in larger caliber axons that appear to terminate in dermal papillae as small Meissner corpuscles. NF200 was rarely detected among the C fiber and A

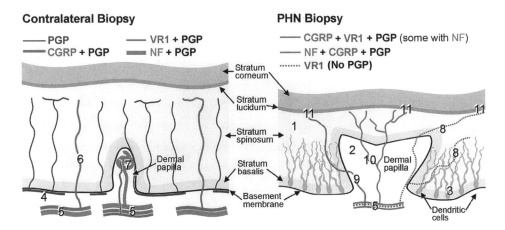

FIGURE 7. Schematic summary of differences between contralateral and post-herpetic neuralgia (PHN) skin. Numbering refers to numbers on the figure. (Original figure is in color.)

1. The epidermis was thinner in the PHN skin.
2. The dermal papillae were larger and more irregularly shaped in PHN skin. Virtually all of the innervation to the epidermis entered via the dermal papillae, whereas most in the contralateral skin entered the epidermis between the dermal papillae (see FIGURES 4 and 5).
3. Only the PHN skin contained numerous anti-protein gene product (PGP) labeled, presumptive dendritic cells concentrated primarily in lamina basalis between the dermal papillae.
4. Innervation that only labels with anti-PGP9.5 is virtually absent in the epidermis of PHN skin. In the contralateral skin, this innervation consisted of axons located immediately subjacent to the basement membrane that terminate as very thin, fairly simple, predominantly radially oriented endings. At least some endings have short T-shaped terminal branches.
5. PHN skin lacked most of the small nerves in the upper dermis that were not in contact with the basement membrane. The remaining nerves were small, with fewer and thinner axons.
6. PHN skin lacked CGRP-positive endings that were supplied directly from the small nerves in the upper dermis and penetrated the epidermis between the dermal papillae.
7. PHN skin lacked axons that terminated like a knot in the dermal papillae. In contralateral skin, this was the only upper dermal and epidermal innervation that labeled with anti-NF and may be myelinated.
8. VR1-positive profiles in PHN skin were present in virtually all dermal papillae, often had several branches, and often had long oblique trajectories into the epidermis. Importantly, about half had little or no detectable anti-PGP 9.5 immunoreactivity. In contralateral skin, VR1-positive profiles was restricted to only a few dermal papillae, had simple profiles, and also had PGP immunoreactivity.
9 and 10. Virtually all of the innervation to PHN epidermis that labeled with anti-PGP 9.5 also labeled with anti-CGRP. This innervation had a more oblique instead of radial orientation, could be highly branched, and may also expresses VR-1 and/or NF immunoreactivity.
11. In contrast to the contralateral skin, most of the endings in the epidermis of PHN skin had long oblique trajectories that reached nearly to the stratum lucidum.

delta fiber endings in the epidermis. In the PHN skin, the Meissner corpuscles were absent in the dermal papillae, but relatively thinner NF200 positive fibers were observed to ascend through the dermal papillae to terminate as highly branched, NF-positive endings in the epidermis. Some of these NF-positive epidermal endings also colabeled with anti-CGRP.

Taken together, the fourth and fifth observations suggest that (1) the levels of some nociceptive-related molecules may be up-regulated in the remaining PHN innervation and may be expressed in abnormal combinations and (2) that Meissner afferents may have sprouted into the epidermis. Alternatively, relatively rare types of innervation may have increased in quantity or sprouted into abnormal locations. These changes may contribute to both hyperalgesia and allodynia in JW's case. An extensive longitudinal study involving 200 patients is underway to follow the progression of innervation changes starting during the onset of acute herpes zoster and following the progression to the recovery of normal cutaneous sensation or the persistent PHN.

CONCLUSION

In summary, the cumulative results of our research and that of many others have revealed that normal cutaneous innervation is supplied by a wide variety of primary sensory neurons. The endings of each type of neuron are morphologically, biochemically, and positionally specialized to preferentially extract a particular feature or set of features among the broad-spectrum cutaneous stimuli that are normally perceived as a seamless continuum constituting our total tactile perception. These varieties of neurons include those that have a capacity to detect a variety of nociceptive stimuli that contribute to our normal range of pain perception in response to injurious or potentially injurious temperatures and physical or chemical trauma as well as acute inflammation. The normal range of tactile perception, including pain, is achieved through a mix of different types of endings whose density and proportion are an equilibrium determined by competition for trophic factors in the skin. In establishing and maintaining the proper mix of endings in this equilibrium, particular types of endings have a unique combination of trophic factor dependencies and response thresholds, in which some trophins can have a promoting effect and others a suppressing effect. Moreover, each type of ending has a unique combination of biochemical characteristics that determine its preferred stimulus and degree of response to other stimuli. Conditions resulting in loss of sensation or pathological pain may cause a disruption in the competition, resulting in a new equilbrium in which some ending types are lost while others increase. Such an imbalance could be referred to as "dysafferentation," as opposed to merely a loss of innervation referred to as deafferentation. Importantly, the increased size and complexity of remaining terminal arbors may result in "irritable nociceptors" that have reduced response thresholds to noxious stimuli that would normally activate the ending as well as reduced attainable thresholds for stimuli that might normally be insufficient to activate the ending.

Although some attempts have been made to prevent loss of innervation or promote regeneration through systemic administration of factors such as NGF (Apfel, 1999), this approach may be far too simplistic given the complex trophic interactions that are known to contribute to the normal mix of cutaneous innervation (Apfel, 2001, 2002). As these factors are better understood, assessments of the mix of aberrant innervation in patients with various peripheral neuropathies may dictate treatment strategies designed to eliminate pain by restoring the normal equilibrium of cutaneous innervation rather than trying to block nociceptive transduction.

REFERENCES FOR ADDITIONAL READING

1. Dyck PJ, Thomas PK, Lambert EH, eds: Peripheral neuropathy. WB Saunders, Philadelphia, 1993.
2. Scadding JW: Peripheral neuropathies. In: Wall PD, Melzack R, eds: Textbook of Pain. Churchill Livingstone, Edinburgh, 1999.
3. Monticelli ML, Beghi E: Chronic symmetric polyneuopathy in the elderly: A field screening investigation in two regions in Italy—background and methods of assessment. The Italian General Practitioner Group. (IGPSG). Neuroepidemiol 12:96–105, 1993.

4. Pirart J: Diabetes mellitus and its degenerative complications: A prospective study of 4400 patients observed between 1947 and 1973. Diabetes Care 1:168–188, 1978.

5. Hughes RAC: Epidemiology of peripheral neuropathy. Editorial review. Curr Opin Neurol 8: 335–338, 1995.

6. Pentland B, Donald SM: Pain in the Guillain-Barré Syndrome: A clinical review. Pain 59:159–164, 1994.

7. Moulin DE, Hagen N, Feasby TE, et al: Pain in Guillan-Barré syndrome [see comments] [Comment in Neurology 1997;49:1474]. Neurology 48:328–331, 1997.

8. Mathews WB: Cryptogenic polyneuropathy. Proc R Soc Med 45:667–669, 1952.

9. Prineas J: Polyneuropathy of undetermined cause. Acta Neurol Scand 46:4–72, 1970.

10. Dyck PJ, Lambert EH: Intensive evaluation of referred unclassified neuropathies yields improved diagnosis. Ann Neurol 10:222–226, 1981.

11. McLeod JG, Pollard JD, Cameron J, et al. Chronic polyneuropathy of undetermined cause. J Neurol Neurosurg Psychiatry 47:530–535, 1984.

12. Fields HL, Rowbotham M, Baron R: Post-herpetic neuralgia: Irritable nociceptors and deafferentation. Neurobiol Dis 5:209–227, 1998.

13. Rowbotham MC, Yosipovitch G, Connolly MK, et al: Cutaneous innervation density in the allodynic form of post-herpetic neuralgia. Neurobiol Dis 3:205–214, 1996.

14. Thomas PK, Tomlinson DR: Diabetic and hypoglycaemic neuropathy. In: Dyck PJ, Thomas PK, Griffin JW, Low PA, Poduslo JF, eds: Peripheral Neuropathy, 3rd edn. WB Saunders, Philadelphia, 1993, pp. 749–774.

15. Vater A: Dissertation de consensu partium corporis humani. Haller, Disputationum anatomicarum selectarum II. Gottingae, 1741.

16. Wagner R, Meissner G: Über das Vorhandensein bisher unbekannter eigenthümlicher Tastkörperchen (corpuscula tactus) in den Gefühlswärzchen der menschlichen Haut und über die Endausbreitung sensitiver Nerven. Nachricht Georg-August-Univ Königl Gesd Wiss Göttingen 2: 17–30, 1852.

17. Ruffini A: Sur un nouvel organe nerveux terminal et sur la présence des corpuscules Golgi-Mazzoni dans le conjonctif sous-cutané de la pulpe des doigts de l'homme. Arch Ital Biol 21:249–265, 1894.

18. Dogiel AS: Die Nervenendigunden in meissnerschen Tastköperen. Mthly Int J Anat Physiol 9: 76–85, 1892.

19. Hoggan G, Hoggan FE: Forked endings in hairs. J Anat 27:224–231, 1892.

20. Retzius G: Biologische Untersuchungen. Neue Follge IV. Samson and Wallin, Stockholm, 1892.

21. Lauria G: Innervation of the human epidermis: A historical review. Ital J Neurol Sci 20:63–70, 1999.

22. Head H, Sherren J: The consequences of injury of the peripheral nerves in man. Brain 28:116–133, 1905.

23. Head H: Studies in Neurology. Oxford University Press, London, 1920.

24. Zotterman Y: Studies in the peripheral nervous mechanism of pain. Acta Med Scand 80:185–242, 1933.

25. Gasser HS: The classification of nerve fibers. Ohio J Sci 41:145–159, 1943.

26. Gasser HS, Erlanger J: The role of fiber size in the establishment of a nerve block by pressure or cocaine. Am J Physiol 88:581–591, 1929.

27. Lewis T, Pickering GW, Rothschild P: Centripetal paralysis arising out of arrested bloodflow to the limb, including notes on a form of tingling. Heart 15:359–383, 1931.

28. Heinbecker P, Bisshop GH, O'Leary J: Pain and the touch fibers in peripheral nerves. Arch Neurol Psychiatry 29:771–789, 1933.

29. Cauna N: Nerve supply and nerve endings in Meissner's corpuscles. Am J Anat 99:315–327, 1956.

30. Cauna N: The free penicillate nerve endings of the human hairy skin. J Anat 115:277–288, 1973.

31. Cauna N: Morphological basis of sensation in hairy skin. Prog Brain Res 43:35–45, 1976.

32. Andres KH: Über die Feinstruktur der Rezeptoren on Sinushaaren. Z Zellforsch 75:335–365, 1966.
33. Andres KH, von Düring M: Morphology of cutaneous receptors. In Iggo A, ed: Handbook of Sensory Physiology. Springer, New York, 1973, pp. 1–28.
34. Patrizzi G, Munger BL: The ultrastructure and innervation of rat vibrissae. J Comp Neurol 26: 423–436, 1966.
35. Chambers MR, Andres KH, Duering M, Iggo A: The structure and function of the slowly adapting type II mechanoreceptor in hairy skin. Q J Exp Physiol 57:417–445, 1972.
36. Perl ER: Myelinated afferent fibres innervating the primate skin and their response to noxious stimuli. J Physiol 197:593–615, 1968.
37. Iggo A, Muir AR: The structure and function of a slowly-adapting touch corpuscle in hairy skin. J Physiol (Lond) 200:763–796, 1969.
38. Chouchkov HN: Ultrastructure of pacinian corpuscles in men and cats. Z Mikrosk Anat Forsch 83:17–32, 1971.
39. Brown AG, Iggo A: A quantitative study of cutaneous receptors and afferent fibres in the cat and rabbit. J Physiol 193:707–733, 1967.
40. Burgess PR, Perl ER: Cutaneous mechanoreceptors and nociceptors. In Iggo A, ed: Handbook of Sensory Physiology: Somatosensory System. Springer-Verlag, Heidelberg, 1973, pp. 29–78.
41. Adrian ED: The messages in sensory nerve fibers and their interpretation. Proc R Soc Lond Ser Br 109:1–18, 1931
42. Gray JAB, Matthews PBC: A comparison of the adaptation of the pacinian corpuscle with the accommodation of its own axon. J Physiol (Lond) 114:454–464, 1951.
43. Sato M: Response of pacinian corpuscles to sinusoidal vibration. J Physiol (Lond) 159:391–409, 1961.
44. Talbot WH, Darian-Smith I, Kornhuber HH, Mountcastle VB: The sense of flutter-vibration: comparison of the human capacity with response patterns of mechanoreceptive afferents from the monkey hand. J Neurophysiol 31:301–334, 1968.
45. Mountcastle VB, Talbot WH, Darian-Smith I, Kornhuber HH: Neural basis of the sense of flutter-vibration. Science 155:597–600, 1967.
46. Werner G, Mountcastle VB: Neural activity in mechanoreceptive cutaneous afferents: Stimulus-response relations, Weber function, and information transmission. J Neurophysiol 28:359–397, 1965.
47. Knibestöl M: Stimulus-response functions of slowly adapting mechanoreceptors in the human glabrous skin area. J Physiol (Lond) 245:63–80, 1975.
48. Witt I, Hensel H: Afferente Impulse aus der Extremitatenhaut der Katze bei thermisher und mechanischer Reizung. Pflug Arch Gesamte Physiol 268:582–596, 1959.
48a. Paré M, Behets C, Cornu O: Paucity of presumptive Ruffini corpuscles in the index finger pads of humans. J Comp Neurol (in press).
49. Paré M, Smith AM, Rice FL: Distribution and terminal arborizations of cutaneous mechanoreceptors in the glabrous finger pads of the monkey. J Comp Neurol 445:347–359, 2002.
50. Johansson O, Fantini F, Hu H: Neuronal structural proteins, transmitters, transmitters enzymes and neuropeptides in humans Meissner's corpuscles: A reappraisal using immunohistochemistry. Arch Dermatol Res 291:419–424, 1999.
51. Paré M, Elde R, Mazurkiewicz JE, et al: The Meissner corpuscle revised: A multiafferented mechanoreceptor with nociceptor immunochemical properties. J Neurosci 21:7236–7246, 2001.
52. Ebara S, Kumamoto K, Mazurkiewicz JE, Rice FL: Substantial differences in the density, types and terminal arborizations among the innervation to the vibrissa follicle-sinus complexes of the rat and cat. J Comp Neurol 449:103–119, 2002.
53. Light AR, Perl ER: Reexamination of the dorsal root projection to the spinal dorsal horn including observations on the differential termination of the dorsal root projection to the spinal dorsal horn icluding observations on the differential termination of coarse and fine fibers. J Comp Neurol 186: 117–131, 1979.

54. Light AR, Perl ER: Spinal termunation of functionally identified primary afferent neurons with slowly conducting myelinated fibers. J Comp Neurol 186:133–150, 1979.

55. Wilson POG, Barber PC, Hamid QA, et al: The immunolocalization of protein gene product 9.5 using rabbit polyclonal and mouse monoclonal antibodies. Br J Exp Path 69:91–104, 1988.

56. Dalsgaard CJ, Rydh M, Haegerstrand A: Cutaneous innervation in man visualized with protein gene product 9.5 (PGP 9.5) antibodies. Histochemistry 92:385–390, 1989.

57. Rice FL, Kinnman E, Aldskogius H, et al: The innervation of the mystacial pad of the rat as revealed by PGP 9.5 immunofluorescence. J Comp Neurol 337:366–385, 1993.

58. Caterina MJ, Rosen TA, Tominaga M, et al: A capsaicin-receptor homologue with high threshold for noxious heat. Nature 398:436–441, 1999.

59. Lewis C, Neldhart S, Holy C, et al: Coexpression of P2X2 and P2X3 receptor subunits can account for ATP-gated currents in sensory neurons. Nature 377:432–435, 1995.

60. Tsuda M, Koizumi S, Kita A, et al: Mechanical allodynia caused by intraplantar injection of P2X receptor agonist in rats: Involvement of heteromeric P2X2/3 receptor signaling in capsaicin-insensitive primary afferent neurons. J Neurosci 200–5, 2000.

61. Tominaga M, Caterina MJ, Malmberg AB, et al: The cloned capsaicin receptor integrates multiple pain-producing stimuli. Neuron 21:531–543, 1998.

62. Caterina MJ, Schumacher MA, Tominaga M, et al: The capsaicin receptor: A heat-activated ion channel in the pain pathway. Nature 389:816–824, 1997.

63. Caterina MJ, Leffler A, Malmberg AB, et al: Impaired nociception and pain sensation in mice lacking the capsaicin receptor. Science 288:306–313, 2000.

64. Torebjörk HE, Lundberg LER, LaMotte RH: Central changes in processing of mechanoreceptive input in capsaicin-induced secondary hyperalgesia in humans. J Physiol (Lond) 448:765–780, 1992.

65. Coggeshall RE, Lekan HA, Doubell TP, et al: Central changes in primary afferent fibers following peripheral nerve lesions. Neuroscience 77:1115–1122, 1997.

66. Moore KA, Baba H, Woolf CJ: Synaptic transmission and plasticity in the superficial dorsal horn. Prog Brain Res 129:63–80, 2000.

67. Paré M, Rice FL, Bodkin NL, Hansen BC: Aging and diabetes related changes in the innervation to glabrous skin in rhesus monkeys [abstract]. Soc Neurosci X:X, 2001.

68. Levi-Montalcini R: The nerve growth factor: 35 years later. EMBO J 6:2856–2867, 1987.

69. Reichardt LF, Fariñas I: Neurotrophic factors and their receptors: Roles in neuronal development and function. In: Molecular and Cellular Approaches to Neural Development (Cowan WM, Jessel TM, Zipursky SL, eds. Oxford University Press, New York, 1997, pp 220–263.

70. Huang EJ, Reichardt LF: Neurotrophins: Roles in neuronal development and function. Annu Rev Neurosci 24:677–736, 2001.

71. Shorey ML: The effect of the destruction of peripheral areas on the differentiation of neuroblasts. J Exp Zool 7:25–63, 1909.

72. Detweiler (1936).

73. Cohen S, Levi-Montalcini R, Hamburger V: A nerve growth-stimulating factor isolated from sarcomas 37 and 180. Proc Natl Acad Sci U S A 40:1014–1018, 1954.

74. Crowley C, Spencer SD, Nishimura MC, et al: Mice lacking nerve growth factor display perinatal loss of sensory and sympathetic neurons yet develop basal forebrain cholinergic neurons. Cell 76: 1001–1011, 1954.

75. Smeyne RJ, Klein R, Schnapp A, et al: Severe sensory and sympathetic neuropathies in mice carrying a disrupted Trk/NGF receptor gene. Nature 368:246–249, 1994.

76. Fundin BT, Silos-Santiago I, Ernfors PJ, et al: Differential dependency of developing mechanoreceptors on neurotrophins, trk receptors and p75 LNGFR. Dev Biol 190:94–116, 1997.

77. Rice FL, Albers KM, Davis BM, et al: Differential effects of various neurotrophin and trk receptor deletions on the unmyelinated innervation of the epidermis in the whisker pad of the mouse. Dev Biol 198:57–81, 1998.

78. Fundin BT, Arvidsson J, Aldskogius H, et al: A comprehensive immunofluorescence and lectin binding analysis of intervibrissal fur innervation in the mystacial pad of the rat. J Comp Neurol 385:185–206, 1997.
79. Fundin BT, Pfaller K, Rice FL: Different distributions of the sensory and autonomic innervation among the microvasculature of the rat mystacial pad. J Comp Neurol 389:545–568, 1997.
80. Rice FL, Fundin BT, Arvidsson J, et al: A comprehensive immunofluorescence and lectin binding analysis of vibrissal follicle sinus complex innervation in the mystacial pad of the rat. J Comp Neurol 385:149–184, 1997.
81. Molliver DC, Wright DE, Leitner ML, et al: IB4-binding DRG neurons switch from NGF to GDNF dependence in early postnatal life. Neuron 19:849–861, 1997.
82. Baloh RH, Enomoto H, Johnson EM Jr, Milbrandt J: The GDNF family ligands and receptors: Implications for neural development. Curr Opin Neurobiol 10:103–110, 2000.
83. McMahon SB, Bennett DLH: Trophic factors and pain. In: Wall PD, Melzack R, eds: Textbook of Pain. Edinburgh, Churchill Livingstone, 1999, pp. 105–128.
84. Petersen KL, Rice FL, Suess F, et al: Relief of post-herpetic neuralgia by surgical removal of painful skin. Pain 2002 (in press).
85. Loeser J: Surgery for post-herpetic neuralgia. In: Watson and Gershon, eds: Herpes Zoster and Post-herpetic Neuralgia, 2nd ed. Eds: 2001, pp. 255–264.
86. Oaklander AL: The density of remaining nerve endings in human skin with and without post-herpetic neuralgia after shingles. Pain 92:139–145, 2001.

Chapter 29

Analgesia in the Periphery

Timothy J. Ness, MD, PhD

Most clinical pain begins in the periphery. Tissue injury, inflammation, and neuropathic pain with characteristics of allodynia and hyperalgesia all are associated with primary afferent activation. Additional *central* processes may perpetuate or magnify peripheral processes, but without some form of input, the pain typically declines. Permanent destruction of nerve endings has not proved to be an effective long-term form of treatment because nerve endings regrow (often in a disorganized fashion), and primary afferent targets in the spinal cord may change in response to altered inputs. One strategy of pain treatment has been the deactivation or desensitization of the afferents that initiate and maintain pain by the use of peripherally administered drugs. There are many forms of peripheral delivery of drugs, ranging from focal injections to topical application to the systemic administration of active agents that are excluded from the central nervous system (e.g., quaternary compounds).

The value of *peripheral* pharmacologic agents is that they may maximize analgesia and minimize side effects. Exclusion from brainstem or cerebral cortical sites limits numerous side effects. Intrathecal or epidural delivery of drugs produces a selective spinal effect of these drugs by physically limiting the amount of the drug that reaches supraspinal structures, but these techniques require invasive procedures. Similarly, conduction blockade of the axons of large nerves using local anesthetics has specificity but requires an invasive procedure and is limited by difficulties associated with sustained delivery of agents and the potential for concurrent motor dysfunction. The most distal form of regional anesthesia is the local application of pharmacologically active agents at the terminals of nerve endings. The intent of this local application is to suppress selectively the generation of action potentials by affecting transduction and sensitization mechanisms occurring within nociceptor transduction sites.

Which primary afferent neurons represent nociceptors is partially open to debate. Various poorly myelinated or unmyelinated (A delta and C) afferent fiber groups have been identified that encode for painful intensities of peripheral stimuli. Some afferents are mechanosensitive but not heat sensitive. Some are activated by certain chemical stimuli but not other stimuli. Some are *silent* and become mechanosensitive only in the presence of certain chemical mediators (for reviews of this topic, see references 48, 61, and 68). All of these afferent fiber groups may represent components of the nociceptive pathway. The neuronal group that has gained the greatest acceptance as the representative nociceptor, is the polymodal nociceptor which encodes for noxious intensities of thermal, mechanical, and chemical stimuli.[38] The sensory endings of these nociceptors have transducer proteins present that are ion channels that are opened by irritant ligands (receptor-type), high-intensity heat, or mechanical distortion of the receptor membrane.[42] Ion flow through these proteins, which are named *VR1, VRL1, P2X₃, DRASIC,* and *mDeg,* causes sufficient membrane depolarization to activate voltage-sensitive sodium channels. The resulting action potential

TABLE 1

Drug Classes With Sites of Action at the Nociceptor Transducer

Classes/Drugs	Presumed Mechanism of Action
Agents Blocking Transduction	
Vanilloids	Deactivation of VR1 and VRL1 receptors
	Neuropeptide depletion
Local anesthestics	Blockade of sodium (SNS/PN3) channels
Antiserotoninergic agents	Blockade of 5-HT$_3$ receptors
Antipurinergic agents	Blockade of P2X$_3$ receptors
Inhibitors of the Transducer Site	
Opioids	Opioid-receptor activation (μ,κ,δ)
Cannabinoids	CB$_1$ receptor activation
Adrenoceptor agonists	α_2 adrenoceptor activation
Agents Blocking Modulation/Modification Processes	
Corticosteroids	Phospholipase A$_2$ inhibition
Nonsteroidal anti-inflammatory drugs	Cyclooxygenase inhibition
Antikinin agents	Blockade of B$_2$ receptors
Antitachykinins	Blockade of NK$_1$ receptor
Anti-neurotrophins	Blockade of trkA receptor

transmits the encoded information along the afferent axon to the central nervous system. Blockade or alteration of these ion channel activities leads to reduced nociceptive transmission and results in analgesia. Candidate pharmacologic agents that affect the activity of these ion channels and that may prove useful as peripheral analgesics include agents that (1) directly block primary transducer activation mechanisms, (2) produce active inhibition of transducer site activity through altered activity of second messenger systems, (3) block the actions of drugs that sensitize the transducer, or (4) block the actions of drugs that modify the nociceptive pathway.[51] Many different drug classes have such actions and have had peripheral receptors or mechanisms described (Table 1). These individual drug classes are discussed separately, with a focus on topically applied analgesics and only minimal discussion of injected agents.

The use of topical analgesics has gained increasing popularity with commercial formulations available for many single (e.g., capsaicin [Zostrix]) or two-agent (e.g., prilocaine/lidocaine [EMLA]) combinations. Patches formulated for transdermal delivery of systemically active agents (e.g., fentanyl [Duragesic], clonidine [Catapres]) similarly have found utility. Combinations of drugs compounded by specialty pharmacies into solutions, gels, or creams have been used by some pain clinicians. A survey[53] identified use of 36 separate drugs in varying concentrations in such compounded formulations (Table 2). Use of such agents was identified throughout most of the United States and Canada and Mexico. The scientific basis for the use of some of these agents via a topical delivery medium is soundly based. For some agents, however, there is no available information. With one exception,[41] there is virtually no information related to combinations of drugs. Given the clinical use of multiagent compounds, it is prudent to review the scientific literature for all potentially used drug classes.

TABLE 2

Agents Reported in Topically Applied Compounds Used for Pain[53]

Local anesthetics	*Nonsteroidal Anti-inflammatories*
Lidocaine 2%, 4%, 5%	Diclofenac
Prilocaine	Ketoprofen 4%, 5%, 10%
Bupivacaine	Aspirin
Tetracaine	Flurbiprofen 5%
	Ibuprofen 2%
Corticosteroids	Piroxicam 0.5% 2%
Dexamethasone 0.15%	
Hydrocortisone 1%, 10%	*Anticonvulsants*
	Carbamazepine 2%
Antidepressants	Gabapentin 6%
Amitriptyline 2%	
Nortriptyline	*Other*
Doxepin	Baclofen 5%
	Orphenadrine
Opioids	Lecithin
Fentanyl	Capsaicin 0.025%, 0.05%
Hydromorphone	Cyclobenzaprine 0.5%, 1%, 2%
Morphine	Clonidine 0.2%
Sufentanil	Diphenhydramine 1%
Loperamide	Nifedipine
	Guanethidine 1%, 2%
NMDA-receptor antagonists	Guaifenesin
Ketamine 5%, 10%, 15%, 20%	Haloperidol
Dextromethorphan	
Amantadine	

VANILLOIDS

Clinical use of vanilloids is predominantly in the form of capsaicin creams available in 0.025% or 0.075% concentrations. Heat, protons, and some algesiogenic chemicals, such as capsaicin, activate transduction mechanisms via the vanilloid receptors (VRs).[36] Recently cloned, the VR1 and VR-like receptor (VRL1) are ligand gated cation (Na^+/Ca^{++}) channels that also are heat and proton activated. The number of VR1 channels present in the transducer increases subacutely in the presence of inflammation as part of an induction process within the dorsal root ganglion cell bodies (a similar induction occurs with sodium ion channels).[47, 72] High-intensity, prolonged, or frequent vanilloid receptor activation may lead to a deactivation of the VR1 receptor by a dephosphorylating calcineurin-linked process. For this reason, the chronic multidaily topical application of capsaicin, the archetype vanilloid receptor agonist, has found utility in the treatment of postherpetic neuralgia, diabetic neuropathy, osteoarthritis, and cluster headache.[23] Depletion of peripheral stores of neuropeptides also has been proposed as a mechanism of action, although studies related to neurokinin antagonists (see later) suggest that this may have limited impact. As an acute therapeutic modality, Robbins et al[63] used high-concentration (5% to 10%) topical capsaicin to desensitize the extremities of patients with the diagnosis of complex regional pain syndrome while receiving regional anesthesia of the affected limb. Of their subjects, 90% reported substantial analgesia lasting for 1 to 18 weeks. Other vanilloid receptor agonists, such as resiniferatoxin, olvanil, and nuvanil, which produce fewer initial symptoms but similar desensitization effects, may have future utility as transducer-desensitizing agents.[16] Apart from the potentially adverse sensory effects of capsaicin, there is little or no toxicity associated with use of these agents in their commercially available forms.

LOCAL ANESTHETICS (SODIUM ION CHANNEL BLOCKERS)

Nociceptor transducer sites have sensory neuron-specific sodium (SNS/PN3) channels that are voltage gated and are responsible for the generation of axonal action potentials. Various inflammatory compounds activate receptors and second messenger systems that lead to increased excitability of these SNS/PN3 channels. After prolonged inflammation, there is an induction of SNS/PN3 channel synthesis similar to that of VR1 induction.[47, 72] The threshold for the generation of action potentials through SNS/PN3 channels is decreased in the presence of sensitizing agents, and spontaneous depolarizations become more common with increased channel number. As a consequence, drugs that block sodium ion channels have obvious effects on sensory transduction and transmission that may be at concentrations that are well below those needed to produce conduction blockade. New formulations of local anesthetics, such as those in colloidal suspensions or as transdermal creams or patches (i.e., EMLA; lidocaine [Lidoderm]), all allow for the new use of an old drug. Potential toxicities are due to systemic levels of medication that may have cardiac or central nervous system effects (e.g., seizures) or effects on methemoglobin generation.

ANTISEROTONINERGIC AGENTS

The pharmacology of serotonin (5-HT) receptors is complex with at least seven main classes of receptors with one to five different subtypes in each class. Receptors are located on primary afferents and at multiple sites within the central nervous system. Peripheral actions of serotonin lead to pain sensation, and central actions are pronociceptive and antinociceptive.[45] Clinically, peripherally restricted $5-HT_3$ receptor antagonists, such as ondansetron or dolasetron, at commonly used doses have not had obvious benefit as analgesics but are used as antiemetics and act to antagonize spinal opioid-induced itching.[7]

ANTIPURINERGIC AGENTS

With cellular injury, there is a release of adenosine triphosphate (ATP) into the intracellular space. ATP is known to bind $P2X_3$ receptor–gated ion channels that are selectively expressed on small-diameter, nonpeptidergic nociceptive sensory neurons.[8] Although there is promise for the use of purinergic antagonists as peripheral analgesics, this potential still awaits basic science laboratory development.

OPIOIDS

Opioids as peripheral analgesics have a long history of use in the treatment of postoperative pain, specifically as localized injections (e.g., > 36 studies of morphine into the knee joint).[32] Opioid receptors become expressed on peripheral afferent nerve terminals in the presence of inflammation,[26] and multiple animal experiments and clinical studies observed that peripheral opioids are more effective in the presence of inflammation.[69] Similar to SNS/PN3 channels and VR1 receptors, the synthesis and peripheral export of κ opioid receptors is increased in response to inflammatory events in the periphery with eventual location at the ends of nerves innervating the site of inflammation.[78, 81] Opioids have been delivered in a topical fashion in the urinary bladder: Duckett et al[18] and Bertschy et al[6] showed excellent postoperative pain control after bladder surgery in children when an intravesical morphine infusion was administered. Topical opioids also have been used in the treatment of painful skin ulcers.[74]

Clinically, in the absence of inflammation or with injection into a site that does not limit systemic redistribution, there seems to be little or no selective peripheral effect of opioids. Picard et al[56] did a systematic review of 26 studies in which opioids were injected into nonarticular sites, including the brachial plexus, perineurally, intrapleurally, intraperitoneally, incisionally, and as part of a Bier block. They found little support for the use of peripheral opioids in nonarticular sites. The peripheral effects of κ opioid receptor agonists are particularly interesting because the systemic administration of peripherally restricted forms of these drugs was proved to have analgesic effects in inflammatory pain models, neuropathic pain models,[33] and visceral pain models.[9, 13, 21, 52] Similarly, peripheral administration of a cream emulsion preparation of loperamide, a mixed opioid agonist that does not cross the blood-brain barrier, was shown to reduce hypersensitivity in animal models.[55] Toxicities associated with opioids are well described and generally are due to central nervous system effects (i.e., nausea, respiratory depression). An exclusion from the central nervous system suggests desirable therapeutic characteristics.

CANNABINOIDS

A novel group of chemical compounds that may prove to have value as peripheral analgesics are the cannabinoids, which interact with the endocannabinoid system.[22, 57, 77] The CB_1 and CB_2 receptors are the molecular targets of Δ^9-THC (tetrahydrocannabinol), a neuroactive agent in cannabis leaves. Both act by G protein–linked mechanisms to produce relatively weak modulatory effects within neuronal systems. In particular, the CB_1 receptors are known to exist on the transducer sites of nociceptive primary afferent neurons, and the local application of a CB_1 receptor agonist results in decreased responses to locally applied formalin or other irritants.[10, 62] Cannabinoids have been reported to have analgesic effects in cancer patients, but these have not been described as due to peripheral actions.[54]

α-ADRENOCEPTOR AGONISTS

After nerve injury, multiple sensory nerves including nociceptors begin to express adrenoceptors on their peripheral extensions, and the use of adrenoceptor agonists becomes logical.[35] The α_2-adrenergic agonist clonidine was shown to have analgesic effects secondary to its actions as a sympatholytic, through central actions on spinal and supraspinal nociceptive processing and more recently as a peripheral analgesic. In patients with sympathetically maintained pain, Davis et al[15] noted a reduction in allodynia in the area immediately surrounding transdermal clonidine patches but no effect on distant sites. Transdermal clonidine also has been used to treat spasticity in patients with spinal cord injury.[79] The limiting factor for use of clonidine has been the hemodynamic consequences of its use.

GLUTAMATE ANTAGONISTS

Glutamate through the activation of N-methyl-D-aspartate (NMDA) receptors has been linked with hypersensitivity processes, acting in the spinal cord and on supraspinal structures. Isolated basic science reports suggested that there could be a role for peripheral NMDA receptors in nociceptive processes.[75] Tverskoy et al[73] reported a beneficial effect of ketamine added to their local anesthetic solution in patients undergoing herniorrhaphy, but it is not clear whether this was a peripheral effect or may have been due, in part, to central effects. Azevedo et al[3] showed reduced pain after gynecologic surgery when a transdermal delivery of 25 mg/d of ketamine was employed, but the drug delivery effect was not site specific. Peripheral NMDA receptors were proposed to interact with peripheral opioid receptors.[34] Toxicities resulting from NMDA-receptor antagonists are mainly due to actions within the central nervous system, with dysphoria, sedation, and hallucinations common after systemic use. Contact dermatitis was noted in 5% of cases treated with tromantadine, a derivative of amantadine.[29]

ANTIINFLAMMATORIES (CORTICOSTEROIDS, NONSTEROIDAL ANTIINFLAMMATORY DRUGS)

When tissue injury occurs, a cascade of biochemical events ensues, resulting in the production of various cytokines and prostaglandins with known sensory effects. A logical strategy to minimize inflammation-related pain would seem to be the inhibition of inflammation itself through the use of steroidal and nonsteroidal antiinflammatories. Inflammation also promotes healing, however. Chemotactic activities, vasodilation, angiogenesis, and fibroblast activation all are activities that are beneficial to the organism and that result in the resolution of the pain-producing process by facilitating and orchestrating the process of healing. The global inhibition of phospholipase activity or cyclooxygenase activity may result in retarded rates or reduced levels of healing[14, 20, 27, 31, 40] and so may be detrimental to the overall goals of a procedural treatment. Use for postoperative pain should include this concern. In the future, it may be possible to alter the specific balance between prostaglandin subtypes in an attempt to maximize their beneficial versus detrimental effects on wound healing.[19] Use of the cyclooxygenase-2 inhibitors does not seem to alleviate the problem, but the use of specific cytokine (anti-interleukin-2) or prostanoid (anti–prostaglandin E_2 or anti–prostaglandin $F_{2\alpha}$) antagonists may allow one to differentiate between good and bad products of inflammation. An alternative strategy to the selective inhibition of detrimental agents is the active addition of agents such as growth factors that counteract detrimental effects of the antiinflammatories.[25, 64, 70]

In the presence of a chronic inflammatory process without an acute injury, there is clearly a role for antiinflammatories. The limitations of specific therapies relate to long-term toxicities of systemically employed agents more than their local effects. Newer forms of nonsteroidal antiinflammatory drugs (NSAIDs) have become available as gels or other topical agents such as patches.[24] A relatively older form of topical medication—aspirin dissolved in diethyl ether—has a long history of pungent and flammable use and has shown analgesic effects on pain associated with herpes zoster with skin levels 80 to 100 times those produced by oral administration of a similar amount of drug.[5] Moore et al[49] did a systematic review of 86 randomized, controlled trials in which topical NSAIDs were used for acute or chronic pains and concluded that the use of these agents for analgesia was superior to placebo in virtually all of the trials. Vaile and Davis[76] were less enthusiastic in their evaluation of topical NSAIDs for the treatment of musculoskeletal pain. Use of topical NSAIDs has resulted in numerous complications,[76] including acute renal failure[37] and exacerbations of asthma.[67] Salicylate toxicity has occurred in children treated with topical agents.[11]

ANTIKININ AGENTS

Bradykinin and kallidin and small amounts of other kinins are produced at sites of injury and inflammation and play a critical role in signaling tissue distress and organizing tissue responses to injury.[17] There are two identified kinin receptors B_1 and B_2, both of which act by G protein–coupled mechanisms. The primary sensory effect of bradykinin is the activation and sensitization of nociceptors through its actions at the B_2 receptor. The corelease of many other sensitizing agents, including prostanoids, histamine, serotonin, nerve growth factor, and cytokines such as interleukin-1, result in an inflammatory *soup*, which further sensitizes the primary afferent neuron transducer terminal. At present, no antikinin agents are clinically available.

ANTITACHYKININS

Although the actions of substance P and associated neuropeptides have been shown to have effects at central nociceptive sites of processing, the role of peripheral effects of these compounds has been less obvious.[58] Human trials of antagonists of the NK_1 receptor (to which substance P binds selectively) have been disappointing with little or no analgesia noted,[28] and so, at present, research related to NK_1 antagonists is of undetermined importance in relation to peripheral analgesia.

ANTINEUROTROPHINS

There is extensive experimental evidence that would support a role for neurotrophic factors in the development of hypersensitivity after the onset of inflammation in peripheral tissues.[44, 46, 60] Consisting of several families of proteins, the neurotrophins are labeled according to their initially identified site of isolation (e.g., brain-derived or glia-derived neurotrophic factors [BDNF and GDNF]) or simply as neurotrophic factors (NT-3, NT-4/5). The neurotrophin that has gained the greatest interest is nerve growth factor (NGF). During development, NGF is necessary for the survival of nociceptors and is truly a growth factor. In adults, NGF acquires actions that lead to the immediate sensitization of nociceptive afferents and delayed phenotypic effects within the dorsal root ganglion.

Neurotrophins act via three different tyrosine kinase receptors (trkA, trkB, and trkC) and by the p75 receptor. The trkA receptor seems responsible for most actions of NGF that lead to hypersensitivity. The sequestration of endogenous NGF through use of an antibody complex seems to dissociate the sensory consequences of inflammation from other measures of inflammation. It would seem that antagonism of NGF effects might have the desired effect of blocking the *bad* sensory effects of inflammation from the *good* healing effects of the many biochemical events. NGF also performs good functions, however, as it is vital for the maintenance of the peripheral nervous system, in particular, the efferent sympathetic nervous system. A global disruption of neurotrophic functions likely would result in neurodegeneration, neuropathies, and potentially cancer. Pharmacologic tools useful in antagonizing NGF effects are limited,[65] but the potentially large size of antagonist polypeptides may prove to be beneficial because they would allow for exclusion from the central nervous system and could allow for localized sequestration in peripheral sites.

ANTIDEPRESSANTS

The tricyclic antidepressant drugs have proven efficacy in virtually every chronic pain disorder. Their effects on pain are believed to be related to their inhibition of reuptake of monoamines within the central nervous system, although peripheral effects also occur. They can be absorbed transdermally;[4] clinically relevant systemic levels of amitriptyline have been reported after use of a transdermal gel.[66] In that case report, the patient had a good effect of the amitriptyline on his depression, but his pain complaints were not improved. No other pain-related cases using topical tricyclic antidepressants have been reported. Antidepressant medications have known, potentially life-threatening toxicities. It is reasonable that because systemic levels of drugs can be obtained from topical application, excessive systemic levels of drug also may be possible, and side effects such as urinary retention and arrhythmias may become manifest. This has been the case for doxepin, which also is prescribed for pruritus.[30, 80]

ANTICONVULSANTS

As shown in Table 2, various anticonvulsants have been compounded into topical forms. A Medline search using the search words *topical, transdermal,* and *anticonvulsants* revealed no clinical literature related to the potential for pain relief with these compounds when administered topically. Clonazepam has been shown to have reasonable transdermal penetration,[50] but no other data related to pharmacokinetics of topical application were identified. Gabapentin, when injected locally, has been shown to have no effect on hypersensitivity caused by a herpesvirus infection in mice.[71] Carbamazepine, when given systemically, is a common cause of rash[59] and has known toxicities with a potential for liver damage, bone marrow suppression, and central nervous system effects. Given the potential dangers associated with their use, the lack of a rationale for their local benefit, and the undetermined pharmacokinetics of their absorption, the topical use of anticonvulsants does not seem logical.

ANTIHISTAMINES

Use of topical agents for pruritus is common, although the efficacy of this treatment has been questioned. Diphenhydramine is available in over-the-counter forms. Despite some reports of systemic toxicity (mental status changes) with its topical use,[12] diphenhydramine is considered safe.

OTHER AGENTS

Numerous other medications have been used in topical formulations. Nifedipine gel has been used on mucosal surfaces, in particular the anal canal because it relaxes the internal anal sphincter and so reduces spasm experienced there.[2] Experiments in mice suggest that transdermal delivery of nifedipine is likely to be minimal.[43] Topical nitroglycerin has effects on chest pain and has been noted to have analgesic effects on cancer pain[39] by a presumed nitric oxide–related mechanism. The transdermal delivery of antipsychotic agents such as chlorpromazine and haloperidol has been investigated[1] but for their central nervous system effects. Muscle relaxants/antispastic agents, such as baclofen, orphenadrine, and cyclobenzaprine, are reported as drugs used in compounded agents, but no identifiable literature supports this route of administration. Some drugs used in compounded agents are intended to improve solubility or penetration characteristics of the other compounds (e.g., lecithin).

SUMMARY

Decisions related to the clinical management of pain are influenced by specificity of the tools physicians have available to treat the pain. The greater the analgesia or the lesser the side effects of treatment, the greater physicians' ability to customize treatment of an individual patient. Peripheral analgesics are an option for pain management that may avoid many of the side effects associated with the use of centrally active drugs. Numerous substances have been noted to have peripheral effects acting on or in the vicinity of the primary nociceptors' transducer sites. These drugs can lead to a reduction of nociceptor activity and stop pain before it is even encoded rather than dealing with its central consequences. Questions related to long-term efficacy of peripheral analgesics, tolerance to their effects, and the toxicity of long-term treatments are yet to be defined. It is likely that in the future, clinicians will have many new specific tools to employ in their treatment of pain that act by peripheral mechanisms, but the use of specific elements of these tools must be driven by scientific evaluation rather than opinion.

ACKNOWLEDGMENTS

The author is supported by grant NIDDK-RO1-DK-51413 from the National Institutes of Health. Thoughtful comments from Dr. Jayne Ness and secretarial assistance of Sandra Roberts are gratefully acknowledged.

REFERENCES

1. Almirall M, Montana J, Escribano E, et al: Effect of D-limonen, alpha-pinene and cineole on in vitro transdermal human skin penetration of chlorpromazine and haloperidol. Arzneimittelforschung 46:676–680, 1996.
2. Antropoli C, Perrotti P, Rubino M, et al: Nifedipine for local use in conservative treatment of anal fissures: Preliminary results of a multicenter study. Dis Colon Rectum 42:1011–1015, 1999.
3. Azevedo VMS, Lauretti GR, Pereira NL, Reis MP: Transdermal ketamine as an adjuvant for postoperative analgesia after abdominal gynecological surgery using lidocaine epidural blockade. Anesth Anal 91:1479–1492, 2000.
4. Bailey DN: Percutaneous absorption of tricyclic antidepressants: Amitriptyline, nortriptyline, imipramine and desipramine. J Analy Toxicol 14:217–218, 1990.
5. Bareggi SR, Pirola R, DeBenedittis G: Skin and plasma levels of acetylsalicylic acid: A comparison between topical aspirin/diethyl ether mixture and oral aspirin in acute herpes zoster and postherpetic neuralgia. Eur J Clin Pharm 54:231–235, 1998.
6. Bertschy C, Aubert D, Lassauge F, et al: Analgesie par morphine intravesicale en Urologie Pediatrique. Progr Urol 9:474–478, 1999.
7. Borgeat A, Stirnemann HR: Ondansetron is effective to treat spinal or epidural morphine-induced pruritis. Anesthesiology 90:432–436, 1999.
8. Burnstock G: P2X receptors in sensory neurones. Br J. Anaesth 84:476–488, 2000.
9. Burton MB, Gebhart GF: Effects of kappa-opioid receptor agonists on responses to colorectal distension in rats with and without acute colonic inflammation. J Pharmacol Exp Ther 285:707–715, 1998.

10. Calignano A, LaRana G, Giuffrida A, Pionelli D: Control of pain initiation by endogenous cannabinoids. Nature 394:277–281, 1998.

11. Candy JM, Morrison C, Paton RD, et al: Salicylate toxicity masquerading as malignant hyperthermia. Paediatr Anaesth 8:421–423, 1998.

12. Chan CY, Wallander KA: Diphenhydramine toxicity in three children with varicella-zoster infection. DICP 25:130–132, 1991.

13. Craft RM, Henley SR, Haaseth RC, et al: Opioid antinociception in a rat model of visceral pain: Systemmic versus local drug administration. J Pharmacol Exp Ther 275:1535–1542, 1995.

14. Dahners LE, Gilbert JA, Lester GE, et al: The effect of a nonsteroidal anti-inflammatory drug on the healing of ligaments. Am J Sports Med 16:641–646, 1988.

15. Davis KD, Treede RD, Raja SN, et al: Topical application of clonidine relieves hyperalgesia in patients with sympathetically maintained pain. Pain 54:361–362, 1993.

16. Dray A: Vanilloids as analgesics. In: Sawyanok J, Cowan A (eds): Novel Aspects of Pain Management: Opioids and Beyond. New York: Wiley-Liss, 1999, pp 117–134.

17. Dray A: Kinins and their receptors in hyperalgesia. Can J Physiol Pharmacol 75:704–712, 1997.

18. Duckett JW, Cangiano T, Cubina M, et al: Intravesical morphine analgesia after bladder surgery. J Urol 157:1407–1409. 1997.

19. Durant S, Duval D, Homo-Delarche F: Effect of exogenous prostaglandins and nonsteroidal anti-inflammatory agents on prostaglandin secretion and proliferation of mouse embryo fibroblasts in culture. Prostaglandins Leukot Essent Fatty Acids 38:1–8, 1989.

20. Eubanks TR, Greenberg JJ, Dobrin PB, et al: The effects of different corticosteroids on the healing colon anastamosis and cecum in a rat model. Am Surg 63:266–269, 1997.

21. Friese N, Diop L, Lambert C, et al: Antinociceptive effects of morphine and U-50,488H on vaginal distension in the anesthetized rat. Life Sci 61:1559–1570, 1997.

22. Fuentes JA, Ruiz-Gayo M, Manzanares J, et al: Cannabinoids as potential new analgesics. Life Sci 65:675–685, 1999.

23. Fusco BM, Giacovazzo M: Peppers and pain: The promise of capsaicin. Drugs 53:909–914, 1997.

24. Galer BS, Rowbotham M, Perander J, et al: Topical diclofenac patch relieves minor sports injury pain: results of a multicenter controlled clinical trial. J Pain Symptom Manage 19:287–294, 2000.

25. Hamon GA, Hunt TK, Spencer EM: In vivo effects of systemic insulin-like growth factor-I alone and complexes with insulin-like growth factor binding protein-3 on corticosteroid suppressed wounds. Growth Regul 3:53–56, 1993.

26. Hassan AHS, Ableitner A, Stein C, Herz A: Inflammation of the rat paw enhances axonal transport of opioid receptors in the sciatic nerve and increases their density in the inflamed tissue. Neuroscience 55:185–195, 1993.

27. Haws MJ, Kucan JO, Roth AC, et al: The effects of chronic ketorolac tromethamine (Toradol) on wound healing. Ann Plas Surg 37:147–151, 1996.

28. Hill RG: NK$_1$ (substance P) receptor antagonists—why are they not analgesic in humans? Trends Pharm Sci 21:244–246, 2000.

29. Jauregui I, Urrutia I, Gamboa PM, Antepara I: Allergic contact dermatitis from tromantadine. J Invest Allergy Clin Immunol 7:260–261, 1997.

30. Jones ME, Skaufle ML: Systemic adverse effects from topical doxepin cream. Ann Pharmacother 35:505–506, 2001.

31. Jones MK, Wang H, Peskar BM, et al: Inhibition of angiogenesis by nonsteroidal anti-inflammatory drugs: Insight into mechanisms and implications for cancer growth and ulcer healing. Nat Med 5:1348–1349, 1999.

32. Kalso E, Tramer MR, Carroll D, et al: Pain relief form intra-articular morphine after knee surgery: A qualitative systematic review. Pain 71:127–134, 1997.

33. Keita H, Kayser V, Guibaud G: Antinociceptive effect of a kappa-opioid receptor agonist that minimally crosses the blood-brain barrier (ICI 204448) in a rat model of mononeuropathy. Eur J Pharmacol 277:275–280, 1995.

34. Kolesnikov YA, Pasternak GW: Peripheral orphanin FQ/nociceptin analgesia. Life Sci 64:2021–2028, 1999.

35. Koltzenberg M: The changing sensitivity in the life of the nociceptor. Pain 6 (suppl): S93–S102, 1999.

36. Kress M, Zeilhofer HU: Capsaicin, protons and heat: New excitement about nociceptors. Trends Pharm Sci 20:112–118, 1999.

37. Krummel T, Dimitrov Y, Moulin B, Hannedouche T: Acute renal failure induced by topical ketoprofen. BMJ 320:93, 2000.

38. Kumazawa T: Primitivism and plasticity of pain: Implications of polymodal receptors. Neurosci Res 32:9–31, 1998.

39. Lauretti GR, Lima IC, Reis MP, et al: Oral ketamine and transdermal nitroglycerin as analgesic adjuvants to oral morphine therapy for cancer pain management. Anesthesiology 90:1528–1533, 1999.

40. Lu KL, Wee WR, Sakamoto T, McDonnell PJ: Comparison of in vitro antiproliferative effects of steroids and nonsteroidal anti-inflammatory drugs on human keratocytes. Cornea 15:185–190, 1996.

41. McCleane G: Topical application of doxepin hydrochloride, capsaicin and a combination of both produces analgesia in chronic neuropathic pain: A randomized, double-blind, placebo-controlled study. Br J Clin Pharmacol 49:574–579, 2000.

42. McCleskey EW, Gold MS: Ion channels of nociception. Ann Rev Physiol 61:835–856, 1999.

43. McDaid DM, Deasy PB: An investigation into the transdermal delivery of nifedipine. Pharm Acta Helv 71:253–258, 1996.

44. McMahon SB: NGF as a mediator of inflammatory pain. Phil Trans R Soc Lond Series B Bio Sci 351: 431–440, 1996.

45. Meller ST, Lewis SJ, Brody MJ, Gebhart GF: The peripheral nociceptive actions of intravenously administered 5-HT in the rat requires dual activation of both 5-HT$_2$ and 5-HT$_3$ receptor subtypes. Brain Res 561:61–68, 1991.

46. Mendell LM, Albers KM, Davis BM: Neurotrophins, nociceptors and pain. Microsc Res Tech 45: 252–261, 1999.

47. Michael GJ, Priestley JV: Differential expression of the mRNA for the vanilloid receptor subtype 1 in cells of the adult rat dorsal root and nodose ganglia and its downregulation by axotomy. J Neurosci 19:1844–1854, 1999.

48. Millan MJ: The induction of pain: An integrative review. Prog Neurobiol 57:1–164, 1999.

49. Moore RA, Tramer MR, Carroll D, et al: Quantitative systematic review of topically applied nonsteroidal anti-inflammatory drugs. BMJ 316:333–338, 1998.

50. Mura P, Faucci MT, Bramanti G, Corti P: Evaluation of transcutols as a clonazepam transdermal permeation enhancer from hydrophilic gel formulations. Euro J Pharm Sci 9:365–372, 2000.

51. Ness TJ: Pharmacology of peripheral analgesia. Pain Practice 3:243–254, 2001.

52. Ness TJ: Kappa opioid receptor agonists differentially inhibit two classes of rat spinal neurons excited by colorectal distension. Gastroenterology 117:388–394, 1999.

53. Ness TJ, Jones L, Smith H: Use of compounded topical analgesics—results of an internet survey. Regional Anesth Pain Med 27:309–312, 2002.

54. Noyes Jr R, Brunk SF, Baram DA, Canter A: Analgesic effect of delta-9-tetrahydrocannabinol. J Clin Pharm 15:139–143, 1975.

55. Nozaki-Taguchi N, Yaksh TL: Characterization of the antihyperalgesic action of a novel peripheral mu-opioid receptor agonist—loperamide. Anesthesiology 90:225–234, 1999.

56. Picard PR, Tramer MR, McQuay HJ, Moore RA: Analgesic efficacy of peripheral opioids (all except intra-articular): A qualitative systematic review of randomized controlled trials. Pain 72: 309–318, 1997.

57. Piomelli D, Giuffrida A, Calignano A, Rodriguez de Fonseca F: The endo-cannabinoid system as a target for therapeutic drugs. Trends Pharm Sci 21:218–224, 2000.

58. Quartara L, Maggi CA: The tachykinin NK1 receptor: Part II. Distribution and pathophysiological roles. Neuropeptides 32:1–49, 1998.

59. Rademaker M, Oakley A, Duffill MB: Cutaneous adverse drug reactions in a hospital setting. N Z Med J 108:165–166, 1995.

60. Rang HP, Bevan S, Perkins MN: Peripherally acting analgesic agents. In: Sawyanok J, Cowan A (eds): Novel Aspects of Pain Management: Opioids and Beyond. New York: Wiley-Liss, 1999, pp 95–115.

61. Reichling DB, Levine JD: The primary afferent nociceptor as pattern generator. Pain 6 (suppl): S103–109, 1999.

62. Richardson JD, Kilo S, Hargreaves KM: Cannabinoids reduce hyperalgesia and inflammation via interactions with peripheral CB_1 receptors. Pain 75:111–119, 1998.

63. Robbins WR, Staats PS, Levine J, et al: Treatment of intractable pain with topical large-dose capsaicin: Preliminary report. Anesth Analg 86:579–583, 1998.

64. Saragas S, Arffa R, Rabin B, et al: Reversal of wound strength retardation by addition of insulin to corticosteroid therapy. Ann Ophthalmol 17:428–430, 1985.

65. Saragovi HU, Gehring K: Development of pharmacological agents for targeting neurotrophins and their receptors. Trends Pharm Sci 21:93–98, 2000.

66. Scott MA, Letrent KJ, Hager KL, Burch JL: Use of transdermal amitriptyline gel in a patient with chronic pain and depression. Pharmacotherapy 19:236–239, 1999.

67. Sharir M: Exacerbation of asthma by topical diclofenac. Arch Ophthalmol 115:294–295, 1997.

68. Snider WD, McMahon SB: Tackling pain at the source: New ideas about nociceptors. Neuron 20: 629–632, 1998.

69. Stein C, Yassouridis A: Peripheral morphine analgesia. Pain 71:119–121, 1997.

70. Suh DY, Hunt TK, Spencer EM: Insulin-like growth factor-I reverses the impairment of wound healing induced by corticosteroids in rats. Endocrinology 131:2399–2403, 1992.

71. Takasaki I, Andoh T, Nojima H, et al: Gabapentin antinociception in mice with acute herpetic pain induced by herpes simplex virus infection. J Pharmacol Exp Ther 296:270–275, 2001.

72. Tate S, Benn S, Hick C, et al: Two sodium channels contribute to the TTX-R sodium current in primary sensory neurons. Nat Neurosci 1:653–655, 1998.

73. Tverskoy M, Oren M, Vaskovich M, et al: Ketamine enhances local anesthetic and analgesic effects of bupivacaine by peripheral mechanisms: A study in postoperative patients. Neurosci Let 215: 5–8, 1996.

74. Twillman RK, Long TD, Cathers TA, Mueller DW: Treatment of painful skin ulcers with topical opioids. J Pain Symptom Manage 17:288–292, 1999.

75. Ushida T, Tani T, Kawasaki M, et al: Peripheral administration of an N-methyl-D-aspartate receptor antagonists (MK-801) changes dorsal horn neuronal responses in rats. Neurosci Lett 260: 89–92, 1999.

76. Vaile JH, Davis P: Topical NSAIDs for musculoskeletal conditions: A review of the literature. Drugs 56:783–799, 1998.

77. Walker JM, Hohmann AG, Martin WJ, et al: The neurobiology of cannabinoid analgesia. Life Sci 65:665–673, 1999.

78. Wilson JL, Nayanar V, Walker JS: The site of anti-arthritic action of the κ-opioid, U-50,488H, in adjuvant arthritis: importance of local administration. Br J Pharmacol 118:1754–1760, 1996.

79. Yablon SA, Sipski ML: Effect of transdermal clonidine on spinal spasticity: A case series. Am J Phys Med Rehabil 72:154–157, 1993.

80. Zell-Kanter M, Toerne TS, Spiegel K, Negrusz A: Doxepin toxicity in a child following topical administration. Ann Pharmacother 34:328–329, 2000.

81. Zhou L, Stein C, Schafer M: Contribution of opioid receptors on primary afferent versus sympathetic neurons to peripheral opioid analgesia. J Pharmacol Exp Ther 286:1000–1006, 1998.

Chapter 30

Peripheral Opioid Analgesia

Wiebke Janson, MD / Christoph Stein, MD

Opioids have long been thought to act exclusively within the central nervous system. In the 1990s, an increasing number of studies reported the existence of opioid receptors outside the central nervous system and suggested that opioids also are able to mediate their analgesic effects in the periphery.[67] Such analgesic effects are particularly prominent under painful inflammatory conditions in animals and in humans.[72] Subsequently, evidence has accumulated suggesting significant involvement of the immune system in the control of pain. During inflammatory processes, opioid receptors are progressively transported along the axon from dorsal root ganglia toward the peripheral sensory nerve endings. Here the increased number of opioid receptors (among other mechanisms) leads to improved analgesia of exogenously administered ligands (e.g., morphine). At the same time, immune cells containing endogenous opioid peptides accumulate within the inflamed tissue. Environmental stimuli (e.g., stress) and releasing agents (e.g., corticotropin-releasing factor, cytokines) can liberate these opioid peptides to interact with the neuronal opioid receptors and elicit local analgesia. Suppression of the immune system (e.g., by irradiation) or blockade of the selectin-dependent extravasation of opioid-containing immune cells and opioid receptor antagonists can abolish these effects. Based on these findings, a current concept proposes that during inflammatory processes, not only the peripheral analgesic effects of exogenous opioids improve, but also endogenous opioid peptides can be secreted from immunocytes, occupy peripheral opioid receptors on sensory nerve endings, and produce analgesia by inhibiting the excitability of these nerves or the release of proinflammatory neuropeptides.[67]

PERIPHERAL OPIOID RECEPTORS

Members of the opioid receptor family are classified as μ, δ, and κ receptors.[2] They belong to the family of seven transmembrane guanine (G-) nucleotide binding protein-coupled receptors and show extensive structural homologies. All three opioid receptors could be identified not only in the central nervous system, but also in peripheral sensory neurons. They have been found on cell bodies in dorsal root ganglia[20, 41] and on central[33] and peripheral terminals of primary afferent neurons in animals[10, 17, 70] and in humans.[71]

The pharmacologic characteristics of these receptors are similar to those in the brain, as shown by saturation and competition experiments.[17] The three opioid receptors identified so far were cloned in the early 1990s, starting with the mouse δ,[13, 28] followed by cloning of μ[7, 8, 14, 75] and κ.[35, 42, 44, 50] When they were cloned, not only the receptors themselves, but also their mRNA could be detected in dorsal root ganglia.[40] The existence of several subtypes of each receptor (μ1, μ2; δ1, δ2; κ1, κ2, κ3) was suggested on the basis of pharmacologic studies, but molecular attempts to identify those subtypes were unsuccessful.[30, 79] Cloning to date revealed only one single receptor of each type. The purported subtypes have been suggested to be splice variants or other posttranslational modifications. Additionally, various opioid receptors show unique functional properties after oligomerization.[22]

Apart from primary afferent neurons, opioid receptors on sympathetic postganglionic neurons were thought to contribute to peripheral opioid analgesia.[74] The evidence was questioned,[32] however, and to date, opioid receptor mRNA could not be found in sympathetic ganglia.[63] δ receptors could not be detected on sympathetic postganglionic neurons in skin, lip, or cornea,[81] and chemical sympathectomy changes neither the expression of opioid receptors in dorsal root ganglia[85] nor the peripheral antinociceptive effects of their ligands in inflammatory pain.[86] Taken together, these results indicate that postganglionic sympathetic neurons do not carry opioid receptors, but whether or not the sympathetic nervous system plays a role in opioid-mediated peripheral analgesia to date is not known.

Opioid binding sites and opioid receptor transcripts also are expressed by immune cells.[4, 17, 66] Stimulatory and inhibitory modulation of immune cell proliferation and function (e.g., chemotaxis, cytokine production, and mast cell degranulation) by opioids was reported.[53] The significance of these effects for the modulation of pain has not been investigated, however.

ANALGESIC EFFECTS OF EXOGENOUS PERIPHERAL OPIOID AGONISTS

The discovery of peripherally expressed opioid receptors changed the traditional view that opioid analgesia could be mediated exclusively within the brain and led to studies with locally applied exogenous opioid agonists. The first hints for a peripheral site of action came from animal studies. To exclude a systemic effect, substances that did not cross the blood-brain barrier[15, 61] or the local-versus-systemic way of application[69] were used. Because the peripherally evoked analgesia showed dose dependency, stereospecificity, and reversibility with antagonists such as naloxone, it was concluded that it is strictly opioid receptor specific. All three members of the opioid receptor family are present and mediate analgesia, depending on the particular circumstances.[69]

Animal studies using different models of inflammation showed that the analgesic effects of locally administered opioids are particularly prominent under inflammatory conditions. One explanation for this phenomenon is the inflammation-dependent up-regulation of opioid receptors in the periphery. Opioid receptors are synthesized in dorsal root ganglia,[39, 63] and after induction of peripheral inflammation, their axonal transport to the nerve endings is strongly enhanced.[17, 19] This enhancement leads to an increase in their number on peripheral nerve terminals. Another explanation is changes in the local milieu of the inflamed tissue (e.g., low pH) that lead to a possible increase in opioid agonist action. This hypothesis is based on the observation that low pH increases opioid agonist efficacy *in vitro* by altering the interaction of opioid receptors with G proteins in neuronal membranes.[9, 57, 65]

In inflamed tissue, opioid agonists also have easier access to their receptors because of disruption of the perineurium, which under normal conditions protects the nerve fiber and is impermeable.[1] The number of sensory nerve terminals and the number of opioid ligand binding sites increase under inflammatory conditions as a result of a phenomenon called *sprouting*.[80]

There are several possible explanations for the improved efficacy of peripherally administered opioids in inflammation. Whether one of them is a dominant factor or whether a combination of all of them is responsible still needs to be clarified.

CLINICAL APPLICATIONS

Many investigators tried to transfer findings from in vitro and animal studies to the clinical setting. Several studies tested local opioid effects in experimentally induced pain. Subcutaneously injected morphine (2 mg) increases heat-pain and pressure-pain thresholds in second-degree burn injury[45] and inhibits capsaicin-induced mechanical hypersensitivity.[29] A study in dental surgery patients revealed that inflammation is advantageous not only in animal models, but also in patients for good effectiveness of peripheral opioid analgesia.[36] Other routes of administration include perineural, intraabdominal, orbital, and topical wound infiltration with opioids.[62] Many studies used the model of postoperative pain after knee surgery, in which morphine was injected intraarticularly. Peripheral analgesia in this model was shown to be opioid receptor specific[68] and of similar potency as conventional analgesia using local anesthetics.[27] To ensure that these effects were strictly peripheral, equal doses of morphine administered intraarticularly and systemically were compared, but the latter was found to be ineffective.[68] Plasma levels of morphine after intraarticular injection were not high enough for central analgesic actions so that systemic effects were excluded.[23] Two systematic reviews revealed that intraarticular morphine has definite analgesic effects in the first 24 to 30 hours after knee arthroscopy.[16, 25] Most studies show encouraging results, and peripheral analgesia seems to be a promising concept for pain treatment in patients.

ANALGESIC EFFECTS OF ENDOGENOUS OPIOID PEPTIDES

After peripheral opioid receptors had been discovered, the question arose whether they play any physiologic role in the cascade answering noxious and painful stimuli. Because there seems to be a connection between infiltrating immune cells and the increased number of opioid receptors in the inflamed peripheral tissue, investigations now have focused on a possible link between the immune system and inflammatory pain.

Many studies undoubtedly show that potent peripheral opioid analgesia can result from the interaction between endogenous opioids derived from immune cells and peripherally expressed opioid receptors.[54, 56, 70, 72] The understanding of the biogenesis of various endogenous opioid peptides, their anatomic distribution, and the characteristics of the receptors with which they interact has progressed in recent decades. Three different precursor proteins from which the classic endogenous opioid peptides are derived were cloned from the late 1970s to the early 1980s:[24, 48, 51] proopiomelanocortin (POMC), prodynorphin (PDYN), and proenkephalin (PENK). These precursor proteins yield three major groups of opioid peptides: PENK is the source of enkephalins (ENK) and several longer peptides; PDYN codes for opioid peptides such as dynorphin A and B (DYN), α- and β-neoendorphin, and several larger proteins; and POMC is the precursor of α- and β-endorphin (END) and several nonopioid peptides, such as melanocyte-stimulating hormone and adrenocorticotropic hormone.

The opioid peptides are the natural ligands for μ (END, ENK), δ (ENK, END), and κ (DYN) opioid receptors. Neurons containing these opioid peptides have been found in brain regions that are involved in nociceptive responses (e.g., thalamus, periaqueductal gray, limbic system, cortex, and spinal cord). Members of all three groups also have been found in immune cells[72] and can be released during inflammation to control pain.[5, 6] In rat paw inflammation, the mRNAs for END and ENK and their transcripts are found within lymphocytes, monocytes, and macrophages. A study showed that different subpopulations of immune cells are responsible for the production of endogenous opioid peptides: In early inflammation, mostly granulocytes produce opioid peptides, whereas later on monocytes and possibly lymphocytes become their main source.[59] The degree of endogenous analgesia is proportional to the number of opioid peptide–producing cells.

Opioid-containing immune cells migrate into inflamed tissue. Environmental stimuli such as stress and releasing agents (e.g., corticotropin-releasing factor, cytokines) can liberate the opioid peptides from these immune cells and elicit local analgesia. Afterward, the depleted leukocytes travel to the regional lymph nodes.[5] The mechanisms underlying this inflammation-triggered immune cell migration are currently under investigation. Adhesion molecules play an important role in the migration process: Extravasation of immune cells involves the activation of a cascade of adhesion molecules, which initially cause the slowing down of circulating immune cells and their rolling on vascular endothelium, a process mediated by selectins on leukocytes (L-selectins) and on endothelial cells (P- and E-selectins). Chemokines then lead to an up-regulation of integrins, which cause a firm adhesion of the immune cells to the endothelial wall. Interruption of this cascade by fucoidin, a selectin blocker, was shown to inhibit immune cell migration into inflamed tissue. Additionally the amount of END-containing cells and of END content in inflamed tissue was decreased significantly, resulting in decreased analgesia.[38] Taken together, these findings indicate an important role of the immune system not only in fighting pathogens, but also in controlling pain in injured tissue.

A novel group of opioid-receptor ligands was discovered in the brain and named endomorphins;[83] this group consists of endomorphin-1 (Tyr-Pro-Trp-Phe-NH$_2$) and endomorphin-2 (Tyr-Pro-Phe-Phe-NH$_2$). Both endomorphins show a characteristic atypical structure and high selectivity for μ receptors.[84] They have a distinct anatomic distribution: Endomorphin-1 is found mainly in the brain, whereas endomorphin-2 can be detected in the spinal cord. Generally, they are localized in circuits involved in the processing of nociceptive information and are thought to play a role in modulating pain as endogenous ligands for presynaptic and postsynaptic spinal μ receptors. Endomorphins inhibit nociceptive transmission in the spinal cord through μ receptor activation.[77] Their exact role in analgesia still needs to be clarified, however.

Another peptide family that was discovered is the orphanin FQ/nociceptin system, comprising the peptides acting on opioid receptor–like (ORL) receptors.[43, 58] The ORL1 receptor is present in neurons distinct from those containing μ opioid receptors at various levels of the neuraxis.[46] In ORL1 receptor knock-out mice, thermal and visceral pain threshold was not altered,[49] the analgesic response to morphine was unchanged, and the development of tolerance was delayed, but the exact role of ORL in pain transmission to date remains unclear.

Taken together, the role of immune cell–derived classic opioid peptides END, ENK, and DYN in peripheral opioid analgesia seems to be established. The role of endomorphins and the nociceptin/ORL system is not yet understood and needs further investigation. Gaining insight into the mechanisms underlying endogenous analgesia would be of great interest for the development of new antinociceptive concepts.

CLINICAL IMPLICATIONS OF PERIPHERAL ENDOGENOUS OPIOID ANALGESIA

The analgesic effect of endogenous opioid peptides is difficult to measure in humans. A study in postoperative patients who underwent knee arthroscopy showed that pain increases after the blockade of the peripheral endogenous opioid system using the intraarticularly injected opioid antagonist naloxone.[69] The endogenous analgesic system also might be important in diseases accompanied by immunosuppression. In particular, the association of increased sensitivity to pain with advancing stages of disease has been shown for immunosuppressed states such as cancer or acquired immunodeficiency syndrome (AIDS).[34, 82] Polyneuropathic pain in patients suffering from AIDS was correlated inversely with reduction in CD4[+] lymphocytes.[18] In a rat model, a decrease in lymphocytes owing immunosuppression by cyclosporine produced complete inhibition of endogenous (stress-induced) peripheral opioid analgesia.[5, 64]

Even though these findings underline the existence of mechanisms producing peripheral endogenous analgesia in humans, clinical experience shows that this form of analgesia is rarely sufficient in patients. Exogenous administration of opioid ligands almost always is needed in moderate-to-severe pain. One potential clinical use of the endogenous opioid system would be improving its efficacy by selectively stimulating the immune system to increase peripheral endogenous analgesia. Further studies are needed to determine whether this approach is reasonable.

SIDE EFFECTS OF PERIPHERAL OPIOID ANALGESIA

An intriguing feature of peripheral analgesia is the lack of the well-known central side effects of systemically administered opioids (e.g., drowsiness, nausea, constipation, dependence, addiction, respiratory depression, and tolerance [loss of analgesic efficacy after repeated or continous application of opioid agonists]). These side effects can restrict the therapeutic use of opioids. It is an important issue whether tolerance also develops at peripheral opioid receptors. Initial hints in animal models without inflammation suggested that tolerance development is possible not only at central but also at peripheral opioid receptors.[31] Because the number, the affinity, and the coupling efficacy of opioid receptors significantly enhance during inflammatory conditions, however, conclusions concerning peripheral opioid analgesia in inflamed tissue cannot be drawn from such studies.

Studies in an inflammation model in mice now postulate a lack of tolerance for peripherally administered opioids,[76, 78] whereas centrally applied ligands led to tolerance development in these mice. For the peripherally selective μ agonist loperamide, lack of tolerance was reported after repeated local administration in a thermal inflammatory model.[52] In the same study, systemically administered morphine produced only partial cross-tolerance with loperamide. These results are underlined by a clinical study in which no cross-tolerance between local morphine-induced and endogenous opioid–induced analgesia could be detected.[71] So far, there seems to be some evidence for a lack of tolerance, but further studies are needed for a definite statement concerning tolerance development in peripheral opioid analgesia.

Another side effect of peripherally administered opioids is their welcome potential for antiinflammatory activity. Opioids are able to inhibit neurogenic inflammation by decreasing substance P release from peripheral terminals of primary afferent neurons, and opioid receptors on immune cells can modulate lymphocyte function and inhibit the synthesis or the release of cytokines.[37] In one study, locally administered endomorphin-1 reduced carrageenan-induced edema,[21] the vascular response to electrical stimulation, and substance P–induced vasodilation and plasma extravasation in the rat.[26] Two novel tetrapeptidic, peripherally selective κ agonists reduced paw volume and histological signs of inflammation in the rat.[3] These findings from animal studies were confirmed in a clinical setting: In patients with chronic arthritis, the number of inflammatory cells in the synovial fluid significantly decreased after intraarticular injection of morphine.[73] Nonopioid proinflammatory effects of morphine were reported.[55] Taken together, there seems to be good evidence that peripherally active μ and κ-agonists have antiinflammatory activity. This evidence underlines their potential therapeutic importance in inflammatory pain because they not only act as analgesics, but also as antiinflammatory drugs and might play an additional role in the suppression of inflammation.

FUTURE IMPLICATIONS

These findings provide new insight into pain associated with a compromised immune system, as in AIDS or in cancer. The inflammation-induced activation of opioid production and the release of exogenous opioids from immune cells may be a novel approach for the development of peripherally acting analgesics. Because the site of action of such drugs is limited strictly to the periphery, these analgesics at best should lack unwanted central side effects typically associated with opioids.

Clinical investigation now is focused on the development of new peripheral opioid agonists and on ways to stimulate the endogenous analgesic system to induce effective analgesia with reduced central side effects. The model of peripheral opioid analgesia seems to offer great opportunities for more specific, side effect–free pain control in patients. Besides using the known opioid agonists, there is potential to improve exogenous opioid analgesia by developing new ligands with a high peripheral opioid receptor affinity and restricted access to the central nervous system. Loperamide, a drug originally known as an antidiarrheal agent, was presented as such a peripherally active, antihyperalgesic μ agonist in a model of thermal injury.[52] Probably owing to loperamide's high affinity to lipids, it accumulates in membranes and is not absorbed systemically.[11] Loperamide shows high affinity and selectivity for the cloned μ receptor, and it is locally active in different inflammation models in rats.[11]

Another approach is based on the inclusion of hydrophilic and hydrophobic properties in molecules, which then preserve peripheral selectivity and high antinociceptive potency.[37] In such a drug, systemic (either oral or parenteral) application would be combined with restriction to a peripheral site of action. Asimadoline (EMD61753) is an example for this concept; it acts as a potent and selective κ agonist with restricted ability to cross the blood-brain barrier after systemic administration. Although asimadoline was well tolerated and absorbed rapidly into the blood in healthy volunteers, oral application of the drug was ineffective in patients with postoperative pain.[37] New peptidic κ ligands were identified by positional scanning of a tetrapeptide combinatorial library screened in opioid receptor radioligand assays.[12] These peptides all exhibit a high selectivity for κ receptors, and they are potent and selective peripheral ligands in vivo.[60] Two members of the second generation of these tetrapeptides (FE200665 and FE200666) were shown to be peripherally selective κ agonists with potent analgesic and antiinflammatory effects.[3]

These investigations show that conventional and novel opioid agonists exist for local administration in painful, inflamed tissue. Preliminary data of peptidic κ agonists suggest that they may be suitable for intravenous application, which offers new opportunities for their use in a clinical setting. Endogenous opioid analgesia theoretically can be stimulated, either by an increase in the number of opioid peptide–producing immunocytes or by an increase in the production or the release of opioid peptides from these cells. Because their site of action is limited strictly to the periphery, these analgesics should lack unwanted central side effects typically associated with opioids. Although this approach is tempting, further studies are needed to investigate whether peripheral endogenous analgesia can be increased without limiting side effects. A detailed understanding of the mechanisms underlying endogenous peripheral opioid analgesia is necessary.

REFERENCES

1. Antonijevic I, Mousa SA, Schäfer M, Stein C: Perineural defect and peripheral opioid analgesia in inflammation. J Neurosci 15:165–72, 1995.

2. Atcheson R, Lambert DG: Update on opioid receptors. Br J Anaesth 73:132–134, 1994.

3. Binder W, Machelska H, Mousa S, et al: Analgesic and anti-inflammatory effects of two novel kappa opioid peptides. Anesthesiology 94:1034–1044, 2001.

4. Bryant HU, Holaday JW: Opioids in immunologic processes. In: Herz A (ed): Opioids II. Berlin: Springer-Verlag, 1993, pp 551–570.

5. Cabot PJ, Carter L, Gaiddon C, et al: Immune-cell derived β-endorphin: Production, release and control of inflammatory pain in rats. J Clin Invest 100:142–148, 1997.

6. Cabot PJ, Carter L, Schäfer M, Stein C: Methionine-enkephalin- and dynorphin-A-release from immune cells and control of inflammatory pain. Pain 93:207–212, 2001.

7. Chen Y, Mestek A, Liu J, Yu L: Molecular cloning of a rat kappa opioid receptor reveals sequence similarities to the mu and delta opioid receptors. Biochem J 295:625–628, 1993.

8. Chen Y, Mestek A, Liu J, et al: Molecular cloning and functional expression of a mu-opioid receptor from rat brain. Mol Pharmacol 44:8–12, 1993.

9. Childers SR: Opiate-inhibited adenylate cyclase in rat brain membranes depleted of G_s-stimulated adenylate cyclase. J Neurochem 50:543–553, 1988.

10. Coggeshall RE, Zhou S, Carlton SM: Opiate receptors on peripheral sensory axons. Brain Res 764:126–132, 1997.

11. DeHaven-Hudkins DL, Burgos LC, Cassel JA, et al: Loperaminde (ADL 2–1294), an opioid antihyperalgesic agent with peripheral selectivity. J Pharmacol Exp Ther 289:494–502, 1999.

12. Dooley CT, Ny P, Bidlack JM, Houghten RA: Selective ligands for mu, delta, and kappa opioid receptors identified from a single mixture based tetrapeptide positional scanning combinatorial library. J Biol Chem 273:18848–18856, 1998.

13. Evans CJ, Keith DE, Morrison H, et al: Cloning of a delta opioid receptor by functional expression. Science 258:1882–1884, 1992.

14. Fukuda K, Kato S, Mori K, et al: Primary structures and expression from cDNAs of rat opioid receptor delta- and mu-subtypes. FEBS Lett 327:311–314, 1993.

15. Giardina G, Clarke GD, Grugni M, et al: Central and peripheral analgesic agents: Chemical strategies for limiting brain penetration in kappa-opioid belonging to different chemical classes. Farmaco 50:405–418, 1995.

16. Gupta A, Bodin L, Holmström B, Berggren L: A systemic review of the peripheral analgesic effects of intraarticular morphine. Anesth Analg 93:761–770, 2001.

17. Hassan AHS, Ableitner A, Stein C, Herz A: Inflammation of the rat paw enhances axonal transport of opioid receptors in the sciatic nerve and increases their density in the inflamed tissue. Neuroscience 55:185–195, 1993.

18. Hewitt DJ, McDonald M, Portenoy RK, et al: Pain syndromes and etiologies in ambulatory AIDS patients. Pain 70:117–123, 1997.

19. Jeanjean AP, Moussaoui SM, Maloteaux JM, Laduron PM: Interleukin-1β induces long-term increase of axonally transported opiate receptors and substance P. Neuroscience 68:151–157, 1995.

20. Ji RR, Zhang Q, Law PY, et al: Expression of μ-, δ-, and κ-opioid receptor-like immunoreactivities in rat dorsal root ganglia after carrageenan-induced inflammation. J Neurosci 15:8156–8166, 1995.

21. Jin S, Lei L, Wang Y, et al: Endomorphin-1 reduces carageenan-induced fos expression in the rat spinal dorsal horn. Neuropeptides 33:281–284, 1999.

22. Jordan BA, Devi LA: G-protein-coupled receptor heterodimerization modulates receptor function. Nature 399:697–700, 1999.

23. Joshi GP, McCarroll SM, Cooney CM, et al: Intra-articular morphine for pain relief after knee arthroscopy. J Bone Joint Surg Br 74:749–751, 1992.

24. Kakidani H, Furutani Y, Takahashi H, et al: Cloning and sequence analysis of the cDNA for porcine beta-neo-endorphin/dynorphin precursor. Nature 298:245–249, 1982.

25. Kalso E, Smith L, McQuay HJ, Moore AR: No pain, no gain: Clinical excellence and scientific rigour—lessons learned from IA morphine. Pain 98(3):269–275, 2002.

26. Khalil Z, Sonderson K, Modig M, Nyberg F: Modulation of peripheral inflammation by locally administered endomorphin-1. Inflamm Res 48:550–556, 1999.

27. Khoury GF, Chen ACN, Garland DE, Stein C: Intraarticular morphine, bupivacaine and morphine/bupivacaine for pain control after knee videoarthroscopy. Anesthesiology 77:263–266, 1992.

28. Kieffer BL, Befort K, Gaveriaux-Ruff C, Hirth CG: The delta-opioid receptor: Isolation of a cDNA by expression cloning and pharmacological characterization. Proc Natl Acad Sci U S A 89: 12048–12052, 1992.

29. Kinnman E, Nygards EB, Hanson P: Peripherally administered morphine attenuates capsaicin-induced mechanical hypersensitivity in humans. Anesth Analg 84:595–599, 1997.

30. Koch T, Schulz S, Schroder H, et al: Carboxyl-terminal splicing of the rat mu opioid receptor modulates agonist-mediated internalization and receptor resensitization. J Biol Chem 273:13652–13657, 1998.

31. Kolesnikov Y, Pasternak GW: Topical opioids in mice: Analgesia and reversal of tolerance by a topical N-methyl-D-aspartate antagonist. J Pharmacol Exp Ther 290:247–252, 1999.

32. Koltzenburg M, Kress M, Reeh PW: The nociceptor sensitization by bradikinin does not depend on sympathetic neurons. Neuroscience 46:465–473, 1992.

33. LaMotte C, Pert CB, Snyder SH: Opiate receptor binding in primate spinal cord: Distribution and changes after dorsal root section. Brain Res 112:407–412, 1976.

34. Lefkowitz M: Pain management for the AIDS patient. J Fla Med Assoc 31:701–704, 1996.

35. Li S, Zhu J, Chen C, et al: Molecular cloning and expression of a rat kappa opioid receptor. Biochem J 295:629–633, 1993.

36. Likar R, Koppert W, Blatnik H, et al: Efficacy of peripheral morphine analgesia in inflamed, non-inflamed and perineural tissue of dental surgery patients. J Pain Symptom Manage 21:330–337, 2001.

37. Machelska H, Binder W, Stein C: Opioid receptors in the periphery. In: Kalso E, McQuay H, Wiesenfeld-Hallin Z (eds): Opioid Sensitivity of Chronic Noncancer Pain. Seattle: IASP Press, 1999, pp 45–58.

38. Machelska H, Cabot PJ, Mousa SA, et al: Pain control in inflammation governed by selectins. Nat Med 4:1425–1428, 1998.

39. Maekawa K, Minami M, Yabuuchi K, et al: In situ hybridization study of mu- and kappa-opioid receptor mRNAs in the rat spinal cord and dorsal root ganglia. Neurosci Lett 168:97–100, 1994.

40. Mansour A, Fox CA, Burke S, et al: Mu, delta, and kappa opioid receptor mRNA expression in the rat CNS: An in situ hybridization study. J Comp Neurol 350:412–438, 1994.

41. Mansour A, Hoversten MT, Taylor LP, et al: The cloned mu, delta and kappa receptors and their endogenous ligands: Evidence for two opioid peptide recognition cores. Brain Res 700:89–98, 1995.

42. Meng F, Xie GX, Thompson RC, et al: Cloning and pharmacological characteristic of a rat kappa opioid receptor. Proc Natl Acad Sci U S A 90:9954–9958, 1993.

43. Meunier JC: Nociceptin/orphanin FQ and the opioid-receptor-like ORL1 receptor. Eur J Pharmacol 340:1–15, 1997.

44. Minami M, Toya T, Katao Y, et al: Cloning and expression of a cDNA for the rat kappa-opioid receptor. FEBS Lett 329:291–295, 1993.

45. Moiniche S, Dahl JB, Kehlet H: Peripheral antinociceptive effects of morphine after burn injury. Acta Anaesthesiol Scand 37:710–712, 1993.

46. Monteillet-Agius G, Fein J, Anton B, Evans CJ: ORL-1 and mu opioid receptor antisera label different fibers in areas involved in pain processing. J Comp Neurol 399:373–383, 1998.

48. Nakanishi S, Inoue A, Kita T, et al: Nucleotide sequence of cloned cDNA for bovine corticotropin-beta-lipotropin precursor. Nature 278:423–427, 1979.

49. Nishi M, Houtani T, Noda Y, et al: Unrestrained nociceptive response and disregulation of hearing ability in mice lacking the nociceptin/orphanin FQ receptor. EMBO J 16:1858–1864, 1997.

50. Nishi M, Takeshima H, Fukuda K, et al: cDNA cloning and pharmacological characterization of an opioid receptor with high affinities for kappa-subtype-selective ligands. FEBS Lett 330:77–80, 1993.

51. Noda M, Furutani Y, Takahashi H, et al: Cloning and sequence analysis of cDNA for bovine adrenal proenkephalin. Nature 295:202–206, 1982.

52. Nozacki-Taguchi N, Yaksh TL: Characterization of the antihyperalgesic action of a novel peripheral mu-opioid receptor agonist—loperamide. Anesthesiology 90:225–234, 1999.

53. Panerai AE, Sycerdote P: β-endorphin in the immune system: A role at last? Immunol Today 18:317–319, 1997.

54. Parsons C, Herz A: Peripheral opioid receptors mediating antinociception in inflammation: Evidence for activation by enkephalin-like opioid peptides after cold water swim stress. J Pharmacol Exp Ther 255:795–802, 1990.

55. Perrot S, Guilbaud G, Kayser V: Effects of intraplantar morphine on paw edema and pain-related behaviour in a rat model of repeated acute inflammation. Pain 83:249–257, 1999.

56. Przewlocki R, Hassan AHS, Lason W, et al: Gene expression and localization of opioid peptides in immune cells of inflamed tissue: Functional role in antinociception. Neuroscience 48:491–500, 1992.

57. Rasenick MM, Childers SR: Modification of G_s-stimulated adenylate cyclase in brain membranes by low pH pretreatment: Correlation with altered guanine nucleotide exchange. J Neurochem 53:219–225, 1989.

58. Reinscheid RK, Nothacker HP, Bourson A, et al: Orphanin FQ: A neuropeptide that activates an opioidlike G protein-coupled receptor. Science 270:792–794, 1995.

59. Rittner HL, Brack A, Machelska H, et al: Opioid peptide-expressing leucocytes: Identification, recruitment, and simultaneously increasing inhibition of inflammatory pain. Anesthesiology 95:500–508, 2001.

60. Riviere PJM, Vanderah TW, Porreca F, et al: Novel peripheral peptidic kappa agonists (abstr). Acta Neurobiol Exp 59:186, 1999.

61. Rogers H, Birch PJ, Harrison SM, et al: GR94839, a kappa-opioid agonist with limited access to the central nervous system, has antinociceptive activity. Br J Pharmacol 106:783–789, 1992.

62. Schäfer M: Peripheral opioid analgesia: from experimental to clinical studies. Curr Opin Anaesth 12:603–607, 1999.

63. Schäfer MKH, Bette M, Romeo H, et al: Localization of kappa-opioid receptor mRNA in neuronal subpopulations of rat sensory ganglia and spinal cord. Neurosci Lett 167:137–140, 1994.

64. Schäfer M, Carter L, Stein C: Interleukin 1 β and corticotropin-releasing factor inhibit pain by releasing opioids from immune cells in inflamed tissue. Proc Natl Acad Sci U S A 91:4219–4223, 1994.

65. Selley DE, Breivogel CS, Childers SR: Modification of G protein-coupled functions by low pH pretreatment of membranes form NG108–15 cells: Increase in opioid agonist efficacy by decreased inactivation of G proteins. Mol Pharmacol 44:731–741, 1993.

66. Sharp BM: Opioid receptor expression and intracellular signaling by cells involved in host defense and immunity. In: Machelska H, Stein C (eds): Immune Mechanisms in Pain and Analgesia. Georgetown: Landes Bioscience, 2002, pp 98–103.

67. Stein C: The control of pain in peripheral tissue by opioids. N Engl J Med 332:1685–1690, 1995.

68. Stein C, Comisel K, Haimerl E, et al: Analgesic effect of intraarticular morphine after arthroscopic knee surgery. N Engl J Med 325:1123–1126, 1991.

69. Stein C, Hassan AHS, Lehrberger K, et al: Local analgesic effect of endogenous opioid peptides. Lancet 342:321–324, 1993.

70. Stein C, Hassan AHS, Przewlocki R, et al: Opioids from immunocytes interact with receptors on sensory nerves to inhibit nociception in inflammation. Proc Natl Acad Sci U S A 87:5935–5939, 1990.

71. Stein C, Pflüger M, Yassouridis A, et al: No tolerance to peripheral morphine analgesia in presence of opioid expression in inflamed synovia. J Clin Invest 98:793–799, 1996.

72. Stein C, Schäfer M, Cabot PJ, et al: Peripheral opioid analgesia. Pain Rev 4:171–185, 1997.

73. Stein A, Yassouridis A, Szopko C, et al: Intraarticular morphine versus dexamethasone in chronic arthritis. Pain 83:525–532, 1999.

74. Taiwo YO, Levine JD: Kappa- and delta-opioids block sympathetically dependent hyperalgesia. J Neurosci 11:928–932, 1991.

75. Thompson RC, Mansour A, Akil H, Watson SJ: Cloning and pharmacological characterization of a rat mu opioid receptor. Neuron 11:903–913, 1993.

76. Tokuyama S, Inoue M, Fuchigami T, Ueda H: Lack of tolerance in peripheral opioid analgesia in mice. Life Sci 62:1677–1681, 1998.

77. Trafton JA, Abbadie C, Marek K, Basbaum AI: Postsynaptic signaling via the (mu)-opioid receptor: Responses of dorsal horn neurons to exogenous opioids and noxious stimulation. J Neurosci 20:8578–8584, 2000.

78. Ueda H, Inoue M: Peripheral morphine analgesia resistant to tolerance in chronic morphine-treated mice. Neurosci Lett 266:105–108, 1999.

79. Uhl GR, Sora I, Wang Z: The mu opiate receptor as a candidate gene for pain: Polymorphism, variations in expression, nociception, and opiate responses. Proc Natl Acad Sci U S A 96:7752–7755, 1999.

80. Weihe E, Nohr D, Millan MJ, et al: Peptide neuroanatomy of adjuvant-induced arthritic inflammation in rat. Agents Actions 25:255–259, 1988.

81. Wenk HN, Honda CN: Immunohistochemical localization of delta opioid receptors in peripheral tissue. J Comp Neurol 408:567–579, 1999.

82. Wyatt SH, Fishman EK: The acute abdomen in individuals with AIDS. Radiol Clin North Am 5:1023–1043, 1994.

83. Zadina JE, Hackler L, Lin-Jun G, Kastin AJ: A potent and selective endogenous agonist for the μ-opiate receptor. Nature 386:499–502, 1997.

84. Zadina JE, Martin-Schild S, Gerall AA, et al: Endomorphins: Novel endogenous mu-opiate receptor agonists in regions of high mu-opiate receptor density. Ann N Y Acad Sci 897:136–144, 1999.

85. Zhang X, Bao L, Arvidsson U, et al: Localization and regulation of the delta-opioid receptor in dorsal root ganglia and spinal cord of the rat and monkey: Evidence for association with the membrane of large-core vesicles. Neuroscience 82:1225–1242, 1998.

86. Zhou L, Zhang Q, Stein C, Schäfer M: Contribution of opioid receptors on primary afferent versus sympathetic neurons to peripheral opioid analgesia. J Pharmacol Exp Ther 286:1000–1006, 1998.

Chapter 31

Topical Analgesic Drugs

Gary McCleane, MD

Historically, the earliest uses of analgesic medication was by topical application. The appeal of applying a substance directly to the site of discomfort is obvious, even if we now know that the origin of that pain may be a location distant to there. Added to this natural appeal is the patient's perception that the topical route of administration is safer than the oral or parenteral route. Although in many cases it may be safer, this is not universally so.

Clearly, accurate dosing is difficult when cream or gel formulations are used, and therefore drugs with a wide margin between the amount needed for therapeutic effect and the amount that causes side effects are desirable. Patch preparations allow a more accurate application of a given dose, but then the vagaries of transdermal absorption and the influences of local blood flow and tissue permeability come into play. In the future, we are promised transdermal delivery substances that will carry the therapeutic agents in a consistent and reliable fashion to their site of action. In the meantime, we are left with a relatively small number of drugs that have a verified analgesic effect when used topically.

NONSTEROIDAL ANTIINFLAMMATORY DRUGS

Topical nonsteroidal antiinflammatory drugs (NSAIDs) are widely used. Much of this use is with over-the-counter preparations, and, despite significant medical scepticism, the quantitative systematic review of topically applied NSAIDs carried out by Moore and colleagues[1] has shown that topical NSAIDs are effective for both acute and chronic pain conditions and are associated with a numbers needed to treat (NNT) of between 3 and 5. This compares favorably with oral analgesics. In their review, they examined the results of 86 trials involving 10,160 subjects. Systemic side effects were rare (less than 0.5% of subjects).

Topical NSAIDs have a lower incidence of gastrointestinal adverse effects than orally administered NSAIDs,[2] probably because plasma concentrations are lower than when given orally.[3] Despite this, deep tissue concentrations are still sufficiently high after topical administration to inhibit the inflammatory enzymes.[4] With so many preparations available in topical and oral formulations, the risk of polypharmacy and consequent side effects is substantial.

GLYCERYL TRINITRATE

For many years, nitrates have been used in the treatment of ischemic heart disease because their smooth muscle relaxant effects induce coronary vasodilatation. This action is caused by release of nitric oxide,[5] which activates guanylate cyclase,[6] leading to an increase in cyclic guanylate monophosphate (cGMP)[7] and hence muscle relaxation. More recently, topical application of glyceryl trinitrate has been used to treat anal fissures.[8–12] In this scenario, it has been postulated that the nitrate causes pain relief by relaxing the smooth muscle anal sphincter.

It seems that topical application of nitrates cause analgesia as well. Ferreira and colleagues[14] demonstrated a blockade of hyperalgesia and neurogenic inflammation with topical glyceryl trinitrate (GTN), and Berrazeuta and colleagues reported a range of trials in which GTN was shown to have an analgesic effect in patients with infusion-related thrombophlebitis,[15] varicose vein sclerosis–induced thrombophlebitis,[16] and supraspinatus tendinitis.[17] Whether this pain relief is caused by an analgesic effect, again mediated by nitric oxide, or by skeletal muscle relaxation (which is also relaxed when cGMP levels are raised[18]) is a matter of speculation. In view of this evidence, one wonders whether the beneficial effect seen when topical GTN is used in patients with anal fissure is due solely to relaxation of the sphincter or whether it is a combined analgesic and relaxant effect.

The attraction of GTN is the potential for achieving analgesia in the absence of risk of gastric irritation or bleeding, renal upset, or platelet dysfunction, all of which are associated with the NSAIDs. With its vasodilatory effects, it is interesting to speculate what effect topical GTN could have on wound healing when used in postoperative patients. However, this same vasodilation can cause "nitrate headache," even if a relatively small quantity is applied peripherally. Furthermore, headache is naturally more frequent if the GTN is applied to more than one site, and consequently its value lies in treating those patients with isolated areas of pain, such as the arthritic joint or isolated painful bone secondary tumor deposit. Tachyphylaxis is also a potential consequence of GTN use. In one study of 200 subjects with musculoskeletal pain, placebo and 2.5% piroxicam had no analgesic effect. GTN produced analgesia that was maximal in the first 3 weeks after commencement of treatment; by week 4, however, pain scores had returned to pretreatment levels.[19]

The analgesia produced by GTN can be augmented by using this agent with other analgesics. In the study just mentioned, when piroxicam 2.5% was used in conjunction with GTN, the analgesia persisted longer, whereas in a study by Lauretti and colleagues[20] in postoperative subjects, it was concluded that although topical GTN had relatively little effect when used alone, it did significantly prolong the analgesic effect of intrathecal sufentanil.

From a clinical perspective, GTN can be obtained in an ointment or patch formulation. With the ever-present risk if nitrate headache, the patch version allows a more measured and consistent use and is less messy for the patient.

CAPSAICIN

More than 150 years ago, a report appeared in the medical literature of alleviation of the pain of chilblains and toothache with capsicum.[21] It is now known that capsaicin, one of the active constituents of capsicum, has a neurotoxic effect when used in high topical concentrations but when used at lower concentrations causes a reversible depletion of substance P from sensory nerves[22,23] and consequent pain relief. This analgesic effect has been demonstrated in the treatment of a wide variety of painful conditions, including osteoarthritis,[24–27] painful diabetic neuropathy,[28–31] post-herpetic neuralgia,[32–34] pain associated with Guillain-Barré syndrome,[35] distal painful polyneuropathy,[36] and surgery-related neuropathic pain.[37]

Naturally, with its chili pepper origins, capsaicin produces a burning, tingling sensation after application, which usually lessens in severity with repeated use. The exacerbation associated with initial application can discourage further use, however, particularly in the subject with allodynia and burning pain as part of their complaint. Furthermore, accidental application close to any moist area, such as the eye, can cause marked discomfort. It has now been shown that the addition of GTN to capsaicin can reduce the discomfort associated with application.[38] The thermal allodynia associated with application of capsaicin is also reduced markedly by GTN.[39]

The potential analgesic effect of GTN has been described. This effect was further supported in a study of 200 subjects with painful arthritic joints. Subjects were randomized to receive placebo, 1.33% GTN, 0.025% capsaicin, and a combination containing 1.33% GTN and 0.025% capsaicin in equal numbers. Baseline (pretreatment) pain scores were recorded, as were pain scores for the entire 4-week treatment period. Placebo had no effect, both GTN and capsaicin alone reduced pain scores, and the combination of GTN and capsaicin seem to have an additive effect in terms of pain reduction. As would also be expected, the tolerability of the capsaicin was enhanced by the addition of GTN.[40] It therefore seems that the addition of a nitrate such as GTN to capsaicin can both enhance its analgesic effect and improve its tolerability. A major drawback is nitrate headache, which prevents the combination from being used in multiple sites. It is intriguing to speculate about the potential effects of other nitrates and whether their use may be associated with fewer headaches than GTN.

When using capsaicin, it may take several weeks before any effect is apparent. Apart from burning or tingling at the site of application side effects are infrequent. Sneezing may occur occasionally and is thought to be caused by small particles of capsaicin that have dried on the skin being inhaled nasally and causing irritation.

TOPICAL LOCAL ANESTHETICS

In recent years, topical application of local anesthetics has gained popularity. An extensively used combination of local anesthetics is a mixture of lidocaine and prilocaine (eutectic mixture of local anaesthetics called EMLA) for incidental pain, such as with venous cannula insertion,[41] and certain postoperative pains, such as pain after circumcision.[42] Some concern exists about the long-term use of such mixtures, with the potential risk of methemoglobinemia associated with the prilocaine component of the mixture. When used excessively, systemic toxicity can occur,[43] although when used more cautiously, toxic systemic levels of the local anesthetics can be avoided.[44]

An alternative to EMLA is topical amethocaine. For the reduction of pain associated with venepuncture, amethocaine is effective[45,46] and may even be superior to EMLA.[47] With cream or gel application, measurement of the dose applied is difficult and inconsistent. Occlusive dressings may be needed to prevent the agent's being wiped off. Lidocaine is now available in a patch preparation (Lidoderm, 5% lidocaine), and with this method of application consistent dosing is achieved. Lidocaine is known to have a systemic mode of action, but given the knowledge that only 5% of the lidocaine is released from the patch, it is likely that its action is that of a local sodium channel blockade. Lidoderm has a verified action in reducing the allodynia and pain associated with post-herpetic neuralgia[48,49] and may be effective in treating other neuropathic pain states.[50,51]

TRICYCLIC ANTIDEPRESSANTS

It is universally accepted that oral tricyclic antidepressants (TCAs) have an analgesic effect in patients with neuropathic pain.[52,53] Amitriptyline,[54–56] imipramine,[57,58] desipramine,[59,60] and clomipramine[61,62] all possess this property, which is not directly related to their antidepressant effect.[63] A variety of explanations are given as to how analgesia is achieved, including a noradrenergic effect,[64] blockade of nicotinic receptors,[65] and sodium channel blockade,[66–68] but it is conventionally accepted that the predominant action is central rather than peripheral.

Doxepin, a TCA, has become available in a topical formulation with an indication for the treatment of itch associated with eczema. Given the prevailing wisdom that TCAs have a central mode of action, it would not be expected that topical application in subjects with neuropathic pain be associated with analgesia. In an initial study of 40 subjects with neuropathic pain randomized in equal numbers to receive either topical placebo or doxepin over a 4-week period, McCleane found that while placebo had no effect on pain scores, topical doxepin reduced pain scores on a 0 to 10 linear visual analog scale by 1.18 ($P < .01$).[69] With the small numbers of subjects in this study and with a lack of supportive data from animal pain models, the results of this study, could be treated with cynicism. However, subsequent to the publication of this study, it has become more apparent from animal experiments that TCAs can have a peripheral mode of action[70–72] and that an adenosine blocking effect of TCAs may, at least in part, be responsible.[73]

In a further human study, McCleane studied 200 subjects with neuropathic pain. They were randomized in equal numbers into four treatment groups: placebo, doxepin, capsaicin, and a combination of doxepin and capsaicin. All agents were applied topically for 4 weeks, and subjects' pain scores on the linear visual analog scale were recorded in the 2 weeks prior to commencement of therapy and for the entire 4-week treatment period (FIGURE 1).

After 4 weeks, the extent of analgesia produced by the three active preparations was equal, although the combination of doxepin and capsaicin produced this analgesia in a more rapid fashion. When subjects were asked about their desire to continue using the preparation they had been using, 2.4% elected to continue with placebo, 25% with the combination, 39%

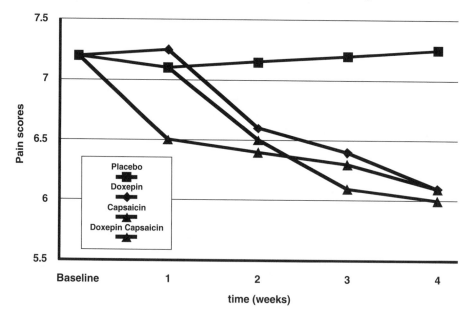

Overall pain as measured by a 0 to 10 visual analogue scale

Placebo
Doxepin
Capsaicin
Doxepin Capsaicin

FIGURE 1. Overall pain as measured by a 0 to 10 visual analog scale.

with capsaicin, and 41% with doxepin alone. The preference for doxepin alone may have been due to the low incidence of side effects associated with its use. Burning discomfort with cream application was reported in 81% of subjects using capsaicin and in only 17% of the doxepin group. Just under 10% of subjects experienced drowsiness with doxepin.

Whereas the analgesia produced by capsaicin and doxepin was equal, doxepin had no effect on the other cardinal symptoms of neuropathic pain; in contrast, capsaicin significantly reduced allodynia and shooting or lancinating pain, whereas capsaicin increased burning pain (probably a reflection of this accepted side effect of capsaicin application rather than an intrinsic effect on the subjects' neuropathic pain).[74]

It therefore seems that TCAs have an analgesic effect on neuropathic pain. Clearly, the use of such a topical preparation would be inappropriate if the area over which the neuropathic pain was felt was large, because application of large volumes of cream could lead to significant systemic absorption and side effects. In the case of smaller areas of pain, the use of topical TCA may achieve analgesia with a lesser risk of side effects than oral administration of the same agent. It seems that the time to analgesic effect may be 2 to 3 weeks, and subjects must therefore be encouraged to persist with application for up to 1 month before they make a judgment as to the efficacy of the preparation.

TOPICAL OPIOIDS

Fentanyl and buprenorphine are now available in transdermal formulations. Patches that deliver 25, 50, and 75 μg per hour of fentanyl and 35, 52.5 and 70 μg per hour of buprenorphine over a 3-day period allow the patient to avoid repetitive oral dosing. The psychological benefit of applying the pain reliever near the primary source of pain offers some advantage, although the effect is a systemic rather than local one.

CONCLUSION

Topical application offers some distinct advantages over oral dosing. Among these are patient preference and a very real therapeutic effect from transdermally delivered drugs. Patients often perceive topical preparations to be safer than their oral equivalents, although in many cases significant systemic concentrations of the drug in question are achieved by topical application and consequently systemic side effects are possible. With some of the available topical preparations, significant evidence exists as to their analgesic effect. With others, such as the TCAs, the available evidence is suggestive of an analgesic effect but requires much further verification. If the initial results are an accurate reflection of the effect of TCAs when applied topically, a significant step forward in our ability to treat neuropathic pain could be achieved.

REFERENCES FOR ADDITIONAL READING

1. Moore RA, Tramer MR, Carroll D, et al: Quantitative systematic review of topically applied non steroidal anti inflammatory drugs. BMJ 1998;316:333–338.
2. Evans JM, McMahon A, McGilchrist M, et al: Topical non steroidal anti inflammatory drugs and admission to hospital for gastrointestinal bleeding and perforation: A record linkage case control study. BMJ 1995;311:22–26.
3. Berner G, Engels B, Vogtle-Junkert U: Percutaneous ibuprofen therapy with Trauma Dolgit gel: Bioequivalence studies. Drugs Exp Clin Res 1989;15:559–564.

4. Treffel P, Gabard B: Feasibility of measuring the bioavailability of topical ibuprofen in commercial formulations using drug content in epidermis and a methyl nicotinate skin inflammation assay. Skin Pharmacol 1993;6:268–275.

5. Feelisch M, Noack EA: Correlation between nitric oxide formation during degradation of organic nitrates and activation of guanylate cyclase. Eur J Pharmacol 1987;139:19–30.

6. Bohme E, Graf H, Schultz G: Effects of sodium nitroprusside and other smooth muscle relaxants on cyclic GMP formation in smooth muscle and platelets. Adv Cycl Nucl Res 1978;9:131.

7. Rapoport RM, Murad F: Endothelium dependent and vaso dilator induced relaxation of smooth muscle: Role of cyclic GMP. J Cycl Nucl Prot Phos Res 1983;9:281.

8. Banerjee AK: Treating anal fissure. BMJ 1997;314:1638–1639.

9. Lund JN, Scholefield JH: A randomised, prospective, double blind, placebo controlled trial of glyceryl trinitrate ointment in treatment of anal fissure. Lancet 1997;349:11–14.

10. Bacher H, Mischinger H-J, Werkgartner G, et al: Local nitroglycerin for treatment of anal fissure: An alternative to lateral sphincterotomy? Dis Colon Rectum 1997;40:840–845.

11. Lund JN, Armitage NC, Scholefield JH: Use of glyceryl trinitrate ointment in the treatment of anal fissure. Br J Surg 1996;83:776–777.

12. Lund JN, Scholefield JH: Glyceryl trinitrate is an effective treatment for anal fissure. Dis Colon Rectum 1997;40:468–470.

13. Loder PB, Kamm MA, Nicholls RJ, Phillips RK: Reversible chemical sphincterotomy by local application of glyceryl trinitrate. Br J Surg 1994;81:1386–1389.

14. Ferreira SH, Lorenzetti BB, Faccioloi LH: Blockade of hyperalgesia and neurogenic oedema by topical application of nitroglycerin. Eur J Pharmacol 1992;217:207–209.

15. Berrazeuta JR, Poveda JJ, Ochoteco J, et al: The anti inflammatory and analgesic action of transdermal glyceryltrinitrate in the treatment of infusion related thrombophlebitis. Postgrad Med J 1993;69:37–40.

16. Berrazueta JR, Fleitas M, Salas E, et al: Local transdermal glyceryl trinitrate has an anti inflammatory action on thrombophlebitis induced by sclerosis of leg varicose veins. Angiology 1994;45:347–351.

17. Berrazueta JR, Losada A, Poveda J, et al: Successful treatment of shoulder pain syndrome due to supraspinatus tendinitis with transdermal nitroglycerin: A double blind study. Pain 1996;66:63–67.

18. Kobzik L, Reid MB, Bredt DS, Stamler JS: Nitric oxide in skeletal muscle. Nature 1994;372:546–548.

19. McCleane GJ: The addition of piroxicam to topically applied glyceryl trinitrate enhances its analgesic effect in musculoskeletal pain: A randomised, double blind, placebo controlled study. Pain Clin 2000;12:113–116.

20. Lauretti GR, Oliveira R, Reis MP, et al: Transdermal nitroglycerine enhances spinal sufentanil postoperative analgesia following orthopaedic surgery. Anesthesiology 1999;90:734–739.

21. Turnbull A: Tincture of capsicum as a remedy for chilblains and toothache. Dublin Med Press 1850; 95:6.

22. Fitzgerald M: Capsaicin and sensory neurones. Pain 1983;15:109–130.

23. Rains C, Bryson HM: Topical capsaicin: A review of its pharmacological properties and therapeutic potential in post herpetic neuralgia, diabetic neuropathy and osteoarthritis. Drugs Aging 1995;7:317–328.

24. Schnitzer T, Morton C, Coker S: Topical capsaicin therapy for osteo arthritic pain: Achieving a maintenance regime. Semin Arthritis Rheum 1994;6:34–40.

25. McCarthy GM, McCarty DJ: Effect of topical capsaicin in the therapy of painful osteoarthritis of the hands. J Rheumatol 1992;19:604–607.

26. Deal CL, Schnitzer TJ, Lipstein E, et al: Treatment of arthritis with topical capsaicin: A double blind trial. Clin Ther 1991;13:383–395.

27. Altman RD, Aven A, Holmberg CE, et al: Capsaicin cream 0.025% as monotherapy for osteoarthritis: A double blind study. Semin Arthritis Rheum 1994;6:25–33.

28. Capsaicin Study Group: Effect of treatment with capsaicin on daily activities of patients with painful diabetic neuropathy. Diabetes Care 1992;15:159–65.

29. Chad DA, Aronin N, Lundstrom R, et al: Does capsaicin relieve the pain of diabetic neuropathy? Pain 1990;42:387–388.

30. The Capsaicin Study Group: Treatment of painful diabetic neuropathy with topical capsaicin. Arch Intern Med 1991;151:2225–2229.

31. Tandan R, Lewis GA, Krusinski PB, et al: Topical capsaicin in painful diabetic neuropathy. Diabetes Care 1992;15:8–13.

32. Bernstein JE, Korman NJ, Bickers DR, et al: Topical capsaicin treatment of chronic postherpetic neuralgia. J Am Acad Dermatol 1989;21:265–270.

33. Watson CPN, Tyler KL, Bickers DR, et al: A randomized vehicle controlled trial of topical capsaicin in the treatment of postherpetic neuralgia. Clin Therapeutics 1993;15:510–526.

34. Watson CPN, Evans RJ, Watt VR: Post herpetic neuralgia and topical capsaicin. Pain 1988;33:333–340.

35. Morgenlander JC, Hurwitz BJ, Massey EW: Capsaicin for the treatment of pain in Guillan-Barre syndrome. Ann Neurol 1990;28:199.

36. Low PA, Opfer-Gehrking TL, Dyck PJ, et al: Double blind, placebo controlled study of the application of capsaicin cream in chronic distal painful polyneuropathy. Pain 1995;450:163–168.

37. Ellison N, Loprinzi CL, Kugler J, et al: Phase III placebo controlled trial of capsaicin cream in the management of surgical neuropathic pain in cancer patients. J Clin Oncol 1997;15:2974–2980.

38. McCleane GJ, McLaughlin M: The addition of GTN to capsaicin cream reduces the discomfort associated with application of capsaicin alone: A volunteer study. Pain 1998;78:149–151.

39. Walker RA, McCleane GJ: The addition of glyceryltrinitrate to capsaicin cream reduces the thermal allodynia associated with the use of capsaicin alone in humans. Neurosci Lett 2002;323;78–80.

40. McCleane GJ: The analgesic efficacy of topical capsaicin is enhanced by glyceryltrinitrate in painful osteoarthritis: A randomized, double blind, placebo controlled study. Eur J Pain 2000;4:355–360.

41. Paut O, Calmejane C, Delorme J, et al: EMLA versus nitrous oxide for venous cannulation in children. Anesth Analg 2001;93:590–593.

42. Ng WT, Ng TK, Tse S, et al: The use of topical lidocaine/prilocaine cream prior to childhood circumcision under local anesthesia. Ambul Surg 2001;9:9–12.

43. Touma S, Jackson JB: Lidocaine and prilocaine toxicity in a patient receiving treatment for mollusca contagiosa. J Am Acad Dermat 2001;44:399–400.

44. Stymne B, Lillieborg S: Plasma concentrations of lignocaine and prilocaine after a 24 h application of analgesic cream (EMLA) to leg ulcers. Br J Dermatol 2001;145:530–534.

45. Arrowsmith J, Campbell C: A comparison of local anaesthetics for venepuncture. Arch Dis Child 2000; 82:309–310.

46. Jain A, Rutter N: Does topical amethocaine gel reduce the pain of venepuncture in new infants? A randomised double blind controlled trial. Arch Dis Child 2000;83:F207.

47. Browne J, Awad I, Plant R, et al: Topical amethocaine (Ametop) is superior to EMLA for intravenous cannulation. Can J Anaesth 1999;46:1014–1018.

48. Galer BS, Rowbotham MC, Perander J, Friedman E: Topical lidocaine patch relieves postherpetic neuralgia more effectively than a vehicle topical patch: Results of an enriched enrollment study. Pain 1999;80:533–538.

49. Comer AM, Lamb HM: Lidocaine patch 5%. Drugs 2000;59:245–249.

50. Dever A, Galer BS: Topical lidocaine patch relieves a variety of neuropathic pain conditions: An open label study. Clin J Pain 2000;16:205–208.

51. Argoff CE: New analgesics for neuropathic pain: The lidocaine patch. Clin J Pain 2000;16:S62–66.

52. McQuay HJ, Moore RA: Antidepressants and chronic pain. BMJ 1997;314:763–764.

53. Watson CPN: The treatment of neuropathic pain: Antidepressants and opioids. Clin J Pain 2000;16: S49–55.

54. Watson CPN, Chipman M, Reed K, et al: Amitriptyline versus naprotiline in postherpetic neuralgia: A randomized, double-blind, crossover trial. Pain 1992;48:29–36.

55. Watson CPN, Evans RJ: A comparative trial of amitriptyline and zimelidine in post-herpetic neuralgia. Pain 1985;23:387–394.

56. Max MB, Schafer SC, Culnane M, et al: Amitriptyline, but not lorazepam, relieves postherpetic neuralgia. Neurology 1988;38:1427–1432.

57. Poulsen L, Arendt-Nielsen L, Brosen K, et al: The hypoalgesic effect of imipramine in different human experimental pain models. Pain 1995;60:287–293.

58. Sindrup SH, Ejlertsen B, Froland A, et al: Imipramine treatment in diabetic neuropathy: Relief of subjective symptoms without changes in peripheral and autonomic function. Eur J Clin Pharmacol 1989;37:151–153.

59. Max MB, Lynch AS, Moiré J, et al: Effects of desipramine, amitriptyline, and fluoxetine on pain in diabetic neuropathy. N Engl J Med 1992;326:1250–1256.

60. Max MB, Kishore-Kumar R, Schafer SC, et al: Efficacy of desipramine in painful diabetic neuropathy: A placebo-controlled trial. Pain 1991;45:3–9.

61. Langohr HD, Stohr M, Petruch F: An open and double-blind crossover study on the efficacy of clomipramine (Anafranil) in patients with painful mono- and polyneuropathies. Eur Neurol 1982; 21:309–17.

62. Sindrup SH, Gram LF, Skjold T, et al: Clomipramine vs desipramine vs placebo in the treatment of diabetic neuropathy symptoms: A double blind cross-over study. Br J Clin Pharmacol 1990;30: 683–691.

63. Max MB, Culnane M, Schafer SC, et al: Amitryptyline relieves diabetic neuropathy pain in patients with normal or depressed mood. Neurology 1987;37:589–596.

64. Ansuategui M, Naharro L, Feria M: Noradrenergic and opioidergic influences on the antinociceptive effect of clomipramine in the formalin test in rats. Psychopharmacology 1989;98:93–96.

65. Park T-J, Shin S-Y, Suh B-C, et al: Differential inhibition of catecholamine secretion by amitriptyline through blockage of nicotinic receptors, sodium channels, and calcium channels in bovine adrenal chromaffin cells. Synapse 1998;29:248–256.

66. Pancrazio JJ, Kamatchi GL, Roscoe AK, Lynch C: Inhibition of neuronal Na^+ channels by antidepressant drugs. J Pharmacol Exp Ther 1998;284:208–214.

67. Habuchi Y, Furukawa T, Tanaka H, et al: Block of Na^+ channels by imipramine in guinea pig cardiac ventricular cells. J Pharmacol Exp Ther 1991;258:1072–1067.

68. Bou-Abboud E, Nattel S: Molecular mechanisms of the reversal of imipramine induced sodium channel blockade by alkalinization in human cardiac myocytes. Cardiovasc Res 1998;38:395–404.

69. McCleane G: Topical doxepin hydrochloride reduces neuropathic pain: A randomized, double blind, placebo controlled study. Pain Clin 2000;12:47–50.

70. Heughan CE, Allen GV, Chase TD, Sawynok J: Peripheral amitriptyline suppresses formalin-induced fos expression in the rat spinal cord. Anesth Analg 2002;94:427–31.

71. Sawynok J, Esser MJ, Reid AR: Peripheral antinociceptive actions of desimipramine and fluoxetine in an inflammatory and neuropathic pain test in the rat. Pain 1999;82:149–158.

72. Su X, Gebhart GF: Effects of tricyclic antidepressants on mechanosensitive pelvic nerve afferent fibres innervating the rat colon. Pain 1998;76:105–114.

73. Sawynok J, Reid AR, Esser MJ: Peripheral antinociceptive action of amitriptyline in the rat formalin test: Involvement of adenosine. Pain 1999;80:45–55.

76. McCleane GJ: Topical application of doxepin hydrochloride, capsaicin and a combination of both produces analgesia in chronic human neuropathic pain: A randomized, double blind, placebo controlled study. Br J Clin Pharmacol 2000;49:574–579.

Chapter 32

Proinflammatory Cytokines in Pain Perception: Implications for Treatment

John P.R. Loughrey, MB, BCh, MRCPI, FCARCSI / Howard S. Smith, MD

Immunity is the state of protection from injury and infectious disease. The immune response is composed of a specific adaptive response (antibodies) and a nonspecific innate response. This innate component, in addition to anatomical barriers, includes phagocytosis and an inflammatory response, which requires migration of cells and infiltration to a site of injury.

Evidence exists for persistent central and peripheral pain states coexisting with exaggerated or prolonged neuroimmune activation.[1] The immune response to neurotropic viruses such as herpes zoster and injury to the spinal cord may be beneficial. If unchecked, however, these responses may contribute to and help maintain chronic pain states. Suppression of the immune responses observed in patients with clinical pain disorders forms the therapeutic rationale behind depot steroid injections and the use of systemic anti-inflammatory medications.

The current rapid evolution of knowledge about the role of cellular and humoral immune responses to noxious stimuli will undoubtedly result in new research and treatment strategies in pain management[2,3] and will also provide a further basis for established practices.

INFLAMMATORY RESPONSE TO PAIN

Glial Cells

Glial cells, which include microglia, astrocytes, and oligodendrocytes, are closely involved in the neuroimmune response that is observed following peripheral or central injury. These cells account for roughly 70% of all brain and spinal cord cells. They perform similar functions to macrophages, and interruption of normal glial function can occur in patients with chronic disease, resulting in cellular dysfunction and death. The initiating signal for microglial induction is poorly understood, but acid-base changes in the environment following neuronal injury appear to play a role.[4] The proposed analgesic effects of inhibitors of glial function have been demonstrated in animal models.[5]

Glial cells, which outnumber neurons, have now been recognized as having important roles in neural function and synaptic transmission. Glia may function to regulate the neural ionic current flux; affect local neural blood flow; contribute to neural metabolic needs; and affect neuronal function and activity by a variety of means.[6] Glia express multiple ion channels and neurotransmitter receptors as well as release neuromodulators such as neurotransmitters (adenosine triphosphate [ATP], glutamate), growth factors (nerve growth factor), and cytokines.[6] It has become apparent that glia may affect neurons and neurons may affect glia; clearly, the entire system of glial-glial interactions, glial-neuronal interactions, and neuronal-neuronal interactions needs to be viewed globally.[6] Glial cells appear to "communicate" with neurons, primarily via intercellular calcium signalling (calcium wave propagation/oscillations) and also play vital roles mediating glutamate clearance (via glial glutamate transporters coupled to Na^+-dependent systems).[6] There appears to be considerable cross-talk between glia cells and neuronal cells.[7]

Glial cells include macroglia (oligodendrocytes and astrocytes) and microglia (cells that seem to be similar to immune cells). The intercellular channels that make up the gap junctions between macroglia contain connexins.[8] Connexins may represent a key target neuroglial communications. Neuronal communication that is synaptic and glial communication via intercellular calcium waves are tightly linked.[8] Also, glial cells seem to function as excitable and appear to serve as active partners in synaptic functions.[6] There exist multiple ion channels in glia (e.g., K+, Cl⁻, Ca^{2+} [L&T], Na^+) as well as numerous receptors for neurotransmitters (e.g., ionotropic, or non-N-methyl-D-aspartate [NMDA], and metabotropic glutamate receptors, as well as calcitonin gene-related protein and substance P receptors).

Glia produce and release neuroactive mediators that may protect (e.g., antioxidants) or insult (e.g., nitric oxide synthase [NOS]-2) neurons and are metabolically active, especially with glutamine metabolism. They may play a role in glia–to-glia communication as well as neuron-to-glia communication. Also, glia may modulate the responsiveness or function, or both, of neighboring neurons, and neurons may modulate the responsiveness or function, or both, of neighboring glia. Activation of glutamate receptors on astrocytes may trigger calcium-dependent glutamate release, which appears sensitive to cyclooxygenase inhibitors (e.g., indomethacin) and blockers of vesicular exocytosis (e.g., tetanus neurotoxins). Glutamine synthase, the enzyme that leads to glutamate formation, is a target of reactive oxygen species and seems to be especially sensitive to peroxynitrite.

It appears that spinal cord glial elements may become activated in response to pathogens (e.g., viruses), mediators released by primary afferent neurons (e.g., substance P, calcium gene-related proteins, ATP, glutamate) and mediators released from neurons in nociceptive pathways (e.g., fractalkine, a protein expressed on the outer surface of neurons that breaks free during strong neuronal exitations;[9] nitric oxide; and prostaglandins).[10] The glial cells may then contribute to the initiation or maintenance of various chronic pain states via release of various substances (e.g., tumor necrosis factor [TNF], interleukin-1, interleukin-6, nitric oxide, reactive oxygen species, arachidonic acid products, excitatory amino acidosis A-(P), which may enhance primary afferent release of substance P and excitatory amino acids and increase the excitability/reactivity of pain transmission neurons.[10,11] Intrathecal fractalkine leads to thermal hyperalgesia and mechanical allodynia, and blockade of the fractalkine receptor (CX3CR-1; expressed on glia but not neurons) may inhibit inflammatory neuropathy–induced pain.[12]

Glia may be involved in contributing to chronic pain states involving neurotropic infectious processes and neural insult as well as extraterritorial pain/mirror-image pain. Extraterritorial pain and mirror image pain may be disrupted by intrathecal administration of a glial metabolic inhibitor or an interleukin-1 receptor antagonist.[13] Propentofylline, a glial modulating agent, exhibits anti-allodynic properties in a rat model of neuropathic pain.[14] Also, spinal administration of CN1–1493 (a p38 mitogen activated protein kinase inhibitor and therefore an inhibitor of proinflammatory cytokine production) has disrupted multiple exaggerated pain states.[10]

Activation of glial α-amino-3-hydroxy-5-methyl-4-isoxazole propionate (AMPA) receptors induce ATP release, which may activate purinergic receptors and coactivation of AMPA, and metabotropic glutamate receptors stimulated calcium-dependent and SNARE protein–

dependent glutamate release that was facilitated by prostaglandin E_2.[7] These glial events may modulate neuronal synaptic transmission.[7]

Chondroitin sulphate proteoglycans (CS-PGs) and tenascin are two classes of axon growth inhibitory extracellular matrix (ECM) constituents that may contribute to the nonpermissive (e.g., impenetrable barrier) nature of glial scar and impede central nervous system (CNS) neuronal regeneration.[15] The neurite inhibitory effects of the CS-PGs (neurocan and phosphacan) seem to be related to their ability to interfere with cell-cell adhesion, whereas versican and brevican as well as the N2 proteoglycan appear to modulate the permissiveness of the ECM.[15] Additionally, versican, which seems to be derived from oligodendrocyte lineage, is upregulated in CNS injury.[16]

It is unknown whether removal of CS-PGs promotes in vivo axon regeneration or may partically restore any dysfunction sustained from neural insult.[15] Of interest is that microglial cells possess receptors for hyaluran (an ECM component), and their motility in vitro is reduced by functional blockage of these receptors.[15]

The ability of glial cells to affect the formation of scar tissue and modulate the neural permissiveness of scar tissue that already exists may have potential utility for chronic pain states with excessive scarring, adhesions, or fibrosis after back surgery.

Tenascin-R is a "neural" member of the tenascin family located in the central nervous system.[17] It is an ECM glycoprotein that may play a role in neuronal protection, stabilization of nerve fiber tracts, neural cell migration, myelination, neuronal maturation, and maintenance of axosomatic synapses.[17]

The expression of tenascin-R is stimulated by soluble factors released by astrocytes (e.g., platelet-derived growth factor and inhibited by growth factors cytokines released from activated microglia (such as TNF-γ).[17] It is conceivable that cytokines (e.g., interleukin-1, interleukin-6, and TNF-γ) interfere with myelination via effects on tenascin-R.[17]

Chemokines

Chemokines are molecules that play a role in altering the integrity of the blood-brain barrier in response to a CNS insult causing local cellular migration. This alteration in the blood-brain barrier appears to occur both centrally and peripherally in response to peripheral inflammatory pain. These molecules are essentially chemotactic cytokines that result in the infiltration into the nervous tissue of lymphocytes and neutrophils. This infiltration to the CNS following injury has been demonstrated following spinal nerve injury.[18] Cell adhesion molecules are proteins found on the cell surface and also determine the route of cell migration. Increased cell adhesion molecule levels may be an earlier indicator of immune activation than cytokines.

Chemokines, or chemoattractant cytokines, play a major role in the processes of leukocyte extravasation and migration. Chemokines are a family of roughly 50 or more small inducible proteins that all have a conserved four-cysteine motif linked by intramolecular disulfide bonds.[19] Although promiscuous in nature, they have their own receptors and may be classified into two main groups according to the relative position of the first two cysteines.[19] The C-x-C or A-chemokine group has an amino acid in between the first two cysteine, whereas in the C–C or B-chemokine group the first two cysteines are located side by side.[19] The C-x-C chemokines are divided into four subgroups, the two 2 major ones of which are a subgroup with a receptor-binding glutamate-leucine-arginine (ELR) sequence and a subgroup without this sequence. The other subgroups seem relatively minor for humans but include the frac-talkine group (known as CX3C).[19] The ELR-C-x-C chemokines recruit predominantly neutro-phils and endothelial cells.[19] The non-ELR-C-x-C chemokines display a wide range of func-tions, including serving as chemoattractants for interleukin-2-activated T-cells.[19] The C-C chemokines mainly attract monocytes, lymphocytes, eosinophils, and basophils.[19]

HIV-1 can enter microglial cells with chemokine receptors (e.g., CCR5, CXCR4, CCR3) and may induce transcription of various cytokines/enzymes or lead to apoptosis via Bax/Bcl2 dys-regulation stimulation of capase 3.[20]

Cytokines

Cytokines are protein molecules released by immune cells in the body in response to infec-tion, inflammation, and trauma and are vital to the host survival response. They have local and systemic effects, both mediated in part by the activation of specific receptors. They are potent molecules, generally acting at picomolar concentrations.[21] They regulate the size and duration of the immune response. These regulatory proteins have been implicated not only in pathological pain states but also in normal brain signalling and processing functions.[22]

The major groupings of cytokines are interleukins, interferons, growth factors, and tumor necrosis factor (formerly known as cachectin). The cytokines interleukin-1, interleukin-6, interleukin-8, and TNF have been the most intensely studied of what are commonly known as the "proinflammatory" cytokines. A cascade-type reaction to noxious stimuli is observed with one cytokine molecule causing induction of another (e.g., TNF leading to interleukin-1 induction).

Watkins and Meyer have identified that cytokine induction leads to pain as a part of a gen-eralized sickness response that includes fever, an endocrine stress response, and energy con-servation behavioral responses.[23,24] Brain and spinal cord cytokine production can occur in response to peripheral noxious stimuli. Pain phenomena such as thermal hyperalgesia, which are mediated by these cytokines, appear to be in part due to prostaglandin production.

Not all cytokines are proinflammatory. A number of cytokines appear to fulfill an anti-inflammatory function (interleukin-4, interleukin-10, interleukin-13), inhibiting further release of the proinflammatory cytokines and also decreasing cyclooxygenase (COX)-2 ex-pression. This function has been shown to reduce interleukin-1 expression and pain behav-ior in an animal model of spinal cord injury.[25]

Mitogen-activated protein (MAP) kinases are a superfamily of serine/threonine phospho-rylating enzymes that play a key role in intracellular signal transduction pathways. There are three major MAP kinases: extracellularly responsive kinases, c-Jun N-terminal kinases, stress-activated protein kinases (JNK/SAPK), and p38.[26] Drugs that inhibit the function of p38, MAP kinase (either by preventing its phosphorylation/activation or by blocking the ATP binding site of phosphorylated p38, thereby preventing it from catalyzing the phosphory-lation of other substrates) have been referred to as cytokine-suppressive anti-inflammatory drugs. The concept of spinal infection (e.g., viral) or other inflammatory processes, even if unilateral in location, causing glial activation in the spinal cord leading to release of proin-flammatory cytokines (e.g., interleukin-1, TNF-α) and subsequent possible exaggerated pain states (e.g., bilateral pain) seems to be particularly supported by the gene therapy work of Milligan, Watkins, and Maier and their colleagues.[10,27–29] The HIV-1 envelope glycoprotein gpl20 binds to and activates glia, leading to activation of protein kinase C, tyrosine kinase, Janus kinase (JAK2), and signal transducer and activator of transcription (STAT-1α).[30] This results in the production or release of interleukin-1 and TNF. Interleukin-1 and TNF each activate p38 MAP kinase, which produces a cascade of signalling effects, including cytokine release and expression of inducible nitric oxide synthase.[27] Potential therapeutic strategies to reverse the chronic pain state animal models that have been employed by the laboratory of Milligan and colleagues have been promising and include interleukin-1 "antagonists," TNF "antagonists," p38 MAP kinase inhibitors (to disrupt interleukin-1/TNF signal transduction cascades), and gene therapy with adenoviral vectors that produce the "anti-inflammatory" cytokine interleukin-10.

Cytokine-induced hyperalgesia may also be mediated in part by bradykinin, substance P, and CGRP. CGRP release appears to be receptor dependent, probably for interleukin-6, interleukin-1B and TNF and may also occur via heat-activated ion channels, which become sensitized after phosphorylation.[31]

Trimeric TNF may also, via receptor-independent means, insert itself into biological membranes and provide ion channel activity.[32]

The actions of cytokines in non-neural tissues are mediated predominantly by two major groups of transcription factors, signal transducers and activators of transcription (STATs) and nuclear factor (NF)–KB.[33] These factors regulate a variety of genes involved in inflammation, cellular adaptation to stress, and cell death.[34] STATs and NF-KB transcription factor may play a crucial role in glial changes of gene expression seen during development; post injury, their target genes include multiple proteins involved in glial cell development and the neuronal and glial response to neural insult, the cytoskeletal protein glial fibrillary acidic protein, the antioxidant proteins metallothioneins, and cell adhesions molecules.[33]

The STAT family of proteins are present in an inactive monomeric form in the cytoplasm.[33] One or several kinases of the family of JAKs may be activated by specific cytokine receptor activation.[33] JAKs will then activate STATs by phosphorylating their tyrosine residues. Growth factor receptors with tyrosine kinase activity may also independently activate JAKs.[33]

Once activated, STAT proteins form homodiners and heterodimers, which translocate to the nucleus and jump-start production of various cytokines by associating with specific DNA regions in the promoters of cytokine-related genes.[35] The JAK-STAT signalling pathway appears to be an integral part of neuronal and glial differentiation in the developing CNS/glial injury response.[36] STAT3, one of the seven described STATs in mammals (STAT1, STAT2, STAT3, STAT4, STAT5a, STAT5b, and STAT6) appears to be a key mediator in the pathway of interleukin-6, a cytokine that seems important in post-neural injury events.[37]

The transcription factor NF-kB is composed primarily of two subunits (p65 and p50), and an inactive form is located in the cytoplasm. Multiple extracellular signals (including receptor-specific signals) promote the activation of a complex cascade of kinases, which results in the phosphorylation of IkB (an inhibitory factor bound to NF-kB).[33] Once IkB is phosphorylated, it becomes ubiquitinated and subsequently degraded by a proteosome. Activated NF-kB is then released and free to translocate to the nucleus, where it may bind to the promoter region of various genes or interact with other transcription factors in neuronal cells of the brain and glial cells of white matter tracts in the CNS.[38]

Activation of the NMDA receptor complex as well as oxidative stress and various other consequences of neural excitotoxic processes may induce or activate NF-kB. NF-kB may then modulate the expression of the c-jun, c-fos, *GFAP* gene, interleukin-1B, TNF-α, and interleukin-6 and may play a role in facilitating inflammatory processes, microglia/astroglia proliferation, scar formation, microglial-astroglial cross-talk, and other events or processes that may result in neuronal or glial insult or damage.[39]

Acarin and coworkers,[40] using afluorated salicylate triflusal (a nonsteroidal anti-inflammatory drug [NSAID]), which blocks in vivo constituitive NF-kB activation in the postnatal brain, have demonstrated that blocking glial NF-kB following a postnatal excitotoxic lesion may provide neuroprotective qualities, leading to down-regulation of glial response as well as reduction of lesion volume. Tepoxalin is also an NSAID with potent analgesic and antiinflammatory properties that inhibits the activation of NF-kB (and therefore interleukin-1 and interleukin-6) in lipopolysaccharide-stimulated microglial cells by preventing the degradation of IkB-X.[41] It is conceivable that transient low-level activation of NKF-kB/TNF-γ or oxidative stress in neurons (but not glia) may induce production of manganese superoxide dismutase and confer some degree of neuroprotection ("preconditioning effect").[39]

Additionally, a significant action of NF-kB is to bolster transcriptional induction of NOS-2 ("inducible" nitric oxide synthase). Agents that inhibit NF-kB activation or prevent NF-kB binding to its gene promoter regions may dampen or inhibit the induction of NOS-2, thereby conferring a potentially neuroprotective role.[39]

There exists some preliminary human data linking cytokine expression to chronic pain. Geiss and coworkers[42] found that post-diskectomy pain correlates with high serum interleukin-6 levels. Empl and coworkers[43] demonstrated that in patients with vasculitic neuropathy, a higher interleukin-6 content on nerve biopsy correlated with more pain.

Goebel and associates were able to diminish pain in a subgroup of patients with chronic pain after administration of intravenous immunoglobulin perhaps due to a decrease in interleukin-1 activity secondary to intravenous immunoglobulin.

Cyclooxygenase

Cyclooxygenase was first purified in 1976 and is the key enzyme involved in the synthesis of prostaglandins from arachadonic acid. COX-2 is an inducible subtype identified in 1991. Because interleukin-1β is a major inducer of central COX-2, this cytokine leads indirectly to the release of prostanoids, which are known to sensitize nociceptor terminals in the periphery and produce localized pain hypersensitivity. As COX-1 is present constitutively in many cell types, the production of selective inhibitors of the inducible COX-2 enzyme has resulted in drugs that reduce inflammation without removing the protective prostaglandins found in the stomach and kidneys. Central inhibition of prostanoid production may be important in reducing centrally generated forms of inflammatory pain hypersensitivity. Another cytokine-mediated enzyme involved in the neuroinflammatory cascade is inducible NOS (iNOS), which has been implicated in the spinal sensitization phenomena associated with chronic pain states.[45]

Lipopolysaccharide induction of NOS-2 in glia involves tyrosine kinases promoting MAP kinases, which activate NF-kB. NF-kB may then induce NOS-2, which increases nitric oxide and soluble gluanyl cyclase activity, leading to increased cyclic guanine monophosphate (cGMP).[45] Dampening mechanisms to sustained cGMP formation or accumulation include down-regulation of soluble gluanyl cyclase by proinflammatory cytokines of inhibitors of transcription and active metabolism of cGMP to GMP by a calcium/calmodulin-dependent (type I) phosphodiesterase. If nitric oxide diffuses to a neigboring cell (e.g., glia to neuron or neuron to glia) in which type I phosphodiesterase is functionally inactive, the cGMP in that cell may accumulate.[45]

ROLE OF CYTOKINES IN PAIN PERCEPTION

Interleukin-1

Interleukin-1 induces hyperalgesia and allodynia when administered subcutaneously.[46] Intraperitoneal administration of interleukin-1 also produces thermal hyperalgesia via production of interleukin-1 in the brain, an effect that is blocked by intracerebroventricular administration of interleukin-1 antagonist. Several animal models of mononeuropathy have demonstrated up-regulation of interleukin-1β expression in the spinal cord.[24] Peripheral noxious stimuli such as formalin subcutaneous injection can also activate spinal cord interleukin-1 production.[47]

A number of modes of action have been proposed for interleukin-1. One is direct binding and activation of sensory nerves, while receptor subtypes have been identified that show partial structural homology. A soluble form of receptor may antagonize and thus regulate interleukin-1 activity, and the antiallodynic effect of interleukin-1 receptor antagonist has also been confirmed.[48] A second mechanism of action is via release of nerve growth factor, which itself can produce hyperalgesia.[49] A third mechanism is via release of prostaglandins, which can cause nerve fiber sensitization.

So it appears that peripheral and central induction of interleukin-1, and in particular interleukin-1β occurs in models of inflammatory and neuropathic pain, and the hyperalgesic and allodynic sequelae can be blocked by central antagonism of interleukin-1. The inhibition of interleukin-1β-mediated hypersensistivity to pain is less effective with systemic as opposed to central administration of interleukin-1 antagonists.[50]

Tumor Necrosis Factor

Both peripheral and central release of TNF have been implicated in the development of inflammatory and neuropathic pain states.[49,51,52] TNF-α expression may be up-regulated in human studies of painful neuropathies. It has also been suggested that systemic soluble TNF-α receptor levels may influence central pain processing mechanisms.[48]

In the brain, TNF can produce fever, sleep, and behavioral changes, and it stimulates osteoclastic activity in bone. Elevation of TNF has been reported in patients with chronic headache.[53] Sickness response functions of the cytokine inflammatory response have been proposed as theoretical mechanisms for clinical phenomena in patients with chronic pain disorders as varied as bone resorption (in complex regional pain syndrome) and sleep disturbance (in fibromyalgia). The TNF gene is controlled by a transcription factor in the nucleus known as NF-κB. TNF and also interleukin-1 are involved in the activation of NF-κB from its latent form, thus amplifying the response. NF-κB also regulates other enzymes involved in eliciting a pain response, and interleukin-6, prostaglandin synthase-2, COX-2, and iNOS are involved. An NF-κB inhibitor has been shown to reduce dynorphin-induced allodynia. Anti-inflammatory agents such as glucocorticoids and aspirin inhibit NF-κB, implicating this as a possible mechanism of analgesic action.

Leem and Bove[54] concluded that TNF can induce ectopic electrogenesis in a minority of nociceptor axons that innervate both deep and cutaneous tissues. Devor[55] has published findings that the ectopic pacemaker hypothesis of neuropathic pain seems to have best held up to scientific scrutiny. It is uncertain whether alterations in sodium channels need to occur concurrently with alterations in cytokine and other mediator activities. Homma and coworkers[56] administered TNF-α to normal uninjured L5 dorsal root ganglia (DRG) and chronically compressed 15 DRG in rats. Their results demonstrated that exogenous TNF-α caused pain and allodynia when deposited at normal DRG and further enhances ongoing allodynia when administered at the compressed DRG, suggesting that endogenous TNF-α may contribute to the early development of mechanical allodynia in rats with chronic DRG compression. They then made a bit of a leap and suggested that inflammatory cytokines (e.g., TNF-α) may contribute to the symptoms of a subgroup of patients with severe low back or lower extremity pain compatible with lumbar radiculopathy but with minimal morphological or anatomical disc abnormalities (e.g., normal magnetic resonance imaging and other objective imaging, laboratory, and electrophysiologic studies).

INFLAMMATORY RESPONSES IN PAIN STATES

Post-Herpetic Neuralgia

In patients with chronic neuropathic pain syndromes following post-herpetic neuralgia, intrathecal elevation of interleukin-8 has been identified as a marker of resistant pain, with a reduction in levels following intrathecal methylprednisolone administration correlating with reduction in pain scores.[57] Herpes zoster is an example of a neurotropic virus. The HIV-1 virus is another that demonstrates a predilection for the central nervous system. A high prevalence of pain symptomatology in up to 80% patients has been observed in HIV-infected individuals. It is known that glial activation and release of neuroexcitatory substances by a portion of the HIV occurs.[10,20] The role of this effect in mediating pain disorders in these patients, however, has yet to be fully elucidated.

Sciatica

Tissues in the area of herniated lumbar discs have been analyzed and confirmed to contain increased levels of inflammatory cytokines, including interleukin-1.[58,59] Furthermore, TNF-α-antagonism prevented the reduction in nerve conduction velocity and also limited intraneural edema formation in an experimental pig model.[51] Phospholipase A2, which is an enzyme that releases arachadonic acid from cell membranes, has been identified and isolated from nucleus pulposis material from patients undergoing diskectomy. Alternative anticytokine strategies may emerge for the treatment of lumbosacral radiculopathies, based on the analgesic effects of nonsteroidal preparations in animal studies.[60]

Spinal Cord Injury

Following traumatic injury to the spinal cord, activation of NF-κB and increased messenger RNA expression for TNF, interleukin-1β, COX-2, and iNOS have been detected. The cellular activation also involves microglia and macrophages, and reduction in the extent of the tissue damage can be observed with antiinflammatory agents such as cyclosporin A.[61]

Cancer Pain

Several cytokines are known to be released from tumor cell lines, including interleukin-1, interleukin-6, and TNF-α.[62] It is possible that these cytokines are synthesized and secreted by tumors affecting the excitability of primary afferent neurons and also causing induction of a central inflammatory response.[63]

Labor Pain

A central inflammatory response with elevation of TNF and interleukin-6 has been identified in the cerebrospinal fluid (CSF) of women in the first stage of labor.[64] The relationship of this finding to the pain of labor has not been elucidated. Similarly, the presence of proinflammatory cytokines in the CSF of postoperative surgical patients[65] has important implications when considering the potential role of NSAIDs as agents in multimodal preemptive analgesic strategies.

CLINICAL APPLICATIONS

The most common clinical application of steroid injection procedures is likely to be in rheumatological disorders, including bursitis, tendinitis, and arthritis, in which an inflammatory basis is established. Steroid applications are also widely used outside the classic inflammatory pain syndromes.

Epidural Corticosteroid

The local application of depot steroid medications in the epidural space has an established basis for the treatment of radicular pain from herniated lumbosacral intervertebral discs.[66] Doses of 80 to 120 mg methylprednisolone acetate diluted in 6 to 10 mL with saline or dilute local anesthetic are commonly employed in monthly series of three applications. The more selective fluoroscopically guided transforaminal approach to the nerve roots exiting the epidural space permits a lower dose of steroid (40 mg methylprednisolone) to be employed.

McQuay and Moore,[67] analyzing data on the effectiveness of epidural corticosteroids for sciatica and back pain found that the number needed to treat (NNT) for short-term (1–60 days), at least 75% pain relief was roughly seven (95% CI, 4.7–16). This means that for every seven patients treated with epidural steroids, one will obtain at least 75% short-term pain relief who would not have achieved this degree of relief had he or she received the control treatment. McQuay and Moore also documented that the NNT for long-term (12 weeks to 1 year), at least 50% pain relief was about 13 (95% CI, 6.6–314). This means that for every 13 patients treated with epidural steroids, one will obtain at least 50% long-term pain relief who would not have achieved this degree of relief had he or she received this control treatment.

Intrathecal Corticosteroid

Recent interest in the central neuroimmune responses observed in patients with spinal cord injury, AIDS-associated pain, and post-herpetic neuralgia has increased. Intrathecal steroid administration has known analgesic effects in different pain disorders. The study by Kotani and colleagues[57] on the analgesic success of intrathecal corticosteroid administration may result in further investigation on the effect of intrathecal methylprednisolone on post-herpetic neuralgia or other pain states with a central inflammatory component. Doses of 60 mg intrathecal methylprednisolone weekly for 4 weeks were administered in that study. However, the early reports of arachnoiditis in patients with multiple sclerosis[68] should provoke caution in the widespread use of this treatment, which is currently likely to be used only for intractable cases.

Cancer Pain. In patients with cancer pain, the systemic effect of corticosteroid is known to be beneficial for symptomatic control and in paticular for bone metastasis-associated pain. The mechanism is thought to be due in part to tumor shrinkage. The wider use of adjuvant agents, including corticosteroids, has been advocated in patients with pain that is poorly responsive to opoids.[69] Dexamethasone 1.5 mg/day was recently shown to produce symptomatic improvement in pain symptoms related to prostate cancer.[70] Local injection of depot preparations at the site of bony metastases that are accessible to fluoroscopically guided injections (such as the sacrum, humerus, scapula, and clavicle) can also produce improvement in pain-related symptoms.

Oral steroids are sometimes given on a short-term basis in an effort to diminish pain and inflammation. On occasion, they may relieve the pain of acute radioculitis, flares of inflammatory arthritis or pain states, and various types of bone pain (e.g., painful osseous metastases). If the treatment of painful osseous metastases is suboptimal with NSAIDs and opioids, oral steroids are an option to add. Some clinicians believe that the steroids are blocking phospholipase 2, which is "proximal" to cyclooxygenase in the arachidonic acid cascade and so it does not make sense to give steroids and NSAID together; however, clinically, they may work better than either alone because the steroid may have multiple actions (e.g., inhibitor/nociceptive inflammatory cytokines altered transcription of various factors).

If a patient is receiving both steroids and NSAIDs, because there is increased risk of gastrointestinal bleeding, or with the administration of steroids in a patient with risk factors for gastrointestinal bleeding, consideration should be given to using budesonide (Entocort), although it is only indicated for Crohn disease. This steroid formulation contains granules that are coated to protect dissolution in gastric juice but that dissolve at a pH greater than 5.5 (i.e., normally when the granules reach the duodenum). Budesonide seems to offer similar efficacy to conventional corticosteroid treatment, with fewer adverse effects, including less adrenal suppression.

Myofascial pain. The addition of dilute steroid to local anesthetic preparations for trigger-point injections in myofascial pain syndromes has its basis in the recognition that local release of allgogenic agents such as histamine, kinins, and the prostaglandins occurs that may be suppressed. These agents may be released as byproducts of anaerobic metabolism secondary to local ischemia. The ischemia is thought to be in part due to excessive contraction precipitated by calcium resease from damaged sarcoplasmic reticulum.

Peripheral and Other Nerve Block Procedures

The ability of corticosteroids to reduce electrical firing in neuromas[71] is often cited as a reason to support the addition of depot steroid preparations to peripheral nerve blocks in the treatment of chronic neuralgias. The ability of a corticosteroid to stabilize neural membranes and to block C fibers[72] may explain the analgesic success of perineural administration. Increased excitation of C fibers is thought to be responsible in part for symptoms of allodynia. Similarly, it is often added to local anesthetic preparations when performing blockade of the medial branch of the dorsal ramus in the treatment of facet joint arthropathy. However, the proximity of the steroid to the affected joint may also explain its effect in this technique.

STEROID INJECTION PREPARATIONS

Methylprednisolone and triamcinolone are the most commonly used corticosterioids in injection preparations. The concentrations of methylprednisolone acetate available are 40 mg/mL or 80 mg/mL and the concentration of triamcinolone is 25 mg/mL. Currently available preparations contain polyethylene glycol and benzyl alcohol. Notwithstanding procedure-related complications such as post–dural puncture headache, the side effects related to their administration in this context can be divided into systemic and neurotoxic.

Systemic Side Effects

The pharmacological effects of glucocorticoids, which include hyperglycemia, weight gain, fluid retention, hypertension, congestive heart failure, and a reversible Cushing syndrome, have all been reported following ESI.[73] Suppression of endogenous adrenal glucocorticoid production following injection of 80 mg methylprednisolone has been observed at 3 weeks following ESI. Relative adrenal insufficiency must be assumed up to 1 month following ESI, and more prolonged adrenal suppression may occur if more than three consecutive monthly ESI procedures are performed.

Neurotoxicity of Steroid Injections

The concern regarding neurotoxicity of these agents arose following reports of arachnoiditis in patients who received repeated intrathecal injections. Nelson and coworkers[68] reported two cases of archnoiditis among 23 patients with multiple sclerosis, and Ryan[74] reported on one case among 108 patients with acute lumbar radiculopathy who all received intrathecal methylprednisolone. It is unclear whether the observed effects were due to the steroid, chemical additives, or an interplay between the demyelinating disease and the injected preparations. Moreover, recent human studies with repeated intrathecal methylprednisolone administration failed to demonstrate any adverse neurological sequelae with prolonged follow-up periods, which included magnetic resonance imaging.[57]

Polyethylene glycol is used as an excipient in concentrations of usually 3% in depot steroid preparations. An excipient is a vehicle used to prepare some pharmaceutical preparations. However, subsequent animal studies failed to provide a basis for explaining the neurotoxic effects observed, and the polyethylene glycol component of the preparation suspected of causing the toxic effects had no effect on a rabbit nerve preparation at clinically relevant concentrations.[75]

Benzyl alcohol is an antibacterial substance found in depot steroid preparations at concentrations of less than 1%. This low concentration is unlikely to cause neurotoxic effects but has been implicated in allergic-type reactions to steroid preparations.[76]

CONCLUSIONS

The responses to many noxious stimuli involve both local and central neuroimmune activation and cytokine release. Persistent activation of these proinflammatory responses are observed in many pain conditions. The potential clinical applications of these observed phenomena include injection of depot steroid preparations and administration of inhibitors of mediators of this inflammation, including the COX-2 enzyme. More specific anticytokine therapies may evolve as the role of these inflammatory mediators in pain states evolves.

REFERENCES FOR ADDITIONAL READING

1. DeLeo JA, Yezierski RP: The role of neuroinflammation and neuroimmune activation in persistent pain. Pain 90:1–6, 2001.
2. Dray A, Urban L: New pharmacological strategies for pain relief. Annu Rev Pharmacol Toxicol 36: 253–280, 1996.
3. Elenkov IJ, Wilder RL, Chrousos GP, Vizi ES: The sympathetic nerve—an integrative interface between two supersystems: the brain and the immune system. Pharmacol Rev 52:595–638, 2000.
4. Caggiano KG, Kraig RP: Eicosanoids and nitric oxide influence induction of reactive gliosis from spreading depression in microglia but not astrocytes. J Comp Neurol 369:93–108, 1996.
5. Sweitzer SM, Schubert P, DeLeo JA: Propentofylline, a glial modulating agent, exhibits antiallodynic properties in a rat model of neuropathic pain. J Pharmacol Exp Ther 297:1210–1217, 2001.
6. Castonguay A, Levesque S, Robitaille R: Glial cells as active partners in synaptic functions. In: Lopez BC, Nieto-Sampedro M, eds. Glial Cell Function: Progress in Brain Research, vol. 132. Elsevier Science BV, Amsterdam, 2001.
7. Bezzi P, Domercq M, Vesce S, et al: Neuron-astrocyte cross-talk during synaptic transmission: Physiological and neuropathological implications. In: Lopez BC, Nieto-Sampedro M, eds. Glial Cell Function: Progress in Brain Research, vol. 132. Elsevier Science BV, Amsterdam, 2001.
8. Rouach N, Giaume C: Connexins and gap junctional communication in astrocytes are targets for neuroglial interaction. In: Lopez BC, Nieto-Sampedro M, eds. Glial Cell Function: Progress in Brain Research, vol. 132. Elsevier Science BV, Amsterdam, 2001.
9. Chapman G, Moores K, Harrison D, et al: Fractalkine cleavage from neuronal membranes represents an acute event in the inflammatory response to excitotoxic brain damage. J Neurosci 20:1–5, 2000.
10. Watkins LR, Milligan ED, Maier SF: Spinal cord glia: New players in pain. Pain 93:201–205, 2001.
11. Oka T, Hori T: Brain cytokines and pain. In: Watkins LR, Maier SF, eds. Cytokines and Pain. Basel, Birkhauser Verlag, 1990, pp 183–204.
12. Twining CM, Milligan ED, Chapman GA, et al: Spinal fractalkine induces allodynia and hyperalgesia. Proc Soc Neurosci 2001;X:27.
13. Watkins LR, Milligan ED, Maier SF: Glial proinflammatory cytokines mediate exaggerated pain states: implication for clinical pain. In: Malchelska H, Stein C, ed: Immune Mechanisms of Pain and Analgesia. Austin, TX, Landes Biosciences, 2001.
14. Sweitzer SM, Schuberf P, DeLeo JA: Propentofylline, a glial modulating agent, exhibits anti-allodynic properties in a model of neuropathic pain. J Pharmacol Exper Ther 297:1210–1270, 2001.
15. Asher RA, Morgensten DA, Moon LDF, Fawcett JW: Chondroitin sulfate proteoglycans: Inhibitory components of the glial scar. In: Lopez BC, Nieto-Sampedro, M, eds. Glial Cell Function: Progress in Brain Research, vol. 132. Elsevier Science BV, Amsterdam, 2001.
16. Asher RA, Morgenstern DA, Shearer MC, et al: Versican is upregulated in CNS injury and is a product of oligodendrocyte lineage cells. J Neurosci. 22:2225–2236, 2002.
17. Pesheva P, Gloor S, Probstmeier R: Tenascin-R as a regulator of CNS glial cell function. In: Lopez BC, Nieto-Sampedro M, eds. Glial Cell Function: Progress in Brain Research, vol. 132. Elsevier Science BV, Amsterdam, 2001.

18. Winkelstein BA, Rutkowski MD, Sweitzer SM, et al: Nerve injury proximal or distal to the DRG induces similar spinal glial activation and selective cytokine expression but differential behavioral responses to pharmacologic treatment. J Comp Neurol 439:127–139, 2001.

19. Anthony DC, Blond D, Dempster R, et al: Chemokine targets in acute brain injury and disease. In: Lopez BC, Nieto-Sampedro M, eds. Glial Cell Function: Progress in Brain Research, vol. 132. Elsevier Science BV, Amsterdam, 2001.

20. Schweighardt B, Atwood WJ: Glial cells as targets of viral infection in the human central nervous system. In: Lopez BC, Nieto-Sampedro M, eds. Glial Cell Function: Progress in Brain Research, vol. 132. Elsevier Science BV, Amsterdam, 2001.

21. Sheeran P, Hall GM: Cytokines in anaesthesia. Br J Anaesth 78:201, 1997.

22. Vitkovic L, Bockaert J, Jacque C: "Inflammatory" cytokines: Neuromodulators in normal brain? J Neurochem 74:457–471, 2000.

23. Watkins LR, Maier SF, Goehler LE: Immune activation: The role of pro-inflammatory cytokines in inflammation, illness responses and pathological pain states. Pain 63:289–302, 1995.

24. Watkins LR, Maier SF: The pain of being sick: Implications of immune-to-brain communication for understanding pain. Annu Rev Psychol 51:29–57, 2000.

25. Plunkett JA, Yu CG, Easton JM, et al: Effects of interleukin-10 (IL-10) on pain behavior and gene expression following excitotoxic spinal cord injury in the rat. Exp Neurol 168:144–154, 2001.

26. Obata T, Brown GE, Yaffe MB: MAP kinase pathways activated by stress: The p38 MAPK pathway. Crit Care Med 28:N67–N77, 2000.

27. Milligan ED, O'Connor KA, Armstrong CB, et al: Systemic administration of CNI–1493, a p38 mitogen-activated protein kinase inhibitor, blocks intrathecal human immunodeficiency virus-1 gp120-induced enhanced pain states. J Pain 2:326–333, 2001.

28. Gazda LS, Milligan ED, Hansen MK, et al: Sciatic inflammatory neuritis (SIN): Behavioral allodynia is paralleled by peri-sciatic proinflammatory cytokine and superoxide production.

29. Chacur M, Milligan ED, Gazda LS, et al: A new model of sciatic inflammatory neuritis (SIN): Induction of unilateral and bilateral mechanical allodynia following acute unilateral peri-sciatic immune activation in rats.

30. Benveniste EN, Benos DJ: TNF-alpha- and IFN-gamma-mediated signal transduction pathways: Effects on glial cell gene expression and fnction. FASEB J 9:1577–1584, 1995.

31. Opree A, Kress M: Involvement of the proinflammatory cytokines tumor necrosis factor-alpha IL-1 beta, and IL-6 but not IL-8 in the development of heat hyperalgesia: Effects on heat evoked calcitonin gene-related peptide release from rat skin. J Neurosci 20:6289–6293, 2000.

32. Baldwin RL, Stolowitz ML, Hood L, et al: Structural changes of tumor necrosis factor alpha associated with membrane insertion and channel formation. Proc Natl Acad Sci U S A 93:1021–1026, 1996.

33. Acarin L, Gonzalez B, Castellano B: Glial activation in the immature rat brain: Implication of inflammatory transcription factors and cutokine expression. In: Lopez BC, Nieto-Sampedro M, eds. Glial Cell Function: Progress in Brain Research, vol. 132. Elsevier Science BV, Amsterdam, 2001.

34. Liu KD, Gaffen SL, Goldsmith MA: JAK/STAT signaling by cytokine receptors. Curr Opin Immunol 10:271–278, 1998.

35. Pelligrini S, Dusanter-Fourt I: The structure, regulation, and function of the Janus kinases (JAK's) and the signal transducers and activators of transcription (STATs). Eur J Biochem 248:615–633, 1997.

36. Cattaneo E, Conti L, DeFraja C: Signalling through the JAK-STAT pathway in the developing brain. Trends Neurosci 22:365–369, 1999.

37. Hirano T: Interleukin 6 and its receptor: Ten years later. Int Rev Immunol 16:249–284; XXXX.

38. Acarin L, Gonzalez B, Castellano B: STAT3 and NFkB activation precedes glial reactivity in the excitatoxically injured young cortex but not in the corresponding distal thalamic nuclei. J Neuropathol Exp Neurol 59:151–163, 2000.

39. Cechetto DF: Role of nuclear factor kappa B in neuropathological mechanisms. In: Lopez BC, Nieto-Sampedro M, eds. Glial Cell Function: Progress in Brain Research, vol. 132. Elsevier Science BV, Amsterdam, 2001.

40. Acarin L, Gonzalez B, Castellano B: Strong down regulation of nuclear factor kappa B activation in glial cells after triflusal treatment. Soc Neurosci Abstr 25:1697, 1999.

41. Fiebich BL, Hofer TJ, Lieb K, et al: The non-steroidal anti-inflammatory drug tepoxalin inhibits interleukin-6 and alpha1-anti-chymotrypsin synthesis in astrocytes by preventing defradation of I kappa B-alpha. Neuropharmacology 38:1325–1333, 1999.

42. Geiss A, Varadi E, Steinbach K, et al: Psychoneuroimmunological correlates of persisting sciatic pain in patients who underwent discectomy. Neurosci Lett 237:65–68, 1997.

43. Empl M, Renaud S, Erne B, et al: TNF-alpha Expression in schmerzhaften und nicht-schmerzhafter Neuropathien. Schmerz 14(Suppl 1):S70, 2000.

44. Goebel A, Netal S, Schedel R, et al: Wirkung von gepoolten humanen Immunglobulinen auf das Schmerzhiveau bei Fibromyalgie patienten. Schmerz 13:573–574, 1999.

45. Baltrons MA, Garcia A: The nitric oxide/cyclic GMP system in astroglial cells. In: Lopez BC, Nieto-Sampedro M, eds. Glial Cell Function: Progress in Brain Research, vol. 132. Elsevier Science B.V., Amsterdam, 2001.

46. Ferreira SH, Lorenzetti BB, Bristow AF, Poole S: Interleukin-1 beta as a potent hyperalgesic agent antagonized by a tripeptide analogue. Nature 334:698–700, 1988.

47. Sweitzer SM, Colburn RW, Rutkowski M, DeLeo JA: Acute peripheral inflammation induces moderate glial activation and spinal IL-1beta expression that correlates with pain behavior in the rat. Brain Res 829:209–221, 1999.

48 Sweitzer S, Martin D, DeLeo JA: Intrathecal interleukin-1 receptor antagonist in combination with soluble tumor necrosis factor receptor exhibits an anti-allodynic action in a rat model of neuropathic pain. Neuroscience 103:529–539, 2001.

49. Woolf CJ, Allchorne A, Safieh-Garabedian B, Poole S: Cytokines, nerve growth factor and inflammatory hyperalgesia: The contribution of tumour necrosis factor alpha. Br J Pharmacol 121:417–424, 1997.

50. Samad TA, Moore KA, Sapirstein A, et al: Interleukin-1b-mediated induction of Cox-2 in the CNS contributes to inflammatory pain hypersensitivity. Nature 410:471–475, 2001.

51. Olmarker K, Rydevik B: Selective inhibition of tumor necrosis factor-alpha prevents nucleus pulposus-induced thrombus formation, intraneural edema, and reduction of nerve conduction velocity: Possible implications for future pharmacologic treatment strategies of sciatica. Spine 26:863–869, 2001.

52. Covey WC, Ignatowski TA, Knight PR, Spengler RN: Brain-derived TNFalpha: Involvement in neuroplastic changes implicated in the conscious perception of persistent pain. Brain Res 859:113–122, 2000.

53. Covelli V, Massari F, Fallacara C, et al: Increased spontaneous release of tumor necrosis factor-alpha/cachectin in headache patients. A possible correlation with plasma endotoxin and hypothalamic-pituitary-adrenal axis. Int J Neurosci 61:53–60, 1991.

54. Leem J-G, Bove GM: Mid-axonal tumor necrosis factor-alpha induces ectopic activity in a subset of slowly conducting cutaneous and deep afferent neurons. J Pain 3:45–49, 2002.

55. Devor M: Neuropathic pain: What do we do with all these theories? Acta Anaesthesiol Scand 45:1121–1127, 2001.

56. Homma Y, Brull SJ, Zhang J-M: A comparison of chronic pain behavior following local application of tumor necrosis factor α to the normal and mechanically compressed lumbar ganglia in the rat. Pain 95:239–246, 2002.

57. Kotani N, Kushikata T, Hashimoto H, et al: Intrathecal methylprednisolone for intractable postherpetic neuralgia. N Engl J Med 343:1514–1519, 2000.

58. Hunt JL, Winkelstein BA, Rutkowski MD, et al: Repeated injury to the lumbar nerve roots produces enhanced mechanical allodynia and persistent spinal neuroinflammation. Spine 26:2073–2079, 2001.

59. Takahashi H, Suguro T, Okazima Y, et al: Inflammatory cytokines in the herniated disc of the lumbar spine. Spine 21:218–224, 1996.

60. Yabuki S, Onda A, Kikuchi S, Myers RR: Prevention of compartment syndrome in dorsal root ganglia caused by exposure to nucleus pulposus. Spine 26:870–875, 2001.

61. Yu CG, Bethea JR, Fairbanks CA, et al: Effects of cyclosporin, interleukin-10 and agmatine on a spontaneous pain-like behavior following excitotoxic spinal cord injury in the rat. Soc Neurosci Abstr 733:8, 2000.

62. Elgert KD, Alleva DG, Mullins DW: Tumor-induced immune dysfunction: The macrophage connection. J Leukocyte Biol 64:275–290, 1998.

63. Arruda JL, Colburn RW, Rickman AJ, et al: Increase of interleukin-6 mRNA in the spinal cord following peripheral nerve injury in the rat: Potential role of IL-6 in neuropathic pain. Brain Res Mol Brain Res 62:228–235, 1998.

64. Klamt JG, Cuhna FQ, Stocche RM, Garcia LV: Cerebrospinal fluid concentrations of Interleukin-6 and tumor necrosis factor of patients in labor pain. Reg Anes Pain Med 24:A38, 1999.

65. Yeager MP, Lunt PL, Arrud J, et al: Cerebrospinal fluid cytokine levels afer surgery with spinal or general anesthesia. Reg Anes Pain Med 24:557–562, 1999.

66. Abram SE: Treatment of lumbosacral radiculopathy with epidural steroids. Anesthesiology 91:1937–1941, 1999.

67. McQuay HJ, Moore RA: An evidence-based resource for pain relief. New York, Oxford University Press, 1998.

68. Nelson DA, Vates TS, Thomas RB: Complications from intrathecal steroid therapy in patients with multiple sclerosis. Acta Neurol Scand 49:176–188, 1973.

69. Mercadante S, Portenoy RK: Opioid poorly-responsive cancer pain. Part 3. Clinical strategies to improve opioid responsiveness. J Pain Symptom Manage 21:338–354, 2001.

70. Saika T, Kusaka N, Tsushima T, et al: Treatment of androgen-independent prostate cancer with dexamethasone: A prospective study in stage D2 patients. Int J Urol 8:290–294, 2001.

71. Devor M, Govrin-Lippmann R, Raber P: Corticosteroids suppress ectopic neural discharge originating in experimental neuromas. Pain 22:127–137, 1985.

72. Johansson A, Hao J, Sjolund B: Local corticosteroid application blocks transmission in normal nociceptive C-fibres. Acta Anaesthesiol Scand 34:335–338, 1990.

73. Abram SE, O'Connor TC: Complications associated with epidural steroid injections. Reg Anesth 21:149–162, 1996.

74. Ryan MD, Taylor TKF: Management of lumbar nerve root pain by intrathecal and epidural injection of depot methylprednisolone acetate. Med J Aust 2:532–534, 1981.

75. Benzon HT, Gissen AJ, Strichartz GR, et al: The effect of polyethylene glycol on mammalian nerve impulses. Anesth Analg 66:553–559, 1987.

76. Verecken P, Birringer C, Knitelius AC, et al: Sensitization to benzyl alcohol: A possible cause of "corticosteroid allergy." Contact Dermatitis 38:106, 1998.

Chapter 33

A Potpourri of Potential Targets for Analgesia

Howard S. Smith, MD

PAIN PROCESSING

The four physiological processes involved with pain are transduction, transmission, modulation, and perception. Mechanical, thermal, and chemical stimuli are *transduced* in primary afferent neurons. The now "electrical" pain signals (produced via ion currents/potentials) are *transmitted* to the central nervous system. Along the way to the brain, pain signals may be *modulated* at various different points. Finally, in the brain, pain *perception* takes place.

The process of transmission involves the ascending pathways. The three major groupings of ascending nociceptive pathways are the spinothalamic tract, the spinobulbar projections—spinoreticular tract and spinomesencephalic tract—and the spinohypothalamic tract.[1] Additionally, three indirect ascending pathways that are integrated and relayed via multiple central nervous system areas toward the brain are the post-synaptic dorsal column system, the spinocervicothalamic tract pathway, and the spinoparabrachial pathways.[1]

Although there seem to be other ways that pain signals can arrive at the brain, it has been proposed that there are two major pain systems (medial and lateral), both feeding the thalamus as a relay center to the brain.[2,3] The medial pain system relays pain signals to the medial (paleo-)thalamus. The medial thalamus is not highly somatotopically organized and is believed to project in a net-like fashion to large areas of the cortex (especially the insula and anterior cingulate cortex). It is believed to be mainly involved in the motivational and affective components of pain.[2] The lateral pain system relays pain signals to the lateral (neo-)thalamus. The lateral thalamus is somatotopically highly organized and is believed to project mainly to the primary and secondary somatosensory areas of the cerebral cortex. It seems to be predominantly involved with the processing and transmission of the discriminative components of nociceptive-type information (i.e., letting the brain know the exact "coordinates" of where the pain is coming from in the body). This is highly complex and possibly somewhat inaccurate, and primary and secondary somatosensory areas are probably involved somewhat in contributing to or shaping the affective aspects of pain; however, these concepts may be useful conceptually.

Functional imaging studies (e.g., functional magnetic resonance imaging and positron emission tomography) have shed some light on higher central nervous system (CNS) areas involved with pain.[4]

Several subcortical sites, including the periaqueductal grey, the hypothalamus, the amygdala, and the cerebellum, may also play a role in contributing to pain perception. Noxious heat and noxious cold stimuli activate four major cortical sites: the region of the central sulcus (referred to as S1), the region of the lateral operculum (referred to as S2), the insula, and the anterior cingulate cortex.[4] Modulation of analgesia can probably occur at numerous areas of the nervous system, but a major role seems to involve the CNS descending (inhibitory) pathways. The descending inhibitory pathways of the CNS seem to converge in a Y-shaped fashion into the dorsolateral funiculus, which terminates in lamina I, II, and V of the dorsal horn of the spinal cord (FIGURE 1).

Targeting on a microlevel as we progress into the so-called decade of pain (2000–2010), future analgesics may differ somewhat from our current agents and may encompass gene therapy, cytokine modulation therapy, antienkephalinase therapy, agents to modulate the balance of the neurotrophic factors in the skin, agents to modulate oncogenes or apoptosis, and reactive oxygen species scavenging analgesics (ROSSA). The future may also see new formulations, such as nonsteroidal anti-inflammatory chewing gum, N-baclofen chewing gum, vanilloid receptor 1 (VR1) antagonist chewing gum, topical patches of VR1 antagonists, topical neurotrophic factors, intranasal or topical ROSSA, intranasal VR1 antagonists, and intranasal or topical calcitonin gene-related protein antagonists.

If certain types of dental pain have VR1 components,[5] VR1 antagonists may be logical therapeutic choice. If ethanol causes an epigastric burning sensation via the VR1 receptor,[6] then an agent such as lafutidine may be very appropriate, since it not only possess an antisecretory effect via histamine H_2-receptor blockade but it also has gastroprotective activities that may be mediated via its modulation of VR1 receptor responses.[7]

Milligan presented her work (as well as that of Watkins and coworkers) on the spinal delivery of adenoviral vectors engineered with the antiinflammatory cytokine interleukin-10 gene for pain control at the 21st annual scientific meeting of the American Pain Society in 2002. Interleukin-10 by blocking the function of proinflammatory cytokines (e.g., interleukin-1, tumor necrosis factor) released from spinal cord glia, was postulated to abolish pain. This seems very foreign compared with approaches of traditional analgesics.

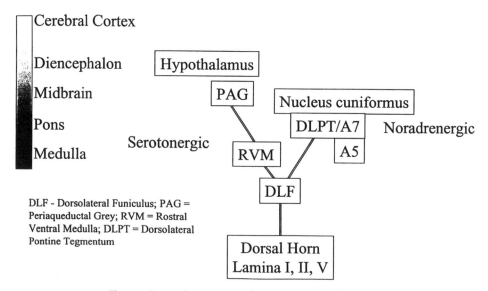

"Y Formation"

Cerebral Cortex

Diencephalon   Hypothalamus

Midbrain   PAG   Nucleus cuniformus

Pons   DLPT/A7   Noradrenergic

Serotonergic

Medulla   RVM   A5

DLF

DLF - Dorsolateral Funiculus; PAG =
Periaqueductal Grey; RVM = Rostral
Ventral Medulla; DLPT = Dorsolateral
Pontine Tegmentum

Dorsal Horn
Lamina I, II, V

Figure 1. Descending pathways of pain modulation, "Y formation"

The brain is extremely important as the final processor, resulting in perception, however, we still are not advanced enough to target specific brain loci. The skin is an organ whose role in pain is first beginning to become appreciated. It is crucial to be able to target molecular/receptor pain generators in efforts to provide optimal analgesia. For example, if there is an overexpression of VR1 in the skin causing pain, then treatment approaches should attempt to zero in on this.

SODIUM CHANNEL BLOCKERS

One of the reasons that antiepileptic drugs can be effective (i.e., analgesic) in treating certain neuropathic pain states is that some of the mechanisms that contribute to neuropathic pain may also play a role in various forms of epilepsy. Four transmembrane currents that have been proposed as contributing to neuropathic pain include sodium channel blockers, calcium channel blockers, and glutamate receptor antagonists. There are certainly other mechanisms at play as well in certain neuropathic pain states. The more we appreciate the contributions of these and other various mechanisms to a specific individual's chronic pain complaints, the better we should be able to devise logical treatment approaches.

Pain transmission from nociceptors generally travels through the dorsal root ganglia (DRG) or trigeminal neurons in a series of action potentials that continue to ascend to the brain where pain perception occurs. Voltage-dependent sodium channels are primarily responsible for the inward transmembrane current leading to depolarization. At least nine functionally distinct voltage-dependent sodium channels (encoded by different genes) exist, with the majority present in the human nervous system.[8]

Three sodium channels—(Navl.7, also termed PN1; Navl.8, also termed SNS (sensory-neuron-specific) or PN3; and Navl.9 also termed NaN or SNS-2—are preferentially expressed in DRG and trigeminal neurons.[8] These three channels are not present at significant levels in other neurons.[8] Navl.7 is a tetrodotoxin-sensitive channel, whereas Navl.8 and Navl.9 are tetrodotoxin resistant.[8]

A fourth channel, Navl.3/type III, normally expressed at very low levels, is significantly up-regulated with various neural insults. These newly formed sodium channels appear to be at least partially responsible for a rapidly repriming tetrodotoxin-sensitive sodium current that occurs after axotomy.[9]

Selective knockdown of Navl.8/SNS using antisense oligodeoxynucleotides prevented and reversed tactile allodynia and thermal hyperalgesia in a sciatic nerve ligation model of neuropathic pain.[10] Also, nerve growth factor–induced hyperalgesia is significantly attenuated in null-mutant mice for the Navl.8/SNS channel.[11]

Cummings and Waxman[9] have proposed that the reduction in persistent tetrodotoxin-resistant current (at least partially attributable to a down-regulation of Navl.9/NaN), which occurs after neural insult, could lead to a hyperpolarizing shift in resting potential, resulting in less resting inactivation of tetradotoxin-sensitive channels. If this is the case, then preventing Nav1.9/NaN down-regulation or actually up-regulating Nav1.9/NaN channels may reduce neuropathic pain. Nav1.3 and Navl.8 channels accumulate close to the tips of injured axons within experimental neuromas.[12]

Lai and associates[13] administered specific antisense oligodeoxynucleotides to the peripheral tetrodotoxin-resistant sodium channel NaV1.8 intrathecally. This led to uptake of oligodeoxynucleotides by DRG neurons, which produced selective decrement of NaV1.8 expression and a reduction in the slow-inactivating, tetrodotoxin-resistant sodium current in the DRG cells.[13] The oligodeoxynucleotide treatment reversed neuropathic pain caused by spinal nerve ligation injury[14] model in rats without affecting nonnoxious sensation.[13] Lai and associates[13] concluded that their results provide direct evidence linking NaV1.8 (which is restricted to sensory neurons) to neuropathic pain.

Additionally, these sodium channels (e.g., Navl.3, Nav1.7, Navl.8, and Navl.9) may be present and altered in neuropathic pain states in second-order,[15] tertiary order, and other neural cell types along the path of pain transmission. Currently, there are no specific analgesic agents that exclusively target specific sodium channels or sodium channel subunits; however, future research efforts may aim toward affecting specific sodium channel subunits.

γ-AMINOBUTYRIC ACID

Another key element in nociceptive neurotransmission is γ-aminobutyric acid (GABA). GABA is the major inhibitory neurotransmitter in the brain. It acts postsynaptically on GABA-A receptors opening anion-premeable channels with an inward movement of chloride ions and resultant hyperpolarization.[16] GABA also acts postsynaptically on G-protein-coupled GABA-B receptors opening channels, which promote potassium conductance and yield a slow inhibitory potentials.[16] Additionally, GABA-B receptors may occur presynaptically and agonists diminish voltage-dependent calcium currents, decreasing the release of GABA and glutamate into the synapes.[16] GABA in the synapse diffuses and is then taken up by the neural elements and glia. Four plasma membrane proteins that act as GABA transporters have been identified: hGAT-1, hGAT-2, hGAT-3, and hBGT-1.[17]

Tiagabine is a derivative of nipecotic acid that selectively inhibits hGAT-1 located primary in the cerebral cortex and hippocampus.[17] The inhibition of the GABA transporter slows the reuptake of synaptically released GABA, thereby prolonging inhibitory post-synaptic potentials.[18]

GABA is synthesized from glutamate by the enzyme glutamic acid decarboxylase (GAD), along with its coenzyme pyridoxine, and degraded by the enzyme GABA-transaminase (GABA-T) to a succinic semialdehyde, which is then further metabolized by succinic semialdehyde dehydrogenase.[19] GABA uptake inhibitors have been synthesized that are tricyclic analog derivatives of nipecotic acid, guvacine, and homo-β-proline and may have some eventual utility in the amelioration of neuropathic pain.[20]

The loss of activity of the inhibitory neurotransmitter GABA in the spinal cord may be one of the factors leading to enhanced pain sensitivity.[21] Endogenous spinal GABA may act tonically to down-regulate thermal responsiveness. Disinhibition of these receptors via GABA antagonists could lead to thermal hyperalgesia.[21] Malan and colleagues[21] demonstrated that GABA-A and GABA-B antagonists can lead to tactile allodynia and thermal hyperalgesia. Additionally, exogenous administration of GABA agonists reversed spinal nerve ligation-induced allodynia and hyperalgesia.

GABA may also play a crucial role in mediating analgesia. Supraspinal (intracerebroventricular) morphine evokes GABA release via the activation of 5-hydroxytryptamine 3 receptors in the spinal cord, leading to antinociceptive effects.[22]

A tonic GABAergic and glycinergic inhibition of low-threshold afferents innervating mechanoreceptors appears to be operating in the normal baseline state (at least in rats); reduced activity in this normal dampening system (especially for GABA)[23] could lead to mechanical allodynia.[24] Intrathecal administration of the GABA-A receptor antagonist bicuculline or the glycine receptor antagonist strychnine produces segmentally localized tactile allodynia-like behavior in conscious rats.[25] Benzodiazepines (e.g., midazolam), which bind to the benzodiazepine site of the GABA-A receptor, are more effective in reducing nociceptive firing in neural injury states (eg spinal nerve ligation model) of enhanced GABA transmission than in normal states.[25] Additionally, Mertens and colleagues[26] suggest that certain chronic pain states may be associated with an imbalance in the levels of excitatory versus inhibitory amino acids (i.e., the ratio of aspartate to GABA and glycine in the spinal dorsal horn).

CALCIUM CHANNEL BLOCKERS

Vanegas and Schaible[96] reviewed the antinociceptive role of high-voltage activated (high-threshold) calcium channel antagonists (L-, N-, and P/Q- type). Strong membrane depolarization activates these calcium channels to allow an influx of calcium ions presynaptically, leading to neurotransmitter release. Calcium channels are expressed throughout the CNS.[27] The N-type voltage-dependent calcium channels (VDCCs) are sensitive to block by omega-conotoxin GVIA.[28] (This toxin is derived from the venom of *Conus geographus*, a fish-hunting cone shell—the G is from *geographus*.)

The N-type channel seems to be concentrated in laminae I and II of the superficial dorsal horn[27] but is also present in deeper laminae. N-type VDCCs are commonly found in neurons that contain substance P[29] and appear to be well positioned to regulate neurotransmitter release (e.g., glutamate) from peptide-containing C fibers.[30]

Tactile allodynia in the spinal nerve ligation model is blocked by intrathecal N-type blockers, SNX-111 (ziconotide), SNX-239, and SNX-159.[31] Also, the combination of blockers of N-type VCGGs and α_2-adrenoceptor agonists (e.g., clonidine) may possess unique synergistic qualities.[32] The P-type VDCCs are sensitive to block by omega-agatoxin IV A and predominantly concentrated in laminae II through VI of the dorsal horn possibly localized to nonpeptide, IB-4 neurons.[28] P-type VDCCs appear to be involved in the initiation of facilitated pain states, mostly associated with inflammation, and seem to be closely associated with N-methyl-D-aspartate (NMDA)-receptor–mediated events.[30] Omega-agatoxin IVA given prior to the application of capsaicin[33] or carrageenan[34] prevents the development of hyperalgesia in animal studies. SNX-230 (a synthetic P/Q-type selective conopeptide homologue) was not used in these studies, but similar results would be expected. L-type VDCC antagonists (e.g., verapamil) seem to enhance morphine analgesia and exhibit analgesic properties.[30]

In contrast to the high-threshold calcium channels, low-voltage activated calcium channels (low-threshold T-type channels) are activated at voltages near the resting membrane potential[35] and, although they would not support neurotransmission alone, may help regulate cell excitability.[30]

The occurrence of subthreshold membrane potential oscillations in DRG neurons appears to increase after spinal nerve ligation,[36] an effect that may be due to increased activity of T-type calcium channels in the remaining afferent neurons serving to increase excitability.[30] Blocking these T-type VDCCs (e.g., ethosuximide) reduces neuronal excitability and creates an environment less favorable for reaching the threshold levels required for membrane depolarization.[30]

Kurtoxin, which belongs to the family of x-scorpion toxins, appears to act as a unique gating modifier that interacts with a broad spectrum of different calcium channel types and affects activation and deactivation of voltage-gated calcium channels.[37]

Vanilloid receptor 1 appears to serve as a polymodal transducer of multiple nociceptive stimuli with underappreciated clinical significance. VR1 may play a role in multiple painful conditions, including diabetic neuropathy[38] and possibly post-herpetic neuralgia and complex regional pain syndrome. Alterations may occur to the state of vanilloid receptors with tissue inflammation or insult that include axonal transport of VR1 mRNA from DRG to central and peripheral axon terminals.[39] VR1 protein expression increases in undamaged DRG neurons after neural insult.[40]

PURINORECEPTORS

Multiple proanalgesic mediators that activate or sensitize (or both) nociceptors evolved during insult to human organ and tissues. Adenosine triphosphate (ATP) is released during various types of insults, including noxious stimulation (e.g., capsaicin), trauma or surgery, and sympathetic varicosities as a cotransmitter with norepinephrine/neuropeptide Y from tumor cells (e.g., vigorous/abrasive insult) and from microvascular endothelial cells (e.g., hyperemia).

Purinoreceptors may be intertwined in the web of inflammatory pain mediators, which may contribute to pain. The purinergic nucleotide receptors have been subclassified into P1 (more responsive to adenosine and adenosine monophosphate [AMP]) and P2 (more responsive to adenosine diphosphate and ATP). Abbracchio and Burnstock[41] proposed that P2 receptors be separated into two major families: a P2X family (ligand-gated [iontropic] cation channels) and a P2Y family (G protein-coupled [metabotropic] receptors). ATP may lead to pain or hyperalgesia by dual mechanisms: (1) direct effects on ionotropic P2X3 receptors on sensory neurons and (2) indirect effects via metabotropic P2Y, receptors in a protein kinase C-dependent pathway leading to VR1 modulation (FIGURE 2).[42]

In the presence of ATP, the temperature threshold for VR1 activation was reduced from $42°C$ to $35°C$ (i.e., thermal allodynia with normally nonpainful stimuli [normal body temperature] were capable of activating VR1).

Inflammation and tissue insult generally give rise to sensitization of nociceptors in the short term via two major avenues, protein kinase A (PKA) or protein kinase C (PKC). Prostaglandins, serotonin, and adenosine are examples of mediators that may activate adenylate cyclase and increase cyclic AMP leading to activation of PKA. PKA phosphorylates a tetrodotoxin-resistant voltage-sensitive sodium channel (TTXRVSNaC) that lowers its threshold and increases the probablility of eliciting an action potential.[41]

Additionally, cyclic AMP may modulate potassium ion currents as well as voltage and cyclic nucleotide-gated conductance.[41] These actions of cyclic AMP probably contribute only a minor role, leading to nociceptor sensitization with the major contribution from the TTXRVSNaC.

A second avenue leading to short-term sensization involves activation of PKC. Sensitization can be reversed by PKC inhibitors or prolonged by phosphatase inhibitors (agents that prevent protein dephosphorylation after it has been phosphorylated by PKC).[43] PKC is known to be activated by a variety of inflammatory mediators (e.g., bradykinin). PKC may affect the NMDA receptor complex and, perhaps more importantly, may play a major role in modulating VR1 via phosphorylation.[44] VR1, located on sensory neurons, is a cation channel that predominantly gates calcium ions.

Phospholipase C or IP3 may directly or indirectly affect VR1, potentially by modulating release of basal phosphatidylinositol-4,5-bisphosphate (without involvement of PKC) (see FIGURE 2). Phosphorylation of VR1, possibly via different mechanisms, promote sensitization. Calcineurin, a calcium-dependent phosphatase may dephosphorylate VR1 and lead to VR1

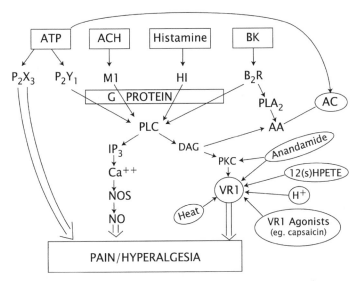

Figure 2. Multiple direct and indirect pathways leading to pain/hyperalgesia.

desinsitization.[43] VR1 is thought to be modulated predominantly by three major means: heat, protons (e.g., acid), and vanilloid agonists (e.g., capsaicin).[45] High concentrations of anandamide appear to activate VR1 (at low concentrations, anandamide may produce inhibitory effects via actions at the cannabinoid CB1 receptor).[46] Modulation probably ultimately takes place via distinctly different pathways. Acid potentiation of VR1 seems to be determined by a key extracellular site.[47] The activation of VR1 leads to a burst increase in neuronal intracellular calcium, which appears to subside more slowly predominantly via mitochondria buffering.[48]

The addition of positive charge to the outer side of the membrane (acid modulation) or the addition of negative charge to the inner side of the membrane (phosphorylation) both may lead to VR1 sensitization.[43]

Purinoreceptors seem to play a significant direct role in certain types of pain states in animal models.[49]

VANILLOID RECEPTORS

The VR1 (now known as TRPV1 [transient receptor potential vanilloid 1]) receptor seems to play a crucial role in the development of thermal hyperalgesia secondary to tissue injury or inflammation.[50] Because the VR1 receptor is responsive to noxious heat,[51] protons, products of the arachidonic acid cascade,[52] (e.g., 12-(S)-HPETE) and other inflammatory analgesic mediators,[53] it may be a key player in inflammatory pain.[54]

The VR1 receptor is present in the majority of both histochemical classes of primary afferent nociceptors in the adult rodent.[55] The VR1 receptor responds to heat and vanilloids (e.g., capsaicin) and may be significantly modulated by protons. It then acts to increase transmembrane cation conductance (e.g., Na^+, Ca^{++}).[55] The increase in intracellular calcium is then buffered by mitochondrial calcium accumulation via the mitochondrial Ca^{++} uniporter.[48] The subsequent release of mitochondrial Ca^{++} into the cytosol via the mitochondrial Na^+/Ca^{++} exchanges occurs very slowly, and this prolonged elevation of mitochondrial and cytoplasmic Ca^{++} via VR1 activation results in desensitization and may reflect "neuronal memory."[48]

Other than the mechanisms discussed, there does not seem to be an obvious prototype endogenous VR1 receptor agonist. However, anandamide, an endogenous lipid metabolite, which normally binds to the cannabinoid receptor CB1 and inhibits the release of CGRP, may also act as a agonist at the VR1 receptor.[56,57]

Other N-acetyl ethanol amines that may be involved during severe inflammation may have even more dramatic potentiating effects at the VR1 receptor.[58] Amides and esters of fatty acids such as anandamide (N-anachidonylethanolamide) and palmitylethanolamide (2-arachidonoylglycerol) are agonists, predominantly at the CB1 and CB2 receptors respectively. Effects of cannabinoid receptor activation by these liquids include inhibition of adenylate cyclase; regulation of ion conductances (e.g., inhibition of voltage-gated calcium channels [L, N, and P/Q], and activiation of potassium channels); activation of focal adhesion kinase, mitogen-activated protein kinase, induction of immediate early gene, and stimulation of nitric oxide synthase.[59]

Effects of anandamide and palmitylethanolamide not mediated via cannibinoid receptors may include inhibition of L-type calcium channels, stimulation of vanilloid receptors (e.g., VR1), altered concentrations of intracellular calcium, and inhibition of gap junction function.[59]

There appears to be partial overlap among the ligand recognition of vanilloid receptors (e.g., VR1), cannabinoid receptors (e.g., CB1), and the anandamide membrane transporter. The two-step process that terminates anandamide activity is reuptake by intact cells via the anandamide membrane transporter and hydrolysis of the amide bond, catalyzed by the enzyme fatty-acid amide hydrolase.[60]

Another potential candidate for an endogenous VR1 agonist is the lipooxygenase metabolite 12-(S)-HPETE.[52] Hwang and coworkers[52] presented evidence for the products of lipoxygenase activating VR1.[52] Three key points are as follows: (1) Lipoxygenase products evoked single-channel currents with the conductance and ion selectivity nearly identical to that produced by capsaicin; (2) Capsazepine, an antagonist of the VR1 receptor, blocked channel activation by lipoxygenase products; and (3) 12-(S)-HPETE, a lipoxygenase product has a three-dimensional structure that superimposes exactly on that of capsaicin.[52]

Premkumar and Ahern[53] propose that the VR1 receptor is phosphorylated by PKC, which produces significant activation. It may then respond maximally to substances such as anandamide, 12-(S)-HPETE, and bradykinin. They hypothesize that these substances induce and enhance VR1 activity in a PKC-dependent fashion.

ADENOSINE AND ADENOSINE RECEPTORS

Adenosine, enzymatically produced from ATP degradation, can mediate inhibition of nerve excitability via A1 adenosine receptors (negatively coupled to cyclic AMP). Also, through cyclic AMP leading to hyperalgesia, adenosine can mediate excitatory effects via A2 adenosine receptors. Adenosine receptors are present on small interneurons and presynaptic afferent nerve terminals in the superficial dorsal horn; however, adenosine may lead to analgesia with spinal administration and intravenous/peripheral administration (topical). Multiple agents (in addition to adenosine itself) may produce analgesia at least in part by stimulating the adenosine receptors (e.g., endogenous adenosine analogs and A1 receptor agonists, amitriptyline, and adenosine kinase inhibitors [such as 5-amino-5' oxyadenosine).[61]

It is conceivable that adenosine-mediated spinal antinociception could result from interactions of adenosine and/or the A1 receptor with the spinal NMDA polysynaptic nociceptive pathway.[62] A complex interplay may exist between ATP metabolism and actions in neuronal cells and synapses and various receptors, which could modulate nociception (FIGURE 3).

FREE RADICALS AND PAIN

Khalil[63] suggests that free radicals contribute to the maintenance of thermal hyperalgia and may be involved in other chronic pain states. Treatment with tirilazad (an antioxidant) significantly alleviated thermal hyperalgesia. Other agents, possibly acting through antioxidant mechanisms, may possess analgesic properties. However, this currently remains anecdotal and speculative.

Oxygen radicals (e.g., superoxide anion) may decrease nerve blood flow by inhibiting nitric oxide synthase and decreasing nitric oxide levels. Spinal nitric oxide has been proposed to mediate the analgesic effects of systemic morphine and intrathecal clonidine.[64,65] Intrathecally administered clonidine is believed to activate α_2-receptors, leading to an increase in acetylcholine, especially in the dorsal horn. It has been proposed that acetylcholine (acting predominantly through muscarinic receptors, especially M1 or M3, and to a lesser extent via nicotinic receptors) produces increased nitric oxide activity, resulting in analgesia. Oxygen radicals may decrease nitric oxide levels, thereby producing antianalgesic effects. In light of this, oxygen radical scavengers may potentially exhibit analgesic properties in this setting.

If evidence mounts to show that oxygen radicals can diminish nitric oxide and yield anti-

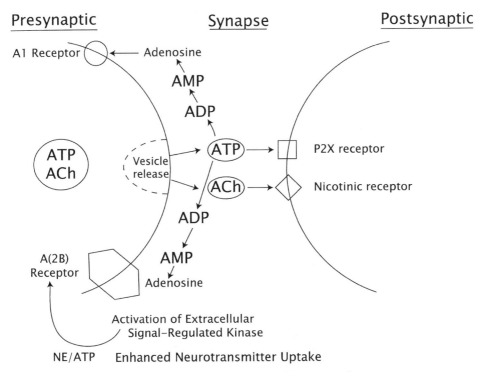

Figure 3. ATP metabolism and potential nociceptive effects.

analgesic effects, then it may be prudent to prophylactically administer antioxidants to patients undergoing revascularization surgery, those with reperfusion injury, or in other settings where oxygen radicals may evolve.

Cannabidiol, a nonpsychoactive constituent of marijuana, and the psychotropic cannabinoid (9-tetrahydro cannabinol), ameliorate glutamate neurotoxicity via NMDA, AMPA, and KA receptors.[66] These effects may be secondary to their potent antioxidant activity. The neuroprotection offered by THC and cannabidiol appears to be independent of cannabinoid receptor activity, and both of these agents may alleviate hyperalgesia and pain. The cannabinoid CB1 and CB2 antagonists may prolong and enhance pain.[67]

Other potent antioxidants (e.g., α-lipoic acid) may replenish glutathione levels and improve symptoms in patients with diabetic neuropathy. In an animal model of diabetic neuropathy, α-lipoic acid increased nerve blood flow, glutathione levels, and digital nerve conduction velocity.[68] In the ALADIN[69] study, an intravenous infusion of α-lipoic acid diminished symptoms of diabetic neuropathy, including pain, burning, paresthesia, and numbness, over the short term.

MISCELLANEOUS POTENTIAL TARGETS FOR ANALGESIA

Mantyh and associates[70] studied the ribosomes-inactivating cytotoxic protein, saporin conjugated to substance P. For saporin to work, it needs to be inside the cell. Entry into the cell is easily accomplished as both substance P and saporin, because the substance P is rapidly internalized upon binding to spinal cord neurons expressing the substance P receptor. Substance P receptors are predominantly located in lamina I.

Potent inhibitors of neuronal nicotine acetylcholine receptors (ABT-594) are other novel analgesic agents with exciting clinical potential. Because they potentially have analgesic activity in models of acute thermal, persistent chemical, and neuropathic pain states, these nonopioid compounds are referred to as broad-spectrum analgesics.[71] AT-594 may have therapeutic potential in ameliorating a wide variety of painful conditions. ABT-594 is somewhat similar to epibatidine, an alkaloid isolated from the skin of Ecuadorian frogs.[71] However, epibatidine is not used as a clinical agent because, like nicotine, it has cardiovascular side effects. As a nonopioid, nonsteroidal antiinflammatory drug, ABT-594 is 30- to 110-fold more potent than morphine, with roughly equal efficacy.[71]

The possibilities for new opioids in the future treatment of pain are immense. A series of phosphinic acid derivatives are currently in development (e.g., RB111). The role of these agents is to inhibit both neutral endopeptidase and aminopeptide, which function as enkephalinases.[72]

KRN5500, a semisynthetic antitumor antibiotic, had significant effects in alleviating mechanical allodynia in two models of neuropathic pain in rats.[73] Another agent that could theoretically exhibit analgesic qualities in certain types of patients (eg pancreatitis) is gabexate mesylate, a synthetic inhibitor of trypsin-like serine proteinases.[74]

Endothelin 1, and possibly via endothelin A receptor-mediated release of calcium in nociceptor-like neurons,[75] may contribute to various pain states.[76]

Malan and colleagues[77] concluded that elevated spinal dynorphin levels resulting from peripheral nerve insult may contribute to the maintenance of neuropathic pain, in part through direct or indirect interactions with the NMDA receptor complex. Targeted therapies that diminish spinal dynorphin in these pain states may potentially ameliorate painful symptoms.

Potential targets could also include modulation of receptor expression (e.g., transcriptional signals/regulators, endocytosis modulators). Some investigators and clinicians have attempted to contrast the relatively rapid endocytotic receptor internalization of fentanyl with morphine (in which internalization is so slow the receptor just seems to sit there on the external membrane side), and they use this contrasting behavior as an explanation of why fentanyl produces less constipation than morphine; however, there are many complex issues, and so the behavior difference in internalization cannot be used to clearly explain clinical differences.

Morphine-induced tolerance does not necessarily involve receptor endocytosis; all opioids lead to some degree of tolerance within various clinical parameters. Morphine seems to require longer exposures and the presence of adequate amounts of B-arrestin-2; however, with these two conditions being met, morphine will eventually lead to MOR endocytosis.[78] It is certainly possible that when opioid receptor reserve is reduced (e.g., altered fractional receptor occupancy) agonist-dependent μ-receptor endocytosis could contribute to regulation of μ-opioid receptor responsiveness to ligand stimulation.[78] This certainly could represent a potential target to affect the responsiveness of receptors. Some therapies may aim to alter inflammatory mediators, cytokines, growth factors, and free radicals in an indirect fashion by attempting to locally modulate the neutrophil accumulation at the painful site (FIGURE 4).

HISTAMINE IN PAIN AND PAIN CONTROL

Histamine is a mediator released from peripheral mast cells as well as the CNS neurons.[79] The release of histamine in the skin following injury is known to result in activation of afferent fibers through the H_1 receptor. This results in the "flare" response (vasodilation in nearby areas that is mediated by the interplay of nerves and mast cells) and also stimulates itching. Specific subsets of primary afferents[80] and spinothalamic lamina I neurons[81] are thought to contribute to itch.

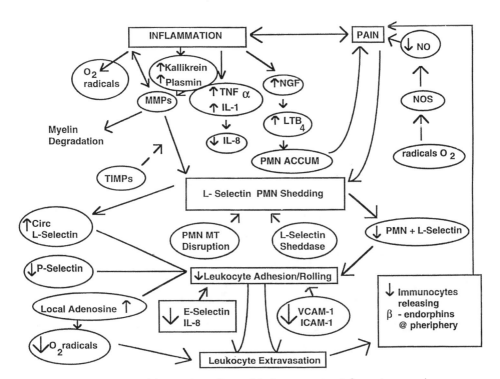

Figure 4. Potential therapeutic mediators of the immune system inflammatory cascade.

In the brainstem, histamine is able to activate antinociceptive (pain-relieving) responses through an action on both H_1 and H_2 receptors.[82,83] Inhibitors of brain histamine breakdown also have analgesic activity,[84] but histamine-releasing drugs such as H_3 antagonists lack this activity.[85] H_1 antagonists block histamine analgesia, but these drugs also have their own analgesic properties, depending on the test and the species. It is not clear to what extent these effects represent actions at peripheral versus CNS H_1 receptors.[79] It is clear that brain H_2 receptor activation is an important component of both opioid and stress-induced nonopioid pain-relieving responses.[86–90]

In doses larger than those needed to block histamine receptors, several (but not all) H_2 and H_3 antagonists induce powerful morphine-like pain relief when injected directly into the brain.[91,92] The prototype analgesic discovered in these studies, called improgan, is derived from the H_2 antagonist cimetidine. In contrast with cimetidine, however, improgan lacks activity at over 50 receptors, including all known histamine and opioid receptors.[93] Chemical derivatives of histamine also induce improgan-like analgesia, suggesting the possibility that these drugs act at an unknown histamine receptor, but this has not been established.[94]

CONCLUSION

Numerous stimuli exist, leading to potential hyperalgesia, and there is complex interplay between various mediators. The simple cartoon in FIGURE 5 displays some of the mechanisms as well as the interplay that may lead to hyperalgesia in inflammation. The patient's recent history, current receptor status (e.g., phosphorylated or dephosphorylated), and local environ-

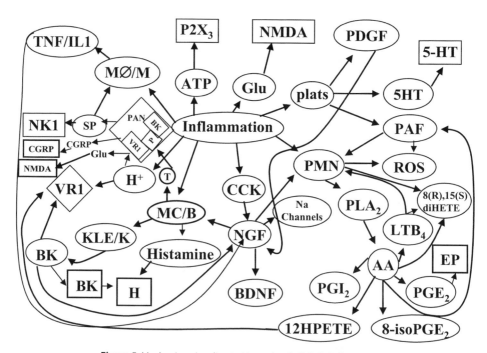

Figure 5. Mechanisms Leading to Hyperalgesia/Pain in Inflammation

ment of receptors may be extremely important in determining the actions of various receptor activation. A delicate balance between the subunit activity of Gs versus $G_{i/0}$ may help modulate nociceptive signals. Additionally, the state of the G proteins are important. The C-terminal tail of the G protein is phosphorylated by G protein–related kinase and, when complexed with a larger unit such as B-arrestin, undergoes endocytic internalization. A constituitive down-regulation process occurs at a low level constantly, and an inducible (mostly via PKCα) down-regulation process also occurs. Once this internalization occurs, receptors and G proteins are recycled; however, they do not all come back (some are degraded). These processes may be extremely important in a patient with chronic pain on long-term medications.

As multiple events transpire in the periphery contributing to nociceptive input, future peripheral analgesic cocktails administered at the site of peripheral tissue injury (e.g., in knee joint after arthroscopy) may include opioids, local anesthetics, α-agonists, VR1 antagonists, inhibitors of CB1/CB2, lipoxygenase inhibitors, and inhibitors of nitric oxide synthase/nitric oxide. Iodoresiniferatoxin is a new potent vanilloid receptor antagonist that may have analgesic utility in the future.[95] Civamide (cis-capsaicin) may have potential as a therapeutic alternative for the treatment of cluster headaches.

REFERENCES FOR ADDITIONAL READING

1. Craig AD, Dostrovsky JO: Medulla to thalamus. In: Wall PD, Melzack R, eds: Textbook of Pain, 4th ed. Limited, London, Churchill Livingston/Harcourt Publishers, 1999.
2. Craig AD, Bushnell MC, Zhang E-T, et al: A thalamic nucleus specific for pain and temperature sensation. Nature 372:770–773, 1994.
3. Melzack R, Casey KL: Sensory motivational, and central control determinants of pain. In: Kenshalo DR, ed: The Skin Senses. Springfield, IL, 1968, pp 423–443.
4. Craig AD, Reiman EM, Evans A, et al: Functional imaging of an illusion of pain. Nature 384:258–260, 1996.
5. Stenholm E, Bongenhielm U, Ahlquist M, et al: VR1 and VRL-1-like immunoreactivity in normal and injured trigeminal dental primary sensory neurons of the rat. Acta Odontol Scand 60:72–79, 2002.
6. Trevisani M, Smart D, Gunthorpe MJ, et al: Ethanol elicits and potentiates nociceptor responses via the vanilloid receptor-1. Nat Neurosci 5:546–551, 2002.
7. Nishihara K, Nozawa Y, Nakano M, et al: Sensitizing effects of lafutidine on CGRP containing afferent nerves in the rat stomach. Br J Pharmacol 135:1487–1494, 2002.
8. Black JA, Dib-Hajj, Cummins TR, et al: Sodium channels as therapeutic targets in neuropathic pain. In: Hansson PT, Fields HL, Hill RG, Marchettini P, eds: Neuropathic Pain: Pathophysiology and Treatment, Progress in Pain Research and Management, Vo. 21. Seattle, IASP Press, 2001.
9. Cummins TR, Waxman SG: Downregulation of tetrodotoxin-resistant sodium currents and up-regulations of a rapidly repriming tetrodotoxin-sensitive sodium current in small spinal sensory neurons after nerve injury. J Neurosci 17:3503–3514, 1997.
10. Porreca F, Lai J, DiBian, Wegert S, et al: A comparison of the potential role of the tetrodotoxin-insensitive sodium channels, PN3/SNS and NaN/SNS2, in rat models of chronic pain. Proc Natl Acad Sci U S A 96:7640–7644, 1999.
11. Kerr B, Souslova V, McMahon S, et al: A role for the TTX-resistant sodium channel NaV1.8 in NGF-induced hyperalgesia, but not neuropathic pain. Neuroreport 12:3077–3080, 2001.
12. Black JA, Cummins TY, Plumpton C, et al: Upregulation of a previously silent sodium channel in axotomized DRG neurons. J Neurophysiol 82:2776 – 2785, 1999.
13. Lai J, Gold M, Kim C-S, et al: Inhibition of neuropathic pain by decreased expression of the tetrodotoxin – resistant sodium channel NaV18. Pain 95:143–152, 2002.

14. Kim SH, Chung JM: An experimental model for peripheral neuropathy produced by segmental spinal nerve ligation in the rat. Pain 50:355–364, 1992.

15. Waxman SG, Cummins TR, Dib-Hajj SD, et al: Voltage-gated sodium channels and the molecular pathogenesis of pain. J Rehab Res 3:517–529, 2000.

16. Bowery NG, Bettler B, Froestl W, et al: International Union of Pharmacology XXXIII. Mammalian gamma–aminobutyric acid (B) receptors: Structure and function. Pharmacol Rev 54:247–264, 2002.

17. Bordeau LA: GABA transporter heterogeneity: pharmacology and cellular localization. Neurochem Int 29:335–356, 1996.

18. Meldrum BD, Chapman AG: Basic mechanisms of gabitril (Tiagabine) and future potential developments. Epilepsia 40:52–56, 1999.

19. Harvey PK, Bradford HF, Davison AN: The inhibitory effect of sodium n-dipropyl acetate on the degenerative enzymes of the GABA shunt. FEBS Lett 52:251–254, 1975.

20. Andersen KE, Lau L, Lundt BF, et al: Synthesis of novel GABA uptake inhibitors. Part 6: preparation and evaluation of N-omega asymmetrically substitued nipecotic acid derivatives. Bioorg Med Chem 9:2773–2785, 2001.

21. Malan TP, Mata HP, Porreca F: Spinal GABA A and GABA(B) receptor pharmacology in a rat model of neuropathic pain. Anesthesiology 96:1161–1167, 2002.

22. Kawamata T, Omote K, Toriyable M, et al: Intracerebroventricular morphine produces antinociception by evoking aminobutyric acid release through activation of 5-hydroxytryptamine 3 receptors in the spinal cord. Anesthesiology 96:1175–1182, 2002.

23. Kontinen VK, Standa LC, Basu A, et al: Electrophysiologic evidence for increased endogenous GABAergic but not glycinergic inhibitory tone in the rat spinal nerve ligation model of neuropathy. Anesthesiology 94:333–339, 2001.

24. Dickenson AH, Chapman V, Green GM: The pharamacology of excitatory and inhibitory amino acid-mediated events in the transmission and modulation of pain in the spinal cord. Gen Pharmacol 28:633–638, 1997.

25. Kontinen V, Dickenson A: Effects of midazolam in the spinal nerve ligatioon model of neuropathic pain in rats. Pain 85:425–431, 2000.

26. Mertens P, Ghaeemmaghami C, Bert L, et al: Amino acids in spinal dorsal horn of patients during surgery for neuropathic pain or spasticity. Neuroreport 11:1795–1798, 2000.

27. Gohil K, Bell JR. Ramachandran J, et al: Neuroanatomical distribution of receptors for a novel voltage-sensitive calcium-channel antagonist. SNX-230 (omega-conopeptive MVIIC). Brain Res 653:258–266, 1994.

28. Olivera BM, Milijanich GP, Ramachandran J, et al: Calcium channel diversity and neurotransmitter release: The omega-conotoxins and omega-agatoxins. Annu Rev Biochem 63:823–867, 1994.

29. Westenbroek RE, Hoskins L, Carrerall WA: Localization of Ca2+ channel subtypes on rat spinal motor neurons, interneurons, and nerve terminals. J Neurosci 18:6319–6330, 1998.

30. Dickenson AH, Matthews EA, Suzuki R: Central nervous system mechanisms of pain in peripheral neuropathy. In: Hansson PT, Fields HL, Hill RG, Marchettini P, eds. Neuropathic Pain: Pathophysiology and Treatment, Progress in Pain Research and Management, vol 21. Seattle, IASP Press 2002, pp 85–106.

31. Bowersox SS, Gadbois T, Singh T, et al: Selective N-type neuronal voltage-sensitive calcium channel blocker, SNX-111, produces spinal antinociception in rat models of acute, persistent and neuropathic pain. J Pharmacol Exp Ther 279:1243–1249, 1996.

32. Horvath G, Brodacz B, Holzer-Petsche U: Role of calcium channels in the spinal transmission of nociceptive information from the mesentery. Pain 93:35–41, 2001.

33. Sluka KA: Blockade of calcium channels can prevent the onset of secondary hyperalgesia and allodynia induced by intradermal injection of capsaicin in rats. Pain 71:157–164, 1997.

34. Sluka KA: Blockade of N- and P/Q-type calcium channels reduces the secondary heat hyperalgesia induced by acute inflammation. J Pharmacol Exp Ther 287:232–237, 1998.

35. Huguenard JR: Low-threshold calcium currents in central nervous system neurons. Annu Rev Physiol 58:329–348, 1996.

36. Liu C-N, Michaelis M, Amir R, Devor M: spinal nerve injury enhances subthreshold membrane potential oscillations in DRG neurons: Relation to neuropathic pain. J Neurophysiol 84:205–215, 2000.

37. Sidach SS, Mintz IM: Kurtoxin, agating modifiers of neuronal high and low–threshold Ca channels. J Neurosci 22:2023–2034, 2002.

38. Kamei J, Zushida K, Morita K, et al: Role of canilloid VR1 receptor in thermal allodynia and hyperalgia in diabetic mice. Eur J Pharmacol 422:83–86, 2001.

39. Tohada, Seraki M, Kanemura T, et al: Axonal transport of VR 1 capsaicin receptor mRNA in primary afferents and its participation in inflammation induced increase in capsaicin sensitivty. J Neurochem 76:1628–1635, 2001.

40. Hudson LJ, Bevan S, Wotherspoon G, et al: VR1 protein expression increases in undamaged DRG neurons after partial nerve injury. Eur J Neurosci 13:2105–2114, 2001.

41. Abbracchio MP, Burnstock G: Purinergic signalling: Pathophysiologic roles. Jpn J Pharmacol 78: 113–145, 1998.

42. Tominaga M, Wada M, Masu M: Potentiation of capsaicin receptor activity by metabotropic ATP receptors as a possible mechanism for ATP-evoked pain and hyperalgesia. Proc Natl Acad Sci U S A 98:6951–6956, 2001.

43. Cesare P, Moriondo A, Vellani V, et al: Ion channels gated by heat. Proc Natl Acad Sci U S A 96; 7658–7663, 1999.

44. Numazaki M, Tominaga T, Toyooka H, et al: Direct phosphorylation of capsaicin receptor VR1 by protein kinase C episilon and identification of two target serine residues. J Biol Chem 277:13378–13378, 2002.

45. Caterina MJ, Rosen TA, Tominga M, et al: A capsaicin-receptor homologue with a high threshold for noxious heat. Nature 398:436–441, 1999.

46. Morisset V, Ahluwalia J, Nagy I, et al: Possible mechanisms of cannabinoid-induced antinociception in the spinal cord. Eur J Pharmacol 429:93–100, 2001.

47. Jordt SE, Tominaga M, Julius D: Acid potentiation of the capsaicin receptor determined by a key extracellular site. Proc Natl Acad Sci U S A 97;8134–8139, 2000.

48. Dedov VN, Roufogalis BD: Mitochondrial calcium accumulation following activation of vanilloid (VR1) receptors by capsaicin in dorsal root ganglion neurons. Neuroscience 95:183–188, 2000.

49. Honore P, Mikusa J, Bianchi B, et al: TNP-ATP, a potent P2X(3) receptor antagonist, blocks acetic acid–induced abdominal constriction in mice: Comparison with reference analgesics. Pain 96:99–105, 2002.

50. Caterina MJ, Leffler A, Malmberg AB, et al: Impaired nociception and pain sensation in mice lacking the capsaicin receptor. Science 288:306–313, 2000.

51. Tominaga M, Caterina MJ, Malmberg AB, et al: The cloned capsaicin receptor integrates multiple pain-producing stimuli. Neuron 21:3;531–543, 1998.

52. Hwang SW, Cho H, Kwak J, et al: Direct activation of capsaicin receptors by products of lipoxygenases: Endogenous capsaicin-like substances. Proc Natl Acad Sci U S A 97;6155–6160, 2000.

53. Premkumar LA, Ahern GP: Induction of vanilloid receptor channel activity by protein kinase C. Nature 408:985–990, 2000.

54. Gauldie SD, McQueen DS, Pertwee R, et al: Anandamide activates peripheral nociceptors in normal and arthritic rat knee joints. Br J Pharmacol 132:617–621, 2001.

55. Tominaga M, Julius D: Capsaicin receptor in the pain pathway [review]. Jpn J Pharmacol 83:20–24, 2000.

56. Smart D, Gunthorpe MJ, Jerman JC, et al: The endogenous lipid anandamide is a full agonist at the human vanilloid receptor (Hvr1). Br J Pharmacol 129:227–230, 2000.

57. Szallasi A: Vanilloid receptor ligands: Hope and realities for the future. Drugs Aging 18:561–573, 2001.

58. Smart D, Jonsson KO, Vandevoorde S, et al: "Entourage": Effects of N-acetyl ethanolamines at human vanilloid receptors. Comparison of effects upon anandamide–induced vanilloid receptor activation and upon anandamide metabolism. Br J Pharmacol 136:452–458, 2002.

59. Howlett AC: The CB1 cannabinoid receptor in the brain. Neurobiol Dis 5:405–416, 1998.

60. DiMarzo V, Griffin G, De Petrocellis L, et al: A structure/activity relationship study on orvanil, an endocannabinoid and vanilloid hybrid. J Pharmacol Exp Ther 300:984–991, 2002.

61. Jarvis MF, Yu H, McGaraughty S, et al: Analgesic and anti-inflammatory effects of A-286501, a novel orally active adenosine kinease inhibitor. Pain 96:107–118, 2002.

62. Reeve AJ, Dickenson AH: The roles of spinal adenosine receptors in the control for acute and more persistent nociceptive responses of dorsal horn neurons in the anaesthetized rat. Br J Pharmacol 116:2221–2228, 1995.

63. Khalil Z, Liu T, Helme RD: Free radicals contribute to the reduction in peripheral vascular responses and the maintenance of thermal hyperalgesia in rats with chronic constriction injury. Pain 79:31–37, 1999.

64. Pan H-L, Chen SR, Eisenach JC: Role of spinal nitric oxide in antiallodynic effect of intrathecal clonidine in neuropathic rats. Anesthesiology 89:1518–1523, 1998.

65. Song HK, Pan H-L, Eisenach JC: Spinal nitric oxide mediates antinociception from IV morphine. Anesthesiology 89:215–221, 1998.

66. Hampson AJ, Grimaldi M, Axelrod J, et al: Cannabidiol and (−)9-tetrahydrocannabinol and neuroprotective antioxidants. Natl Acad Sci 95:8286–8273, 1998.

67. Calignano A, La Rana G, Giuffrida A, et al: Control of pain initiation by endogenous cannabinoids. Nature 394:277–281, 1998.

68. Nagamatsu M, Nickander KK, Schmelzer JD, et al: Lipoic acid improves nerve blood flow, reduces oxidatice stress, and improves distal nerve conduction in experimental diabetic neuropathy. Diabetes Care 18:1160–1167, 1995.

69. Ziegler D, Hanefeld M, Ruhnau KJ, et al: Treatment of symptomatic diabetic peripheral neuropathy with the antioxidant α-lipoic acid: A 3-week multicenter randomized controlled trial (ALADIN study). Diabetologia 38:1425–1433, 1995.

70. Mantyh PW, Rogers SD, Honore P, et al: Inhibition of hyperalgesia by ablation of lamina I spinal neurons expressing the substance P receptor. Science 278:275–279, 1997.

71. Bannon AW, Decker MW, Hollada MW, et al: Broad-spectrum, non-opioid analgesia activity by selective modulation of neuronal nicotinic acetylcholine receptors. Science 279:77–81, 1998.

72. Smith H: Neuropathic pain mechanisms and potential future pharmacotherapeutic strategies. Cur Rev Pain 2:217–219, 1998.

73. Abdi S, Vilassova N, Decosterd I, et al: The effects of KRN5500, a spicamycin derivative, on neuropathic and nociceptive pain models in rats. Anesth Analg 91:955–959, 2000.

74. Erba F, Fiorucci L, Pascarella S, et al: Selective inhibition of human mast cell tryptase by gabexate mesylate, and antiproteinase drug. Biochem Pharmacol 61:271–276, 2001.

75. Zhou QL, Strichartz G, Davar G: Endothelin-1 activates ET (A) receptors to increase intracellular calcium in model sensory neurons. Neruoreport 12:3853–3857, 2001.

76. Davar G, Hans G, Fareed MU, et al: Behavioral signs of acute pain produced by application of endothelin–1 to rat sciatic nerve. Neuroreport 9:2279–2283, 1998.

77. Malan TP, Ossipav MH, Gardell LR, et al: Extraterriotorial neuropathic pain correlates with multi-segmental elevation of spinal dynorphin in nerve-injured rats. Pain 86:185–194, 2002.

78. Sternini C, Brecha NC, Minnis J, et al: Role of agonist-dependent receptor internalization in the regulation of mu opioid receptrs. Neuroscience 98:233–241, 2000.

79. Hough LB, Leurs R: Structure and Function of GPCRs in the Nervous System. Oxford, Oxford University Press, 2002.

80. Schmelz M: Itch: Mediators and mechanisms. J Dermatol Sci 28:91–96, 2002.

81. Andrew D, Craig AD: Spinothalamic lamina I neurones selectively responsive to cutaneous warming in cats. J Physiol 537:489–495, 2001.

82. Glick SD, Crane LA: Opiate-like and abstinence-like effects of intracerebral histamine administration in rats. Nature 273:547–549, 1978.

83. Thoburn KK, Hough LB, Nalwalk JW, Mischler SA: Histamine-induced modulation of nociceptive responses. Pain 58:29–37, 1994.

84. Malmberg-Aiello P, Lamberti C, Ipponi A, et al: Effects of two histamine-N-methyltransferase inhibitors, SKF 91488 and BW 301U, in rodent antinociception. Naunyn Schmiedebergs Arch Pharmacol 355:354–360, 1997.

85. Li BY, Nalwalk JW, Barker LA, et al: Characterization of the antinociceptive properties of cimetidine and a structural analog. J Pharmacol Exp Ther 276:500–508, 1996.

86. Barke KE, Hough LB: Characterization of basal and morphine-induced histamine release in the rat periaqueductal gray. J Neurochem 63:238–244, 1994.

87. Hough LB, Nalwalk JW: Modulation of morphine antinociception by antagonism of H_2 receptors in the periaqueductal gray. Brain Res 588:58–66, 1992.

88. Hough LB, Nalwalk JW, Battles AM: Zolantidine-induced attenuation of morphine antinociception in rhesus monkeys. Brain Res 526:153–155, 1990.

89. Gogas KR, Hough LB, Eberle NB, et al: A role for histamine and H_2 receptors in opioid antinociception. J Pharmacol Exp Ther 250:476–484, 1989.

90. Gogas KR, Hough LB: Inhibition of naloxone-resistant antinociception by centrally-administered H_2 antagonists. J Pharmacol Exp Ther 248:262–267, 1989.

91. Hough LB, Nalwalk JW, Barnes WG, et al: A third life for burimamide: Discovery and characterization of a novel class of non-opioid analgesics derived from histamine antagonists. In: Glick SD, Maisonneuve IM, eds. New Medications for Drug Abuse New York, New York Academy of Science, 2000, pp 25–40.

92. Hough LB, Nalwalk JW, Li BY, et al: Novel qualitative structure-activity relationships for the antinociceptive actions of H2 antagonists, H3 antagonists and derivatives. J Pharmacol Exp Ther 283:1534–1543, 1997.

93. Hough LB, Nalwalk JW, Barnes WG, et al: A third legacy for burimamide: Discovery and characterization of improgan and a new class of non-opioid analgesics derived from histamine antagonists. In: Watanabe T, Timmerman H, Yanai K, eds. Histamine Research in the New Millenium Elsevier, Amsterdam, 2001, pp 237–242.

94. Hough LB, Nalwalk JW, Leurs R, et al: Antinociceptive activity of impentamine, a histamine congener, after CNS administration. Life Sci 64:PL79–PL86, 1999.

95. Wahl P, Foged C, Tullin S, et al: Iodo-resiniferatoxin, a new potent vallinoid receptor anatagonist. Mol Pharmacol 59:9–15, 2001.

Chapter 34

Analgesic Use in Acute Pain Management

Andreas Grabinsky, MD / Mark V. Boswell, MD, PhD

BASIC CONSIDERATIONS

Acute pain provides a warning of impending or actual tissue injury. Heeding the warning may prevent further tissue damage. Over time, as the normal healing process occurs, the injury usually becomes less painful. Conventional wisdom suggests that there may be a survival advantage afforded by the acute pain system. This advantage is evident in the rare individual who lacks nociceptive fibers that transduce painful stimuli. Many pain-producing injuries are not caused by accidents, however, but willfully during the course of surgeries or other medical procedures. In these cases, acute pain does not serve any useful therapeutic purpose because the cause of the pain is well defined. Obvious causes of acute pain include tissue injury to skin, muscles, bones, and joints; distention or stretch of hollow abdominal or pelvic organs; and irritation of pleura and peritoneum. Painful conditions not caused specifically by otherwise well-intentioned therapeutic endeavors also may occur postoperatively, including sickle cell pain, headache, herpes zoster, renal colic, ischemic pain, gallstones, gastritis, and esophagitis. In most of these cases, a diagnosis is established quickly.

After surgery, untreated or poorly treated pain may impede the healing process and increase the risk of other medical problems, such as myocardial infarction, congestive heart failure, and infection. Pain has a negative influence on multiple organ systems. The reflex responses to acute pain are responsible for increased catecholamine and cortisol levels, which are manifestations of a hypermetabolic state, with protein catabolism, gluconeogenesis, lipolysis, and hypercoagulability. Pain also negatively affects the immune system, which makes patients with acute pain more prone to postoperative infections. Muscle tone is increased, resulting in higher oxygen demands. Stimulation of the sympathetic system causes hypertension, tachycardia, increased cardiac workload, and a higher cardiac oxygen demand. This negative influence on the cardiovascular system, especially in older patients with underlying coronary or cerebral artery disease, increases the risk of perioperative ischemia, myocardial infarction, and stroke.

Postoperative pain after upper abdominal and thoracic surgery can result in reduced vital capacity, tidal volume, residual volume, and functional residual capacity and an increased respiratory rate. Pain secondary to thoracic or abdominal procedures results in a guarding and muscle splinting, the so-called positive pillow sign, where the patient sits in a half-upright position in bed, pressing a pillow against the abdomen. Such patients are at increased risk for pulmonary complications, such as atelectasis, decreased clearance of bronchial secretions, pneumonia, and respiratory failure. Patients who are not able to get out of bed because of pain are at risk for deep venous thrombosis and possible pulmonary embolism. Adverse effects of acute pain also may affect the cost of health care, in the form of prolonged hospital stays and more frequent readmissions to the hospital because of pain or related complications.

The importance of treating pain is underscored by the standards on pain management developed by the Joint Commission on Accreditation of Healthcare Organizations (JCAHO).[3] Pain management now is recognized as a patient right: "Health care facilities now must recognize the right of patients to appropriate assessment and management of pain; identify pain in patients during their initial assessment and, where required, during ongoing, periodic reassessments; and educate patients and their families about pain management."

The physiologic consequences of poorly treated pain are well defined[10] and frequently cited as reasons for providing pain management. As addressed by the JCAHO standards,[3] humanitarian issues mandate quality pain medicine. Good pain management is a relatively simple endeavor, with the proper tools. The basic skills needed to provide competent pain management include the commitment to provide good medical care, the ability to assess a patient's medical condition and include the patient in the decision-making process, a basic understanding of analgesic pharmacology, and the willingness to titrate a few good analgesics to achieve satisfactory pain relief.

Achieving satisfactory pain relief requires some sort of pain measuring scale, against which the success of therapy can be gauged. A typical scale used on rounds is the *verbal analog scale*, a modification of the visual analog scale used in research, with 0 being no pain and 10 being the worst pain imaginable. Either scale is satisfactory, but the verbal scale is easier to administer on rounds (but may have less scientific value). Examples of printed scales and pain rulers are available in textbooks on pain management. It is appropriate to ask about pain on rounds and in the clinic. The clinician should make sure that his or her institution has adopted some form of pain measurement tool or standard. Although some patients may not be able to understand the pain scale, with creative questioning the clinician should be able to determine whether or not a patient is in excruciating pain. After determining the pain score, the findings should be documented in the patient's medical record.

Satisfactory pain relief implies that pain is at a level agreeable to the patient. This also means that the patient has been informed adequately as to what good pain control is. Good pain control is a pain level that has minimal effects on physiologic functions and does not impair activities of daily living. If the patient can watch television, talk on the telephone, and do a crossword puzzle, it is safe to say that pain is not at a level of 8 to 10. Pain still may be at a level of 4 or 5, however. Reducing the pain level to less than 4 is a reasonable goal. Complete pain relief usually is not necessary or appropriate because pain relief does come at a cost. Although subtherapeutic doses of morphine usually do not cause clinically significant respiratory depression in healthy patients, aggressive doses of morphine may impair breathing in a feeble patient or one with chronic obstructive pulmonary disease. The clinician should be on the *conservative* side when titrating pain relief. Another dose of morphine always can be given, but it may be awkward to have to give a dose of naloxone. (Do not hesitate to titrate naloxone to effect when needed, starting with 0.04 mg. An emergency department dose of naloxone of 0.4 mg is seldom warranted.)

Pain management begins with the history and physical examination. Taking the *pain history* is similar to taking other components of the medical history. The first questions asked should inquire about the characteristics of the pain, including location, quality (e.g., sharp, dull, aching, throbbing, burning), duration, and modifying factors. The past medical and surgical history should be reviewed to identify conditions that may interfere with pain management, such as pulmonary disease, renal insufficiency, or hepatic disease. Previous back surgery may make epidural catheter placement more difficult, but usually is only an inconvenience. More importantly, how a patient responded to a previous surgery may provide clues to how the patient will fare this time around. A patient who has had previous surgery may help plan appropriate pain management; the clinician should not miss the opportunity to gain from the patient's previous experience.

There is no *pain-free* surgery, and even an operation performed for pain control (such as a total knee arthroplasty) takes some time to show results. It happens quite often that patients who were on large doses of opioids before surgery receive a *standard* patient-controlled analgesia (PCA) order by the surgery intern for postoperative pain control. In such cases it is not long until the Pain Service is called because "the PCA is not working" or the patient is perceived as a potential drug abuser.

After surgery, acute postoperative pain not only is normal, but also is easy to identify and treat. New-onset acute pain or exacerbation of preexisting acute pain must be evaluated for a possible underlying cause, however, distinct from the expected postoperative condition. This statement seems obvious, but in some cases the only action taken in response to an acute pain exacerbation is to call the Pain Service. In such instances, the tendency may be just to increase the PCA dose. This action may delay the diagnosis of an underlying problem, such as a perforated viscus, wound infection, or abscess. It is unlikely, however, that the analgesic would mask the underlying problem completely when the physician is attentive to the patient's condition.

It is still a common misconception that a patient in acute pain should not receive pain medications until the underlying medical or surgical condition is diagnosed. Even with an acute, life-threatening medical or surgical crisis, every patient deserves reasonable attempts at pain control. In ancient times, when a correct diagnosis relied solely on the physical examination (and the physician's ability to reproduce the pain with palpation), withholding pain medication might have been an acceptable practice. Today, it is unlikely that appendicitis would be diagnosed solely on the physical examination, without a complete blood, and computed tomography scan or ultrasound of the abdomen. If there is any doubt about the effects of the analgesics, opioids are reversed easily with low doses of naloxone.

The physical examination must include vital signs (blood pressure, heart rate, respiratory rate, temperature, pulse oximetry reading), pain score, auscultation of the heart and lungs, and a focused examination including a look at the surgical dressing and a check of the intravenous catheter and the epidural catheter. Follow-up visits should include vital signs; pain score; description of improvement regarding pain, mobility, or psychological condition; an overall impression; and the formulation of a treatment plan. All changes in the treatment plan should be explained either in the progress note or by directly contacting the primary service responsible for the patient (i.e., the intern). The goals and plan of care should be discussed with the patient, and appropriate instructions should be given. The patient should be followed daily or twice daily as guided by his or her condition. If pain control is not optimal, appropriate steps must be taken to diagnose and treat the pain.

Mild-to-moderate pain may be treated with a nonsteroidal anti-inflammatory drug (NSAID) such as ibuprofen or acetaminophen (considered to be an NSAID for this discussion). If the patient is unable to take oral medications, ketorolac, 15 to 30 mg intravenously every 6 hours for 3 to 5 days, may be used. If treatment with an NSAID is insufficient to control the pain (which is often the case), an opioid should be added. Fixed combination drugs, such as acetaminophen and hydrocodone or oxycodone, may be used to supplement the NSAID. Alternatively an opioid preparation may be used first, particularly if there is concern about bleeding or hematoma formation. The analgesic effects of opioids and NSAIDs are at least additive. Adult doses of NSAIDs are shown in Table 1 and equianalgesic doses of opioids in Table 2.[2]

With moderate-to-severe pain, which is expected after major abdominal and thoracic sur-

TABLE 1

NSAIDs: Dosing Data for Adult Patients

Drug	Usual Adult Dose	Comments
Oral NSAIDs		
Acetaminophen	650–975 mg q 4h	Acetaminophen lacks the peripheral antiinflammatory activity of other NSAIDs
Aspirin	650–975 mg q 4 h	The standard against which other NSAIDs are compared. Inhibits platelet aggregation; may cause postoperative bleeding
Choline magnesium trisalicylate (Trilisate)	1,000–1,500 mg bid	May have minimal antiplatelet activity; also available as oral liquid
Celecoxib	100 qd to Bid	COX-2 selective NSAID with improved platelet and gastrointestinal profile
Diflunisal (Dolobid)	1,000 mg initial dose followed by 500 mg q12 h	Equivalent in strength to codeine, 60 mg, plus acetaminophen; fewer platelet effects than aspirin
Etodolac (Lodine)	200–400 mg q6–8 h	
Fenoprofen calcium (Nalfon)	200 mg q4–6 h	
Ibuprofen (Motrin, others)	400 mg q4–6 h	Available as several brand names and as generic; also available as oral suspension
Ketoprofen (Orudis)	25–75 mg q6–8 h	
Magnesium salicylate	650 mg q4h	Many brands and generic forms available
Naproxen (Naprosyn)	500 mg initial dose followed by 250 mg q6–8h	Also available as oral liquid
Naproxen sodium (Anaprox)	550 mg initial dose followed by 275 mg q6–8h	
Relecoxib	25 mg qd	COX-2-selective NSAID; approved for acute pain (25 mg bid for 5 d)
Salsalate (Disalcid, others)	500 mg q4h	May have minimal antiplatelet activity
Sodium salicylate	325–650 mg q3–4h	Available in generic form from several distributors
Parenteral NSAID		
Ketorolac tromethamine (Toradol)	30 or 60 mg IM/IV initial dose followed by 15 or 30 mg q6hr. Oral dose following IM dosage: 10 mg q6–8h	Use not to exceed 5 days

NSAIDs, nonsteroidal anti-inflammatory drugs; COX-2, cycloxygenase-2.

Modified from Carr DB, Jacox AK, Chapman RC, et al: Clinical Practice Guideline: Acute Pain Management: Operative or Medical Procedures and Trauma. Rockville, MD: Agency for Health Care Policy and Research, U.S. Department of Health and Human Services, 1992.

geries, higher doses of pure opioid agonists, such as morphine or oxycodone, must be used. The decision to use an oral or parenteral opioid depends on whether the patient can tolerate oral medications. The intravenous route of administration is not always better, but parenteral dosing achieves therapeutic blood levels more rapidly. In some cases, it may be more expeditious to use a PCA pump, after calculating the opioid dosage likely to provide adequate pain relief, to get the pain under control as fast as possible. When using a PCA pump (discussed in detail subsequently) the loading dose (also called a *bolus dose*) must not be forgotten. This is equivalent to giving a loading dose of esmolol before starting an esmolol infusion; the infusion will not

TABLE 2

Opioids: Dosing Data for Adult Patients

	Approximate Equianalgesic Doses		Recommended Starting Dose (Adults Weighing > 50 kg)	
	Oral	Parenteral	Oral	Parenteral
Opioid agonist Drug				
Morphine	30 mg q3–4h	10 mg q3–4h	30 mg q3–4h	10 mg q3–4h
Codeine	130 mg q3–4h	75 mg q3–4h	60 mg q3–4h	60 mg q2h (IM/SC)
Hydromophone (Dilaudid)	7.5 mg q3–4h	1.5 mg q3–4h	6 mg q3–4h	1.5 mg q3–4h
Hydrocodone (in Lorcet, Lortab, Vicodin, others)	30 mg q3–4h	Not available	10 mg q3–4h	Not available
Levorphanol (Levo-Dromoran)	4 mg q6–8h	2 mg q6–8h	4 mg q6–8h	2 mg q6–8h
Meperidine* (Demerol)	300 mg q2–3h	100 mg q3h	Not recommended	100 mg q3h
Oxycodone (Roxicodone; also in Percocet, Percodan, Tylox)	15–20 mg q3–4h	Not available	10 mg q3–4h	Not available
Opioid agonist-antagonist and partial agonist				
Buprenorphine (Buprenex)	Not available	0.3–0.4 mg q6–8h	Not available	0.4 mg q6–8h
Butorphanol (Stadol)	Not available	2 mg q3–4h	Not available	2 mg q3–4h
Nalbuphine (Nubain)	Not available	10 mg q3–4h	Not available	10 mg q3–4h
Pentazocine (Talwin, others)	150 mg q3–4h	60 mg q3–4h	50 mg q4–6h	Not recommended

Note: The oral to parenteral ratio of morphine with long-term dosing is 3:1. The oral-to-parenteral ratio for hydromorphone is 5:1.

*See caveats with imeperidine, listed in Table 35–3.

Modified from Carr DB, Jacox AK, Chapman RC, et al: Clinical Practice Guideline: Acute Pain Management: Operative or Medical Procedures and Trauma. Rockville MD: Agency for Health Care Policy and Research, U.S. Department of Health and Human Services, 1992.

achieve a therapeutic blood level without a loading dose. Severe pain requires the early use of potent opioids, preferably by the intravenous route, although an NSAID should be included in the treatment regimen for its additive effect, as long as there is no contraindication.

Intramuscular administration should be avoided because injections hurt. Arguments also can be made that drug uptake is unpredictable after intramuscular injection. In any case, there is little to recommend the routine use of intramuscular injections for pain management. Subcutaneous infusions may be useful, when intravenous access is unavailable or impractical (e.g., opioid infusions for hospice patients). Uptake of morphine, hydromorphone, and fentanyl is predictable with subcutaneous injection, and concentrated solutions may be used for continuous infusions (e.g., morphine or hydromorphone at $\geq$ 10 mg/mL).

A note of caution is necessary regarding controlled-release formulations of opioids (e.g., MS Contin, Oramorph, OxyContin, and Duragesic) for acute pain management. Controlled-release opioids are not recommended during the first 24 hours after surgery because dose requirements are not well defined in the early postoperative period. Opioid requirements generally decrease over time. Thereafter, it may be reasonable to consider a long-acting opioid, to avoid the peaks and valleys in blood levels associated with immediate-release formulations, if the patient will require an opioid for more than a few days. Fentanyl patches are not recommended for postoperative pain management in opioid-naive patients because of the long apparent half-life of the release system. If a patient was receiving a controlled-release opioid before surgery, however, continuation of the controlled-release drug may be appropriate. (See subsequent section regarding patients taking long-term opioids.) The student and experienced physician alike should refer to current textbooks for more detailed information regarding drugs, dosages, and specific treatment techniques.[1, 4–9]

SPECIAL PAIN MANAGEMENT TECHNIQUES

Patient-Controlled Analgesia

PCA is a popular opioid delivery system for acute pain management. There are many studies proving the effectiveness and safety of PCA pumps. PCA consists of a microprocessor-driven pump that is capable of delivering a programmed amount of pain medication with each push of a button and a constant basal rate infusion at a predetermined hourly rate. The safety of the technique rests on the premise that the patient pushes the button and not well-meaning family members. If a patient self-administers a dose that causes sedation, he or she will not push the button again until the unwanted effect dissipates. Although PCA pumps programmed with reasonable dosage settings, based on patient age, weight, and physical condition, rarely cause injury, occasionally patients have clinically significant respiratory depression. Available evidence suggests, however, that PCA is at least as safe as parenteral administration of opioids. Postoperative hypoxemia is fairly common after major surgery, from the surgical trespass and not the opioids, at least in the unsedated patient. In high-risk patients, particularly elderly patients or patients with concomitant medical diseases that may affect cognition or pulmonary function, an appropriate rule of thumb is to start low and titrate to effect. Appropriate monitors on the floor include the medical and nursing staff, patient care assistants who help collect vital signs, and judiciously applied pulse oximetry.

Pump programming varies with individual makes and models, but generally four parameters have to be programmed into the PCA pump. When initiating PCA, unless the patient has received an opioid within 30 minutes or so of starting the PCA, a bolus dose of opioid must be given. PCA should be considered a form of maintenance therapy. Patient-administered doses alone (discussed later) are unlikely to achieve pain relief because the individual doses are subtherapeutic. A typical bolus (loading) dose in the range of 5 to 10 mg of morphine is appropriate for the average 70-kg young adult. If doses of opioid were given recently, the bolus dose may be less, in the range of 2 to 4 mg of morphine. Clinical judgment is indicated here. If in doubt, titrate to effect.

Next, one must program the demand dose, which is the amount of drug that the patient will receive with each press of the button. With some devices, this is called the *bolus dose*, but it should not be confused with the bolus (loading) dose described previously. For the average patient, the usual demand dose is 1.0 mg of morphine. The lockout interval should be programmed, which prevents the patient from self-administering another dose shortly after a previous dose. Generally, lockout intervals are 6 to 10 minutes in length, which strikes a balance between allowing the patient rapid access to the analgesic and letting enough time elapse for the dose to have full therapeutic effect. See Table 3 for standard PCA settings for commonly used opioids. Contraindications for PCA are listed in Table 4.

A basal infusion at night may be used in some cases, based on the premise that the patient will awaken in pain if a small amount of drug is not administered continuously when the patient sleeps. This may or may not be true. We provide a basal infusion on the first postoperative night for otherwise healthy patients. A basal infusion slightly increases the risk of respiratory depression, however, with PCA-delivered opioids. If the physician is uncertain

TABLE 3

Standard Patient-Controlled Analgesia Settings for Commonly Used Opioids

	Morphine	Hydromorphone	Meperidine
Concentration	1 mg/mL	0.2 mg/mL	10 mg/mL
Demand dose	1 mg	0.2 mg	10 mg
Lockout interval	10 min	10 min	10 min
Basal rate	1 mg/h	0.2 mg/h	10 mg/h
Hourly limit	7 mg	1.4 mg	70 mg

Note: Meperidine should not be used in patients with renal insufficiency or for longer than 48 hours. The total 24-hour dose of meperidine should not exceed 600 mg in the average adult. Morphine metabolites also may accumulate with renal insufficiency. Morphine is not dialyzable. Hydromorphone generally is considered to be safe for patients with poor renal function.

about the risks in a given patient, the basal infusion should be omitted. A typical basal rate for morphine is 1.0 mg/h in the average 70-kg young adult.

Most patients obtain good pain control with PCA receiving two to three demand doses per hour, with or without a basal infusion. This works out to approximately 10 mg of morphine in a 4-hour period, which is about what one would expect, based on the *standard* 4-hour parenteral dose of morphine typically recommended for the average adult.

A built-in safety factor with PCA is the hourly limit (in some devices there is a 4-hour limit). The hourly limit is the total amount of drug that the patient will be allowed to receive in 1 hour, including that delivered by demand doses, the basal infusion, and any bolus doses administered. When the hourly limit is reached, the pump is inactivated until restarted by the nurse or physician. The hourly limit does not have to be set to the total amount of drug that is possible to get. If there is concern about the patient overusing the pump, the hourly limit can be set lower than otherwise would be calculated. The patient should be monitored and the limit increased as necessary. For elderly patients, the calculated doses should be reduced by 50%.

Example: A 75-year-old man is scheduled for a total knee arthroplasty. He has been taking NSAIDs for pain control. Program the PCA as follows:

Basal infusion: Morphine, 0.5 mg/h (consider not using a basal infusion)

Demand dose: Morphine, 0.5 mg

TABLE 4

Absolute and Relative Contraindications for Patient-Controlled Analgesia in Pain Management

Absolute	Relative
Patient refusal	Extremes of age
Patient unable to understand patient-controlled analgesia	
Untrained staff	

Lockout: 10 minutes

Hourly limit: 3 mg

The objective is to reduce the opioid dose for elderly patients. In this case, a good argument can be made to use a postoperative epidural, which may obviate the need for opioids, at least during the first postoperative day.

One of the advantages of PCA is that it calculates the patient's requirement for pain medication. Most PCAs are capable of saving the patient's requested demand doses (attempted doses) and the doses administered. The optimal settings of the PCA should allow the patient to be in a comfortable state with fewer than three to four demand doses per hour. If the patient presses the button many times more than the number of doses administered (e.g., 20 attempts in 1 hour and only 2 delivered doses), the demand dose is too low, or the patient does not understand how to use the pump.

With PCA, it is possible for the patient to be independent from a fixed drug schedule mandated by staffing considerations on the ward. Doses administered often are not different from what would have been delivered in the ideal PRN situation, with properly written orders and timely administration of analgesic. The requirements for patient monitoring are not reduced with PCA. Although a subtherapeutic dose of morphine is unlikely to cause clinically significant respiratory depression, a therapeutic dose is associated with some inherent risk, which must be balanced with the needs of the patient. A PCA pump does not obviate the need for the intensive care unit in patients needing a higher level of monitoring. In some patients, aggressive pain management may warrant the higher level of monitoring available only in the intensive care unit. In most patients, however, thoughtfully programmed PCA pumps are used safely on the wards.

Epidural Infusions

The epidural catheter should be inserted in the operating room or the preoperative holding area before induction of general anesthesia so that the catheter can be placed and tested safely. An additional benefit of the preoperative placement of the epidural catheter is the opportunity to use the catheter intraoperatively, reducing anesthetic requirements.

In contrast to epidural opioids, which work by a receptor-mediated mechanism spinally (and supraspinally), epidural local anesthetics act primarily on spinal nerve roots. Opioid effects may involve many spinal segments, whereas the maximal effect of the local anesthetic is near the level of the epidural catheter tip. Particularly after thoracic or upper abdominal surgeries, epidural infusions for postoperative pain control provide excellent pain relief, provided that the catheters are placed at the spinal level closest to the dermatomal level of the incision.

Because opioids and local anesthetics have different mechanisms of action, their effects are at least additive. This additive effect has the benefit of reducing the total dose of each type of agent and reducing the side effects of both. Standard epidural infusions used at University Hospitals of Cleveland are shown in Table 5 and 6. Contraindications to epidural techniques are listed in Table 7.

In some cases, a local anesthetic is used as the sole agent in the epidural infusion. In these cases, we usually supplement the epidural with an intravenous PCA. This approach is particularly useful when the local anesthetic alone causes hypotension or lower extremity weakness. Failure to achieve pain relief with an epidural infusion is usually due to improper

TABLE 5

Standard Epidural Infusion Mixtures Used at University Hospitals of Cleveland

Name	Mixture
Bupivacaine/hydromorphone	250 mL preservative-free normal saline 225 mg bupivacaine (0.1%) 2 mg hydromorphone (0.01 mg/mL) 4–6 mL/h
Bupivacaine/morphine (low dose)	250 mL preservative-free normal saline 112.5 mg bupivacaine (0.05%) 2.5 mg morphine (0.01 mg/mL) 8–10 mL/h
Morphine	200 mL preservative-free normal saline 10 mg morphine 0.05 mg/mL 4–8 mL/h
Bupivacaine	250 mL preservative-free normal saline 225 mg bupivacaine (0.1%) 4–6 mL/h

Note: Hydromorphone is used more often than morphine. User preference or side effects, such as nausea, may suggest use of the alternate opioid. The bupivacaine/morphine infusion shown is used for lower extremity procedures. Despite the low opioid concentrations, pruritus is still fairly common (15%). Incidence of lower extremity weakness is less than 5%.

TABLE 6

Examples of Epidural Infusions Used, Depending on the Surgery and Spinal Level of Epidural Catheter Insertion

Surgery	Epidural Catheter Insertion Level	Infusion Type
Thoracotomy	T5–T10	Bupivacaine/hydromorphone at 4–8 mL/h Bupivacaine at 4–8 ml/h plus PCA
	L1–L5	Morphine at 4–8 ml/h
Upper abdominal procedure	T8–T12	Bupivacaine/hydromorphone at 4–8 mL/h Bupivacaine at 4–8 mL/h plus PCA
	L1–L5	Morphine at 4–8 mL/h
Abdominal hysterectomy	T12–L1	Bupivacaine/hydromorphone at 4–8 mL/h Bupivacaine at 4–8 mL/h plus PCA
Knee replacement	L3–L4	Bupivacaine at 4–8 mL/h plus PCA Bupivacaine/morphine at 6–12 mL/h

Note: see Table 35–3 for components of the infusions. These are approximate infusion rates, titrated to effect. With local anesthetic–only epidural infusions, morphine or hydromorphone intravenous PCA is used to supplement the epidural. This facilitates discontinuation of the epidural infusion without compromising pain control. Patients with total joint replacements have the epidural removed the day after surgery because all are started on warfarin the night of surgery.

PCA, patient-controlled analgesia.

TABLE 7

Absolute and Relative Contraindications for Use of Epidural Catheters in Pain Management

Absolute	Relative
Patient refusal	Hypovolemia
Inability of patient to take or maintain position for epidural placement	Preexisting neurologic disease
Coagulopathy	
Bacteremia	
Infection at insertion site	

catheter placement, migration of the epidural catheter, or an excessively long interval between the last epidural dose in the operating room and the start of the epidural infusion in the postanesthesia care unit (PACU). For this reason, the epidural infusion should be started in the operating room or as soon as possible after arriving in the PACU.

If an epidural catheter does not give the expected pain relief, a test dose of a local anesthetic should be given. A test dose of 5 mL of 1% to 2% lidocaine gives significant pain relief within 5 minutes, if the catheter is placed correctly in the epidural space. Epidural infusions can be used safely for 1 week, if proper attention is given to aseptic technique with catheter placement and the dressing is inspected daily.

The PCA concept has been applied to epidural infusions. Instead of giving a continuous infusion rate, the patient receives a lower basal epidural infusion and a demand capability, as used with traditional intravenous PCA. This approach may offer the same advantages as intravenous PCA and the superior pain relief possible with epidural infusions.

COMMON CLINICAL SETTINGS

In the Postanethesia Care Unit

Postoperative pain in the PACU is most often taken care of by PACU nurses, following standing orders written by the surgeon or anesthesiologist. The Pain Service may be called, however, when the *standard doses* are not working. In these cases, reviewing the patient's history may reveal previous use of pain medications that was not considered by the primary team when ordering analgesics for postoperative pain control. A focused examination is necessary to rule out other painful conditions, such as pain secondary to urinary retention, ileus, myocardial ischemia, intraoperative positioning, and corneal abrasion. If there are signs that the pain may not be the *normal* postoperative pain expected, the surgical team and the anesthesiologist should be informed immediately.

Postoperative pain usually responds to intermittent doses of opioids, given at frequent intervals until pain is controlled. For an opioid-naive patient, assuming opioids were given intraoperatively (the anesthesia record should be consulted), intravenous doses of morphine in 5-mg aliquots every 5 minutes may suffice. Higher doses are needed if intraoperative analgesics were not given; remember the loading dose concept. If a patient requires 30 mg of morphine in the early PACU period, the physician may wish to consult with the anesthesiologist who did the case. The surgeon and anesthesiologist share responsibility for the patient while in the PACU and should be able to offer some suggestions. (The attending physician may have some recommendations regarding appropriate analgesic administration.)

In some cases, the opioid of choice may not be working as well as anticipated. Some patients seem to be resistant to some opioids. Hydromorphone may work better than morphine for a particular patient (and vice versa), because of theoretical receptor or pharmacodynamic factors. This phenomenon has been seen in cancer patients. In this case, a different opioid should be tried. Although meperidine is losing favor because of well-known toxic effects of its metabolite, normeperidine, which accumulates in renal insufficiency (morphine metabolites also accumulate with renal insufficiency), in some cases it may be a reasonable alternative to morphine, particularly if morphine is suspected to be causing nausea.

Although analgesic doses of opioids may contribute to nausea and vomiting in the PACU, this is difficult to assess when blood levels of anesthetic agents are still present. If not contraindicated (such as in plastic surgery, eye surgery, tonsillectomy, renal or hepatic disease, or hypovolemia), intravenous ketorolac may provide significant pain relief. Use of an NSAID should be considered early on if the opioid is not working.

Except when the intravenous catheter "fell out" and there are no plans to replace the it, intramuscular injections should be avoided because of the unpredictable uptake of drug and delay in achieving therapeutic blood levels (it may take 30 minutes for the full effect of the intramuscular injection to be apparent). PCA pumps are considered the standard of care in many institutions. When a parenteral dose of opioid is anticipated for more than 12 hours, a PCA pump should be provided, assuming the patient can understand and use the pump appropriately. Preoperative teaching should include instruction on pain management and use of the PCA pump. The PCA should be started early enough to allow appropriate titration and evaluation of pain relief before discharge to the floor.

Postoperative patients in the PACU are at increased risk for respiratory depression with opioids, which may compound postoperative respiratory problems resulting from inadequate pain relief, such as splinting and poor inspiratory effort. Because of residual effects of anesthetics and muscle relaxants, even small doses of opioids can depress respiratory rates and tidal volumes in postoperative patients. Generally speaking, opioids result first in increased sedation followed by decreased respiratory rates or tidal volumes and a regularization of the respiration pattern. Increasing sedation usually precedes life-threatening respiratory depression, but this is not always the case. Aggressive pain management demands vigilance on the part of physicians and nurses.

Respiratory rates may remain in the normal range when tidal volumes are depressed. As a result, the minute ventilation is depressed (the definition of respiratory depression). Because a single dose of morphine given intravenously can take 15 minutes to reach peak effect, the physician should ensure that the patient is monitored adequately after bolus administration. Supplemental oxygen by nasal canula should be used until the patient meets requirements for discharge from the PACU. After major abdominal surgery or thoracotomy, consideration should be given to continuing nasal oxygen overnight because episodes of desaturation are common on the first postoperative night, even in otherwise healthy patients.

On the Ward

In the ideal world, postoperative pain management on the ward is a seamless continuation of the excellent pain control provided by the PACU team. Despite best intentions, however, this may not be the case in some instances. The rules of engagement for acute pain management on the floor are essentially the same as in the PACU. First, the physician must assess the patient, determine what has and has not worked, and plan a reasonable course of action. For patients having had major abdominal procedures or thoracotomies, PCA is the most expeditious way of achieving reliable pain relief.

Sometimes patients are admitted to the hospital for pain control. Efforts at pain management on an outpatient basis or in the emergency department may have failed, resulting in admission to the hospital as a last resort. Some of these patients may be suffering an acute exacerbation of chronic medical conditions, such as cancer, pancreatitis, sickle cell pain, herpes zoster or other chronic, poorly defined painful conditions. The physician should not forget that these patients might be taking chronic pain medications. It may be necessary to treat these patients aggressively and start intravenous opioids early in the course of treatment. Use of PCA with an appropriate basal rate and demand dose should allow rapid titration of an opioid and determine quickly what dose of opioid provides good pain relief. This approach avoids the inevitable delay associated with titrating oral opioids in the hospital setting. Our experience with postoperative pain management gives us confidence that we can evaluate and treat patients with chronic disorders admitted to the hospital for pain control.

PCA pumps record the number of demand attempts by the patient and the number of doses the patient received. With this information, the PCA pump can be adjusted to meet the patient's needs. If the patient has required more than four or five demand doses per hour, consideration should be given to raising the demand dose by 50%. Some patients manage to push the button on the PCA more than several hundred times per hour and yet are underdosed. These patients need to be reeducated about the proper use of the pump or switched to nurse-administered analgesia. If the patient pushes the button only once every couple of hours, the demand dose usually can be reduced or the basal rate stopped. In most cases, after the appropriate dose for a given patient has been found, PCA usage *stabilizes* and gradually declines over subsequent days.

When it is time to switch to an oral opioid, previous PCA usage helps guide the transition. If pain is likely to continue for some time (for cancer patients or after major orthopedic surgery), it is a relatively easy task to calculate the patient's hourly requirement for pain medication. Totaling the basal rate plus the average number of hourly demand doses yields the total hourly dose needed to provide adequate pain relief. This can be converted to an equivalent oral 4-hour or 12-hour dose, if a controlled-release formulation will be used. The physician must remember to factor in the parenteral-to-enteral conversion ratio.

A patient obtaining good pain relief with usual PCA settings (e.g., 1-mg demand morphine dose and no basal) generally can be switched to a fixed combination drug, such as acetaminophen and codeine, when taking liquids. If considering a controlled-release drug, an hourly morphine requirement of 1.0 mg/h is approximately equal to 30 mg of MS Contin administered every 12 hours. When planning to use a controlled-release preparation, the physician should make sure that ongoing pain justifies that decision.

Switching a patient from a parenteral to an oral opioid or from one opioid to another is not a predictable mathematical exercise. Conversion table are just recommendations, often based on single dose studies obtained in the research setting. Although conversion tables do give an approximate dose with which to start, in most cases doses need to be adjusted up or down. From a safety standpoint, it is better to underestimate the requirements for a given patient and make up the difference with breakthough doses (particularly when using a controlled-release formulation).

In the Office

Acute pain is a common reason for a patient to consult a physician. The underlying disease is evaluated and diagnosed. Nevertheless, every patient in acute pain expects not only diagnostic studies, but also efficient pain management. Most commonly, patients receive NSAIDs as a first-line treatment or a fixed combination NSAID and opioid. Although many minor acute pain conditions are treated effectively with NSAIDs or combination preparations, some conditions, such as cancer pain, pancreatitis, sickle cell disease, and herpes zoster, may be difficult to manage in the outpatient setting.

SPECIAL CLINICAL SITUATIONS

Patients on Long-Term Opioids

Of special interest are patients on long-term opioids (the clinician must determine as accurately as possible how much drug and for how long). Such patients often require their usual daily amount of opioid in addition to that needed for postoperative pain control. Typically the daily dose of the long-term controlled–release opioid (e.g., MS Contin or Oramorph) should be converted to an hourly parenteral dosage. This can be provided as an hourly basal infusion using PCA. If there is concern that the postoperative condition of the patient (e.g., pulmonary disease) may increase the risk associated with aggressive pain management, the calculated infusion rate should be reduced by about 50%. An equal amount of opioid also is required on demand for adequate control of pain (in addition to the basal infusion).

Total opioid requirements may be reduced by using an epidural or by adding an NSAID. If an epidural local anesthetic infusion is planned, consider giving a supplemental opioid at appropriate intervals (e.g., one third of the usual 24-hour dose of opioid divided into six doses and given at 4-hour intervals) to prevent withdrawal. Signs of withdrawal include restlessness, irritability, flulike symptoms, tachycardia, hypertension, dilated pupils, and diarrhea. Even if the epidural contains an opioid, withdrawal symptoms still may occur, and the clinician should be prepared to give supplemental systemic opioid as needed.

Example: A 50-year-old woman undergoing a total knee replacement has been taking 90 mg of controlled-release morphine twice a day for several months before the operation. She will be allowed liquids and oral medications the first night after surgery. Calculate the PCA settings as follows:

Calculate the basal opioid requirement:

180 mg oral morphine/24 h

60 mg intravenous morphine equivalent/24 h (3:1 oral-to-parenteral ratio)

2.5 mg/h morphine basal infusion; as a fudge factor, this may be reduced by 50%

Program a demand dose of 2.5 mg with a lockout of 10 minutes. The hourly limit should be about 15 mg (this allows five demand doses per hour). This patient also may do well with a postoperative epidural bupivacaine infusion for pain control. Plan on giving 10 to 20 mg of oral morphine every 4 hours postoperatively to prevent withdrawal symptoms. When the epidural is discontinued, restart the controlled-release morphine at the preoperative dosage, and continue the oral morphine for breakthrough pain. Thereafter, the opioid can be tapered as tolerated. If a patient does not act the way you anticipated during the postoperative period, investigate, recalculate the doses, and make the necessary midcourse corrections.

The key to success is planning, assessment and reassessment, vigilance, and a willingness to be flexible. Some patients may require higher doses of their controlled-release preparation for the first several days to weeks postoperatively, particularly if they are going to participate effectively in physical therapy.

Patients Abusing Opioids

A history of drug abuse often complicates patient management but rarely presents unsurmountable obstacles to treatment. Although there is some concern that postoperative opioids may place the patient at risk for drug relapse, in many cases, postoperative opioids cannot be avoided. In this situation, a frank discussion with the patient about risks and benefits may illuminate a clear course of action. In some instances, a postoperative epidural may obviate the need for opioids.

Patients with ongoing drug abuse also present problems; however, the issues are often simple and revolve around how much analgesic to administer postoperatively. This may require some guess work on the part of the physician because dose equivalents of street drugs, such as heroin, are unknown, and drug purity is not available. Whether or not a patient who is currently abusing drugs (e.g., a heroin addict) has a low *tolerance to pain* is immaterial and is probably not the case anyway. In any case, there is little to be gained by underdosing the patient.

In these cases, a pure agonist such as morphine or hydromorphone is appropriate, to avoid inducing withdrawal, which may occur with a partial agonist or agonist-antagonist drug such as nalbuphine or pentazocine. More important is the fact that the patient will have a higher than normal opioid requirement because of opioid tolerance from previous drug use. This acquired tolerance necessitates a reasonable starting dose of opioid (morphine or hydromorphone) and subsequent dose-titration to achieve adequate pain control.

The first step is to calculate how much opioid to provide by basal infusion to prevent opioid withdrawal. It is unlikely to arrive at the correct dosage the first time around. The clinician should start by estimating how much drug (i.e., heroin) the patient typically uses in a 24-hour period, and convert this to an hourly parenteral morphine dose. Heroin also is known as diacetylmorphine and is a prodrug for morphine. Heroin is approximately twice as potent as morphine. This serves as the basal opioid requirement, to which must be added the therapeutic analgesic dose required for pain control. In this situation, a PCA pump may be the most expeditious route to satisfactory dose titration and pain control. The approach is similar to that used for the patient taking prescribed opioids preoperatively.

Example: A 30-year-old man has undergone an exploratory laparotomy and will be NPO postoperatively. He admits to using about 200 mg of heroin on a daily basis. Purity is unclear, but assume that the drug is about 50% pure. Calculate the basal infusion for the PCA as follows:

200 mg of street heroin/24 h

100 mg of pure heroin/24 h

200 mg of morphine/24 h (heroin is twice as potent as morphine)

8 mg/h morphine by basal infusion; as a fudge factor, reduce this calculated value by 50%:

    4 mg/h is a reasonable starting dose

Based on the calculated hourly requirement, 4 mg is a reasonable demand dose of morphine, with a lockout of 10 minutes. The hourly limit should be about 28 mg. Make adjustments up or down as necessary to provide adequate pain control. Arrangements need to be made for discharge. Referral to a drug treatment program for methadone maintenance is a consideration.

PCA can be used safely with drug-addicted patients, although occasional patients may attempt to manipulate or reprogram the PCA pump or remove the syringe. This is an uncommon event, however, when appropriate doses of opioids are prescribed. For patients who are tolerant to opioids, PCA doses must be titrated to achieve pain relief.

Calculating the opioid conversion doses for patients on methadone also can be a daunting problem. The same pharmacologic issues apply whether the patient is on a methadone maintenance program or taking methadone for control of chronic pain. (The legal differences are important from a prescribing standpoint, but not in the acute care setting, where pain management is the main consideration.) Single dose studies with methadone indicated that methadone has about the same potency as morphine, with a slightly better oral bioavailability. For example, 20 mg of oral methadone is equivalent to 30 mg of oral morphine, and the parenteral doses are the same. With long-term dosing with methadone, however, potency is unpredictable. The problem is related to the prolonged terminal elimination half-life of methadone, which may be more than 24 hours. Unpredictable pharmacodynamic effects cloud the picture further. For safety reasons, with long-term dosing, it is helpful to think of methadone as being as potent as intravenous hydromorphone, whether the methadone is given orally or parenterally (methadone has a high bioavailability when given orally).

Example: A 45-year-old patient who is taking 50 mg of methadone daily on a long-term basis (for pain control or through a methadone maintenance program) presents for thoracotomy and refuses an epidural catheter for pain management. Calculate PCA settings for this patient as follows:

Basal infusion: 50 mg of oral methadone/d (25 mg/12 h)

2 mg of oral methadone/h

2 mg of intravenous hydromorphone every 4 hours. Note the differences in duration of action between the two drugs. This is at best a rough approximation of the actual potency equivalents of the two drugs.

12 mg hydromorphone/24 h

0.5 mg of hydromorphone/h

Based on the basal dose of 0.5 mg of hydromorphone per hour, a demand dose of 0.5 mg of hydromorphone may be a reasonable starting dose. The hourly limit should be about 3.0 mg. These calculations involve a lot of assumptions. It is better to underdose, however, than overdose the patient. You can always go up on the doses. If you prefer to use morphine instead of hydromorphone, multiply by 5, which is the approximate potency ratio of hydromorphone to morphine (the tables suggest 6.7, but 5 is an easier number to work with).

Before PCA is ordered for a patient with history of drug abuse, the physician should make it clear to the patient that any manipulation of the PCA by the patient will result in the PCA being discontinued. In complicated cases, it is often beneficial to consult Psychiatry, Psychology, or Addiction Medicine colleagues for guidance. All patients, whether they have a history of drug abuse or not, show so-called drug-seeking behavior when their pain is undertreated. In many cases, it is enough for the patient to ask the nurse one or two times for more pain medication to be labeled as a drug addict. In some cases, the patient just has to fit the stereotype of a drug addict (e.g., unshaven, tattoos) for requests for additional pain medication to result in being branded an addict, resulting in inappropriate withdrawal of all opioids and terrible pain control. It is no wonder that opioid abusers seem to have a low pain tolerance; they are often woefully underdosed when medically appropriate analgesics are prescribed.

Patients With Cancer Pain

Although the tendency is to think of cancer pain as a form of chronic pain, in most circumstances, the same principles apply to acute noncancer pain and pain secondary to malignancy. Acute pain is often a reason why a patient with cancer first sees a physician. Later in the course of the disease, an acute pain exacerbation may be a sign of progression of disease or development of metastasis. Acute pain also can be caused by cancer treatment (e.g., skin irritation or radiation injury, esophagitis, myalgias, postherpetic neuralgia) or surgery. The main point is that patients often have a history of previous opioid use, sometimes at quite large daily doses. This history mandates higher than otherwise expected doses to treat acute exacerbations of pain. In this situation, controlled-release preparations may be converted to hourly intravenous equivalents of morphine or hydromorphone and provided by PCA. This approach may allow faster titration of drug to achieve adequate pain relief. If the patient can take oral opioids, it may be appropriate to continue the controlled-release opioid and to add an immediate-release preparation to the regimen. The breakthrough dose should be at least one third of the 12-hour controlled-release dose. Satisfactory pain relief may require aggressive dose titration. An NSAID should be used if not contraindicated.

Geriatric Patients

More medical specialties have begun to focus on the treatment of the geriatric patient. In most Western countries, the geriatric population is the fastest-growing segment of the population. Just as children are not *small adults*, geriatric patients are not just *wrinkled adults*. The body composition of geriatric patients differs from younger adult patients. Geriatric patients have less body water and lean muscle mass and a higher fat mass and may have reduced liver and kidney function, which affect drug metabolism. Elderly patients have a higher incidence of systemic diseases and a more advanced stage of those diseases. Because of their reduced cardiac and pulmonary reserve, geriatric patients are more prone to side effects of pain medication, including respiratory depression, renal failure, gastric ulcerations, and cognitive effects. Cognitive or memory deficits may prevent the use of PCA, particularly if the patient cannot remember how to use the pump.

Besides the increased sensitivity of older patients to opioids, opioids have a longer circulation time because of reduced metabolism and clearance. Opioids must be titrated carefully in elderly patients. Calculated PCA doses should be reduced by 50% for elderly patients. Epidural doses of opioids must be reduced as well because of enhanced pharmacodynamic effects. NSAIDs can be beneficial in elderly patients because of their opioid-sparing effect, but coexisting renal or hepatic insufficiency can be worsened by the use of NSAIDs.

Patients With Renal or Hepatic Disease

NSAIDs should be avoided in patients with underlying liver or kidney disease. NSAIDs can induce or worsen renal insufficiency and often are contraindicated in patients with hepatic or renal dysfunction.

Opioid analgesics are metabolized by the liver and excreted by the kidneys. Hepatic impairment can lower the clearance of morphine, prolong its elimination, and cause an apparent increase in bioavailability with oral dosing. Renal disease also increases the apparent bioavailability of morphine and its active metabolite, morphine-6-glucuronide. Continuous infusions of opioids can result in accumulation of the parent compound or its active metabolites.

Toxic effects of meperidine and its active metabolite, normeperidine, are well known. Mild renal insufficiency can result in significant accumulation of normeperidine. Meperidine should not be used in patients with renal insufficiency. Toxic effects can be seen, however, even in patients with normal renal function, so meperidine should not be used for more than several days or at doses higher than 600 mg/24 h.

In cases of renal impairment, opioids without active metabolites should be used to improve their margin of safety. Hydromorphone and fentanyl do not seem to have active metabolites that are renally excreted. The use of a PCA pump is permissible but with lower basal rates, or no basal rate at all, and longer lockout intervals. Even with PCA, the risk of drug accumulation is not eliminated, and patients must be assessed frequently. In general, epidural opioids have a smaller risk of side effects simply because they are given in much lower doses than with enteral or parenteral routes of administration. Epidural catheter insertion may be risky in patients with renal or hepatic failure because of coagulopathy.

REFERENCES

1. Ashburn MA, Ready LB: Postoperative pain. In: Bonica's Management of Pain, 3rd ed. Philadelphia: Lippincott Williams & Wilkins, 2001, pp 765–779.
2. Carr DB, Jacox AK, Chapman RC, et al: Clinical Practice Guideline: Acute Pain Management: Operative or Medical Procedures and Trauma. Rockville, MD: Agency for Health Care Policy and Research, U.S. Department of Health and Human Services, 1992.
3. Joint Commission on Accreditation of Healthcare Organizations Pain Standards for 2001. Available at http://www.jcaho.org/trkhco_frm.html.
4. Liu SS, and Benzon HT: Outcomes and complications of acute pain management. In: Raj PP (ed): Practical Management of Pain, 3rd ed. St Louis: Mosby, 2000, pp 871–889.
5. Macintyre PE, Ready LB: Acute Pain Management: A practical guide, 2nd ed. London: WB Saunders, 2001.
6. Max MB, Payne R: Principles of Analgesic Use in the Treatment of Acute Pain and Cancer Pain, 4th ed. American Pain Society, 1999.
7. Narinder R: Spinal opioids for acute pain management. In: Raj PP (ed): Practical Management of Pain, 3rd ed. St Louis: Mosby, 2000, pp 689–709.

8. Ready, LB: Acute perioperative pain. In: Miller RD (ed): Anesthesia, 5th ed. Edinburgh: Churchill Livingstone, 2000.

9. Ready LB, Ashburn M, Caplan RA, et al: Practice guidelines for acute pain management in the perioperative setting: A report by the American Society of Anesthesiologists task force on pain management, acute pain section. Anesthesiology 82:1071, 1995.

10. Sinatra RS: Acute pain management and acute pain services. In: Cousins MJ, Bridenbaugh PO (eds): Neural Blockade in Clinical Anesthesia and Management of Pain, 3rd ed. Philadelphia: Lippincott-Raven, 1998, pp 793–835.

Chapter 35

Potential Analgesic Interactions

Howard S. Smith, MD

Drug interactions have been defined as "the possibility that one drug may alter the intensity of pharmacological effects of another drug given concurrently."[1] Although drug interactions (producing synergistic, additive, or antagonistic effects) can involve environmental chemicals and nutrients or nutritional supplements as well as "alternative" and over-the-counter medications, this chapter primarily focuses on prescription drug–drug interactions.[1,2] The incidence is difficult to estimate but may vary from roughly 3% to 5% (with few medications), up to 20% in hospitalized patients taking 10 to 20 medications.[1]

Interactions that are believed to be clinically significant may be significantly less frequent. Drug-drug interactions have been classified into pharmacokinetic (in which one drug affects the disposition of another), pharmacodynamic (in which one drug affects the way in which the body responds to another drug), or pharmaceutical (in which there are physical incompatibilities between drugs).[1,2]

Pharmacokinetic interactions seem to be the most common type and may occur due to changes in absorption, alteration in protein binding or changes in distribution (amount of free drug that gains access to binding sites), or changes in biotransformation or excretion. Changes in bioavailability, which determine dose adjustments or conversion between intravenous and oral dosing, can markedly alter the final serum concentration of a medication.

Medical conditions and factors that may affect the amount of free circulating drug (e.g., decreased plasma protein concentration) include liver disease (decreased protein synthesis), trauma or surgery (increased protein catabolism), burns (altered distribution of albumin into extravascular space), and renal disease (excessive elimination of protein).

The elimination half-life of a medication, which essentially determines the dosing interval, depends on drug distribution and clearance:

$$T\frac{1}{2} = \frac{0.693 \text{ (Volume of Distribution)}}{\text{Clearance}}$$

The half-life multiplied by 3.3 yields the time in hours that it takes for the drug to reach 90% of steady state concentration. This number of hours can be used to determine a general guideline between dose adjustments. Biotransformation can usually be considered in two phases. Phase I reactions involve conversion of the parent compound to a more polar substance (e.g., cytochrome p450 system), and phase II reactions involve conjugation to a glucuronide, sulfate, acetate, and so on. Biotransformation can be modified by age, other drugs, "enzyme inducers," hepatic disease, and genetic polymorphism in the cytochrome p450 system.

Once a drug reaches its site of action, usually a receptor (ligand-gated ion channel, G protein-coupled receptor, voltage-gated ion channel, or transcriptional regulator) or an enzyme, it can bind to a specific site, with varying binding strength and affinity constants. Then, the ability of the bound medication to iniate cell changes leading to an effect determines efficacy.

CYTOCHROME P450 SYSTEM

The cytochrome p450 enzymes are a group of heterogeneous heme-thiolate proteins present in many tissues of numerous organisms (usually in the endoplasmic reticulum). These hemoproteins, which have a spectral absorbance maximum produced at or near 450 nm, are in close association with another membrane protein, NADPH-cytochrome p450 reductase. Cytochrome p450 (CYP450) and cytochrome p450 reductase form the major pillars of the CYP450 system and appear to be in a ratio of about the CYP450 molecules per one reductase. The CYP450 enzyme system is also known as a mixed-function oxygenase because one atom of molecular oxygen is incorporated into a drug in the form of a hydroxyl(-OH) moiety and the other oxygen atom is incorporated into water. Reduced nicotinamide dinucleotide phosphate provides the reducing equivalents. The p450 nomenclature is as follows: CYP stands for cytochrome; the number after P identifies the enzyme family; the letter after the number is the subfamily designation; and the number after the letter identifies the individual enzyme. Enzymes with greater than 40% amino acid sequence homology are included in the same family, and enzymes with greater than 55% homology are included in the same subfamily.

There appears to be potential pharmacological and toxicological impact of CYP450 screening. Widespread CYP450 screening may help establish large databases in efforts to provide rationales for individualized therapy.[34] Clinicians should keep in mind that although pharmacokinetic drug-drug interactions may change blood levels of a drug, this tends to be subclinical in 85% to 90% of patients, with significant interactions occurring only in 10% to 15% of patients. Severely ill or debilitated patients may tolerate only a small margin of error in the metabolism of drugs (most human studies enlist relatively healthy individuals). The CYP450 Drug Ineraction Table, which is updated monthly, is maintained by David A. Flockhart, MD, PhD, in the Division of Clinical Pharmacology at Georgetown University Medical Center and can be found at *dflock02@medlib.georgetown.edu.*

Pharmacokinetics and Pharmacodynamics

Human drug-metabolizing systems can vary dramatically in different individuals and can be induced or activated or inhibited by a variety of exogenous agents, including drugs, alcohol, dietary factors, and cigarette smoke, as well as by endogenous factors.[3] This incredible complexity makes it extremely difficult to predict the clinical impact of any one particular medication dose via a specific route in any one individual. Inducers are agents that "rev up" the cytochrome system, leading to increased metabolism and less drug effect (e.g., withdrawal, lack of efficacy/analgesia). Inhibitors are agents that impair the cytochrome system's ability to normally metabolize the drug, which could lead to increased drug effect (e.g., oversedation) (TABLES 1 and 2).

Although many of these potential interactions affecting various combinations of medications are more hypothetical than real, there are also some that achieve clinical significance.

Many drugs are metabolized by more than one CYP450 system, and an inducer of one system may inhibit another; therefore, in a patient on 10 medications, the interactions and metabolic modulation may be extremely complex.

Genetic polymorphism may occur in several CYP450 systems, affecting drug metabolism and the individual effects of a particular agent. It was this significant interindividual variability and the concern for drug toxicity that lead the Food and Drug Administration to rec-

TABLE 1

Drug Metabolizing Systems

Metabolism	Inhibitors	Inducer
CYP2D6		
Codeine ——→Morphine	Methadone	Carbamazepine
Hydrocodone —→Hydromorphone	Selective serotonin reuptake inhibitors	
Tramadol ——→M1	(e.g., fluoextine)	
Tricyclic anti- —→Inactive metabolites		
depressants		
Mexiletine——→Inactive metabolites		

ommend that all drugs be evaluated for CYP450 activity during their development before marketing. More than 70 single nucleotide polymorphisms (allelic variants) have been described for the CYP2D6 gene.[4] Four phenotype metabolizer exists: poor, intermediate, extensive, and ultrarapid.[4] A deficiency of the CYP2D6 enzyme is inherited as an autosomal recessive trait; these patients (roughly 7% of people of European descent and 1% of people of Asian descent) qualify as poor metabolizers.[4]

In most patients, codeine is metabolized predominantly via O-demethylation by the CYP2D6 system, with a lesser amount via N-demethylation by the CYP3A system.[5,6] In extensive metabolizers this holds true; however, poor metabolizers have a predominance of N-demethylation.[5] There is an almost complete loss of codeine's analgesic effects when quinidine is present due to CYP2D6 inhibition by quinidine and resultant lack of morphine formation.[7]

Caraco and associates,[8] in a double-blind study, administered 120 mg of codeine phosphate, codeine and quinidine, or quinidine alone to healthy volunteers known to be poor or extensive metabolizers in the CYP2D6 system. Clearance by the extensive metabolizers

TABLE 2

Drug Metabolizing Systems

Substrates	Inhibitors	Inducers
CYP2D6		
Codeine	Quinidine	
Tramadol		Carbamazepine
Meperidine	Cimetidine	Phenobarbitol
Propoxyphene	Ritonavir	Phenytoin
Oxycodone		
Hydrocodone		
Detromethorphan (*O*-demethylation)	Methadone	Rifampin
Cyclobenzaprine	Fluoextine (QT prolongation)	
Mexiletine		
Nortriptyline		
Doxepin		

(*continued*)

TABLE 2

Drug Metabolizing Systems (*Continued*)

Substrates	Inhibitors	Inducers
CYTOCHROME 3A4		
Alfentanil	Erythromycin	
	Indinavir	
Fentanyl	Nelfinavir	
	Ritonavir ($\downarrow$ Fentanyl/clearance by 67%)	
	Saquinavir	Rifampin
Sufentanil	Grapefruit juice	
	(Naringenin, a component of the juice)	
	Ketocanazole	
	Fluvoxamine	Corticosteroids
		Carbamazepine
		Phenobarbital
Methadone	Quinine	Methadone
	Norfluoxetine	Rifampin (can precipitate withdrawal)
Dextromethorphan (*N*-demethylation)		
CYP1A2		
Amitriptyline		Smoking/polycyclic aromatic hydro-carbons (present in cigarette smoke)
		Charcoal-broiled food
		Rifampin
Desipramine	Fluvoxamine	Carbamazepine
	Ciproflaxacin	Phenytoin
	Cimetidine	Phenobarbital
	Paroxetine	
Acetaminophen		
Caffeine		
Phenothiazine		
CYP2C19		
Barbiturates	Fluoxamine	Rifampin
Mephenytoin		
Topiramate	Fluoxetine	Phenobarbitol
	Omeprazole	Phenytoin
CYP2C9		
Warfarin		Rifampin
Phenytoin	Amiodarone	Phenobarbital
Naproxen	Zafirlukast	Carbamazepine
	Cimetidine	

was roughly 200-fold greater than by the poor metabolizers. Pharmacodynamic effects (respiration, papillary diameter) were much greater in the extensive metabolizer group. In the presence of quinidine, the extensive metabolizer group was similar to the poor metabolizer group; this has been called phenocopying.

This illustrates the importance of an appreciation of pharmacokinetics and pharmcodynamics as well as the use of principles of titration in efforts to avoid undertreating poor metabolizers or extensive metabolizers receiving CYP2D6 inhibitors.

Effects and Interactions of Various Drugs

Oxycodone may be affected by the cytochrome p450 system in the gut, where its absorption (both sustained-release tablets and immediate-release solution) in healthy volunteers seems to be affected by the ingestion of a fatty meal.[9] Although this may not be clinically significant in healthy volunteers, the clinical significance of this in patients with advanced chronic illness is unclear. In the liver oxycodone is metabolized by CYP2D6 to noroxycodone.[10]

The significance of oxymorphone, another metabolite, is unclear.[11] Although oxymorphone may contribute to oxycodone analgesic effects in rats, Poyhia and coworkers[11] could not demonstrate clinical significance of oxymorphone after intravenous oxycodone (this form is not available in the United States) in humans. It is still conceivable, however, that oxymorphone or another oxycodone metabolite may contribute to oxycodone's analgesic effects in humans, although this remains elusive. If oxycodone metabolites were to contribute to analgesia, poor metabolizers or patients receiving inhibitors might be expected to have poor efficacy or inadequate analgesia from oxycodone.

Meperidine is one of the worst choices of opioids in elderly patients because it seems to affect mental status more than most other opioids, it is a negative inotrope, it is a positive chronotrope, and its toxic metabolite accumulates in renal insufficiency. Meperidine has a local anesthetic-type action and is metabolized to normeperidine (about half as analgesic as meperidine), which lowers the seizure threshold and may induce central nervous system excitability.

A commonly used "weak" opioid is propoxyphene, which is most often used with acetaminophen (Darvocet) or with aspirin (Darvon). Propoxyphene is an odorless, white crystalline powder with a bitter taste and a molecular weight of 375.94. Chemically, it is (2S,3R)–(+)–4–(dimethylamino)–3–methyl–1,2–diphenyl–2–butanol propionate (ester), and it is structurally somewhat related to methadone. Both are somewhat "linear" as opposed to the "ringed" opioids. Five rings distinguish the phenanthrenes (e.g., morphine) and two rings distinguish the phenylpiperidines (e.g., fentanyl). Peak plasma concentrations of propoxyphene are reached in about 2 to 2 ½ hours after oral administration. Propoxyphene (half-life, ~ 6–12 hours) is metabolized in the liver to norpropoxyphene (half-life, ~ 30–36 hours). Norpropoxyphene has significantly fewer central nervous system depressant effects than propoxyphene but a greater local anesthetic effect, which may lead to prolonged intracardiac conduction times (PR and QRS intervals).[12] This strong local anesthetic effect may explain why propoxyphene (and, similarly, meperidine) may be analgesic in situations in which other opioids have "failed."

Propoxyphene has a *Physician's Desk Reference* black box warning that states

- Do not prescribe propoxyphene for patients who are suicidal or addiction-prone.
- Prescribe propoxyphene with caution for patients taking tranquilizers or antidepressant drugs and patients who use alcohol in excess.

- Tell your patients not to exceed the recommended dose and to limit their intake of alcohol.

In a 1975 survey of deaths due to overdosage, in roughly 20% of the fatal cases death occurred within the first hour (5% occurred in 15 minutes).

Propoxyphene comes in two forms, propoxyphene hydrochloride (Darvon compound-65, with 65 mg of propoxyphene hydrochloride) and propoxyphene napsylate (Darvocet-N 50 or Darvocet-N 100 with 100 mg of proproxyphene napsylate). Following administration of 65, 130, or 195 mg of propoxyphene hydrochloride, the bioavailability of propoxyphene is equivalent to that of 100, 200, or 300 mg, respectively, of propoxyphene napsylate. The napsylate salt tends to be absorbed more slowly than the hydrochloride. The maximum recommended daily dose of propoxyphene hydrochloride is 390 mg/day, and the maximum recommended dose of propoxyphene napsylate is 600 mg/day.

Smith[13] reported that the analgesic activity of propoxyphene was less than that of aspirin. Propoxyphene is the other opioid that may demonstrate potent local anesthetic properties at clinical doses. As a result, it may lead to depression of the cardiac conduction system in cases of overdose.[14] Propoxyphene toxicity is a real concern in patients with liver disease because of significant first-pass metabolism to norpropoxyphene (propoxyphene may facilitate hepatic insult). Rare instances of jaundice have occurred in patients without known preexisting liver disease.[15] In patients with renal failure, high blood levels of both propoxyphene and norpropoxyphene can accumulate, which tend not to be removed well by hemodialysis secondary to high protein binding.[16] Propoxyphene should be avoided in renal insufficiency. Subacute painful myopathy has occurred following chronic propoxyphene overdosage.[16]

Meperidine should never be used in combination with monoamine oxidase (MAO) inhibitors, because it could lead to a potentially lethal serotonin syndrome. Coadministration of cimetidine 1200 mg/day with meperidine decreased meperidine clearance by up to 22%.[12] Morphine is cleared essentially by glucuronidation; significant interactions at the cytochrome level are not seen.

A CYP3A4-mediated interaction is that of erythromcycin (a CYP3A4 inhibitor) given before surgery and fentanyl intraoperatively, leading to prolonged respiratory depression.[17] Administration of cimetidine with fentanyl doubles the latter's elimination half-life, thus potentially enhancing its pharmacological effects and duration of action.[17]

Caution should be used when giving propoxyphene to patients taking carbamazepine since propoxyphene inhibits carbamazepine metabolism to the point of potentially inducing toxicity.[18]

Since smoking affects certain CYP450 systems, it could conceivably affect the metabolism or effects of various analgesic agents.

Methadone is primarily metabolized by CYP3A4 (with perhaps a small contribution from CYP1A2). Ciprofloxacin (which inhibits CYP3A4 and CYP1A2) was administered to a patient who was treated with a stable dose of methadone with no problems for 6 years, with resultant profound sedation, confusion, and respiratory depression.[19] Antiviral agents may greatly affect methadone metabolism. A patient experienced methadone withdrawl symptoms when nevirapine (an inducer of CYP3A4) was added to his regimen.[20] Rifampin can cause the same effect.[21] Other agents can also affect methadone metabolism: Phenytoin lowers methadone concentration by about half in 3 to 4 days.[22] Phenobarbital and carbamazepine increase methadone metabolism.[22] Zidovudine may increase methadone levels.[22] Plasma levels of methadone increase by 20% to 100% in the presence of fluvoxamine.[22] Although there is certainly no evidence of any untoward effects, it seems prudent, if a patient is being treated with methadone or fentanyl, to avoid drinking liters of grapefruit juice and tonic water (quinine), both of which are CYP3A4 inhibitors.

The benzodiazepine-methadone combination can lead to significant respiratory depression.[22] Chronic alcoholism can reduce methadone levels and acute alcohol intake may increase levels. Chronic methadone administration (20–50 mg/d) may lead to chronic inhibition of certain cytochrome p450 enzyme systems.[23]

Methadone can also affect the metabolism of other agents, as it is a strong inhibitor of CYP2D6, which metabolizes codeine, oxycodone, and so on.[23] Therefore, if oxycodone and methadone are administered concurrently, the methadone may potentially lead to increases in the oxycodone levels or effect.

Additionally, if two substrates of the same cytochrome are given together, one may act as an extremely strong preferable substrate, essentially monopolizing all the cytochromes metabolic activities; therefore, it would be essentially functioning as a competative cytochrome inhibitor with the potential of leading to toxicity or side effects of the other substrate. Other interactions certainly need to be considered as well, such as additive or synergistic effects, pharmacodynamic interactions, and protein-binding effects.

The levels of free methadone may be altered by an inhibition of α_1-acid glycoprotein synthesis by alkylating substances.[7] Still another potential effect on administered methadone activity in the inhibition of P-glycoprotein by anticancer drugs, which may lead to altered transmembrane transport of morphine, methadone, or fentanyl. The clinical significance of such events remains unclear.

Buprenorphine (Buprenex), a partial μ-receptor agonist has been used by various clinicians in opioid withdrawl protocols, in a similar fashion to clonidine. The usual clinical doses of buprenorphine for analgesia are 0.3 mg, 0.45 mg, and 0.6 mg. In the United States, buprenorphine is clinically available only as a parenteral preparation to be given by intramuscular injection or intravenously. To give a bolus dose subcutaneously, a continuous infusion must be administered; otherwise, as with fentanyl, if lipid stores are not saturated it will not be effective via the subcutaneous route. A 7-day matrix transdermal system containing buprenorphine, called buprenorphine transdermal system, may eventually have a role in alleviating the pain of osteoarthritis.[24] In Europe, it is available in a sublingual preparation. In fact, there may still be a small number of patients in the United States who are taking it this way because of receiving the drug on a compassionate-use basis via a US study of sublingual buprenorphine. Bose and associates[25] are looking at the potential for electrically assisted transdermal delivery of buprenorphine.

Buprenorphine binds very avidly to the μ-receptor and is not "knocked off" very easily. In fact, if a patient has respiratory depression from buprenorphine, some clinicians advocate that the pharmacological treatment (aside from mechanical support of ventilation as appropriate) is not naloxone, which may not be as effective as is needed in usual doses, but is actually more buprenorphine. However, I do not know any nurses who would follow this protocol.

Large overdoses or intravenous misuse of buprenorphine may lead to hepatitis.[26] Buprenorphine is N-dealkylated to norbuprenorphine by CYD3A.[26] The parent compound apparently may concentrate in mitochrondria, where it may collapse the mitochrondrial membrane potential, inhibit β-oxidation, and uncouple and inhibit mitochrondrial respiration and adenosine triphosphate formation. Inducers of CYP3A attenuate and inhibitors of CYP3A aggravate this insult and transaminase increases.[26]

Hydromorphone (Dilaudid) may offer significant advantages in essentially being the opioid of choice in renal failure and having one of the least problems of all the opioids with drug interactions. Hydromorphone has not been reportd to have any major clinically significant interactions with tricyclic antidepressants, selective serotonin reuptake inhibitors, macrolide antibiotics, and so on.[10]

P-GLYCOPROTEIN

N-glycoprotein (P-gp) is a 170 kd transmembrane glycoprotein that functions as an adenosine triphosphate–dependent efflux pump, thereby exporting drugs and endogenous metabolites out of the cell.[27] It is expressed in the capillary endothelium of the blood-brain barrier as well as cell membrances of intestinal enterocytes and biliary and renal epithelial cells.

Expression of P-gp in major organs associated with absorption, distribution, and elimination lead to the hypothesis that P-gp evolved as a protective mechanism against a wide variety of potentially toxic substances, restricting distribution and facilitating elimination of P-gp substrates.[28]

Following the absorption of P-gp substrate from the intestinal lumen into the enterocyte, the substrate must be absorbed from the enterocyte into the circulation to have systemic effects. P-gp in the intestinal wall functions as a gastrointestinal "bouncer" to spit back out various undesirable substrates from the enterocyte into the intestinal lumen to be eliminated with the feces. P-gp can be induced or inhibited by many of the same agents that induce or inhibit various CYP450 systems

Some pharmacologists seem to be paying less attention to the cytochrome p450 systems and more attention to P-gp. One reason for this may be that P-gp can offset or reverse or augment the effects of the CYP450 system. CYP450 enzymes are not just in the liver. P-gp and CYP3A4 share various substrates and inhibitors and are located in many of same places.[29] CYP3A4, which accounts for roughly 70% of the total cytochrome activity in the intestine, may "help" P-gp in reducing systemic exposure to particular xenobiotics.[30] A substrate of both P-gp and CYP3A4 upon entering the enterocyte may encounter one of three fates: (1) direct absorption into the systemic circulation, (2) metabolism by CYP3A4 in the enterocyte, or (3) secretion back into the intestinal lumen by P-gp.[31] Substrates that are secreted back into the intestinal lumen may be reabsorbed at a more distal site and then may again undergo absorption, metabolism, or secretion.[31] This could lead to a cycling effect (enteroeneteric recycling), increasing mean residence time in the intestinal lumen.[31]

Morphine seems to be a P-gp substrate, and therefore morphine P-gp may play a role in limiting morphine entry into the brain. Morphine has been shown to increase analgesia in P-gp knockout mice compared with wild-type mice.[32] Wandel and associates[33] found that fentanyl, sufentanil, and alfentanil did not behave as P-gp substrates and concluded that opioids have a wide spectrum of P-gp activity, acting as both substrates and inhibitors, and this may contribute to their varying central nervous system effects.

Drug Interactions

The interaction of MAO inhibitors with opioids should not be taken lightly. Meperidine seems to be the worst, perhaps owing to issues that include the fact that MAO inhibitors (e.g., phenelzine) may inhibit meperidine demethylase,[35] meperidine may block neuronal uptake of 5-HT,[36] and an N-hydroxy derivative normeperidine may lead to a similar type reaction.[37]

The opioid that has been used safely with MAO inhibitors the most in the literature is morphine,[38] however, there was a severe interaction between morphine (6 mg) MAO inhibitor (tranylcypromine 40 mg/g) in a patient who became unconscious and hypotensive. The situation resolved after 2 minutes.[39]

Clinicians should be advised that dextromethorphan-MAO inhibitor interactions have led to death.[40] This needs to be kept in mind as combination products of morphine and dextromethorphen become available. Fentanyl also seems to be a reasonably safe alternative with MAO inhibitors.[41]

Zhan and coworkers[42] reported the finding from the 1996 Medical Expenditure Panel Survey and listed drugs to be avoided in elderly patients or those believed to be rarely appropriate based largely on 1997 Beers Criteria[43] and Expert Panel concerns. The original 1991 Beers criteria[44] and 1997 updated version[43] continue to be somewhat debated, since they cannot capture all the factors that define appropriate decision making,[45] such as weighing risk/benefit ratios. They may be considered as a screening test in assessing inappropriate use, however.[43] The 11 drugs Zhan's group listed to always avoid in the elderly were barbiturates, flurazepam, meprobamate, chlorpropamide, meperidine (removed from the formulary of at least one hospital), pentazocine, trimethobenzamide, belladonna alkaloids, dicyclomine, hyoscyamine, and propantheline.[42] The eight drugs classified as rarely appropriate in the elderly were chlordiazepoxide, diazepam, propoxyphene, carisoprodol, chlorzoxazone, cyclobenzaprine, metaxalone, and methocarbamol.[42] According to John R. Horn, PharmD. presenting at the 11th Annual Meeting of the Academy of Managed Care Pharmacy, "With the present system, pharmacists and physicians are placed on guard against far too many DDIs [drug-drug interactions] . . . In vitro studies and knowledge of metabolic pathways are helpful to predict potential DDIs, but they won't tell you much about what will [actually] happen in a specific patient . . . Clinical observations, rather than theoretical and in vitro information, should be used as the basis for flagging DDIs."

REFERENCES FOR ADDITIONAL READING

1. Nies A, Spielberg SP: Principles of therapeutics. In: Hardman J, Limbird LE, Morlinoff PB, eds: Goodman and Gilman's the Pharmacological Basis of therapeutics, 9th ed. McGraw-Hill, New York, 1996, pp 43–52.

2. Crowther N, Holbrook AM, Kenwright R, et al: Drug interactions among commonly used medications: Chart simplified data from critical literature review. Can Fam Physician 43:1972–1976, 1979–1981, 1997.

3. Park BK, Kitteringham NR, Pirmohamed M, et al: Relevance of induction of human drug-metabolizing enzymes: Pharmacological and toxicological implications. Br J Clin Pharmacol 41: 477–491, 1996.

4. Bertilsson L, Dahl ML, Dalen P, et al: Molecular genetics of CYP2D6: Clinical relevance with focus on psychotropic drugs. Br J Clin Pharmacol 53:111–122, 2002.

5. Mortimer O, Persson K, Landona MG, et al: Polymorphic formation of morphine from codeine in poor and extensive metabolizers of dextromethorphan: Relationship to the presence of immuno-identified cytochrome P-450 IIDI. Clin Pharmacol Ther 47:27–35, 1990.

6. Ladona MG, Lindstrom B, Thyr C, et al: Differential fetal development of the O and N-demethylation of codeine and dextromethorphan in man. Br J Clin Pharmacol 32:295–302, 1991.

7. Lotsch J, Sharke C, Tegeder I, et al: Drug interactions with patient-controlled analgesic. Clin Pharmacokinet 41:31–57, 2002.
8. Caraco J, Sheller J, Wood AJJ, et al: Pharmacogenetic determination of the effects of codeine and prediction of drug interactions. J Pharmacol Exp Ther 278:1165–1174, 1996.
9. Benziger D, Kaiko RF, Miotto JB, et al: Differential effects of food on the bioavailability of controlled-release oxycodone tablets and immediate-release oxycodone solution. J Pharm Sci 85:406–410, 1996.
10. Bernard SA, Bruera E: Drug interactions in palliative care. J Clin Oncol 18:1780–1799, 2000.
11. Poyhia R, Olkkola KT, Seppala T, et al: The pharmacokinetics of oxycodone after intravenous injection in adults. Br J Clin Pharmacol 32:516–518, 1991.
12. Nicklander R, Smits S, Steinberg M: Propoxyphene and norpropoxyphene: Pharmacology and toxic effects in animals. JPET 200:245–253, 1977.
13. Smith R: Federal government faces painful decision on Darvon. Science 203:857–858, 1971.
14. Holland D, Steinberg M: Electrophysiological properties of propoxyphene or norpropoxyphene in canine cardiac conducting tissues in vitro and in vivo. Toxicol Appl Pharmacol 47:123–133, 1979.
15. Giacomini K, Giacomini JC, Gibson TP, et al: Propoxyphene and norpropoxyphene plasma concentrations after oral propoxyphene in cirrhotic patients with and without surgically constructed porta caval shunt. Clin Pharmacol Ther 28:417–424, 1980.
16. Mather L: Clinical pharmacokinetics of analgesic drugs. In: Ray PP, ed: Practical Management of Pain, 2nd ed. Mosby, St. Louis, 1992.
17. Maurer PM, Bartkowski RR: Drug interactions of clinical significance with opioid analgesics. Drug Saf 8:30–48, 1993.
18. Hansen B, et al: Influence of dextropropoxyphene on steady state serum levels and protein binding of three antiepileptic drugs in man. Acta Neurol Scand 61:357–367, 1980.
19. Herrlin K, Segerdahl M, Gustafsson LL, et al: Methadone, ciprofloxacin, and adverse drug reactions. Lancet 356:2069–2070, 2000.
20. Heelon MW, Meade LB: Methadone withdrawal when starting an antiretroviral regimen including nevirapine. Pharmacotherapy 19:471–472, 1999.
21. Michalets EL: Update: Clinically significant cytochrome P-450 drug interactions. Pharmacotherapy 18:84–112, 1998.
22. Schlatter J, Madras JL, Saulnier JL, et al: Drug interactions with methadone. Presse Med 28:1381–1384, 1999.
23. Wu D, Otton SV, Sproulee BA, et al: Inhibition of human cytochrome P450 2D6 (CYP2D6) by methadone. Br J Clin Pharmacol 35:30–34, 1993.
24. Spyker D, St. Ville J, Lederman M, et al: Analgesic efficacy and safety of buprenorphine transdermal system (BTDS) in patients with osteoarthritis. J of Pain 3:(Suppl 12), 2002.
25. Bose S, Ravis WR, Lin YJ, et al: Electrically-assisted transdermal delivery by buprenorphine. J Control Release 73:197–203, 2001.
26. Berson A, Fau D, Fornacciari R, et al: Mechanisms for experimental buprenorphine hepatotoxicity: Major role of mitochondrial dysfunction versus metabolic activation. J Hepatol 34:261–269, 2001.
27. Hansten PD, Levy RH: Role of P-glycoprotein and organic anion transporting polypeptides in drug absorbtion and distribution: Focus on H1 receptor antagonists. Clin Drug Invest 21:587–596, 2001.
28. Schinkel AH: The physiological function of drug transporting P-gylcoproteins. Sem Cancer Biol 8:161–170, 1997.
29. Wacher VJ, Wu CY, Benet LZ: Overlapping substrate specificies and tissue distribution of cytochrome P450 3A and P-glycoprotein: Implications for drug delivery and activity in cancer chemotherapy. Mol Carcinogen 13:129–134, 1995.

30. Hall SD, Thummel KE, Watkins PB, et al: Molecular and physical mechanisms of first-pass excretion. Drug Metab Dispos 27:161–166, 1999.

31. Matheny CJ, Lamb MW, Brouwer KLR, et al: Pharmacokinetic and pharmacodynamic implications of P-glycoprotein modulation. Pharmacotherapy 21:778–796, 2001.

32. Thompson SJ, Koszdin K, Bernards CM: Opiate-induced analgesia is increased and prolonged in mick lacking P-glycoprotein. Anesthestiology 92:1392–1399, 2000.

33. Wandel C, Kim R, Wood M, et al: Interaction of morphine, fentanyl sufentanil, alfentanil, and loperamide with the efflux drug transporter P-glycoprotein. Anesthesiology 96:913–920, 2002.

34. Riley RJ: The potential pharmacological and toxicological impact of P450 screening. Curr Opin Drug Discov Devel 4:45–54, 2001.

35. Eade NR, Renton KW: The effect of phenelzine and tranylcypromine on the degradation of meperidine. J Pharmacol Exp Ther 173:31–36, 1970.

36. Carlsson A, Lindgvist M: Central and peripheral monoaminergic membrane-pump blockade by some addictive analgesics and antihistamines. J Pharm Pharmacol 21:460–464, 1969.

37. Yeh SY: Metabolism of meperidine in several animal species. J Pharm Sci 73:1783–1787, 1984.

38. Taylor DC: Alarming reaction to pethidine in patients on phenelzine. Lancet 2:401–402, 1962.

39. Barry BJ: Adverse effects of MAO inhibitors with narcotics reversed with naloxone [letter]. Anesth Intens Care 7:194, 1979.

40. Rivers N, Homer B: Possible lethal reaction between nardil and dextromethorphan [letter]. Can Med Assoc J 103:85, 1970.

41. Rossiter A, Souney PF: Interaction between MAOIs and opioids: Pharmacologic and clinical considerations. Hosp Formul 28:692–698, 1993.

42. Zhan C, Sangl J, Bierman AS, et al: Potentially inappropriate medication use in the community-dwelling elderly. Findings from the 1996 Medical Expenditure Panel Survey. JAMA 286:2823–2829, 2001.

43. Beers MH: Explicit criteria for determining potentially inappropriate medication use by the elderly: An update. Arch Intern Med 157:1531–1536, 1997.

44. Beers MH, Ouslander JG, Rollingher I, et al: Explicit criteria for determining inappropriate medication use in nursing home residents. Arch Intern Med 151:1825–1832, 1991.

45. Anderson G, Beers M, Kerluk K: Auditing prescription practice using explicit criteria and computerized drug benefit claims data. J Eval Clin Pract 3:283–294, 1997.

Chapter 36

Basic Pharmacotherapeutics of Migraine

K. M. A. Welch, MD

INTRODUCTION

Specific treatments for migraine should be based on understanding its pathogenesis. Research has identified a cerebral cortical origin of migraine aura and the trigeminovascular system and its central projections as the origin of headache pain. Drug therapies for migraine, both current and potential targets for future development, are reviewed in this chapter, prefaced in each section by a discourse on migraine pathophysiology. Basic concepts of migraine pathogenesis underlying drug action are addressed for stages of the migraine attack and its consequences. These include (1) neuronal hyperexcitablity during the interictal phase, (2) cortical spreading depression (CSD) as the basis of aura, (3) trigeminal nerve activation at a peripheral or central origin that accounts for headache, and (4) progressive damage to the periaqueductal grey matter (PAG) that may explain some aspects of central sensitization or change in phenotypic expression of the disorder. At each stage, opportunities are present for therapeutic targets.

Preventive medications are discussed that focus on diminishing brain excitability and blocking triggers of the aura. Successful intervention might involve drugs that delay aura propagation or interfere with the aura-trigeminal interface at which aura induces headache. Drugs that terminate trigeminal activation from either a peripheral or a central location are effective against pain. Drugs that modulate trigeminal activity might counteract the central sensitization of the trigeminal pain pathways that accounts for prolonged pain of headache. Finally, this review addresses the newest concept in migraine therapy, that the central nociceptive systems might require protective medications to prevent repeated attacks of migraine, altering the phenotypic expression of the illness from episodic to chronic.

INTERICTAL PHASE AND PREVENTIVE DRUGS

The concept that the migraine attack originates in the brain and can be triggered by various factors under various conditions argues in favor of a threshold that governs the triggering of attacks. The nature of the final common pathway with which these factors interact probably constitutes the true cause of migraine. Neurophysiological, cerebral blood flow (CBF), and metabolic measurements have suggested neuronal and neurovascular instability between migraine attacks. One recently proposed model to explain these physiological shifts is transient or persistently exaggerated excitability of neurons in the cerebral cortex, especially occipital.[1] Although the pathways mediating headache pain may be the same in all individuals, these pathways may be more easily triggered in patients with episodic migraines. As an example of interictal differences in brain activity between normal subjects and migraine sufferers, transcranial magnetic stimulation to the occipital cortex required to produce phosphene generation was significantly lower in patients with migraines with aura between their headaches than it was in normal control subject.[2]

Differing cellular mechanisms may underlie increased central neuronal hyperexcitability in migraine. In a rare autosomal-dominant subtype of migraine, familial hemiplegic migraine, mutation of a gene involved in the production of a brain-specific P/Q-type calcium channel was identified in about 50% of families.[3] This indicates that at least this uncommon form of migraine results from a calcium channelopathy and possibly more typical migraine, at least in some cases of families studied subsequently.[4] A channelopathy might explain the efficacy of certain prophylactics, such as the calcium channel blockers flunarizine and verapamil, and anticonvulsants, such as sodium valproate, gabapentin, and topiramate, which alter the properties of ion channels and excitability. In fact, as TABLE 1 shows, preventive drugs previously used to prevent migraine by virtue of multiple and different mechanisms of action, all have a common property of diminishing excitability, albeit by differing mechanisms.

Other possible sources of neuronal hyperexcitability are a mitochondrial defect or a disturbance in magnesium metabolism.[5] Intracellular magnesium stores may be low in migraine sufferers; this deficiency could affect mitochondria function, or it could alter membrane stability by receptor gating or binding to membrane phospholipids. In support of this, FIGURE 1 shows low magnesium levels in phosphorus-31 spectroscopic images of members of a family with hemiplegic migraine. Trials of riboflavin and magnesium in migraine prevention have provided evidence of modest benefit only, however.[6,7]

MECHANISM UNDERLYING AURA AND DRUGS THAT PREVENT HEADACHE ACTIVATION

One fifth of migraine sufferers experience aura prior to headache onset,[8,9] which is predominantly visual.[10] Cortical spreading depression, first observed by Leao in 1944,[11,12] is considered the basis of the aura. Cortical neuronal excitation followed by depression of normal neuronal activity spreads slowly from the site of initiation at rates between 2 and 6 mm/min. Spreading depression does not follow vascular boundaries, although pial arterial and venous dilation occur simultaneously with the first activated neural activity.[13] A brief increase in regional CBF is followed by decreased regional CBF to oligemic values, lasting approximately 1 hour after the passage of the wave of neuronal inhibition.[14] Like spreading depression, this cortical oligemia does not follow vascular boundaries. Advances in brain imaging, including regional CBF measured by xeno-133, diffusion/perfusion magnetic resonance imaging (MRI), functional MRI-BOLD, and magnetoencephalography have allowed investigators to observe CSD during migraine aura.[15–20] Cao and colleagues[17] studying the properties of migraine attacks induced by visual stimulation using fMRI noted that transient

TABLE 1

Sites at Which Standard Preventive Drugs Regulate Neuronal Hyperexcitability

Site	Antiserotonin	β-lock	Ca²⁺ Blocker	NSAIDs	Valproate
Na⁺ channel					+
Ca²⁺ channel	?		+		+/?
EAA Receptor			+		
GABA REC/Cl⁻					+/?
5HT/NE NT	+	+	+	+	

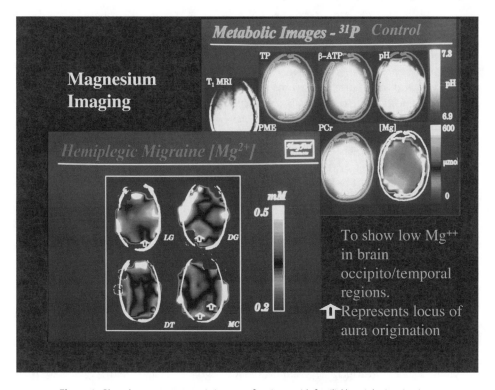

Figure 1. Phosphorus spectroscopic images of patients with familial hemiplegic migraine.

activation followed by a spreading suppression of neuronal activity was accompanied by vasodilation and hyperoxygenation.[17]

The mechanism by which aura transduces the headache of migraine is unclear. Spreading depression causes stimulation of the trigeminal nucleus caudalis,[21] a region believed to be part of the central pathway mediating migraine pain. This might be secondary to involvement of cortical-subcortical connections to nociceptive centers recruited by the wave of cortical excitation and suppression. Alternatively, the wave of spreading depression may invade cortical trigeminal terminals, setting up a cascade of events leading to inflammation as a persistent source of trigeminal stimulation and headache. Recent evidence has implicated both the trigeminal and the parasympathetic systems through brainstem connections, accounting for vasodilatation and inflammatory change of the extracerebral circulation, particularly meningeal vessels, during and after CSD.[22]

Most studies of spreading depression in migraine sufferers have focused on the aura phase of migraine. Woods and associates[19] observed spreading oligemia in association with spontaneous headache in a patient with migraine but no aura, however. Changes in regional CBF resembled those observed during aura by other investigators.[16,18] Cao and colleagues[17] reported a spreading suppression of neural activity in the occipital cortex prior to headache in migraine patients with or without aura.[17] Results of these studies suggest that the same neuronal events may precede the initiation of migraine in all patients, although CSD and changes in CBF remain clinically silent in migraine without aura. On the other hand, other investigators have not observed changes in blood flow in patients with migraine without aura, raising the alternative possibility that the trigeminal system may be activated by noncortical mechanisms, such as changes in pain modulation.[23]

Preventing activation of headache by interfering with the initial triggering or propagation of CSD might be a viable approach to migraine management. For example, migraine sine hemicrania, aura without headache, presumably is an example of a case in which CSD does not spread into regions where cortical-subcortical connections can activate brainstem nociceptive networks or fails to activate the trigeminovascular system. Although CSD is considered an "all or nothing" phenomenon, magnesium and glutamate or N-methyl-D-aspartate (NMDA) antagonists can block CSD. The potential exists for magnesium preparations, glutamate antagonists, nitric oxide inhibitors (L-NMMA), or drugs that provide dendritic gap junction blockade to avoid activation of headache mechanisms. Such therapeutic approaches are in various stages of development.

HEADACHE AND THE ACTION OF CONTEMPORARY ABORTIVE DRUGS

Migraine headache may originate from dilation of the large cranial vessels and dura mater, innervated by the trigeminal nerve as part of the trigeminovascular system.[25-27] Stimulation of trigeminal sensory neurons induces inflammation and plasma protein extravasation (PPE).[28] The vasoactive peptides substance P and neurokinin A, released by the trigeminovascular system, cause PPE from the vessels, mast cell degranulation, platelet adherence and aggregation, and endothelial activation.[29,30] The result is meningeal inflammation that persists for minutes to hours, possibly the principal mechanism for the prolonged intense headache pain. The antimigraine agents sumatriptan, ergotamine, dihydroergotamine, and methysergide have been shown to block this plasma extravasation, thereby reducing neurogenic inflammation.[31] However, not all drugs that block PPE have an antimigraine effect,[32,33] a point of controversy when attributing mechanisms of migraine headache, since it is unclear whether PPE and meningeal inflammation occur in humans during migraine.[34] For example, CP-122,288, a potent PPE inhibitor without vasoconstrictor effects,[35] is ineffective in aborting migraine.[32] TABLE 2 summarizes the PPE data versus migraine effect.

The vasodilator peptides calcitonin gene-related peptide (CGRP), substance P, and neurokinin A are found in the cell bodies of trigeminal neurons.[36-38] CGRP has been implicated most in the headache of migraine.[39] CGRP is present in nonmyelinated fibers in the trigeminal ganglion,[40] and CGRP-like immunoreactivity has been identified in regions of the trigeminal nuclei known to receive primary afferent terminals.[41] The sensory role of CGRP in the trigeminal system is unclear but possibly involves vascular nociception. Electrical stimulation of the ganglion released CGRP in cat and humans,[39] and CGRP was detected in jugular venous blood during a migraine attack, but not substance P.[42] The neurogenic inflammation theory of migraine proposed that CGRP released from trigeminal sensory afferents causes vasodilation and plasma extravasations from dural vessels.[43] Triptans, acting as 5-HT$_{1B/D}$ agonists, block these responses.[44] Infusion of CGRP to susceptible individuals can elicit migraine-like headache.[45] It remains to be determined whether specific CGRP antagonists are effective in alleviating migraine attacks.

Triptans are 5-HT$_{1B/1D}$ receptor agonists with potent antimigraine effects.[46] They block transmission in the trigeminovascular system, similar to the nonspecific ergotamine derivatives.[47] These agonists include sumatriptan,[48,49] naratriptan,[50,51] rizatriptan,[52] zolmitriptan,[53] almotriptan, and eletriptan. Triptans do not block peripheral (nontrigeminal) pain processing.[50,54] It is unclear whether the benefit of the 5-HT agonists in relieving migraine headache

TABLE 2

Plasma Protein Extravasation and Antimigraine Effect

Plasma Protein Extravasation	Migraine Effect	No Effect
Ergots/DHE	Yes	~
Triptan 1-B/D	Yes	~
$5HT_{1D}$	~	Yes
ASA	Yes	~
CP228228	~	Yes
En/SP/NK antag	~	Yes
$5HT_{1F}$	Yes? Central	~
CGRP antag.	Yes	~

En, endothelin; SP, substance P; NK, neurokinin Y; DHE, dihydroergotamine

is through a peripheral or a central action, or both. Further, it is unclear whether any peripheral action is by vasoconstriction or inhibition of peptide release, or both. Sumatriptan does not cross the blood-brain barrier[55] but can inhibit the trigeminal nucleus activation when disrupted.[48,49] Since, in theory, the blood-brain barrier may be altered during migraine,[56–58] a central action cannot be ruled out for sumatriptan. In support, sumatriptan must be administered after the onset of headache to be efficacious. All second-generation triptans developed after sumatriptan readily penetrate the blood-brain barrier.

The vasoconstrictive action of the triptans extends to the coronary vasculature, although they are active only at concentrations well below those attained in clinically aborting migraine headache. Nevertheless, cardiovascular complications have occurred with the use of these drugs, although rarely.[59] Restricting the patient population that can receive these drugs to those without coronary or cerebrovascular diseases or the risk thereof is an undesirable element of clinical practice. Although the effectiveness of the triptans is generally of high order, it is far from absolute and this, plus the adverse event profile, demands the continued search for new drug targets, new drugs, and new approaches to understanding migraine mechanisms.

NOVEL ASPECTS OF MIGRAINE MECHANISMS AND THE SEARCH FOR NEW DRUG STRATEGIES

The brainstem may play a pivotal role in the pathophysiology of migraine. In a study of acute migraine without aura using positron emission tomography, an area of the contralateral rostral brainstem covering the dorsal pons and midbrain, particularly the PAG, dorsal raphe nucleus, and locus ceruleus, was activated during the attack and after effective treatment by sumatriptan.[60] Further, iron levels were abnormal in the midbrain PAG of patients with episodic and chronic migraine.[61] These areas, especially PAG, may produce migraine-like headache when stimulated in humans[62,63] or triggered by certain structural pathologies.[64,65] Thus, episodic dysfunction of brainstem neurons may have a key role in migraine pain, through either aberrant activation or impaired modulation of impulse flow in the trigeminal system. Since the PAG is the center of a powerful antinociceptive system in the brain, this offers new approaches to acute migraine drugs acting as neuromodulators via this system. The PAG itself is a site of triptan binding and an alternative or additional explanation for the action of these drugs.[59] Of interest, PAG modulation of trigeminovascular nociceptive afferent signals in experimental animals[66] is blocked after local blockade of the P/Q voltage-gated calcium channel with agatoxin-IVA.[67] As noted previously, missense mutations in the CaV2.1 subunit of this channel was found in families with familial hemiplegic migraine[3] and may account for more typical migraine as well.[4]

Evidence for central neuronal hyperexcitability has been observed in a study of cutaneous allodynia during migraine in humans, findings indicating central sensitization at a second- or third-order neuron level.[68] Abnormal supraspinal pain modulation is in keeping with PAG dysfunction and aberrance of its balanced nociceptive facilitatory or inhibitory functions.[69] This, plus abnormal sensitization at a second-order neuron level, introduces numerous drug targets that might restore normal modulation of pain or reduce pain severity and duration once the trigeminal system is activated.[69] For example, since the main receptor involved in sensitization appears to be the NMDA, trials of NMDA antagonists seem logical. Other approaches, such as $\alpha2$-receptor agonist use, known to be effective in chronic pain management, might prove to be beneficial adjunctive therapies during migraine attacks.[69]

Recently, we documented increased iron in the PAG of episodic and chronic migraine patients.[61] One possible explanation this is that repeated hyperoxia accompanying PAG activation, or of other like nociceptive centers with high metabolic activity and high iron turnover, might result in progressive free radical–mediated cellular damage. The strong associations of the burden of illness with this marker iron deposition of PAG damage might explain why episodic migraine becomes chronic over time in some patients. Accordingly, rapid and effective abortive treatment and aggressive preventive measures seem essential in those patients with frequent migraine attacks. The potential for even subtle but cumulative free radical damage during attacks suggests the importance of combining treatment with a free radical scavenger, for example vitamin E.

For future drug discovery, mouse models of gene-based diseases have become an established mode of investigation in contemporary biomedical research. Although no singular genetic basis for the prevalent forms of migraine is known, much information can be obtained by examining gene regulation during events known to be involved in migraine pathogenesis.[70] Molecular targets for migraine mechanisms probably are many; a mouse experimental model has the dual advantages of screening multiple genes and studying the effects of these genes by genetic manipulation. Adopting this approach, we recently identified the vigorous up-regulation of antioxidant genes during CSD in a mouse model, supporting the need for the brain to protect itself from free radical damage during migraine attacks.[70] Further, this approach provided information on atrial natriuretic peptide as a potential target to prevent CSD activation of headache and identified changes in neuropeptide Y. Since estrogen is a neuronal modulator and a key factor in migraine pathogenesis, we also took this approach in the mouse, using the female estrus cycle as an opportunity to model ovarian steroid changes associated with triggering attacks of menstrual and ovulatory migraine.[71] In trigeminal ganglia, we discovered that the level of neuropeptide Y rose and fell with estrogen levels, unlike CGRP or atrial natruiretic peptide, which were also present. Since neuropeptide prevents CGRP release from trigeminal neurons, its fall with estrogen levels might be linked to triggering menstrual migraine. This illustrates how using such models can assist in choosing an appropriate and narrowed focus for future clinical research.

CONCLUSION

Current knowledge of migraine mechanisms as they underpin the pharmacotherapeutics of the disorder were reviewed. Migraine preventive drugs need to be developed that specifically target mechanisms of increased neuronal excitability. This will be difficult to achieve with any specificity, since the cause of excitability is probably multifactorial. Specific blockade of CSD initiation or propagation might prove a more effective approach. Current abortive migraine drugs such as the triptans are effective, but adverse safety profile limits their ideal use in some patients. Since experience with the triptans also has shown the need for greater effectiveness, ongoing drug discovery seems appropriate. Drugs that target modulation of pain pathways as well as primary pain mechanisms should be explored. Attention also should be directed to long-term consequences of repeated migraine attacks when crafting novel therapeutic strategies.

Disclosures

K. Michael Welch, MD has been a consultant/scientific advisor for AstraZeneca Pharmaceuticals, GlaxoSmithKline, and Pharmacia.

REFERENCES FOR ADDITIONAL READING

1. Welch KMA, D'Andrea G, Tepley N, Barkeley GL, Ramadan NM. The concept of migraine as a state of central neuronal hyper excitability. Headache 1990;8:817–828.
2. Aurora SK, Ahmad BK, Welch KMA, Bhardhwaj P, Ramadan NM. Transcranial magnetic stimulation confirms hyper excitability of occipital cortex in migraine. Neurology 1998; 50:1111–1114.
3. Ophoff RA, Terwindt GM, Vergouwe MN, et al. Familial hemiplegic migraine and episodic ataxia type-2 are caused by mutations in the Ca2+ channel gene CACNLA4. Cell 1996; 87:543–552.
4. Nyholt DR, Lea RA, Goadsby PJ, et al: Familial typical migraine: Linkage to chromosome 19p13 and evidence for genetic heterogeneity. Neurology 50:1428–1432, 1998.
5. Welch KM, Ramadan NM: Mitochondria, magnesium and migraine. J Neurol Sci 134:9–14, 1995.
6. Peikert A, Wilimzig C, Kohne-Volland R: Prophylaxis of migraine with oral magnesium: Results from a prospective multi-center, placebo-controlled and double blind randomized study. *Cephalalgia* 16:257–263, 1996.
7. Schoenen J, Jacquy J, Lenaerts M: High-dose riboflavin is effective in migraine prophylaxis: Results from a double blind, randomized, placebo-controlled trial. *Neurology* 48:A86–A87, 1997.
8. Russell MB, Rassmussen BK, Fenger K, Olesen J: Migraine without aura and migraine with aura are distinct clinical entities: A study of four hundred and eight-four male and female migraineurs from the general population. Cephalalgia 16:239–245, 1996.
9. Stewart WF, Sechter A, Rasmussen BK: Migraine prevalence: A review of population-based studies. Neurology 44:S17–S23, 1994.
10 Russell MB, Olesen J: A nosographic analysis of the migraine aura in a general population. Brain 119:355–361, 1996.
11. Leao AAP: Spreading depression of activity in cerebral cortex. J Neurophysiol 7:359–390, 1944.
12. Leao AAP: Pial circulation and spreading activity in the cerebral cortex. J Neurophysiol 7:391–396, 1944.
13. Lauritzen M, Jorgensen MB, Diemer NH, et al: Persistent oligaemia of rat cerebral cortex in the wake of spreading depression. Ann Neurol 12:469–474, 1982.
14. Lauritzen M: Long-lasting reduction of cortical blood flow of the rat brain after spreading depression with preserved autoregulation and impaired CO_2 response. J Cereb Blood Flow Metab 4:546–554, 1984.
15. Olesen J: Cerebral and extracranial circulatory disturbances in migraine: Pathophysiological implications. Cerebrovasc Brain Metab Rev 3:1–28, 1991.
16. Olesen J, Larsen B, Lauritzen M: Focal hyperemia followed by spreading oligemia and impaired activation of rCBF in classic migraine. Ann Neurol 9:344–352, 1981.

17. Cao Y, Welch KMA, Aurora S, Vikingstad EM: Functional MRI-BOLD of visually triggered headache in patients with migraine. Arch Neurol 56:548–554, 1999.

18. Cutrer FM, Sorensen AG, Weisskoff RM, et al: Perfusion-weighted imaging defects during spontaneous migrainous aura. Ann Neurol 43:25–31, 1998.

19. Woods RP, Iacoboni M, Mazziotta JC: Bilateral spreading cerebral hypoperfusion during spontaneous migraine headache. N Engl J Med 331:1689–1692, 1994.

20. Hadjikhani N, Sanchez del Rio M, Wu O, et al: Mechanisms of migraine aura revealed by functional MRI in human visual cortex. Proc Nat Acad Sci USA 98:4687–4692, 2001.

21. Moskowitz MA, Nozaki K, Kraig RP: Neocortical spreading depression provokes the expression of C-fos protein-like immunoreactivity within the trigeminal nucleus caudalis via trigeminovascular mechanisms. J Neurosc 13:1167–1177, 1993.

22. Bolay H, Reuter U, Dunn AK, et al: Intrinsic brain activity triggers trigeminal meningeal afferents in a migraine model. Nat Med 8:136–142, 2002.

23. Goadsby PJ: The pathophysiology of headache. In: Silberstein SD, Lipton RB, Solomon S, eds: Wolff's Headache and Other Head Pain, 7th ed. Oxford University Press, Oxford, 2001, pp 57–72.

24. Feindel W, Penfield W, McNaughton F: The tentorial nerves and localization of intracranial pain in man. Neurology 10:555–563, 1960.

25. Goadsby PJ, Hoskin KL: The distribution of trigeminovascular afferents in the non-human primate brain Macaca nemestrina: A c-fos immunocytochemical study. J Anat 190:367–375, 1997.

26. Hoskin KL, Zagami A, Goadsby PJ: Stimulation of the middle meningeal artery leads to bilateral Fos expression in the trigeminocervical nucleus: A comparative study of monkey and cat. J Anat 194:579–588, 1999.

27. May A, Goadsby PJ: The trigeminovascular system in humans: Pathophysiological implications for primary headache syndromes of the neural influences on the cerebral circulation. J Cerebr Blood Flow.

28. Moskowitz MA: Basic mechanisms in vascular headache. Neurol Clin 8:801–815, 1990.

29 Dimitriadou V, Buzzi MG, Moskowitz MA, Theoharides TC: Trigeminal sensory fiber stimulation induces morphological changes reflecting secretion in rat dura mater mast cells. Neuroscience 44: 97–112, 1991.

30. Dimitriadou V, Buzzi MG, Theoharides TC, Moskowitz MA: Ultrastructural evidence for neurogenically mediated changes in blood vessels of the rat dura mater and tongue following antidromic trigeminal stimulation. Neuroscience 48:187–203, 1992.

31. Moskowitz MA, Cutrer FM: Sumatriptan: A receptor-targeted treatment for migraine. Annu Rev Med 44:145–154, 1993.

32. Roon KI, Olesen J, Diener HC, et al: No acute antimigraine efficcy of CP-122, 288, a highly potent inhibitor of neurogenic inflammation: Results of two randomized double-blind placebo-controlled clinical trials. Ann Neurol 47:238–241, 2000.

33. Goadsby PJ: The pharmacology of headache. Prog Neurobiol 62:509–525, 2000.

34. Goadsby PJ, Hoskin KL: Differential effects of low dose CP122, 288 and eletriptan on Fos expression due to stimulation of the superior sagittal sinus in the cat. Pain 82:15–22, 1999.

35. Lee WS, Moskowitz MA: Conformationally restricted sumatriptan analogues, CP-122, 288 and CP-122, 638, exhibit enhanced potency against neurogenic inflammation in dura mater. Brain Res 626: 303–305, 1993.

36. Uddman R, Edvinsson L, Ekman R, et al: Innervation of the feline cerebral vasculature by nerve fibers containing calcitonin gene-related peptide: Trigeminal origin and co-existence with substance P. Neurosci Lett 62:131–136, 1985.

37. Liu-Chen L-Y, Gillespie SA, Norregaard TV, Moskowitz MA: Co-localization of retrogradely transported wheat germ agglutinin and the putative neurotransmitter substance P within trigeminal ganglion cells projecting to cat middle cerebral. J Comp Neurol 225:187–192, 1984.

38. Edvinsson L, Brodin E, Jansen I, Uddman R: Neurokinin A in cerebral vessels: Characterization, localization and effects in vitro. Regulatory Peptides 20:181–197, 1988.

39. Goadsby PJ, Edvinsson L, Ekman R: Release of vasoactive peptides in the extracerebral circulation of man and the cat during activation of the trigeminovascular system. Ann Neurol 23:193–196, 1988.

40. Alvarez FJ, Morris HR, Priestley JV: Sub-populations of smaller diameter trigeminal primary afferent neurons defined by expression of calcitonin gene-related peptide and the cell surface oligosaccharide recognized by monoclonal antibody LA4. J Neurocytol 20:716–731, 1991.

41. Sugimoto T, Fujiyoshi Y, Xiao C, et al: Central projection of calcitonin gene-related peptide (CGRP)- and substance P (SP)-immunoreactive trigeminal primary neurons in the rat. J Comp Neurol 378:425–442, 1997.

42. Gallai V, Sarchielli P, Floridi A, et al: Vasoactive peptides levels in the plasma of young migraine patients with and without aura assessed both interictally and ictally. Cephalalgia 15:384–390, 1995.

43. Buzzi MG, Bonamini M, Moskowitz MA: Neurogenic model of migraine. Cephalalgia 15:277–280, 1995.

44. Goadsby PJ, Edvinsson L: Sumatriptan reverses the changes in calcitonin gene-related peptide seen in the headache phase of migraine. Cephalalgia 11(Suppl 11):3, 1991.

45. Lassen LH, Jacobsen VB, Petersen P, et al: Human calcitonin gene-related peptide (hCGRP)-induced headache in migraineurs. Eur J Neurol 5(Suppl 3):S63, 1998.

46. Ferrari MD: Migraine. Lancet 351:1043–1051, 1998.

47. Nozaki K, Moskowitz MA, Boccalini P: CP-93, 129, sumatriptan, dihydroergotamine block c-fos expression within the rat trigeminal nucleus caudalis caused by chemical stimulation of the meninges. Br J Pharmacol 106:409–415, 1992.

48. Kaube H, Hoskin KL, Goadsby PJ: Sumatriptan inhibits central trigeminal neurons only after blood-brain barrier disruption. Br J Pharmacol 109:788–792, 1993.

49. Shepheard SL, Williamson DJ, Williams J, et al: Comparison of the effects of sumatriptan and the NK1 antagonist CP-99, 994 on plasma extravasation in the dura mater and c-fos mRNA expression in the trigeminal nucleus caudalis of rats. Neuropharmacology 34:255–261, 1993.

50. Goadsby PJ, Knight YE: Inhibition of trigeminal neurons after intravenous administration of naratriptan through an action at the serotonin ($5HT_{1B/1D}$) receptors. Br J Pharmacol 122:918–922, 1997.

51. Cumberbatch MJ, Hill RG, Hargreaves RJ: Differential effects of the 5HT1B/1D receptor agonist naratriptan on trigeminal versus spinal nocicep5 3tive responses. Cephalalgia 18:659–664, 1998.

52. Cumberbatch MJ, Hill RG, Hargreaves RJ: Rizatriptan has central antinociceptive effects against durally evoked responses. Eur J Pharmacol 328:37–40, 1997.

53. Goadsby PJ, Hoskin KL: Inhibition of trigeminal neurons by intravenous administration of the serotonin (5HT)-1-D receptor agonist zolmitriptan (311C90): Are brain stem sites a therapeutic target in migraine? Pain 67:355–359, 1996.

54. Harrison SD, Balawi SA, Feinmann C, Harris M: Atypical facial pain: A double-blind placebo-controlled crossover pilot study of subcutaneous sumatriptan. Eur Neuropsychopharmacol 7:83–88, 1997.

55. Humphrey PPA, Feniuk W, Perren MJ, et al: Serotonin and migraine. Ann NY Acad Sci 600:587–598, 1990.

56. Bahra A, Matharu MS, Buchel C, et al: Brainstem activation specific to migraine headache. Lancet 357:1016–1017, 2001.

57. Raichle ME, Hartman BK, Eichling JO, Sharpe LG: Central noradrenergic regulation of cerebral blood flow and vascular permeability. Proc Nat Acad Sci U S A 72:3726–3730, 1975.

58. Harik SI, McGunigal T: The protective influence of the locus ceruleus on the blood-brain barrier. Ann Neurol 15:568–574, 1984.

59. Welch KM, Mathew NT, Stone P, et al: Tolerability of sumatriptan: Clinical trials and post-marketing experience. Cephalalgia 20:687–695, 2000.

60, Weiller C, May A, Limmroth V, et al: Brain stem activation in spontaneous human migraine attacks. Nat Med 1:658–660, 1995.

61. Welch KMA, Nagesh V, Aurora SK, Gelman N: Periaqueductal gray matter dysfunction in migraine: Cause or the burden of illness? Headache 41:629–637, 2001.

62. Raskin NH, Hosobuchi Y, Lamb S: Headache may arise from perturbation of brain. Headache 27: 416–420, 1987.

63. Veloso F, Kumar K, Toth C: Headache secondary to deep brain implantation. Headache 38:507–515, 1998.

64. Haas DC, Kent PF, Friedman DI: Headache caused by a single lesion of multiple sclerosis in the periaqueductal gray area. 33:452–455, 1993.

65. Goadsby PJ: Neurovascular headache and a midbrain vascular malformation: Evidence for a role of the brainstem in chronic migraine. Cephalalgia 2002 (in press).

66. Knight YE, Goadsby PJ: The periaqueductal gray matter modulates trigeminovascular input: A role in migraine? Neuroscience 106:793–800, 2001.

67. Knight YE, Bartsch T, Kaube H, Goadsby PJ: P/Q-type calcium channel blockade in the PAG facilitates trigeminal nociception: A functional genetic link for migraine? J Neurosci 2002 (in press).

68. Burstein R, Yarnitsky D, Goor-Aryeh I, et al: An association between migraine and cutaneous allodynia. Ann Neurol 47:614–624, 2000.

69. Millan MJ: Descending monoaminergic modulation of pain: Basic principles, novel insights from receptor multiplicity, and therapeutic perspectives. Neurosci News 4:19–34, 2001.

70. Choudhuri R, Cui L, Yong C, et al: Cortical spreading depression and gene regulation: relevance to migraine. Ann Neurol 51:499–506, 2002.

71. Berman NE, Puri V, Cui L, et al: Trigeminal ganglion neuropeptides cycle with ovarian steroids in a model of menstrual migraine. Proc Am Headache Soc, 2002.

Chapter 37

Clinical Pharmacotherapeutics of Headache

Pradeep Chopra, MD / Howard S. Smith, MD / Zahid Bajwa, MD

In 1988, the International Headache Society in 1988 formulated a classification system for headache disorders. The diagnostic criteria have been endorsed by the World Health Organization and have been included in the International Classification of Diseases (ICD-10).[4] Headaches are classified into primary and secondary headache disorders. The primary headache disorders consist of the following:

1. Migraine with aura
2. Migraine without aura
3. Tension-type headache—chronic and episodic
4. Cluster headache—chronic and episodic

Primary headaches such as migraine with or without aura, tension-type, and cluster headache account for about 90% of all headaches.[1,5,6] Secondary headaches are symptomatic of an underlying disease such as infection, increased intracranial pressure, brain tumor or bleeding. Migraine, as defined by the International Headache Society, is an idiopathic, recurring headache disorder manifesting in attacks lasting 4 to 72 hours. The diagnostic criteria for migraine are given in Table 1.

PATHOGENESIS OF MIGRAINE HEADACHE

Patients with migraines have a central neuronal hyperexcitable state. Activation of the trigeminal nerve and vasodilation of the intracranial cerebral blood arteries and vessels in the dura set off a state of perivascular inflammation. Serotonin receptors[22,23,46,47] on the intracranial blood vessels have predominantly 5-HT_{1A} and 5-HT_{1B} receptors. Specific agonists for the 5-HT_{1A} and 5-HT_{1B} receptors are now being used to treat migraines. Stimulation of the post-synaptic 5-HT_{1B} receptor causes vasoconstriction. Activation of the 5-HT_{1D} presynaptic receptor on the trigeminal nerve reduces neurogenic inflammation by inhibiting the release of substance P and calcitonin gene-related peptide.

DIAGNOSIS OF MIGRAINE

A careful history and physical examination are key to determining the type of most headaches. A diagnosis of migraine is made based on identifying triggers, headache patterns, and the natural history of the headache. A typical migraine consists of some or all of the four components: prodromal phase, aura, headache, and recovery. Prodrome and aura are not always present. The prodromal phase may consist of hyperactivity, irritability, or depression. Aura is more easily identified, and visual aura is present in 75% of the patients. Migraine headaches usually start with moderate intensity and soon become severe. They tend to be throbbing and

TABLE 1

Diagnostic Criteria for Migraine Without and With Aura

Migraine Without Aura

A. At least five attacks fulfilling criteria B through D.

B. Headache attacks lasting 4 to 72 hours (untreated or unsuccessfully treated).

C. Headache that has at least two of the following characteristics:

   1. Unilateral location
   2. Pulsating quality
   3. Moderate or severe intensity (inhibits or prohibits daily activities)
   4. Aggravation by walking stairs or similar routine physical activity

D. During headache, at least one of the following is present:
   5. Nausea and/or vomiting
   6. Photophobia and phonophobia

E. At least one of the following is present:

   1. History, physical, and neurological examinations do not suggest headaches secondary to organic or systemic metabolic disease.
   2. History and/or physical and/or neurological examinations do suggest such disorder, but it is ruled out by appropriate investigations.
   3. Such a disorder is present, but migraine attacks do not occur for the first time in close temporal relation to the disorder.

Migraine With Aura

A. At least two attacks fulfilling criterion B.

B. At least three of the following four characteristics are present:

   1. One or more fully reversible aura symptoms indicating focal cerebral cortical and/or brainstem dysfunction.
   2. At least one aura symptom develops gradually over more than 4 minutes or two or more symptoms occur in succession.
   3. No aura symptom lasts more than 60 minutes. If more than one aura symptom is present, accepted duration is proportionally increased.
   4. Headache follows aura with a free interval of less than 60 minutes. (It may also begin before or simultaneously with the aura).

C. At least one of the following is present:

   1. History, physical, and neurological examinations do not suggest headaches secondary to organic or systemic metabolic disease.
   2. History and/or physical and/or neurological examinations do suggest such disorder, but it is ruled out by appropriate investigations.
   3. Such a disorder is present, but migraine attacks do not occur for the first time in close temporal relation to the disorder.

unilateral. The headache may start one side and switch sides or may become global. Any activity such as bending forward, sneezing, or coughing that increases intracranial pressure will increase the intensity of the headache.[6–8] Associated symptoms with a migraine are nausea, vomiting, phonophobia, photophobia, diaphoresis, and orthostatic hypotension. Migraines are recurring and have a moderate to severe intensity. They can be triggered by certain well-known factors like certain foods, weather, smoke, hunger, and stress. The International Headache Society has established a set of diagnostic criteria for the diagnosis of migraine.

MANAGEMENT OF MIGRAINE

Broadly, treatment of headaches is based on the type of headache, migraine, tension or cluster. Each of these classes of headaches can be managed with abortive treatment or preventive treatment.

Abortive Treatment

The key to aborting a migraine depends on the choice of medication as well as its route of delivery. The sooner the medication is taken, the more effective it is. It is much better to take a large single dose than several smaller doses. Most migraines are associated with nausea, which limits the use of oral medications.

The triptans are considered very effective abortive medications for migraines. The commonly used triptans are sumatriptan, naratriptan, rizatriptan, zolmitriptan, eletriptan, almatriptan, and fravotriptan. All the clinically used triptans are selective $5-HT_1$ agonist. They possess a basic indole ring with different side chains, which is responsible for some of their pharmacokinetic properties.

Sumatriptan (Imitrex). This is a selective $5-HT_1$ agonist. It is available in the form of a nasal spray (5 mg, 20 mg), tablets (25 mg, 50 mg, 100 mg), and subcutaneous injection (6 mg). This was the first triptan introduced into clinical practice, and it is considered to be the gold standard in the treatment of migraines with triptans. The time to maximum blood level (T_{max}) is 2 hours, and the half-life is 5 to 6 hours. Sumatriptan tablets have a low bioavailability of only 14%, which explains the inconsistency in response with repeat doses. The subcutaneous form has 96% bioavailability with the most rapid onset of action of all the triptans. This rapidity of onset of action may explain some its side effects, such as heaviness in the chest and throat, chest discomfort, anxiety, jaw tightness, and paresthesias of the head, neck, and extremities. These symptoms are not as obvious with the oral and nasal form.

Sumatriptan[24,25,41] does not cross the blood-brain barrier and is not associated with central nervous system (CNS) effects such as asthenia, somnolence, and dizziness. All of the triptans are contraindicated in patients with history or symptoms of coronary artery disease, peripheral vascular disease, or cerebrovascular disease. Sumatriptan tablets have been used in elderly patients, but caution should be exercised.

The recommended starting dose is 50 mg. Patients may repeat the dose every 3 to 4 hours for a maximum of 200 mg in 24 hours. Recurrence of headaches is a problem with all triptans. The dose may be repeated, but repeating it too often may lead to rebound headaches.

The indications for using sumatriptan are (1) acute treatment of migraine attacks with or without aura; and (2) acute treatment of cluster headache episodes (injection form). Sumatriptan is not indicated in the management of hemiplegic or basilar migraine or for the prophylactic treatment of migraine. It is avoided in patients with uncontrolled hypertension and those on monoamine oxidase (MAO) inhibitors. It should not be taken within 24 hours of any ergotamine-containing medication (e.g., dihydroergotamine or methysergide). It is not to be used during pregnancy and in nursing mothers.

The injection form should not be given intravenously because of its potential for causing coronary artery vasospasm. It comes with an autoinjector. The needle penetrates approximately one quarter of an inch. The injection must be given subcutaneously only. Patient education is essential to avoid intramuscular or intravenous injection. The maximum single dose is 6 mg subcutaneously. No clear benefit has been demonstrated with repeating the dose. However, if a dose has to be repeated, it should be done not before 1 hour of the last dose.

The nasal form of sumatriptan has more rapid onset of action than the oral form. It is indicated for the treatment of acute migraine with or without aura. It is especially useful in patients with migraines associated with nausea. The nasal spray is administered as a single dose of 20 mg in one nostril. A 10 mg dose may be achieved by administering 5 mg into each nostril. A 20 mg dose maybe repeated not before 2 hours if the headache recurs. A maximum of 40 mg in 24 hours may be administered.

Naratriptan (Amerge). Naratriptan[27] has an affinity for 5-HT_{1D} and 5-HT_{1B} receptors. By activating the 5-HT_{1D} and 5-HT_{1B} receptors located on the intracranial blood vessels, it produces vasoconstriction, which has been correlated with relief of migraines. It is available as a tablet form only. The oral bioavailability is 70%. The T_{max} is 3 to 4 hours.

Naratriptan (Amerge) is available as 1 mg and 2.5 mg tablets. It is indicated for the treatment of moderate to severe acute onset migraines with or without aura. In clinical studies, a better response was obtained after a single dose of 2.5 mg. If the headache recurs or a partial response is seen, then a second 2.5 mg tablet may be taken after 4 hours. Recurrence with naratriptan is the lowest of all the triptans. There is no advantage to taking a dose greater than 5 mg in 24 hours. Naratriptan has a longer onset of action and a longer duration of action and has been found to be useful in patients with prolonged, slowly developing migraines.

The side effects with naratriptan are relatively milder and are the same as with the other triptans. The contraindications are the same as with sumatriptan. It should be restricted in patients with coronary artery disease.

Rizatriptan (Maxalt). Rizatriptan has a high affinity for 5-HT_{1D} and 5-HT_{1B} receptors. It is available as a tablet form and as an oral disintegrating form. The mean oral bioavailability is 45% and the T_{max} is 1 to 1.5 hours.

In clinical studies, there was a decrease in the incidence of migraine-associated photophobia, phonophobia, and nausea. Rizatriptan is indicated in the treatment of acute-onset migraine with or without aura. It should not be used in the prophylactic treatment of migraines. Side effects with rizatriptan are the same as with other triptans and have the same restrictions or in its use.

Rizatriptan is available as 5 mg and 10 mg tablets and as the Maxalt-MLT oral disintegrating (5 mg, 10 mg) tablets. Clinical studies have shown that 10 mg is more effective than 5 mg. If the headache recurs or there is partial relief, redosing should be separated by at least 2 hours, and no more than 30 mg maybe taken in 24 hours. The Maxalt-MLT oral disintegrating tablet can be placed on the tongue, where it dissolves easily. Should not be used to treat more 4 headaches in 30 days.

Zolmitriptan (Zomig). Zolmitriptan[31,32] is a selective 5-HT_{1D} and 5-HT_{1B} receptor agonist. It has a modest affinity for 5-HT_{1A} receptors. The therapeutic effects of zolmitriptan can be explained by its action of the 5-HT_{1D} and 5-HT_{1B} receptors of the intracranial blood vessels and the trigeminal nerve, resulting in constriction of the blood vessels and inhibition of release of proinflammatory neuropeptides.

The T_{max} for the oral tablet is 1.5 hours. The bioavailability is approximately 40%. The metabolite of zolmitriptan is an active N-desmethyl product that has a potency two to six times that of the parent drug. Thus, the metabolite may contribute a substantial portion of the overall effect of zolmitriptan administration. The side effect profile and contraindications are similar to those of sumatriptan and all the other triptans.

Zolmitriptan is available in 2.5 mg and 5 mg tablets and as disintegrating (2.5 mg, 5 mg) tablets. Clinical studies have shown that the 2.5 mg is better tolerated, and no added benefit is seen compared to the 5 mg dose. The dose maybe repeated after 2 hours with a maximum of 10 mg in 24 hours. May not be used to treat more than 3 headaches in 30 days.

Other Abortive Medications. Midrin. Midrin is composed of isometheptene, dichloralphenazone and acetaminophen 325 mg. Isometheptene is a sympathomimetic amine;[2] it acts by vasoconstricting the dilated cranial blood vessels. Dichloralphenazone is a mild sedative, helping reduce anxiety associated with pain, and acetaminophen acts by raising the threshold to painful stimuli.

Midrin[21] is contraindicated in patients with hypertension, glaucoma, and coronary artery disease and in those on MAO inhibitors. It may be a reasonably effective medication for the relief of acute migraine and/or tension headaches. It is administered in a dose of two capsules followed by one capsule every hour until relief, with a maximum of 6 per day and 20 per week. Patients taking the drug for the first time are advised to take 1 capsule at a time to avoid excessive sedation. For tension headaches 1 to 2 caps every 4 hours with a maximum of 8 caps per day may be administered.

Butalbital Compounds. These are various compounds containing butalbital. They are Fiorinal (butalbital 50 mg, aspirin 325 mg, caffeine 40 mg); Fioricet and Esgic (butalbital 50 mg, acetaminophen 325 mg, caffeine 40 mg); Esgic Plus (butalbital 50 mg, acetaminophen 500 mg, caffeine 40 mg); and Phrenilin (butalbital 50 mg, acetaminophen 325 mg).

These drugs may be reasonably effective in the treatment of acute migraine. They can be habit forming. Compounds containing aspirin seem to be more effective than the ones containing acetaminophen.

Some of the side effects seen are lethargy, lightheadedness, and nausea. These drugs have potential for abuse because of the anxiolytic effect of butalbital. Phrenilin may be useful for patients who cannot take aspirin or caffeine.

Nonsteroidal Anti-inflammatory Drugs (NSAIDs). These are good drugs for the short-term treatment of migraine headaches such as menstrual migraines. Their use is limited by their potential side effects on the renal and gastrointestinal systems. The mechanism of action of NSAIDs[26] is reduction of perivascular neurogenic inflammation and prostaglandin synthesis inhibition.

The commonly used drugs from this class are naproxen (Aleve) and tolfenamic acid. Naproxen is an arylacetic NSAID. It possesses both analgesic and antipyretic action. Each tablet of Aleve contains 220 mg of naproxen. To start with, two tablets maybe taken. The dose maybe repeated in 3 to 4 hours for a maximum of six tablets per day.

Ketorolac (Toradol) is an injectable NSAID. It may be useful as an abortive medication and is usually well tolerated. It may be given as a 30 mg or 60 mg intramuscular or intravenous injection with a maximum of 120 mg in 24 hours; however, lower doses (10 mg–30 mg) may be efficacious as well. It is contraindicated in patients with hepatic and renal impairment.

Ergotamines. The ergotamines seem to have partial agonist activity at α-adrenergic (clinically predominantly at the alpha-2 adrenergic receptor), tryptaminergic, and dopaminergic receptors. The α-adrenergic effect is mild and the vasoconstrictive effect is by its direct effect on the serotonin receptors. Ergotamines[29,33,34] also decrease the firing rate of serotonergic neurotransmission in the brainstem. Their usefulness in treating migraines also depends on their property to cause vasoconstriction of the extracranial blood vessels, decreasing the amplitude and blood flow in the cranial arteries. They are effective in controlling up to 70% of acute migraine attacks.

Bioavailability is much higher with the rectal than the oral form. The bioavailability of the oral form is less than 5%. The T_{max} is about 1 hour after both oral and rectal administration. The elimination half-life of the drug is 2 hours. It is stored in the tissues, and that may explain its long effect. Ergotamine (as well as DHE) bind avidly to their receptors with a long occupancy time before they dissociate (after a single dose of ergotamine drug elimination could be up to 72 hours).

Ergotamines are available in oral, and sublingual forms and as rectal suppositories. The commonly available preparations are Ergostat, Ergomar sublingual (ergotamine tartrate, 2 mg); Cafergot, Wigraine tablet (ergotamine 1 mg, caffeine 100 mg); and Cafergot, Wigraine suppository (ergotamine 2 mg, Caffeine 100 mg).

Nausea and vomiting are the most common side effects, occurring in 10% of patients after oral administration. The nausea is a central effect and is usually the limiting factor in taking this drug. The rectal form causes less nausea and is much more effective. Other side effects seen are precordial pain, tingling and numbness in the extremities, muscle pains, insomnia and dizziness. Ergotamines are contraindicated in patients with peripheral vascular disease, peptic ulcer, coronary artery disease, and hypertension.

Ergotamine is best taken at the onset of a migraine headache. The initial dose is 2 mg tablet sublingual. It maybe repeated at half-hourly intervals, up to a maximum of 6 mg in any 24-hour period. No more than 10 mg must be taken in any one week. Rebound headaches may occur if ergotamine is taken consecutively for 2 days. The suppositories are far more effective and are especially useful in patients with nausea. The starting dose for the suppository preparation (supp) may be one half supp and must be titrated to effect. The dose may be repeated after 1 hour, but is limited to two supp in any 24-hour period. If no relief is seen after the first dose of either an oral or a rectal dose, it is unlikely that patients will respond to a second dose.

Dihydroergotamine (DHE) Nasal Spray. DHE is derived from ergotamine by it being reduced at the 9–10 double bond on the D-lysergic acid moiety. DHE has a high affinity for the $5\text{-HT}_{1D\alpha}$ and $5\text{-HT}_{1D\beta}$ receptors. It also binds to the 5-HT_{1A}, 5-HT_{1B}, 5-HT_{1F}, noradrenaline, and dopamine receptors. Activation of the 5-HT_{1D}^{35} receptors on the intracranial blood vessels causes them to vasoconstrict. DHE is a moderate arterial vasoconstrictor (weaker than ergotamine) but a potent venoconstrictor. Both DHE and ergotamine have a similar profile of receptor interactions but differ in the degree of various receptor-mediated effects (e.g., DHE is much less emetic and has less uterine effects than ergotamine). Activation of $5\text{-HT}_{1D}{}^{35}$ receptors on the trigeminal nerves results in inhibition of the release of inflammatory neuropeptides.

DHE[36,37,38,39,40] has a very poor oral bioavailability, but the mean bioavailability after intranasal administration is 32%. It is given either as an intramuscular injection or as an intranasal spray (Migranal). It is very effective when given intravenously. Nausea and vomiting are its most common side effects. Chest and throat tightness, muscle pain in the legs, tingling or numbness in the fingers and toes, flushed feeling in the head, and diarrhea after intravenous administration are some of its other side effects. On rare occasions, serious side effects such as angina, vascular insufficiency, and arrhythmias have been noted. It is contraindicated in patients with pregnancy, peripheral vascular disease, hypertension, and coronary artery disease.

For the nasal spray (Migranal), each ampul contains one complete dose of DHE. One spray will deliver 0.5 mg of DHE. One spray should be administered in each nostril. It maybe repeated 15 minutes later. No additional benefit is obtained with more than four sprays (2 mg). For acute intractable migraine attacks, one protocol is to give prochlorperazine 5 mg intravenously followed by 0.75 mg to 1mg of DHE administered intravenously over 2 or 3 minutes. It may be repeated after 1 hour. Intravenous DHE is very valuable in treating intractable migraines.

Steroids. Corticosteroids have been used in the treatment of acute migraines especially those associated with menstrual periods. Dexamethasone seems to be the most effective. Prednisone and intramuscular adrenocorticotropic hormone have also been used. The dose is either dexamethasone 4 mg or prednisone 20 mg taken orally and repeated every 3 to 4 hours. If used judiciously and tapered rapidly, the side effects are generally minimal. The total dose must be restricted and limited to treatment of severe migraine attacks.

Preventive Medications

Migraine prophylactic[49] therapy is indicated in situations in which patients have two or more attacks per month and are disabled for 3 or 4 days, require abortive medication more than twice a week, or have no sustained relief with symptomatic medications or under special circumstances in which a migraine headache may cause a risk of permanent neurological injury or hemiplegic migraine. The aim of preventive therapy is to lessen the severity of the pain, make abortive medications more effective, and decrease the number of attacks to less than 50%.

Patients with migraines have a state of central neuronal hyperexcitability.[42,43,44] There is evidence to show that activation of central serotonin receptors may precipitate an acute attack. Preventive medications involve one or several of these mechanisms: modulation of central neurotransmitters, antagonists to 5-HT receptors, and augmentation of central α-aminobutyric acidergic inhibition.

The choice of drugs for prophylaxis depends primarily on the severity and frequency of the attacks, impact on the quality of life, and disability and side effect profile of the drug. Together with pharmacotherapy, patients must also use nonpharmacological methods such as biofeedback, avoid triggering agents, adjustments to their diet, and physical therapy.

Prophylactic therapy is started with low doses and gradually built up. This helps patients tolerate these drugs better and avoids side effects. For any medication, a trial of at least 3 to 4 months is undertaken before rejecting it. Most prophylactic medications need to be withdrawn slowly.

Medications used for the prevention of migraine include the following:

1. Tricyclic antidepressants (TCAs)
   - Amitriptyline
   - Nortriptyline
   - Protriptyline
   - Desipramine
   - Doxepin
2. β-Adrenergic blockers
   - Propranlol
   - Metoprolol
   - Nadolol
   - Atenolol
   - Timolol
3. Calcium-channel blockers
   - Verapamil
   - Diltiazem
   5-HT$_2$ antagonists
   - Methysergide
   - Cyproheptadine
5. Anticonvulsant agents
   - Sodium valproate
   - Gabapentin[63,64,65,66]
6. Magnesium[45,68]
7. Selective serotonin receptor inhibitor (SSRIs)[58]

Tricyclic Antidepressants (TCAs). The most widely used TCA for migraine is amitriptyline.[54] The mechanism of action is believed to be modulation of the 5-HT and norepinephrine effects. The anti-migraine effect of the TCAs is independent of the antidepressant effect, although the antidepressant effect may add to the clinical benefit. Sedation, weight gain, dry mouth, tachycardia, and constipation are common. Because of its side effect profile, it is to be used with caution in the elderly. Nortriptyline has fewer cardiac side effects and can be used in the elderly.

Tricyclic antidepressants are helpful for treating migraines as well as chronic daily headaches. They must be started at the lowest dose and slowly titrated up. This helps patients tolerate the side effects and improves patient compliance. Because of its sedative effect, amitriptyline is given at bedtime. It can be started with either a 5 mg or a 10 mg tablet at night and slowly increased to 50 mg over several weeks. It can be titrated at doses up to 200 mg a day.

β-Adrenergic Blockers. β-Blockers are very effective in patients with migraines and hypertension. Their mechanism of action has been postulated to be blockage of nitric oxide activity or 5-HT$_{2B}$ antagonists, or both. Some of the side effects of β-blockers are orthostatic hypotension, fatigue, diarrhea, insomnia, depression, memory disturbance, and male impotence. They are contraindicated in patients with asthma and congestive cardiac failure.

Propranlol[57,63] is effective between 40 to 160 mg/day. When the drug is stopped; it must be slowly tapered off. Timolol is given up to 20 mg twice daily. It is started at a very low dose of 5 mg twice daily and slowly increased. Metoprolol is also administered twice daily. The dose is 50 mg to 100 mg per day. The dose for nadolol is 40 mg to 160 mg a day. It is less sedating than propranolol.

MANAGEMENT OPTIONS FOR TENSION-TYPE HEADACHES

According to the IHS classification, the terms *muscle contraction headache, tension headache* and *chronic daily headache* have been replaced by *tension-type headache*. Patients often describe their headaches as a band-like tightness with a deep to dull ache.[3,67] The pain waxes and wanes throughout the day. Tension-type headaches do not have the same features as migraines. They occur more frequently, and are not throbbing or associated with an aura. Many patients with tension-type headaches also have migraines. There is a very high incidence of overuse of over-the-counter analgesics, aspirin, acetaminophen, barbiturates, benzodiazepines, and caffeine.

The exact pathophysiology of tension-type headache is unclear. Increased muscle contraction, the trigeminal neurovascular system, and serotonergic neuromodulators as well as vascular changes may all contribute to tension-type headaches. Patients with tension-type headaches often present with scalp tenderness and cervical muscle tension, but this may be the result of other ongoing processes in the central nervous system and not the primary cause of their headaches.

The treatment of tension-type headaches involves reducing medication overuse, relaxation and biofeedback techniques, and stress management. When treating patients with tension-type headaches the clinician should ask about analgesics the patients have been using. Biofeedback and relaxation techniques are often very effective and best learned by motivated patients.

Medications for tension-type headaches can be taken either as abortive or preventive agents. For patients with intermittent episodes of tension-type headaches, an abortive agent will suffice. Patients who suffer from more frequent headaches tend to overuse analgesics, and those in whom quality of life is decreased need to be on preventive therapy.

Nonsteroidal antiinflammatory drugs are effective for tension-type headaches as well as migraines. Many of them are available over the counter. Their side effects are mostly gastrointestinal disturbance, live toxicity, and renal damage. NSAIDs that are effective include: indomethacin, ibuprofen, flubiprofen and naproxen. The newer cyclooxygenase-2 inhibitors (Celebrex, Vioxx, Valdecoxib) may have less significant gastrointestinal side effects, but renal and hepatic dysfunction may occur.

Aspirin[26] is a very effective abortive for tension-type headaches. Its use is limited by its side effects, such as gastrointestinal bleeding, hepatic dysfunction, and platelet dysfunction. Acetaminophen overuse can worsen tension-type headaches. Acetaminophen is very effective for moderate to severe headaches, but should be limited to 4 g per day. Caffeine is effective for moderate intensity headaches, and when taken in combination with aspirin or acetaminophen, may be effective in treating severe headaches. Its mechanism of action seems to be its effects on the intracranial blood vessels.

MANAGEMENT OPTIONS FOR CLUSTER HEADACHES

Cluster headaches[71,72,73,74,75] are periodic, excruciatingly painful attacks lasting from 30 minutes to 1.5 hours, with an average of 45 minutes for each attack. They are more common in males (1:4) and start between the ages of 25 and 45 years. They are localized around the eye, temple, frontal area, and cheek. Lacrimation, nasal drainage, conjunctival injection and facial sweating often accompany an attack. The onset is sudden without any premonitory symptoms or aura. Cluster headaches come on in cycles. Each cycle may last from several days to months, mostly between 4 weeks and 8 weeks. The interim period maybe from months to years. Patients who have had cluster headaches for a long time tend to lose them in their 40s.

The treatment of cluster headaches is very similar to the treatment of migraines. They respond well to abortive and preventive medications. Since the attacks are sudden and severe, oral medications are of little help. Abortive medications used for cluster headaches are oxygen therapy, triptans, ergotamines, and intranasal lidocaine. Oxygen therapy is very effective. Patients are advised to breathe 100% oxygen at 7 to 8 L/min through a mask. This can be used in conjunction with other treatments, such as nasal DHE, injectable and nasal sumatriptan (Imitrex), ergotamines, ketorolac, and intranasal lidocaine.

Preventive therapy for cluster headaches is recommended because of the intensity of the pain. They are started when a cluster cycle starts and need not be maintained all year. Drugs used for preventive therapy include steroids, lithium, and verapamil. Steroids used for preventive treatment are triamcinolone, prednisone, or dexamethasone. They may be started with a high dose and then maintained on a low dose. Because of the short time they are taken, side effects are unusual. Lithium carbonate is given in low doses and is generally well tolerated. It is given as 300 mg once a day and may be increased to three times a day depending on the response. Most patients tolerate the low doses, and side effects are unusual. Verapamil is usually very well tolerated and can be given with steroids and lithium, if the headaches are severe. Some clinicians have used verapamil in conjunction with valproic acid for certain patients with refractory cluster headaches.

REFERENCES FOR ADDITIONAL READING

1. Stewart WF, Lipton RB: Work-related disability: Results from the American Migraine Study. Cephalalgia 16:231–238, 1996.
2. Robbins DL: Management of Headache and Headache Medications, 2nd ed. Springer-Verlag, New York, 2000.
3. Pryse-Phillips W, Findlay H, Tugwell P, et al: A Canadian population survey on the clinical epidemiologic and societal impact of migraine and tension-type headache. Can J Neurol Sci 19: 333–339, 1992.
4. International Headache Society: Classification and diagnostic criteria for headache disorders, cranial neuralgias, and facial pain. Cephalalgia 8(suppl 7):1–96, 1988.
5. Stewart WF, Lipton RB, Celentano DD, et al: Prevalence of migraine headache in the United States: Relation to age, income, race and other sociodemographic factors. JAMA 267:64–69, 1992.
6. Monzon MJ, Lainez MJA: Quality of life in migraine and chronic daily headache patients. Cephalalgia 18:638–643, 1998.
7. Linet MS, Stewart WF: Migraine headache: Epidemiologic perspectives. Epidemiol Rev 6:107–139, 1984.
8. Stewart WF, Lipton RB, Liberman J: Variation in migraine prevalence by race. Neurology 16: 231–238, 1996.
9. Silberstein SD: Evaluation and emergency treatment of headache. Headache 32:396–407, 1992.
10. Silberstein SD: Preventive headache treatment. Cephlalgia 17:67–72, 1997.
11. Stang PE, Yanagihara T, Swanson JW, et al: Incidence of migraine headaches: A population-based study in Olmstead County, Minnesota. Neurology 42:1657–1662, 1992.
12. Lipton RB, Stewart WF, Celentano DD, et al: Undiagnosed migraine: A comparison of symptom-based and self-reported physician diagnosis. Arch Intern Med 152:1273–1278, 1992.
13. Dahlof C: Assessment of health-related quality of life in migraine. Cephalalgia 13:233–237, 1993.

14. Lipton RB, Stewart WF: Migraine in the United States: Epidemiology and health care use. Neurology 43(suppl 3):6–10, 1993.
15. Peroutka SJ, Wilhoit T, Jones K: Clinical susceptibility to migraine with aura is modified by dopamine D2 receptor (DRD2) NCOI Alleles. Neurology 49:201–206, 1997.
16. Fisher CM: Painful states: A neurological commentary. Clin Neurosurg 31:32–53, 1984.
17. Joutel A, Bousser MG, Biousse V, et al: A gene for familial hemiplegia migraine maps to chromosome 19. Nat Genet 5:40–45, 1993.
18. Raskin NH: Headache, 2nd ed. Churchill Livingstone., New York, 1988.
19. Torelli P, Colgno D, Mazoni GC. Weekend headache: Retrospective study in migraine without aura and episodic tension-type headache. Headache 3911–20, 1999.
20. Mathew NT, Reuveni U, Perez F: Transformed or evolutive migraine. Headache 27:102–106, 1987.
21. Mathew NT, Kurman R, Perez F: Drug induced refractory headache: clinical features and management. Headache 30:634–638, 1990.
22. Lauritzen M: Links between cortical spreading depression and migraine: Clinical and experimental aspects. In: Migraine and Other Headaches: The Vascular Mechanisms, Vol 1. Olesen J, ed: Raven Press, New York, 1991, pp 143–151.
23. Weiller C, May A, Limmroth V, et al: Brain stem activation in spontaneous human migraine attacks. Nat Med 1:658–660, 1995.
24. Humphrey PPA, Feniuk W: Mode of action of the anti-migraine drug sumatriptan. Trends Pharmacol Sci 12:444–446, 1991.
25. Ferrari MD, Saxena PR: On serotonin and migraine: a clinical and pharmacological review. Cephalalgia 13:151–165, 1993.
26. Peters BH, Fraim CJ, Masel BE: Comparison of 650 mg aspirin and 1000 mg acetaminophen with each other, and with placebo in moderately severe headache. Am J Med 74:36–42, 1983.
27. Mathew NT, Asgharnejad M, Peykamian M, Laurenza A: On behalf of the naratriptan treatment of migraine: Results of a double-blind, placebo controlled, crossover study. Neurology 49:1485–1490, 1997.
28. Stewart WF, Shechter A, Lipton RB: Migraine heterogeneity: Disability, pain intensity, and attack frequency and duration. Neurology 44:S24–S39, 1994.
29. Sanders SW, Haering N, Mosbert H, Jaeger H: Pharmacokinetics of ergotamine in healthy volunteers following oral and rectal dosing. Eur J Clin Pharmacol 30:331–334, 1986.
30. Ferrari MD: The Triptan War. Anno 1998. Presented at the annual meeting of the American Academy of Neurology, April 1998.
31. Lipton RB, Stewart WF: Clinical applications of zolmitriptan. Cephalalgia 17:53–59, 1997.
32. Goadsby PJ: A triptan too far? J Neurol Neursurg Psychiatry 64:143–147, 1998.
33. Perrin VL: Clinical pharmacokinetics of ergotamine in migraine and cluster headache. Clin Pharmacokinet 10:334–352, 1985.
34. Ibraheem JJ, Paalzow L, Tfelt-Hansen P: Low bioavailability of ergotamine tartrate after oral and rectal administration in migraine sufferers. Br J Clin Pharmacol 16:695–699, 1983.
35. .Muller-Schweinitzer E: Studies on the 5-HT receptor in vascular smooth muscle. Res Clin Stud Headache 6:6–12, 1978.
36. Muller-Schweinitzer E: Pharmacological actions of the main metabolites of dihydroergotamine. Europ J Clin Pharmacol 26:699–705, 1984.
37. Aghajanian GK, Wang RY: Physiology and pharmacology of central serotonergic neurons. In: Psychopharmacology: A Generation of Progress. Lipton MA, Dimascio A, Kollan KF, eds: Raven Press, New York, 1978, pp 171–183.
38. Aellig WH: Investigation of the venoconstrictor effect of 8'hydroxydihydro-ergotamine, the main metabolite of dihydroergotamine, in man. Eur J Clin Pharmacol 26:239–242, 1984.
39. Callaham M, Raskin NH: A controlled study of dihydroergotamine in the treatment of acute migraine headache. Headache 26:168–171, 1986.

40. Raskin NH: Repetitive intravenous dihydroergotamine as treatment for intractable migraine. Neurology 36:995–997, 1986.

41. Tfelt-Hansen P: Sumatriptan for the treatment of migraine attacks: A review of controlled clinical trials. Cephalalgia 13:238–244, 1993.

42. Golla FL, Winter AL: Analysis of cerebral responses to flicker in patients complaining of episodic headache. Electroenceph Clin Neurophysiol 11:539–549, 1959.

43. Nyrke T, Kangasniemi P, Land AH: Difference of steady-state visual evoked potentials in classic and common migraine. Electroenceph Clin Neurophysiol 73:285–294, 1989.

44. Welch KMA, D'Andrea G, Tepley N, et al: The concept of migraine as a state of central neuronal hyperexcitability. Neurol Clin 8:817–828, 1990.

45. Ramadan NM, Halvorson H, Vande-Linda A, et al: Low brain magnesium in migraine. Headache 29:416–419, 1989.

46. Curran DA, Hinterberger H, Lance JW: Total plasma serotonin, 5-hydroxyindoleacetic acid and P-hydroxy-M-methoxymandelic acid excretion in normal and migrainous subjects. Brain 88:997–1010, 1965.

47. Anthony M, Hinterberger H, Lance JW: Plasma serotonin in migraine and stress. Arch Neurol 16:544–552, 1967.

48. Kimball RW, Friedman AP, Vallejo E: Effect of serotonin in migraine patients. Neurology (Miorwap) 1960; 10:107–111, 1960.

49. Tfelt-Hansen P, Welch KMA: Migraine: Prioritizing prophylactic treatment. In: Olesen J, Tfelt-Hansen P, Welch KMA, eds: The Headaches. Raven Press, New York, 1993, pp 403–404.

50. Jensen R, Brinck T, Olesen J: Sodium valproate has a prophylactic effect on migraine without aura: a triple-blind, placebo-controlled crossover study. Neurology 44:647–651, 1994.

51. Cutrer FM, Moskowitz MA: Actions of valproate and neurosteroids in a model of trigeminal pain. Headache 36:285, 1996.

52. Peatfield RC, Olesen J: Migraine: Precipitating factors. In: Olesen J, Tfelt-Hansen P, Welch KMA, eds: The Headaches. Raven Press, New York, 1993, p 243.

53. Limmorth V, Lee WS, Cutrer FM, et al: Meningeal GABAA receptors located outside the blood-brain barrier mediate sodium valproate blockade of neurogenic and substance P-induced inflammation: Possible mechanism in migraine. Cephalalgia 15:102, 1995.

54. Couch JR, Ziegler DK, Hassaneur R: Amitriptyline in the prophylaxis of migraine: Effectiveness and relationship of antimigraine and antidepressant effects. Neurology 26:121–127, 1976.

55. Hering R, Kuritzky A: Sodium valproate in the prophylactic treatment of migraine double-blind study versus placebo. Cephalalgia 12:81–84, 1992.

56. Newman LC, Lipton RB, Solomon S, Stewart WF: Daily headache in a population sample: Results from the American Migraine Study. Headache 34:295, 1994.

57. Kaniecki RG: A comparative study of propranolol and divalproex sodium in the prophylaxis of migraine. Arch Neurol 54:1141–1144, 1997.

58. Saper JR, Silberstein SD, Lake AE, Winters ME: Double-blind trials of fluoxetine: Chronic daily headache and migraine. Headache 34:497–502, 1994.

59. Manna V, Bolino F, DiCicco L: Chronic tension-type headache, mood depression and serotonin: Therapeutic effects of fluvoxamine and mianserine. Headache 34:44–49, 1994.

60. Nishikawa T, Scatton B: Inhibitory influence of GABA on central serotoninergic transmission: Raphi nuclei as the neuroanatomical site of GABAergic inhibition of cerebral serotoninergic neurons. Brain Res 331–391, 1985.

61. Fisher CM: Late-life migraine accompaniments: Further experience. Stroke 17:1033–1042, 1986.

62. Silberstein SD, Lipton RB, Goadsby PJ: Headache in Clinical Practice. Isis Medical Media, Oxford, 1998.

63. Girowell A, Kulisevsky J, Barbanog M, et al: A double-blind placebo controlled comparative trial of gabapentin and propranolol in patients with essential tremor. Neurology 50:A71–A72, 1988.

64. Magnus-Miller L, Podolnick P, Mathew NTM, Saper J: Efficacy and safety of gabapentin (Neuron-

tin) in migraine prophylaxis. [abstract] Paper presented at the American Pain Society Annual Meeting, 1998.

65. Mathew NT: Gabapentin in migraine prophylaxis. Cephalalgia 16:367, 1996.

66. Gorson KG, Schott C, Rand WM, et al: Gabapentin in the treatment of painful diabetic neuropathy: A placebo controlled double-blind, crossover trial. Neurology 50:A103, 1998.

67. Silberstein SD, Lipton RB: Overview of diagnosis and treatment of migraine. Neurology 44:6–16, 1994.

68. Pfaffenrath V, Wessely P, Meyer C, et al: Magnesium in the prophylaxis of migraine: a double-blind placebo controlled study. Cephalalgia 16:436–440, 1996.

69. Mauskop A, Altura BT, Cracco RQ, Altura BM: Intravenous magnesium sulfate relieves acute migraine in patients with low serum ionized magnesium levels. 45:A379, 1995.

70. Welch KMA, Levine SR, D'Andrea G, et al: Preliminary observations on brain energy metabolism in migraine studied by in vivo 31-phosphorus NNMR spectroscopy. Neurology 39:538–541, 1989.

71. Gabe IJ, Speierings ELH: Prophylactic treatment of cluster headache with Verapamil. Headache 29:167–168; 1989.

72. Anderson P, Jespersen L: Dihydroergotamine nasal spray in the treatment of attacks of cluster headache. Cephalalgia 6:51–54; 1986.

73. Couch JR, Ziegler D: Prednisone therapy for cluster headache. Headache 17:15–18, 1977.

74. Manzoni GC, Micieli G, Granella F, et al: Award Lecture, Vth International Headache Congress, Washington, DC, 1991.

75. Mathew NT: Cluster headache. Neurology 42(Suppl 2):22–31, 1992.

Chapter 38

Novel Analgesic Approaches to Painful Bone Metastases

Howard S. Smith, MD / Sajid Kahn, MD

The mechanisms of bone pain in osseous metastatic lesions remain unclear but are almost certain to be multifactorial. Bone metastases may lead to pain via stimulation of nociceptors by algesic mediators (e.g., cytokines, prostaglandin E, bradykinin, serotonin, substance P). Involvement or invasion, stretching, or compression of pain-sensitive structures such as nerves, vasculature, and periosteum and microfractures of various joint structures may also lead to pain. Pain from osseous metastatic lesions may also occur from mechanical instability of "weakened bone" or high intraosseous pressures (>50 mm Hg).[1]

In addition to osseous and tumor origins for the pain of bone metastases, proalgesic substances may contribute, such as cytokines, inflammatory mediators, vasoactive intestinal peptide (VIP), matrix metalloproteinases, endothelin 1 binding to endothelin A, osteoclasts, and the acidic environment of bone resorption (e.g., protons activating the vanilloid receptor-1 and/or acid sensing ion channel receptors) (FIGURE 1 and TABLE 1).

THE BALANCE OF MAKING AND BREAKING BONE

The major culprit in bone destruction is the osteoclast. A second minor and later mechanism is tumor-mediated osteolysis. Additionally, tumor involvement can compromise osseous vascular supply, leading to bone necrosis or destruction. Bone formation can occur by multiple mechanisms. Certain tumor cells may induce ossification of fibrous stroma (e.g., osteoblastic metastases with abundant stroma). Reactive bone formation (e.g., the usual response of bone to fracture) occurs more commonly.[2]

Widespread metastases occur after the primary tumor has seeded the lymphatic and vascular channels to carry tumor cells to distant osseous sites. The tumor cells undergo endothelial attachment and are then able to make their way into the substance of the bone. Once the tumor cell is situated in bone and has established itself, growth can occur through tumor angiogenesis factors attracting new vasculature.[2]

Bone destruction takes place predominantly via vigorous osteoclast activity. Several tumors (e.g., breast, prostate, lung) produce and secrete osteoclastic activators, including transforming growth factor, and prostaglandins, interleukins, tumor necrosis factor, and platelet-derived growth factor. Also, granulocyte-macrophage colony-stimulating factors, parathyroid hormone–related protein, procathepsin D, and 5-lipoxygenase metabolites (e.g., 5-hydroxy eicosatetraenoic acid and leukotrienes) stimulate isolated osteoclasts to resorb bone in vitro.

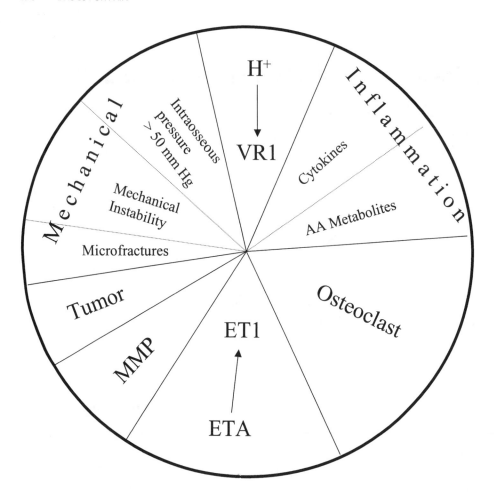

FIGURE 1. Potential Mechanisms of Pain in Bone Metastases

PATHOPHYSIOLOGY OF BONE RESORPTION

Although numerous contributing factors lead to the pain of osseous metastases, a significant portion of the pain seems to be related to osteoclstic bone resorption. Osteoclasts solubilize the mineral (e.g., hydroxyapatite) and degrade the organic matrix (e.g., type 1 collagen) with cysteine-proteinases. The bone resorption occurs in an acidic microenvironment produced by proton secretion via vacular H^+ ATPases in osteoclastic membranes. The first step in the process of bone resorption is that the osteoclast adheres to the bone surface. This adherence is mediated by specific membrane receptors. Podosomes are osteoclastic processes, that become the primary attachment sites to bone. The podosomes are made up of integrins and cytoskeletal proteins: actin microfilaments surrounded by vinculin and talin.[3]

The predominant attachment site is the vitronectin receptors (e.g., α, β_3 integrin), which recognizes the RGD (Arg-Gly-Asp) amino acid sequence in various bone matrix proteins (osteopontin, vitronectin, bone sialoprotein).[3]

TABLE 1

Potential Analgesic Treatment Strategies

Mechanism:	Treatment:
Mechanical	Brace / immobilize
	Steroids
	Radiation
	Surgery
Tumor	Chemotherapy
	Radiation
	Surgery
ET1:	ETB via local opioid effects
AA Metabolites:	Steroids
	NSAIDs (especially if penetrate acid environment)
Inflammatory (Cytokines) Growth Factors	Steroids
	VIP
MMPs:	IIMPs
	Tetracyclines
	CMT (Chemically Modified Tetracyclines)
	VIP
	Other
Osteoclasts	OPG (Osteoprotegerin)
	Bisphosphonates
	Radiation
	Calcitonin
	Interferon-γ
H^+	VR1 Antagonists (Iodo-resiniferators)
	ASIC
	mDEG

A highly convoluted membrane area termed the ruffled border and sealing zone appear in the osteoclast during bone resorption. The accumulation of podosomes at the bone surface occurs first with ligand binding to the vitronectin receptor.[3] Subsequently, a tight sealing zone is formed where osteoclastic acid and proteases are secreted to resorb bone. The sealing zone is completed as actively resorbing osteoclasts reorganize elements to form a "double circle" of vinculin and talin around a core of F-actin.[3]

Other potential strategies that may impair osteoclastic function include bafilomycin A1 (specific inhibitor of vacuolar, H^+-ATPase), peptides with the RGD sequence, and other agents that may interfere with vinculin, talin, and/or F-actin (e.g., colchinine). Decoy RGD sequence peptides or agents adversely affecting vinculin, talin, or F-action may inhibit osteoclast attachment to the bone surface.

The osteoclast is normally affected by two major influences. The first is a ryanodine receptor-like molecule on the cell surface, which acts as a divalent cation sensor.[3] A transient rise in cytosolic calcium results from this receptor binding divalent cations, which then contributes to osteoclast regulation. The second major means of osteoclast regulation is via its calcitonin receptor, which couples two G proteins. Additionally, osteoclasts are also inhibited by phosphonates,[4] calcitonin,[5] and calcitonin gene-related peptide.[5]

Osteoblasts seem to be able to stimulate osteoclastic bone resorption indirectly. Parathyroid harmone, $1,25$-dihyroxyvitamin D_3, and tumor necrosis factor-α (TNF-α) require osteoblasts to produce osteolysis. It is thought that following binding of the above ligands to their osteoblastic receptors, the osteoblast releases a factor known as osteoclast-resorption stimulating activity (ORSA).[6]

RADIATION-INDUCED ANALGESIA

The majority of patients with osseous metastases obtain analgesia from locally delivered radiation (external beam radiotherapy or systemic radiopharmaceutical therapy).[7] The mechanism of radiation-induced analgesia to metastatic bone lesions remains unknown, although there are a number of possibilities to explain this phenomenon. Early pain relief with wide-field radiation therapy is so rapid that tumor cell kill cannot be a viable explanation. Pain relief, which occurs later and is persistent, certainly may be at least partially related to tumor cell kill. Also, radiation has a direct action on osteoclastic formation via effects on proliferating progenitor cells, but this would also not account for early pain relief.

It is conceivable that osteoblastic processes contribute to pain in metastatic osseous lesions. If this were so, then this direct early inactivation of osteoblasts by radiation could lead to analgesia. Most evidence would not support this hypothesis. However, it is conceivable that osteoblasts may have a significant influence on osteoclastic activity in metastatic lesions. As the activity of the osteoclast may contribute significantly to the pain of metastatic osseous lesions, any intervention, that directly or indirectly interferes with osteoclastic function has potential usefulness as part of an analgesic treatment regimen.

External beam radiotherapy rapidly inactivates radiosensitive osteoblasts. It thereby impairs osteoblastic function, including ORSA release/function, which secondarily results in impaired osteoclastic stimulation/function.[8] Additionally, late effects include direct injury to radiosensitive proliferating osteoclast progenitor cells.[8] Alpha-particle emitting "surface-seeking" bone-seekers (e.g., actinides) such as plutonium deliver a proportionally much larger dose to osteoclasts than to osteoblasts (which are shielded by newly formed bone). These agents, such as radium-223, can selectively radiate osteoblasts, thereby impairing osteoclastic function.[9]

A delicate balance between Th1 cytokines and Th2 cytokines maintain a neutral environment. When the Th1 cytokines overshadow the Th2 cytokines, a proinflammatory effect predominates. Conversely, when Th2 cytokines over shadow the Th1 cytokines, an antiinflammatory effect predominates.[10]

Interleukin-12 is the key monocyte-derived cytokine that induces interferon-γ via activation of the stat-4 gene.[10,11] Interleukin-10 is the key monocyte-derived cytokine inducing interleukin-4 via activation of the Stat-6 gene.[10,12,13] Interleukin-4 may be the key player in the Th1/Th2 balance and may have a direct protective effect against cartilage bone degradation.[14] Daily interleukin-4/interleukin-10 treatment has been demonstrated to be efficacious in animal models of arthritis.[10,15] These apparent synergistic results of the interleukin-4/interleukin-10 combination may stem from better suppression of TNF-α and interleukin-1 production as well as a marked increase interleukin-1 receptor antagonist interleukin-1 ratio.[10,15] Conversely, as far as the proinflammatory effects of Th1 cytokines, interleukin-12 seems to be critical. Interleukin-12 markedly enhanced the collagen-induced arthritis response in a murine model,[16] whereas anti-interleukin-12 treatment prevented arthritis onset.[17]

Of interest is the potential role of employing misoprostol, which by supressing mitogen-stimulated Th-1 and Th-2 cytokine production (in a dose-dependent manner) may exert a stabilizing force in efforts to maintain a baseline Th-1/Th-2 balance.[18] Potential therapeutic targets to achieve analgesia include tipping the Th1 and Th2 balance in favor of Th2 cytokine predominance (e.g., VIP); osteoprotegerin ligand (OPGL) inhibitors (e.g., osteoprotegerin, TNF-α inhibitors (e.g., entanercept), antagonists to the RANK receptor, impairing the proton pump mechanism, cyclooxygenase inhibitors (especially if they work well in an acidic microenvironment), agents that shut down osteoclast functions, matrix metalloproteinase inhibitors; (e.g., minocycline, chemically modified tetracyclines [e.g., col-3], diacerein),[19] antagonists to various receptors on sensory neurons and vanilloid receptor-1, acid sensing ion channel, and prostaglandin E_2 receptors (EP receptors). Conventional agents and local anesthetics may act on usual targets (e.g., neural elements) as well as inhibiting the EP1 receptors (where prostaglandin$_2$ acts). Combinations of therapies may be synergistic.[20]

Vasoactive intestinal peptide appears to possess significant antiinflammatory effects. VIP may tip the Th1/Th2 cytokine balance toward Th2, promoting Th2 function and differentiation and inhibiting Th1 responses by modulating macrophages and probably interleukin-2/interferon production.[14,21]

Treatment with may suppress proinflammatory cytokines and matrix metalloproteinases.[22] Additionally, VIP exhibits direct and indirect effects on macrophages, primarily via the macrophage VPAC1 receptor, which is also present on T lymphcytes (although VIP effects on T lymphocytes are probably less significant than on macrophages). VIP may also decrease via the increase in interleukin-4, leading to a significant boost in the interleukin-4–mediated induction of osteoprotegerin.[22,23]

If much of the pain from metastatic bone lesions results from the effects of osteoclastic activity, then "shutting down" the osteoclasts is paramount to analgesic treatment. Osteoclast bone-resorbing activity is dependent on the binding of the (TNF family molecule osteoprotegerin ligand (OPGL),[21] which is expressed on activated T cells and osteoblasts, to a receptor termed *receptor activator of nuclear factor* κB (NF-κB), abbreviated RANK.[21] RANK is expressed on osteoclast precursors and mature osteoclasts.[24] Any treatment that impedes the OPGL-RANK interaction will impair RANK activation and therefore impair osteoclastic activity and bone resorption. Osteoprotegerin (OPG) is a soluble tumor necrosis factor receptor molecule that is secreted and binds to the RANK activating site of OPGL, acting as a "dummy" or "decoy" receptor and preventing OPGL from binding to and activating the osteoclast RANK receptor (FIGURE 2).[21,25,26]

Other terminology has been used for some of the above-mentioned factors. Terms that have been used in the literature for OPGL include osteoclast differentiation factor, TNF-related activation- induced cytokine, and NF-κB, ligand (RANKL).[27] A term that has been used in the literature for RANK is osteoclast differentiation and activation receptor. Also, osteoprotegerin has been named osteoclastogenesis inhibitor factor.

In a series of elegant experiments, Mantyh's laboratory demonstrated that osteoprotegerin

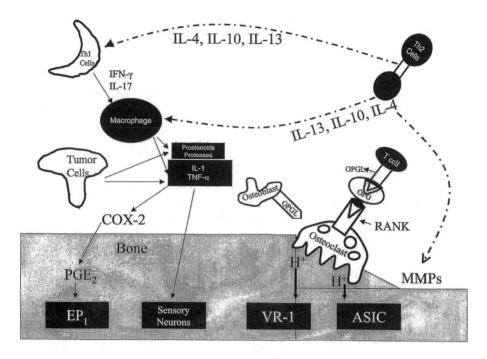

Figure 2. Algesic mediators of painful bone metastases.

does shut down osteoclast activity, resulting in analgesia and significant improvement in pain behavior.[28–30] Additionally, much work is being done on the potential role of osteoprotegerin in modulating rheumatoid arthritis.[31,32]

Bisphosphonates may actually inhibit osteoclastic activity through stimulating osteoprotegerin production (although that may only account for a small part of bisphosphonate actions).[33] Phytoestrogens (e.g., soy) may also stimulate osteoprotegerin production and may be a natural alternative to inhibiting osteoclastic activities.[34]

Platelet products may stimulate osteoclast-like cells via prostaglandin/RANK dependent mechanism,[35] thus making platelets a potential player and therapeutic target in certain situations of inflammatory bone pain.

Agents other than osteoprotegerin or VIP that may potentially contribute to shutting down osteoclasts include bisphosphonates (e.g., CGP 42' 446)[4] and interleukin-18, which is a product of osteoblast-like cells and activated macrophages.[36] Interleukin-18 inhibits osteoclast formation by inducing T cells to produce granulocyte-macrophage colony-stimulating factor.[36]

The Smith theory of radiation-induced analgesia proposes that a significant mechanism is via osteoblast insult, which essentially takes out available or functional OPGL so that it cannot activate the osteoclast by binding to the RANK receptor. In the absence of osteoclast stimulation, it is effectively as if osteoclasts were functionally shut down in terms of being pro-algesic.

Multicenter studies are in progress to evaluate the therapeutic role of radiofrequency ablation in treating patients with painful bone metastases.

The use of rational polypharmacy employing various therapeutic combinations such as the hypothetical VOID therapy—**V**IP (which may promote Th2 cytokines, inhibit Th1 cytokines, function as an MMP-2 inhibitor, inhibit macrophage function, and promote/induce OPG via IL-4), **O**PG, and an **I**nhibitor of cyclooxygenase (COX) 2, and **D**iacerein (which may inhibit interleukin-1 and function as a matrix metalloproteinase inhibitor)[37]—may be one of the future analgesic cocktails for attempts to achieve optimal analgesia with minimal side effects.

Lumiracoxib (Cyclooxygenase-189) is in phase III clinical trials and may be considered for the treatment of osteoarthritis, rheumatoid arthritis, and pain. It is a highly selective COX-2 inhibitor developed by Novartis and is expected to be at least as effective as nonselective nonsteroidal antiinflammatory drugs, with an improved side effect profile. Compared with diclofenac, COX-189 has substantially reduced affinity for COX-1, being 300-fold less potent. COX-189 is predicted to be more effective in a low pH environment. This would be beneficial for pain relief in sites of metastatic bone lesions, where the local environment is acidic in nature. The pKa of COX-189 is 4.3.

Although the clinical impression has been that COX-2 inhibitors should be beneficial for bone pain, in the rat model of bone cancer pain, it was demonstrated that although morphine is effective in reducing bone cancer–related pain behaviors at least at advanced stages of bone destruction, inhibitors of COX-2 were not effective.[38]

In conclusion, by understanding some of the mechanisms leading to painful osseous metastases and launching a multifaceted treatment plan, we may be better equipped to achieve optimal analgesia.

REFERENCES FOR ADDITIONAL READING

1. Hungerford DS: Bone marrow pressure and intromedullary venography. In: Owen R, Goodfellow J, Bullough P (eds): Scientific Foundations of Orthopedics and Traumatology. London, Heinmann 1980, pages 357–360.
2. Garrett RI: Bone destruction in cancer. Semin Oncol 20:4–9, 1993.
3. Galasko CSB: Mechanisms of lytic and blastic metastatic disease of bone. Clin Orthop 169:20–27, 1982.
4. Coleman RE: Bisphosphonate treatment of bone metastases and hypercalcemia of malignancy. Oncology 5:55–65, 1991.
5. Houston SJ, Rubens RD: The systemic treatment of bone metastases. Clin Orthop 312:95–104, 1995.
6. Bullough PG: Atlas of Orthopaedic Pathology with Clinical and Radiologic Correlations, 2nd ed. New York, Gower Medical Publishing, 1992, pages 6, 17–29.
7. Bates T, Yarnold JR, Blintzerr P, et al: Bone metastasis consensus statement. Int J Radiat Oncol Biol Phys 23:215–216, 1992.
8. Emani B, Lyman J, Brown A, et al: Tolerance of normal tissue to therapeutic irradiation. Int J Radat Oncol Biol Phys 21:109, 1991.
9. Larsen RH, Salberg G, Borch KW, et al: Treatment of skeletal metastases with alpha emitting 223 Ra: Blood clearance pattern in patients with advanced breast and prostate cancer [abstract]. JNM 43(Suppl):160P, 2002.
10. Miossec P, Van den Berg W: Th1/Th2 cytokine balance in arthritis. Arthrit Rheuma 40:2105–2115, 1997.
11. Thierfelder WE, van Deursen JM, Yamamoto K, et al: Requirement for stat 4 in interleukin-12-mediated responses of natural killer and T cells. Nature 382:171–174, 1996.

12. Hou J, Schindler U, Henzel WJ, et al: An interleukin-4-induced transcription factor: IL-4 stat. Science 265:1701–1706, 1994.

13. Iakeda K, Tanaka T, Shi W, et al: Essential role of stat 6 in IL-4 signalling. Nature 380:627–630, 1996.

14. Boyle DL, et al: Intra-articular IL-4 gene therapy in arthritis: Anti-inflammatory effect and enhanced Th2 activity. Gene Ther 6:1911–1918, 1999.

15. Joosten LAB, Lubberts E, Durez P, et al: Role of interleukin-4 and interleukin-10 in murine collagen-induced arthritis: Protective effect of interleukin-4 and interleukin-10 treatment on cartilage destruction. Arthrit Rheum 40:249–260, 1997.

16. Germann T, Szeliga J, Hess H, et al: Administration of interleukin-12 in combination with type II collagen induces severe arthritis in DBA/1 mice. Proc Natl Acad Sci U S A 92:4823–4827, 1995.

17. Joosten LAB, Lubberts E, Helsen MMA, et al: Dual role of interleukin-12 in early and late stages of murine collagen type 1 arthritis. J Immunol 19:4090–4102, 1997.

18. Rus V, Nguyen P, Chevrier M, et al: Preliminary studies of in vitro and in vivo effects and misoprostol on Th-1 and Th-2 cytokine production. Am J Ther 2:911–916, 1995.

19. Lokeshwar BL, Selzer MG, Zhu BQ, et al: Inhibition of cell proliferation, invasion, tumor growth and metastasis by an oral-antimicrobial tetracycline analog (COL-3) in a metastatic prostate cancer model. Int J Cancer 98:297–309, 2002.

20. Llavaneras A, Ramamurthy NS, Heikkila P, et al: A combination of a chemically modified doxycycline and a bisphosphonate synergistically inhibits endotoxin-induced periodontal breakdown in rats. J Periodontol 72:1069–1077, 2001.

21. Kong Y-Y, Felge U, Sarosi I, et al: Activated T cell regulate bone loss and joint destruction in adjuvant arthritis through osteoprotegerin ligand. Nature 402:304–308, 1999.

22. Firestein GS: VIP: A very important protein in arthritis. Nat Med 7:537–538, 2001..

23. Delgado M, Abad C, Martinez C, et al: Vasoactive intestinal peptide prevents experimental arthritis by down regulating both autoimmune and inflammatory components of the disease. Nat Med 7:563–568, 2001.

24. Hsu H, Lacey KL, Dunstan CR, et al: Tumor necrosis factor receptor family member RANK mediates osteoclast differentiation and activation induced by osteoprotegerin ligand. Proc Natl Acad Sci U S A 996:3540–3545, 1999.

25. Simonet WS, Lacey DL, Dunstan CR, et al: Osteoprotegerin: A novel secreted protein involved in the regulation of bone density. Cell 89:309–319, 1997.

26. Thompson SWN, Tonge D: Bone cancer gain without the pain. Nat Med 6:504–505, 2000.

27. Yasuda H, Shima N, Nakagawa N, et al: Osteoclast differentiation factor is a ligand for osteoprotegerin/osteoclastogenesis-inhibitory factor and is identical to TRANCE/RANKL. Proc Natl Acad Sci U S A. 95:3597–3602, 1998.

28. Luger NM, Honore R, Sabino MAC, et al: Osteoprotegerin diminishes advanced bone cancer pain. Cancer Res 61:4038–4047, 2001.

29. Honore P, Luger NM, Sabino MA, et al: Osteoprotegerin blocks bone cancer – induced skeletal destruction, skeletal pain and pain-related neurochemical reorganization of the spinal cord. Nat Med 6:521–528, 2000.

30. Schwei MJ, Honore P, Rogers SD, et al: Neurochemical and cellular reorganization of the spinal cord in a murine model of bone cancer pain. J Neurosci 19:10886–10897, 1999.

31. Redlich K, Hayer S, Maier A, et al: Tumor necrosis factor alpha-mediated joint destruction is inhibited by targeting osteoclasts with osteoprotegerin. Arthrit Rheum 46:785–792, 2002.

32. Goldring SR, Gravallese EM: Pathogenesis of bone lesions in rheumatoid arthritis. Curr Rheumatol Rep 4:226–231, 2002.

33. Viereck V, Emons G, Lauck V, et al: Bisphosphonates pamidronate and zoledronic acid stimulate osteoprotegerin production by primary human osteoblasts. Biochem Biophys Res Commun 291: 680–686, 2002.

34. Viereck V, Grundker C, Blaschke S, et al: Phytoestrogen genistein stimulated the production of osteoprotegerin by human trabecular osteblasts. J Cell Biochem 84:725–735, 2002.

35. Gruber R, Karerth F, Fischer MB, et al: Platelet–released supernatants stimulate formation of osteoclast–like cells through a prostaglandin/RANKL–dependent mechanism. Bone 30:726–732, 2002.

36. Gravallese EM, Goldring SR: Cellular mechanisms and the role of cytokines in bone erosions in rheumatoid arthritis. Arthrit Rheum 43:2143–2157, 2000.

37. Pelletier J-P, Yaron M, Haraoui B, et al: Efficacy and safety of diacerein in osteoarthritis of the knee: A double-blind, placebo-controlled trial. Arthrit Rheum 43:2339–2348, 2000.

38. Medhurst SJ, Walker K, Bowes M, et al: A rat model of bona cancer pain. Pain 96:129–140, 2002.

Chapter 39

Assessing Analgesic Therapeutic Outcomes

Howard Smith, MD / Joseph Audette, MA, MD / Alan Witkower, EdD

THE TREATMENT OUTCOMES IN PAIN SURVEY TOOL

Assessing individual outcomes during outpatient multidisciplinary chronic pain treatment is often an extremely challenging task. There are many tools and instruments currently available, but the Treatment Outcomes in Pain Survey tool (TOPS) has been specifically designed to assess and follow outcomes in the chronic pain population.[1,2] TOPS has been described as an augmented SF-36.[1,2] The Medical Outcomes Study Short (MOS) Form 36—item questionnaire (SF-36) compares the health status of large populations without a preponderance of one single medical condition.[3] The SF-36 assesses eight domains, but it has not been found to be especially useful for following the changes in function and pain seen in chronic pain populations.

The eight domains of the SF-36 are bodily pain (BP), general health (GH), mental health (MH), physical functioning (PF), role emotional (RE), social functioning (SF), role physical (RP), and vitality (VT). The TOPS scale initially had nine domains, but one (satisfaction with outcomes) was modified in subsequent versions. The nine domains of TOPS are Pain Symptom, Family/Social Disability, Functional Limitations, Total Pain Experience, Objective Work Disability, Life Control, Solicitous Responses, Passive Coping, and Satisfaction with Outcomes. This enhanced SF-36 (TOPS scale) was constructed by obtaining patient data from the SF-36 with 12 additional role functioning questions. These additional questions were taken in part from the 61-item Multidimensional Pain Inventory (MPI)[4] and the 10-item Oswestry Disability Questionnaire,[5] with four additional pain-related questions that are similar to those found in the MOS pain-related questions,[6] the Brief Pain Inventory,[7] and a six-item coping scale from the MOS.[6]

The questions adapted from the Oswestry Disability Questionnaire (designed for back pain patients) includes questions that relate to impairment (pain), physical functioning (how long the patient can sit and/or stand), and disability (ability to travel or have sexual relations).[5]

Although the TOPS instrument is an extremely useful tool, it is time-consuming, is based entirely on the patient's subjective responses, and requires that the clinician has access, either by computer or by sending forms away, for scoring. As a result, it may not an ideal instrument to use in every clinic and may not provide the clinician with an answer immediately of how the patient is doing relative to previous visits (although it has that potential with adequate time, scanning equipment, and computer software.)

One system that has been promoted by Passik and Portenoy and that may be helpful to clinicians in the office who are prescribing chronic opioids for pain is to document the four As.[8,9] The four As are Analgesia (pain relief), Activities of daily living (psychosocial functioning), Adverse effects (side effects), and Aberrant drug taking (addiction-related outcomes). Sample questions include the following:

Analgesia

1. What was your pain level on average during the past week? (0–10)
2. What was your pain level at its worst during the past week? (0–10)
3. Compare your average pain during the past week with the average pain you had before you were treated with your current pain relievers. What percentage of your pain has been relieved? (0–100)
4. Is the amount of pain relief you are now obtaining from your current pain relievers enough to make a real difference in your life? (yes/no)
5. (For the health care provider to answer) Is the pain relief clinically significant? (yes/no)

Activities of Daily Living

Compare your usual functioning during the past month with your usual functioning before you were treated with your current pain relievers in the following areas (for each area circle one (better/same/worse): Physical functioning; mood; family relationships; social relationships; sleep patterns; overall functioning.

Adverse Side Effects

1. Are you able to tolerate your current pain relievers? (yes/no)
2. Are you experiencing any side effects from your current pain relievers? (yes/no)
3. What is the severity of the constipation you are experiencing? (none/mild/moderate/severe)
4. (For the health care provider to answer) Are the side effects tolerable for the patient? (yes/no/unsure)

Aberrant Behaviors Assessed in Checklist

Circle the frequency of each of the following behaviors (0/1/2/3/≥4):

- *Adverse consequences possibly resulting from drug use:* purposeful oversedation, negative mood change, decline in psychological function, decline in social function, appearing intoxicated, decline in physical function, increasingly unkempt or impaired, worrisome drug effects ("getting high"), involvement in motor vehicle or other accident, engages in sale of sex to obtain drugs.

- *Possible loss of control or division of medications:* Requests frequent early renewals, increases dose without authorization, reports lost or stolen prescriptions, requests higher doses in worrisome manner, successfully obtains prescriptions from other doctors, attempts to obtain prescriptions from other doctors, uses medication for purpose other than prescribed (e.g., to help sleep), engages in staff splitting, changes route of administration.

- *Preoccupation with opioids or other drugs:* Asks for medication by name, does not comply with other recommended treatments, reports no effects of other medications, misses appointments except for medication renewal, contact with street culture, abusing alcohol and street drugs, hoarding of medication.

- *Other occurrences of potential concern:* Patient arrested or detained by police, patient a victim of abuse, associates arrested or detained by police.

Passik and associates[8] analyzed responses from 282 patients on chronic opioid therapy. Ninety percent of patients believed that the pain relief improved their quality of life. More than 93% were able to tolerate their medication. Constipation was frequent, experienced by 80.7%; however, it was severe in only 9.6%, with other adverse effects being infrequent. Overall functioning improved in 78.2% of patients. Physical functioning and mood improved in more than 70% of patients, and aberrant drug–taking behavior was rare.[8]

Passik and Weinreb[9] concluded that their four As checklist was a valuable instrument for tracking outcomes in patients receiving long-term opioid therapy for chronic pain.

Use of chronic opioid analgesic therapy (COAT) for chronic noncancer pain continues to be controversial.[10,11] The challenging and controversial nature of this treatment approach has induced professional organizations and regulatory agencies to develop consensus statements and guidelines to direct clinicians in this arena.[12,13] Included in these principles for appropriate use of opioids for chronic noncancer pain are the requirement for periodic review of the efficacy of treatment and documentation substantiating continuation of COAT. Yet these are areas where physicians may have the most difficulty complying, given the pace of practice in the current health care environment. The four As checklist is time consuming and cumbersome: if you do not have the checklist, you may not remember it or be able to write it down quickly in the chart on a progress note. Additionally, it is not quantitative and therefore more difficult to compare visit-to-visit progress or to track trends.

THE SAFE SCORE

Another tool, that has been advocated to help with this purpose is called the SAFE Score.[14,15] Although it has not yet been rigorously validated, it is simple and practical and may possess clinical utility. It is a score generated by the health care provider that is meant to reflect a multidimensional assessment of outcome to COAT. It is not meant to replace more elaborate patient-based assessment tools but could possibly serve as an adjunct and possibly in the future shed some light on the differences between patients' perception of how they are doing on opioid treatment versus the physician-based view of outcome.

The SAFE Tool is both practical in its ease of use and clinically useful. (FIGURE 1). The goals of the SAFE tool are to

- Demonstrate that the clinician has routinely evaluated the efficacy of the treatment from multiple perspectives.
- Guide the clinician toward a broader view of treatment options beyond adjusting the medication regimen.
- Document the clinician's rationale for continuation, modification, or cessation of COAT.

Scoring System for the SAFE Tool

At each visit, the clinician rates the patient's functioning and pain relief in four domains. The domains assessed are the following:
S = Social (social functioning)
A = Analgesia (pain relief)
F = Function (physical functioning)
E = Emotional (emotional functioning)

FIGURE 1

Sample S.A.F.E. Form

Rating					Criterion
Social Marital, family, friends, leisure, recreational	1 supportive harmonious socializing engaged	2	3	4	5 conflictual discord isolated bored
Analgesia Intensity, frequency, duration	1 comfortable effective controlled	2	3	4	5 intolerable ineffective uncontrolled
Function Work, ADL's, home manage- ment, school, training, phys- ical activity	1 independent active productive energetic	2	3	4	5 dependent unmotivated passive deconditioned
Emotional Cognitive, stress, attitude, mood, behavior, neuro- vegetative signs	1 clear relaxed optimistic upbeat composed	2	3	4	5 confused tense pessimistic depressed distressed
Total Score					

The patient's status in each of the four domains is rated as follows:

1 = Excellent
2 = Good
3 = Fair
4 = Borderline
5 = Poor

The ratings in each of the four domains are then combined to yield a SAFE score. The SAFE score can range from 4 to 20.

Interpretation of scores

The green zone is a SAFE score of 4 to 12 and/or a decrease of 2 points in total score from baseline. With a score in green zone, the patient is considered to be doing well and the plan would be to continue with the current medication regimen or consider reducing the total dose of the opioids.

FIGURE 2

Green zone cases using the SAFE scoring tool

Example A		Example B	
Social	3	Social	2
Analgesia	2	Analgesia	4
Function	3	Function	3
Emotional	3	Emotional	1
Green zone SAFE score	11	Green zone SAFE score	10

The *yellow zone* a SAFE score of 13 to 16 and/or a rating of 5 in any category and/or an increase of 2 or more from baseline in the total score. With a score in the yellow zone, the patient should be monitored closely and reassessed frequently.

The *red zone* is a SAFE score greater than or equal to 17. With a score in the red zone, a change in the treatment would be warranted.

Treatment options depend on the pattern of scores. If attempts are made to address problems in specific domains and the patient is still not showing an improvement in the SAFE score, then the patient may not be an appropriate candidate for long-term opioid therapy.

FIGURE 2 illustrates green zone cases. In example A, there is good analgesic response to opioids, with a fair response in the other domains. No change in treatment would be necessary unless adverse reactions to the medications required an adjustment or discontinuation. In example B, there is borderline analgesic response but good social and emotional responses and a fair physical functioning response. Some pain specialists may determine that the medication regimen should be optimized. For others, this pattern of ratings may reflect a reasonable improvement in quality of life for the patient. Therefore, continuing the present medication regimen would be a reasonable option.

FIGURE 3 illustrates how the SAFE tool can be used to track changes in the status of the same patient on two consecutive visits. In the change in scores from example C to example

FIGURE 3

Tracking a change in status using the SAFE scoring tool

Example C		Example D	
Social	5	Social	3
Analgesia	3	Analgesia	4
Function	5	Function	3
Emotional	5	Emotional	3
Red zone SAFE score	18	Green zone SAFE score	13

FIGURE 4

Tracking change in status using the SAFE scoring tool

Example E		Example F	
Social	3	Social	3
Analgesia	2	Analgesia	2
Function	3	Function	4
Emotional	3	Emotional	4
Green zone SAFE score	11	Yellow zone SAFE score	13

D, although analgesia deteriorates from fair to borderline, there is significant improvement in the other domains. The clinician may feel this is satisfactory for this particular patient and continue with the current medication regimen. Once again, too narrow a focus on analgesic response may lead to unnecessary dose escalation. This case also illustrates the situation in which even though the total score at visit D is greater than 12 and would be a *yellow zone*, it is assigned as a *green zone* because there was a decrease of more than 2 in the total score. Alternately, the clinician may determine that a borderline analgesic response is not optimal. The choices for intervention may include rotating to another opioid agent, increasing the current opioid dose, adding adjuvant medications, referring for nonpharmacological treatment, or discontinuing high-dose opioids.

FIGURE 4 again illustrates a single patient on two consecutive visits. Here, analgesia has remained good over time, but there has been a negative impact on the domains of function and emotion. Pain specialists who are focused on the pain scores of such a patient may be comfortable with continuing the established treatment plan. However, using SAFE, an expanded view of the patient's overall status will alert the clinician to monitor the patient's physical and emotional functioning in future visits. If the ratings in the psychological and physical domains persist, then the clinician may recommend that the patient pursue psychosocial treatment or physical rehabilitation in addition to maintaining the medication regimen.

SAFE Data

In efforts to confirm the clinical utility of the SAFE assessment tool, 60 patients were prospectively enrolled (25 male and 35 female) with 140 evaluation scores. The subjects made multiple visits involving 6 different evaluators. Of the 35 female patients who were evaluated, 23 were in the green zone, 10 in yellow zone, and 1 in red zone. For the 25 male patients, 17 were in the green zone, 9 in the yellow zone, and 0 in the red zone (FIGURE 5).

Patients ranged from 21 to 88 years of age, with an average age of 49 years (FIGURE 6). FIGURE 7 illustrates the breakdown of the diagnostic categories and FIGURE 8 displays the opioid dose ranges. The average SAFE scores in each domain as well as the average total score are given in FIGURE 9. FIGURE 10 illustrates the breakdown of SAFE scores relative to opioid dose. The opioids used in the clinic included Oxycontin, MS Contin, Duragesic, Levo-

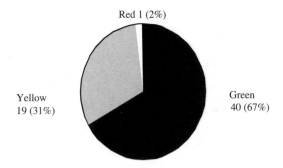

Figure 5. Distribution of patients with Green, Yellow, and Red SAFE scores

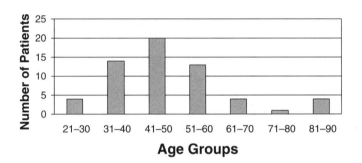

Figure 6. Age distribution of patients assessed by SAFE.

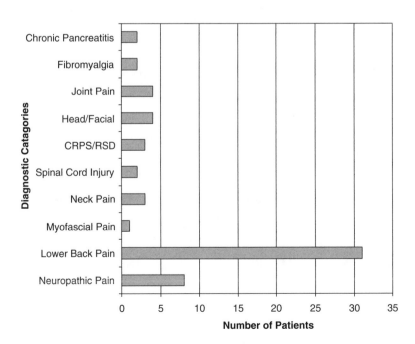

Figure 7. Distribution of diagnostic categories in patients assessed by SAFE.

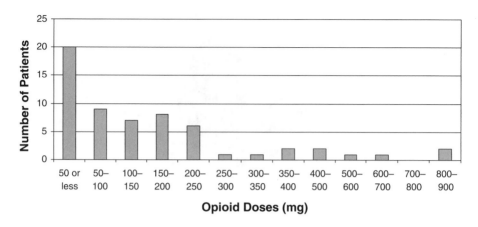

Figure 8. Distribution of opioid dose ranges among patients.

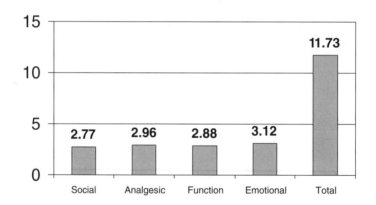

Figure 9. Average SAFE scores in each domain and average total score.

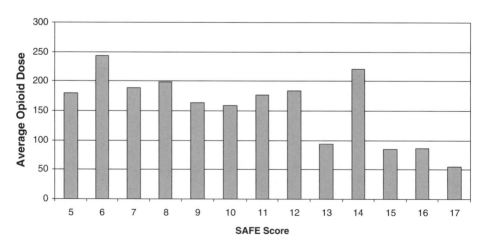

Figure 10. Distribution of opioid doses relative to SAFE scores.

dromoran, Kadian, methadone, and various short-acting agents with oxycodone, hydro-codone, and codeine.

CONCLUSIONS

The SAFE score is a multidimensional, global monitoring tool for assessing patients' response to chronic opioid analgesic therapy. The tool is Simple to use in a busy practice and is easily Adapted to diverse clinical situations. The tool Facilitates documentation of treatment response in multiple dimensions. Finally, the tool can be used as an Effective method to review the progress of the patient over time.

We want to make it clear that the SAFE tool requires further study to determine reliability and validity and therefore should be used with caution at this time. We are not making any recommendations about what treatment action should be taken based on the score. The score is meant only to highlight to the clinician that consideration for some change in treatment plan may be indicated if the score changes as outlined in the above discussion.

In the future, the simplicity of the SAFE tool may lend itself to application on handheld devices such as the palm pilot for convenient use in a pain clinic setting for assessing trends on any given patient followed over time.

REFERENCES FOR ADDITIONAL READING

1. Rogers WH, Wittink H, Wagner A, et al: Assessing individual outcomes during outpatient multidisciplinary chronic pain treatment by means of an augmented SF-36. Pain Med 1:44–54, 2000.
2. Rogers WH, Wittink H, Ashburn MA, et al: Using the "TOPS," and outcomes instrument for multidisciplinary outpatient pain treatment. Pain Med 1:55–67, 2000.
3. Ware JE Jr, Sherbourne CD: The MOS 36-item short-form health survey (SF_36). I. Conceptual Framework and Item Selection. Med Care (Phila) 30:473–483, 1992.
4. Kerns R, Turk D, Rudy T: The West Haven-Yale Multidimensional Pain Inventory (WHYMPI). Pain 23:345–346, 1985.
5. Fairbanks J, Couper J, Davies J et al: The Oswestry low back pain disability questionnaire. Physiotherapy 66:271–273, 1980.
6. Tarlor A, Ware J Jr, Greenfield S, et al: The Medical Outcomes Study: An application of methods for monitoring the results of medical care. JAMA 262:925–930, 1989.
7. Daut R, Cleeland C, Flannery R: Development of the Wisconsin Brief Pain Questionnaire to assess pain in cancer and other diseases. Pain 17:197–210, 1983.
8. Passik SD, Whitcomb LA, Dodd S, et al: Pain outcomes in long-term treatment with opioids: Preliminary results with a newly developed physician checklist. Presented at the Fourth Conference on Pain Management and Chemical Dependency, Washington, DC, December 7–9, 2000.
9. Passik SD, Weinreb HJ: Managing chronic non-malignant pain: Overcoming obstacles to the use of opioids. Adv Ther 17:70–83, 2000.
10. Hardon RN: Pain, psychological status, and functional recovery among patients on daily opioids. Curr Rev Pain 3:18–23, 1999.
11. Jamison RN, et al: Opioid therapy for chronic noncancer back pain: A randomized prospective study. Spine 23:2591–2600, 1998.
12. The use of opioids for the treatment of chronic pain. A consensus statement from the American Academy of Pain Medicine and the American Pain Society. Clin J Pain 13(1):6–8, 1997.

13. Model Guidelines for the Use of Controlled Substances for the Treatment of Pain. The Federation of State Medical Boards of the United States. SD J Med 52(1): 25–27, 1999.

14. Smith H, Audette J, Witkower A: Chronic opioid therapy for chronic non-malignant pain: Pain relief, functional improvement, quality of life? Presented at the 20th Annual Scientific Meeting of the American Pain Society, Phoenix, AZ, April 19–22, 2001.

15. Audette J, Smith H, Witkower A: Development of a novel physician assessment tool for monitoring patient on opioids with chronic non-cancer pain. Am J Phys Med Rehabil 81(7):547, 2002.

Index

Page numbers in *italics* indicate figures; page numbers followed by t indicate tables.